PHYSIOLOGY OF INFLAMMATION

THE AMERICAN PHYSIOLOGICAL SOCIETY
METHODS IN PHYSIOLOGY SERIES

PHYSIOLOGY

OF

INFLAMMATION

Edited by

Klaus Ley, M.D.

Department of Biomedical Engineering
University of Virginia School of Medicine

OXFORD
UNIVERSITY PRESS

2001

OXFORD
UNIVERSITY PRESS

Oxford   New York
Athens   Auckland   Bangkok   Bogotá   Buenos Aires   Calcutta
Cape Town   Chennai   Dar es Salaam   Delhi   Florence   Hong Kong   Istanbul
Karachi   Kuala Lumpur   Madrid   Melbourne   Mexico City   Mumbai
Nairobi   Paris   São Paulo   Shanghai   Singapore   Taipei   Tokyo   Toronto   Warsaw
and associated companies in
Berlin   Ibadan

Copyright © 2001 the American Physiological Society

Published by Oxford University Press, Inc.
198 Madison Avenue, New York, New York 10016
http://www.oup-usa.org

Library of Congress Cataloging-in-Publication Data
Physiology of inflammation / edited by Klaus Ley.
p. ; cm.—(Methods in physiology series)
Includes bibliographical references and index.
ISBN 0-19-512829-X (cloth : paper)
1. Inflammation.   I. Ley, Klaus, 1957- II. Series.
[DNLM: 1. Inflammation– immunology.
2. Inflammation–physiopathology.
3. Inflammation Mediatiors.
[QW 700 P578 2000]
RB131 .P496 2000
616'.0473—dc21   00-035946

2 4 6 8 9 7 5 3 1

Printed in the United States of America
On acid-free paper

Acknowledgments

This book would not have been possible without the commitment and energy of all contributors. I would like to thank all authors for delivering their manuscripts and figures on time and for responding to all requests for revisions at the different stages. I thank Helen Mallory of Biomedical Engineering at the University of Virginia for tirelessly reminding everyone to be on target, and especially for her invaluable help in preparing the index. I gratefully acknowledge the help and encouragement by the Technical Books Committee of the American Physiological Society and by Jeff House of Oxford University Press. Also, I would like to thank Susan Hannan, Nancy Wolitzer, and Edith Barry of Oxford University Press for their editing work.

Contents

Contributors

DAVID H. ADAMS, PH.D., F.R.C.P.
Liver Research Laboratories
MRC Centre for Immune
    Regulation
The University of Birmingham
Institute of Clinical Science
Birmingham
United Kingdom

DARIO C. ALTIERI, M.D.
Department of Pathology
Boyer Center for Molecular
    Medicine
Yale University School of Medicine
New Haven, Connecticut

BERNARD M. BABIOR, M.D., PH.D.
Department of Molecular and
    Experimental Medicine
The Scripps Research Institute
La Jolla, California

CHRISTOPHER D. BUCKLEY,
    D.PHIL., M.R.C.P.
Division of Immunity and Infection
MRC Centre for Immune Regulation
Department of Rheumatology
University of Birmingham
Birmingham
United Kingdom

DANIEL C. BULLARD, PH.D.
Department of Comparative
    Medicine
The University of Alabama at
    Birmingham
Birmingham, Alabama

MYRON I. CYBULSKY, M.D.
Department of Laboratory Medicine
    and Pathobiology
University of Toronto
Toronto General Hospital Research
    Institute
Toronto, Ontario
Canada

MICHAEL L. DUSTIN, PH.D.
Department of Pathology
Center for Immunology
Washington University
School of Medicine
St. Louis, Missouri

TOMAS GANZ, M.D., PH.D.
Department of Medicine
University of California, Los
    Angeles
School of Medicine
Los Angeles, California

D. NEIL GRANGER, PH.D.
Department of Molecular and
    Cellular Physiology
Louisiana State University Medical
    Center
Shreveport, Louisiana

NORMAN R. HARRIS, PH.D.
Bioengineering Program
Pennsylvania State University
University Park, Pennsylvania

CHRIS HASLETT, M.R.C.P. (UK),
F.R.C.P. (EDINBURGH), F.R.C.P.
(LONDON)
Centre for Inflammation Research
Department of Clinical and
  Surgical Sciences (Respiratory
  Medicine)
University of Edinburgh Medical
  School
United Kingdom, Edinburgh

PER HEDQVIST, M.D.
Department of Physiology and
  Pharmacology
Karolinska Institutet
Sweden, Stockholm

CAROLYN R. HOYAL, PH.D.
Sequenom, Inc.
La Jolla, California

VIRGINIA HUXLEY, PH.D.
Department of Physiology
University of Missouri Medical
  School
Columbia, Missouri

SHARON J. HYDUK, PH.D.
Department of Laboratory Medicine
  and Pathobiology
University of Toronto
Toronto General Hospital Research
  Institute
Toronto, Ontario
Canada

BRENT JOHNSTON, PH.D.
Department of Physiology and
  Biophysics
The University of Calgary
Faculty of Medicine
Calgary, Alberta
Canada

GEOFFREY S. KANSAS, PH.D.
Department of Microbiology and
  Immunology
Northwestern University Medical
  School
Chicago, Illinois

YEESIM KHEW-GOODALL, PH.D.
Division of Human Immunology
Hanson Centre for Cancer
  Research
Adelaide, South Australia
Australia

PAUL KUBES, PH.D.
Department of Physiology and
  Biophysics
The University of Calgary
Faculty of Medicine
Calgary, Alberta
Canada

MICHAEL B. LAWRENCE, PH.D.
Department of Biomedical
  Engineering
University of Virginia
School of Engineering and Applied
  Science
Charlottesville, Virginia

ALLAN M. LEFER, PH.D.
Department of Physiology
Jefferson Medical College
Thomas Jefferson University
Philadelphia, Pennsylvania

ROBERT I. LEHRER, M.D.
Department of Medicine
University of California, Los
  Angeles
School of Medicine
Los Angeles, California

MARCEL LEVI, PH.D., M.D.
Center of Hemostasis, Thrombosis,
  Atherosclerosis and Inflammation
  Research
Academic Medical Center
University of Amsterdam
Amsterdam
The Netherlands

KLAUS LEY, M.D
Department of Biomedical
  Engineering
University of Virginia
School of Medicine
Charlottesville, Virginia

LENNART LINDBOM, PH.D.
Department of Physiology and
  Pharmacology
Karolinska Institutet
Stockholm,
Sweden

JOEL LINDEN, PH.D.
Department of Internal Medicine
University of Virginia
Health Sciences Center
Charlottesville, Virginia

FRANCIS W. LUSCINSKAS, PH.D.
Department of Pathology
Brigham and Women's Hospital
Harvard Medical School
Boston, Massachusetts

ANDREW D. LUSTER, M.D., PH.D.
Department of Infectious Disease
Massachusetts General Hospital
Harvard Medical School
Boston, Massachusetts

JAMES MACLEAN, M.D.
Department of Allergy and
  Immunology
Massachusetts General Hospital
Harvard Medical School
Boston, Massachusetts

B. PAUL MORGAN, PH.D.,
  F.R.C.PATH., M.R.C.P.
Department of Medical Bio-
  chemistry
University of Wales
College of Medicine
Cardiff,
United Kingdom

ROLANDO E. RUMBAUT, M.D.,
  PH.D.
Departments of Medicine and
  Pediatrics
Baylor College of Medicine & Houston
  Veterans Affairs Medical Center
Houston, Texas

JOHN SAVILL, PH.D., F.R.C.P.
  (LONDON), F.R.C.P. (EDIN-
  BURGH), F.M.E.D.SCI.
Centre for Inflammation Research
Department of Clinical and Surgical
  Sciences (Internal Medicine)
University of Edinburgh Medical
  School
Edinburgh,
United Kingdom

ROSARIO SCALIA, M.D., PH.D.
Department of Physiology
Jefferson Medical College
Thomas Jefferson University
Philadelphia, Pennsylvania

ROLAND SEIFERT, M.D.
Department of Pharmacology and
  Toxicology
The University of Kansas
Lawrence, Kansas

DAVID L. SIMMONS, PH.D.
Molecular Neurobiology Group
SmithKline Beecham
Essex
United Kingdom

BRIAN STEIN, F.R.A.C.P.
Division of Human Immunology
Hanson Centre for Cancer Research
Adelaide, South Australia
Australia

MATHEW A. VADAS, PH.D.,
  F.R.A.C.P., F.R.C.P.A.
Division of Human Immunology
Hanson Centre for Cancer Research
Adelaide, South Australia
Australia

SANDER VAN DEVENTER, PH.D.,
  M.D.
Center of Hemostasis, Thrombosis,
  Atherosclerosis and Inflammation
  Research
Academic Medical Center
University of Amsterdam
Amsterdam,
The Netherlands

TOM VAN DER POLL, M.D., PH.D.
Center of Hemostasis, Thrombosis,
  Atherosclerosis and Inflammation
  Research
Academic Medical Center
University of Amsterdam
Amsterdam,
The Netherlands

IRVING L. WEISSMAN, M.D.
Departments of Pathology and
  Developmental Biology
Stanford University
School of Medicine
Stanford, California

KATHARINA WENZEL-SEIFERT,
  M.D.
Higuchi Biosciences Center
Department of Pharmacology and
  Toxicology
The University of Kansas
Lawrence, Kansas

DOUGLAS E. WRIGHT, PH.D.
Departments of Pathology and
  Developmental Biology
Stanford University
School of Medicine
Stanford, California

PHYSIOLOGY OF
INFLAMMATION

1

History of Inflammation Research

KLAUS LEY

To understand the inflammatory response and the state of inflammation research today, it is useful to consider the roots of our knowledge. Inflammation must have caught the eye of prehistoric medicine men and women as one of the fundamental responses of the mammalian organism to injury. The physicians of antiquity began to develop much of the nomenclature still used for the classification of the macroscopic signs of inflammation. The groundwork for our mechanistic understanding of the inflammatory process was laid by the careful and detailed morphologic and microscopic investigations of the 18th and 19th centuries. With limited tools for the study of cause–effect relationships, those investigators used their imagination to fill in the blanks between the phenomena they observed. Fruitful controversies resulted from different interpretations of the same observations, and critical experiments were designed to resolve such conflicts productively.

A historic perspective on such controversies is useful in at least two ways. First, it illustrates that scientific progress is not continuous, but often requires thesis and antithesis to arrive eventually at an accepted resolution. Second, the history of inflammation research illuminates how science is influenced by the personalities of the scientists conducting the investigations. Inconvenient and unsatisfactory as they may be, today's enigmas and scientific controversies are probably necessary ingredients to bring forth tomorrow's new paradigms.

Classic Greece Through the Middle Ages

Signs and consequences of inflammation were known to doctors in the ancient Sumerian and Egyptian cultures. For example, the Egyptians described abscesses and ulcers, and the Code of Hammurabi (2000 BC) contains instructions on how to treat abscesses of the eye (Eisen, 1977). However, it was not until the Greek physician and scientist, Hippocrates of Cos, introduced words like *edema* and *erysipelas* that the vocabulary describing symptoms of inflammation began to be developed. Hippocrates may also have been the first to regard inflammation as the beginning of a healing process, a view that resonates with the modern perspective on the resolution of inflamma-

1

tion (Chapter 24). The first comprehensive description of inflammatory symptoms can be found in the writings of Aulus Celsus (died AD 38). In his *De Medicina*, he introduced four of the five cardinal symptoms of inflammation: *rubor, tumor, color,* and *dolor* (redness, swelling, heat, and pain). Interestingly, he was neither a physician nor a scientist, but an encyclopedist who wrote on various subjects.

Galen of Pergamon (born AD 129) added a fifth sign of inflammation, *functio laesa,* (impaired function; Anonymous, 1978). He was a successful physician and surgeon to Roman Emperor Marcus Aurelius. Galen introduced the concept of the four vital humors: *sanguis* (blood), *pituita* (phlegm), *chole* (yellow bile), and *melaine chole* (black bile). Inflammation was considered a maladjustment of the ratios of these four humors. He did not consider pus to be harmful, which gave rise to the concept of "laudable pus," which must be allowed to exit through an incision. Galen advised against chilling an inflammatory swelling, because chilling would turn the tissue livid and into a *scirros* (bad scar). He thought that blood permeated the artery walls during inflammation and would percolate throughout the tissue. Galen's writings were influential for at least a millennium, and physicians throughout the Middle Ages were educated based on his texts.

Early Descriptive Pathology

Although the medical description of symptoms and treatments of inflammation was developed much earlier, inflammation research did not start until the invention of the compound microscope by Dutch scientist Zacharias Jansen in 1590. The physician Hermann Boerhaave (1663–1738) used the microscope to see blood vessels in inflamed tissues. He concluded that the smallest blood vessels were too narrow to carry all the blood flow in inflammation, and thus heat was generated due to friction (Jarcho, 1970b). Boerhaave's student Hieronymus Gaubius (1705–1780) became an influential teacher in Europe and found that inflammation can increase the "disposition to coagulation" (Jarcho, 1970a), an interesting foreshadowing of the modern recognition that inflammation and coagulation are interrelated. Antoni van Leeuwenhoek (1719) built the first microscope with sufficient optical resolution to see individual red blood cells moving in small blood vessels, but the white cells appear to have escaped his attention.

The first description of inflammatory cells can be found in Dutrochet (1824), who reported that individual blood corpuscles could escape sideways from the vessel wall and slowly move into the clear portion (of the preparation), where the speed of motion was very slow, in marked contrast to that of the blood stream from which the globule came. He speculated about the nature of leukocyte transmigration and suggested that vessels may have orifices in their walls that allow blood elements to enter the tissues. Rudolf Wagner (1839, Tab. XIV, Fig. IV) is credited with the first description of leukocyte rolling: *"In dem hellen Raum zwischen dem Blutkörperchenstrom und den von mehrerern parallelen Fäden eingefaßten Gefäßwandungen sieht man die runden,*

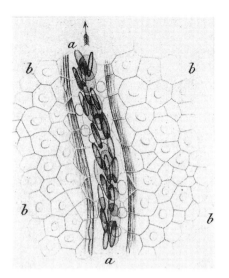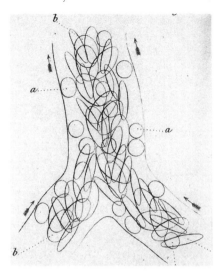

Fig. 1.1. Rolling leukocytes in venules of the frog *Rana temporaria*, reproduced from *Icones Physiologicae* by Rudolf Wagner (1839, Table 14, legend translated). Left: a vein stem at 350-fold magnification and near the surface of the epidermis, whose cobblestone-like, connected, mostly hexagonal, flat cells, usually with a nucleus b, b, b, b are spread over the vessel. The blood corpuscles are visible in several rows, some lying on their flat side, others on edge; in the bright space between the flowing blood and the vessel wall, which is surrounded by several parallel fibers, round, bright, and slowly moving lymphocytes can be seen. The image is shown at weak illumination. Right: A contour drawing of the situation at a bifurcation in the same tissue; a: leukocytes, b: erythrocytes. Direction of blood flow indicated by arrows.

hellen, viel langsamer sich bewegenden Lymphkörperchen." (In the bright space between the flowing blood and the vessel wall, which is surrounded by several parallel fibers, round, bright, and slowly moving lymphocytes can be seen; see Fig. 1.1). This observation was later confirmed by Rudolf Virchow (1871), who added more precision, noting that rolling leukocytes could become transiently adherent and sometimes reenter the blood flow. He also observed leukocyte transmigration, but attributed a nutritive rather than an inflammatory function to this phenomenon. Similar observations were made by Augustus Volney Waller (1814–1870; Jarcho, 1971a) and William Addison (1802–1881), who gave a very clear description of leukocyte transmigration and erythrocyte diapedesis in inflammation induced by scalding or trauma (Jarcho, 1971b). Addison and Waller both discovered that pus was composed of white blood cells. Waller reported that leukocytes could transmigrate after the death of the experimental animal, thus showing that their movement was not driven by blood pressure.

The most important contributions to inflammation research in the 19th century were made by Elie Metchnikoff (1893) and Julius Cohnheim (1877,

1889). Cohnheim gave a detailed description of the leukocyte adhesion cascade, including leukocyte transmigration: "First, in a vein with typical margination of white blood cells, one sees a pointed edge in the outer vessel wall. This (white blood cell) moves further away to the outside and is finally connected only through a thin, long stalk. Finally, this stalk is detached, and now a colorless, matte-shining, contractile corpuscle is sitting outside, a white blood cell" (Cohnheim, 1889, p. 198, translated from German). Remarkably, Cohnheim assumed that a molecular change of the vascular endothelium must underlie this process.

Max Schultze (1865; Brewer, 1994) was the first to report that white blood cells were not a uniform class of cells, but have different shapes. Metchnikoff (1893) extended those observations and defined lymphocytes, monocytes (*macrophages*), and granulocytes (*microphages*). He distinguished neutrophils from eosinophils (Paul Ehrlich) and recognized that plasma cells (Wilhelm Waldeyer) and mast cells (Paul Ehrlich) were also inflammatory cells. Metchnikoff (1893) wrote: "The essential and primary element in typical inflammation consists in a reaction of the phagocytes against the harmful agent" (p. 187). For his groundbreaking work, Metchnikoff, the founder of the cellular theory of inflammation, shared the Nobel prize with Paul Ehrlich, who had worked on complement and antibodies and is generally credited with founding the humoral school of immunity. With these developments, the general concepts of endothelial activation, leukocyte adhesion, phagocytic activity, and immunity had been introduced.

In vivo Models of Inflammation

In the first half of the 20th century, several important in vivo models of inflammation were developed. Arthus realized that severe inflammation could be induced by injecting antigen into the skin of immunized animals. Intravital microscopic models of inflammation were developed in mammals. E. R. Clark and E. L. Clark (1935) developed a chamber that they inserted into the ears of rabbits and observed the adhesion and transmigration of leukocytes. An important addition was made by Sir Henry Dale (1929), who had worked on synaptic transmission and recognized that inflammation must also be brought about by chemical mediators; he identified histamine as the first inflammatory mediator. This discovery was followed by that of serotonin and bradykinin (Rocha e Silva, 1978). An elegant model of microcirculation was developed in the bat wing that did not require surgery for the observations (Nicoll and Webb, 1946); however, that model was not used for inflammation studies until much later (Mayrovitz et al., 1977).

Early studies into leukocyte rolling and adhesion in the mesenteric membranes of rabbits, guinea pigs, and cats were conducted by Vejlens (1938), who infused gelatin and other colloids and observed erythrocyte aggregation and, at the same time, increased leukocyte rolling. Vejlens (erroneously) concluded that increased red cell aggregation caused the phenomenon of leukocyte rolling, but considered that increased adhesiveness could be an alternative explanation. Vejlens had trained with Robin Fåhraeus (1929), who made seminal contributions to the relation between erythrocyte and blood flow velocity and realized that the velocity of a blood particle is inversely related to its local concentration.

With the advent of electron microscopy, detailed morphological studies on the nature of leukocyte transmigration became possible. Perhaps the most important contributions were made by Marchesi, Florey, and Gowans, who elucidated the relationship between leukocytes and endothelial cells during transmigration (Marchesi and Gowans, 1964; Marchesi and Florey, 1960).

The quantitative understanding of the movement of blood cells in microvessels was advanced by modeling the movement of a sphere in a fluid-filled tube, pioneered by Happel (Happel and Byrne, 1954) and later extended by Goldman and colleagues (1967). These studies became invaluable for understanding the movement of free-flowing and rolling leukocytes in flow chambers and microvessels. To achieve a more complete understanding of leukocyte adhesion under the dynamic conditions of blood flowing in microvessels and to take full advantage of Happel's and Goldman's studies, it was necessary to develop means to measure the blood flow velocity. This was achieved by the dual-slit method combined with autotracking correlation (Baker and Wayland, 1974). A second requirement was the ability to record images from the microcirculation, first by means of film (Atherton and Born, 1972) and later through videotape. Atherton and Born (1973) were the first to measure the velocity of rolling leukocytes in microvessels and systematically relate rolling velocity to blood flow velocity. Goldman's studies paved the way for a quantitative understanding of the "critical" or "hydrodynamic" velocity that separates rolling cells engaged in adhesive interaction from freely flowing cells in vitro (Lawrence and Springer, 1991) and in vivo (Ley and Gaehtgens, 1991).

In vitro Models of Inflammation

A very early in vitro study of blood cells described the electrophoresis of horse leukocytes (Abrahamson, 1927). Those experiments suggested that a decreased surface charge on white blood cells may aid their adhesion to the endothelium under inflammatory conditions. The reliable isolation of leukocytes and, more specifically, neutrophils from peripheral blood (Böyum, 1968) was a second important step toward putting together in vitro adhesion assays. Blood cell isolation was rapidly improved and extended for a broader spectrum of cells (English and Anderson, 1974).

A key development for the advancement of inflammation research in general, and leukocyte adhesion research in particular, was the advent of cell culture systems for vascular cells. Jaffe and coworkers (1973) pioneered the culture of endothelial cells from human umbilical veins, which formed the basis for the discovery of most endothelial–leukocyte adhesion molecules.

During the same period, haptotaxis was discovered as the tendency of motile and adherent cells to migrate to an area of greater adhesiveness (Carter, 1965). One of the first leukocyte adhesion assays reported that macrophages migrated less rapidly when they adhered to the substrate more firmly (Weiss and Glaves, 1975). The first in vitro leukocyte–endothelial adhesion assay was reported by Hoover et al. (1978), who found that neuraminidase treatment increased the number of adherent leukocytes. One year later, the effect of chemoattractants on neutrophil adhesion was discovered (Fehr and Dahinden, 1979).

A seminal contribution to in vitro adhesion assays was the introduction of the Stamper–Woodruff assay for lymphocyte adhesion in the presence of shear stress (Stamper and Woodruff, 1976; Woodruff et al., 1977). In this assay, a cryostat section obtained from a peripheral lymph node is overlaid with a suspension of lymphocytes that are allowed to adhere to the section under mild rotation. Specific adherence to high endothelial venules could be shown, which ultimately led to the discovery of L-selectin and other lymphocyte homing receptors. The Stamper–Woodruff assay was eventually refined to adhesion assays with defined wall shear stress. The first successful design was the parallel-plate flow chamber (McIntire and Eskin, 1984) that was developed into a leukocyte adhesion assay (Lawrence et al., 1987). Although tube flow assays were developed even earlier (Goldsmith, 1971), these systems were not used for leukocyte adhesion and detachment assays until much later (Bargatze et al., 1994). In the last two decades, other adhesion, aggregation, and detachment assays using shear flow have been developed and are treated in detail in Chapter 11.

Molecular Understanding of Inflammation

It is always dangerous for the author of a history chapter to get too close to the present, because many controversial issues have not yet been resolved to the satisfaction of all investigators. However, today's knowledge of the inflammatory process is so heavily dependent on molecular insights that this chapter would be incomplete without mentioning a few milestones.

The inflammatory cytokines IL-1β (Auron et al., 1984) and TNF-α (Liu et al., 1987; Ruddle et al., 1987) were discovered in the 1980s and were soon used to activate endothelial cells and to induce them to support leukocyte adhesion (Bevilacqua et al., 1985). These experiments led to the identification of E-selectin as an important leukocyte adhesion molecule (Bevilacqua et al., 1987).

Based on morphological and functional studies, it had been suspected that specific adhesion molecules might be involved in the homing of naive lymphocytes to secondary lymphatic organs (Gowans and Knight, 1964; Stamper and Woodruff, 1976). Using a B-cell lymphoma that bound to peripheral lymph node, but not Peyer's patch high endothelial venules in the Stamper–Woodruff assay, Gallatin et al. (1983) generated a monoclonal antibody to a 90 kDa antigen that later became known as L-selectin.

Three independent lines of investigation led to the identification of the leukocyte β_2 integrins. A rare human disease, leukocyte adhesion deficiency was discovered in the early 1980s (Anderson et al., 1981) and later related to the absence of a family of cell surface glycoproteins (Buchanan et al., 1982; Arnaout et al., 1984; Dana et al., 1984; Springer et al., 1984), which became known as the CD18 or β_2 integrins. One of the β_2 integrins was initially identified as lymphocyte function-associated antigen, or LFA-1, because it participated in T-cell mediated killing (Davignon et al., 1981). LFA-1 is identical to CD11a/CD18. At the same time, a complement receptor (CR3) was identified as a cell surface heterodimer (Beller et al., 1982, Wright et al., 1983), which turned out to be the CD11b/CD18 member of the β_2 integrin family.

The first member of the α_4 family of integrins, also important in leukocyte adhesion, was initially identified as very late antigen-4, or VLA-4 (Hemler et al., 1987). Integrin ligands on inflamed endothelial cells were functionally characterized by Springer's (1984) group as molecules that were inducible by inflammatory cytokines, leading to the discovery of intercellular adhesion molecule-1 (ICAM-1; Dustin et al., 1986) and ICAM-2 (Dustin and Springer, 1988; Staunton et al., 1989). The first endothelial ligand for α_4 integrins, vascular cell adhesion molecule-1 (VCAM-1) was independently discovered by two groups (Osborn et al., 1989; Rice and Bevilacqua, 1989)

In the late 1980s, the new technology of gene targeting and homologous recombination became available (Capecchi, 1989). The introduction of positive and negative markers to select for and against induced mutations allowed the production of gene-targeted "knockout" mice. In rapid succession, gene-targeted mice were made for many molecules important in inflammation, including inflammatory cytokines and their receptors (Durum and Muegge, 1998), leukocyte and endothelial adhesion molecules (Ley, 1995), and chemokines and their receptors (Schwarz and Wells, 1999). The availability of these mice has revolutionized in vivo experimentation and led to a revival of in vivo physiology in general, and inflammation physiology in particular. With gene-targeted mice, the intact mammalian organism now can be interrogated at the molecular level in unprecedented ways.

Conclusion

The history of inflammation research stretches over 2000 years, with 200 years of research at the cellular level and 20 years of research at the molecular level. The amazing insights that have been obtained have not only led to a better understanding of the inflammatory phenomena, but have also benefited the diagnosis and treatment of patients with inflammatory disorders. There is no evidence that the pace of discoveries in inflammation research will slow down as the inflammatory components of chronic diseases like atherosclerosis and diabetes are recognized and investigated.

References

Abrahamson, H. A. (1927) The mechanism of the inflammatory process. I. The electrophoresis of the blood cells of the horse and its relation to leukocyte emigration. *J. Exp. Med.* 46:987–1002.

Anderson, D. C., Hughes, B. J., and Smith, C. W. (1981) Abnormal mobility of neonatal polymorphonuclear granulocytes. Relationship to impaired redistribution of surface adhesion sites by chemotactic factors or colchicine. *J. Clin. Invest.* 68:863–874

Anonymous. (1978) Galen on abnormal swellings. *J. Hist. Med. Allied Sci.* 33:531–549.

Arnaout, M. A, Spits, H, Terhorst, C., Pitt, J, and Todd, R. F. (1984) Deficiency of a leukocyte surface glycoprotein (LFA-1) in two patients with Mo 1 deficiency. Effects of cell activation on Mo 1/LFA-1 surface expression in normal and deficient leukocytes *J. Clin. Invest.* 74:1291–1300.

Atherton, A., and Born, G.V.R (1972) Quantitative investigations of the adhesiveness of circulating polymorphonuclear leukocytes to blood vessels. *J. Physiol. (Lond.)* 222:447–474.

Atherton, A., and Born, G.V.R. (1973) Relationship between the velocity of rolling granulocytes and that of the blood flow in venules *J. Physiol. (London)* 233:157–165.

Auron, P. E., Webb, A. C., Rosenwasser, L. J., Mucci, S. F., Rich, A, Wolff, S. M., and Dinarello, C. A. (1984) Nucleotide sequence of human monocyte interleukin 1 precursor cDNA *Pro. Nat. Acad. Sci. USA* 81:7907–7911

Baker, M, and Wayland, H (1974) On-line volume flow rate and velocity profile measurement for blood in microvessels *Microvasc. Res.* 7:131–143

Bargatze, R. F, Kurk, S., Butcher, E. C, and Jutila, M. A. (1994) Neutrophils roll on adherent neutrophils bound to cytokine-induced endothelial cells via L-selectin on the rolling cells *J. Exp. Med.* 180:1785–1792.

Beller, D. I, Springer, T. A., and Schreiber, R. D. (1982) Anti-Mac-1 selectively inhibits the mouse and human type three complement receptor. *J. Exp. Med.* 156:1000–1009.

Bevilacqua, M. P., Pober, J. S., Wheeler, M. E., Cotran, R. S., and Gimbrone, M. A Jr. (1985) Interleukin 1 acts on cultured human vascular endothelium to increase the adhesion of polymorphonuclear leukocytes, monocytes, and related leukocyte cell lines.*J. Clin. Invest.* 76:2003–2011.

Bevilacqua, M. P., Pober, J. S, Mendrick, D. L., Cotran, R. S., and Gimbrone, M. A. Jr. (1987) Identification of an inducible endothelial-leukocyte adhesion molecule. *Proc. Natl. Acad. Sci. USA* 84:9238–9242.

Böyum, A. (1968) Isolation of mononuclear cells and granulocytes from human blood *Scand. J. Lab. Invest.* 21:77–89.

Brewer, D. B. (1994) Max Schultze and the living, moving, phagocytosing leucocytes: 1865. *Med. Hist.* 38:91–101.

Buchanan, M. R., Crowley, C. A., Rosin, R. E., Gimbrone, M. A., Jr., and Babior, B. M. (1982) Studies on the interaction between GP-180–deficient neutrophils and vascular endothelium. *Blood* 60:160–165

Capecchi, M. R. (1989) Altering the genome by homologous recombination. *Science* 244:1288–1292

Carter, S. B. (1965) Principles of cell motility: The direction of cell movement and cancer invasion. *Nature* 208:1183–1187.

Clark, E. R., and Clark, E. L. (1935) Observations on changes in blood vascular endothelium in the living animal. *Am. J. Anat.* 57:385–438.

Cohnheim, J. (1877) *Vorlesungen über allgemeine Pathologie*. Berlin: August Hirschwald Verlag.

Cohnheim, J. (1889) *Lectures on General Pathology: A Handbook for Practitioners and Students*. London: The New Sydenham Society.

Dale, H. H. (1929) Some chemical factors in the control of the circulation *Lancet* 1:1233–1237.

Dana, N., Todd, R. F, Pitt J., Springer, T. A, and Arnaout, M. A. (1984) Deficiency of a surface membrane glycoprotein (Mo 1) in man *J. Clin. Invest.* 73:153–159.

Davignon, D., Martz, E, Reynolds, T., Kurzinger, K, and Springer, T. A. (1981) Lymphocyte function-associated antigen 1 (LFA-1): A surface antigen distinct from Lyt-2,3 that participates in T-lymphocyte mediated killing. *Proc. Natl. Acad. Sci. USA* 78:4535–4539.

Durum, S. K., and Muegge, K. (1998) *Cytokine knockouts*. Totowa, NJ: Humana Press.

Dustin, M. L., Rothlein, R., Bhan, A. K., Dinarello, C. A., and Springer, T. A. (1986) Induction by IL-1 and interferon-gamma: Tissue distribution, biochemistry, and function of a natural adherence molecule (ICAM-1) *J. Immunol.* 137:245–254.

Dustin, M. L, and Springer, T. A. (1988) Lymphocyte function-associated antigen-1 (LFA-1) interaction with intercellular adhesion molecule-1 (ICAM-1) is one of at least three mechanisms for lymphocyte adhesion to cultured endothelial cells *J. Cell Biol.* 107:321–331.

Dutrochet, H. (1824) *Recherches anatomiques et physiologiques sur la structure intime des animaux et des végetaux, et sur leur motilité.* Paris: Ballière et Fils.

Eisen, V (1977) Past and present views of inflammation. *Agents & Actions Suppl.* 3:9–16.

English, D., and Anderson, B. R. (1974) Single step separation of red blood cells, granulocytes and mononuclear leukocytes on discontinuous density gradients of Ficoll-Hypaque *J. Immunol. Meth.* 5:249–254.

Fåhraeus, R. (1929) The suspension stability of the blood. *Physiol. Rev.* 9:241–274.

Fehr, J., and Dahinden, C. (1979) Modulating influence of chemotactic factor-induced cell adhesiveness on granulocyte function *J. Clin. Invest.* 64:8–16.

Gallatin, W. M., Weissman, I. L., and Butcher, E. C. (1983) A cell-surface molecule involved in organ-specific homing of lymphocytes. *Nature* 304:30–34

Goldman, A. J., Cox, R. G., and Brenner, H. (1967) Slow viscous motion of a sphere parallel to a plane wall. II Couette flow *Chem. Eng. Sci.* 22:653–660

Goldsmith, H. L. (1971) Red cell motions and wall interactions in tube flow. *Fed. Proc.* 30:1578–1588.

Gowans, J. L., and Knight, J. L (1964) The route of recirculation of lymphocytes in the rat. *Proc. R. Soc. Lond. (Biol.)* 159:257–282.

Happel, J, and Byrne, B. J. (1954) Motion of sphere and fluid in a cylindrical tube. *Ind. Eng. Chem.* 46:1181–1186

Hemler, M. E., Huang, C., Takada, Y., Schwarz, L., Strominger, J. L., and Clabby, M. L. (1987) Characterization of the cell surface heterodimer VLA-4 and related peptides. *J. Biol. Chem.* 262:11478–11485.

Hoover, R., Briggs, R., and Karnovsky, M. (1978) The adhesive interaction between polymorphonuclear leukocytes and endothelial cells in vitro. *Cell* 14:423–428.

Jaffe, E. A., Nachman, R. L., Becker, C. G., and Minick, C. R. (1973) Culture of human endothelial cells derived from umbilical veins: Identification by morphologic and immunologic criteria *J. Clin. Invest.* 52:2745–2756.

Jarcho, S. (1970a) Gaubius on inflammation. I. *Am. J. Cardiol.* 26:192–195.

Jarcho, S. (1970b) Boerhaave on inflammation. II. *Am. J. Cardiol.* 25:480–482.

Jarcho, S. (1971a) Augustus Volney Waller on blood vessels and inflammation II *Am. J. Cardiol.* 28:712–714.

Jarcho, S. (1971b) William Addison on blood vessels and inflammation (1841–43). *Am. J. Cardiol.* 28:223–225.

Lawrence, M. B., McIntire, L. V., and Eskin, S. G. (1987) Effect of flow on polymorphonuclear leukocyte/endothelial cell adhesion. *Blood* 70:1284–1290.

Lawrence, M. B., and Springer, T. A. (1991) Leukocytes roll on a selectin at physiologic flow rates. Distinction from and prerequisite for adhesion through integrins. *Cell* 65:859–873.

Ley, K, and Gaehtgens, P. (1991) Endothelial, not hemodynamic differences are responsible for preferential leukocyte rolling in venules. *Circ. Res.* 69:1034–1041.

Ley, K. (1995) Gene-targeted mice in leukocyte adhesion research *Microcirc.* 2:141–150.

Liu, C. C., Steffen, M., King, F., and Young, J. D. (1987) Identification, isolation, and characterization of a novel cytotoxin in murine cytolytic lymphocytes *Cell* 51:393–403.

Marchesi, V. T, and Florey, H. W. (1960) Electron micrographic observations on the emigration of leukocytes. *J. Exp. Physiol. Cog. Med. Sci.* 45:343–348.

Marchesi, V. T., and Gowans, J. L. (1964) The migration of lymphocytes through the endothelium of venules in lymphnodes: An electron microscopic study *Proc. R. Soc. Lond. (Biol.)* 159:282–290.

Mayrovitz, H. N., Wiedeman, M. P., and Tuma, R. F. (1977) Factors influencing leukocyte adherence in microvessels. *Thromb. Haemostas. (Stuttgart)* 38:823–830.

McIntire, L. V., and Eskin, S. G. (1984) Mechanical and biochemical aspects of leukocyte interactions with model vessel walls. In. *White Cell Mechanics: Basic Science and Clinical Aspects.* H. J. Meiselman, M. A. Lichtman, and P. L. LaCelle, eds. New York: A. R. Liss, pp. 202–219.

Metchnikoff, M. E. (1893) *Lectures on the Comparative Pathology of Inflammation.* London: Kegan Paul, Trench & Truebner.

Nicoll, P. A, and Webb, R. R. (1946) Blood circulation in the subcutaneous tissue of the living bat's wing. *Ann. NY Acad. Sci.* 46:697–711.

Osborn, L., Hession, C., Tizard, R., Vassallo, C., Luhowskyj, S., Chi-Rosso, G., and Lobb, R. R. (1989) Direct expression cloning of vascular cell adhesion molecule 1, a cytokine-induced endothelial protein that binds to lymphocytes. *Cell* 59:1203–1211.

Rice, G. E., and Bevilacqua, M. P. (1989) An inducible endothelial cell surface glycoprotein mediates melanoma adhesion. *Science* 246:1303–1306.

Rocha e Silva, M. (1978) A brief survey of the history of inflammation. *Agents & Actions* 8:45–49.

Ruddle, N. H., Li, C. B., Tang, W. L., Gray, P. W., and McGrath, K. M. (1987) Lymphotoxin cloning, regulation and mechanism of killing. *Ciba Found. Symp.* 131:64–82.

Schultze, M. (1865) Ein heizbarer Objecttisch und seine Verwendung bei Untersuchungen des Blutes. *Archiv. F. Mikroskop. Anatomie* 1:1–42.

Schwarz, M. K., and Wells, T. N. C. (1999) Interfering with chemokine networks—the hope for new therapeutics *Curr. Opinion Chem. Biol.* 3:407–417.

Springer, T. A., Thompson, W. S., Miller, L. J., Schmalstieg, F. C., and Anderson, D. C. (1984) Inherited deficiency of the Mac-1, LFA-1, p 150,95 glycoprotein family and its molecular basis. *J. Exp. Med.* 160:1901–1918.

Stamper, H. B., and Woodruff, J. J. (1976) Lymphocyte homing into lymph nodes: in vitro demonstration of the selective affinities of recirculating lymphocytes for high-endothelial venules. *J. Exp. Med.* 144:828–833.

Staunton, D. E., Dustin, M. L., and Springer, T. A. (1989) Functional cloning of ICAM-2, a cell adhesion ligand for LFA-1 homologous to ICAM-1. *Nature* 339:61–64.

van Leeuwenhoek, A. (1719) *Epistolae ad societatem regiam anglicam.* Leiden: Joh. Arnold.

Vejlens, G. (1938) The distribution of leukocytes in the vascular system. *Acta Pathol. Microbiol. Scand.* Suppl. 33:1–239.

Virchow, R. (1871) *Die Cellularpathologie in Ihrer Begründung auf Physiologische und Pathologische Gewebelehre,* 4th ed. Berlin: August Hirschwald Verlag.

Wagner, R. (1839) *Erläuterungstafeln zur Physiologie und Entwicklungsgeschichte.* Leipzig: Leopold Voss, Table XIV.

Weiss, L., and Glaves, D. (1975) Effects of migration inhibiting factor(s) on the in vitro detachment of macrophages. *J. Immunol.* 115:1362–1365.

Woodruff, J. J., Katz, I. M., Lucas, L. E., and Stamper, H. B. (1977) An in vitro model of lymphocyte homing. II. Membrane and cytoplasmic events involved in lymphocyte adherence to specialized high-endothelial venules of lymph nodes. *J. Immunol.* 119:1603–1610.

Wright, S. D., Rao, P. E., Van Voorhis, W. C., Craigmyle, L. S., Iida, K., Talle, M. A., Westberg, E. F., Goldstein, G. W., and Silverstein, S. C. (1983) Identification of the C3bi receptor of human monocytes and macrophages by using monoclonal antibodies. *Proc. Natl. Acad. Sci. USA* 80:5699–5703.

2

Formation and Differentiation of Leukocytes

DOUGLAS E. WRIGHT and IRVING L. WEISSMAN

Inflammatory responses often involve the selective accumulation in tissues of complex mixtures of leukocytes. In order to understand the processes governing migration and accumulation of mature leukocytes, it is useful to begin by considering the development of leukocytes in adult bone marrow, as well as the earliest migrations made by hematopoietic cells during prenatal development.

In adult mammals, bone marrow is the direct or indirect source of all lineages of hematopoietic cells that mediate inflammation. These lineages arise from rare self-renewing, pluripotent hematopoietic stem cells (HSC) through a series of intermediate progenitors with restricted self-renewal capacity, restricted developmental potential, or both. These intermediate progenitors either differentiate to mature effector cells in the bone marrow, or leave the marrow and mature elsewhere.

Till and McCulloch (1961) were the first to provide evidence for the existence of multipotent cells such as HSC: HSC are defined as cells individually capable of giving rise to all lineages of hematopoietic cells (erythrocytic, megakaryocytic, and numerous subsets of lymphocytic and myelomonocytic cells) as well as self-renewal. In the early 1960s they brought the concept of limiting dilution and clonogenic assays to hematopoietic cell biology, and provided direct evidence that a clonal precursor exists at the single cell level that can give rise to all myeloerythroid blood cell types (Till and McCulloch, 1961; Becker et al., 1963), as well as self-renew (Siminovitch et al., 1963). Later, Wu et al. (1968) provided evidence that at least a subset of clonogenic myeloerythroid precursors could also give rise to lymphocytes, (Wu et al., 1968) and that they could self-renew (Wu, 1983). Collectively, these cells were radioprotective, in that they could rescue lethally irradiated animals.

In the years following the Till and McCulloch studies, fetal and adult HSC, as well as other key progenitors developmentally downstream from HSC, have been enriched to near homogeneity by flow cytometry and other methods. Isolation of HSC and these intermediate progenitors has opened the door to research on the control of hematopoiesis at the level of regulatory genes, soluble and membrane-bound factors that promote differentiation of certain lineages, and interactions among hematopoietic cells and bone marrow stromal cells.

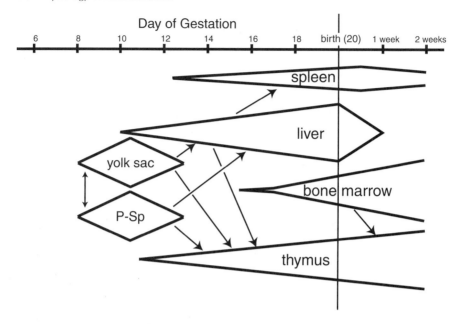

Fig. 2.1. Ontogeny of hematopoietic progenitors: Because blood cells are needed in the fetus prior to development of the bone marrow, fetal hematopoiesis is an itinerant function, as shown. It is likely that the first intraembryonic site where stem cells are found, the P-Sp, is not actually a site of hematopoiesis per se, but is instead a site of HSC maturation, E, embryonic day; P-Sp, paraaortic splanchnopleura. (Figure adapted from Ikuta et al., 1992).

Prenatal Hematopoietic Ontogeny

Hematopoiesis during prenatal development is an itinerant function, in that the locations where blood production occurs change several times before birth (Fig. 2.1). This is necessary because the site of most adult hematopoiesis (the bone marrow) develops later in gestation than the need for circulating blood cells. Blood-forming stem cells may undergo specific stages of development in different locations, leading ultimately to the adult HSC, although the relationship between fetal and adult HSC is not yet clear. The establishment of new sites of hematopoiesis in embryonic and fetal life is thought to be driven by successive migrations of pluripotent stem cells.* These early

*The notion that precisely timed migrations of multipotent hematopoietic progenitor cells are responsible for the establishment of new hematopoietic sites is often assumed to be correct, although evidence for such migrations is indirect, owing to the difficulty of labeling specifically and tracking rare cells in vivo that at present can be distinguished only by combinations of markers. Indeed, the possibilities that HSC may be constitutively released into the circulation, or that they arise de novo in each location from totipotent cells or from mesodermal progenitors more primitive than HSC have not been excluded.

movements may share mechanisms with migrating effector cells in inflammatory lesions in adults.

Early Sites of Hematopoiesis

In mammals, the earliest hematopoiesis is extraembryonic, occurring in the yolk sac blood islands, which appear at embryonic day (E) 7.5 in the mouse. Yolk sac blood production is termed *primitive* hematopoiesis, in that mostly nucleated erythrocytes with fetal-type hemoglobin are made, in contrast to the enucleated erythrocytes with adult-type hemoglobin that arise from *definitive* hematopoiesis. The earliest cells able to give rise to definitive erythropoiesis in culture do, however, originate in the precirculation yolk sac (Wong et al., 1986; Palis et al., 1999). Stem cells capable of lymphoid and myeloid engraftment in adult recipients have been isolated from the yolk sacs of chicks (Moore and Owen, 1967) and from mice at E11 (Moore and Metcalf, 1970). Adult mice, injected as E8–9 embryos in their yolk sac cavity with E8–9 yolk sac blood islands, contained in their bone marrow donor-derived cells capable of yielding colony-forming-units-spleen (CFU-S, clonogenic colonies described by Till and McCulloch, 1961, that form in the spleens of irradiated mice following intravenous injection of hematopoietic progenitors). The thymi of these adults had donor-derived T-lineage cells (Weissman et al., 1978). Cells capable of reconstituting all adult blood lineages when injected into conditioned neonatal recipients have been obtained from the aorta–gonad–mesonephros (AGM) region and from yolk sacs of E9 embryos (Yoder, et al., 1997a, 1997b).

The site of the earliest intraembryonic hematopoiesis, first identified in chick-quail chimeras in a series of grafting experiments by Dieterlen-Lievre, was shown to be the para-aortic splanchnopleura (P-Sp), an area of dorsal mesoderm (Dieterlen-Lievre, 1975; Carpenter and Turpen 1979; Dieterlen-Lievre and Martin, 1981; Turpen et al., 1981). In E10 (but not E9) mouse embryos, the AGM region, derived from the mammalian P-Sp, contains pluripotent stem cells that, after 2 days of in vitro culture, are capable of reconstituting irradiated adults in all hematopoietic lineages (Medvinsky and Dzierzak, 1996).

At E8–E9 the intraembryonic circulation in the mouse is established, and at E10 hematopoiesis begins in the liver, which becomes the main source of blood cell production in mid to late gestation (Fig 2.1), with a gradual shift to definitive hematopoiesis. The spleen is colonized by E12.5, and contains HSC by E14.5 (Godin et al., 1999). Bone marrow is colonized by E15– E16 (Ogawa et al., 1988; Delassus and Cumano, 1996), albeit with small numbers of cells; B lymphopoiesis begins in bone marrow at E17 (Delassus and Cumano, 1996).

Early Migrations of Hematopoietic Stem Cells

HSC migration appears to occur at least twice during prenatal development, and both of these migrations are likely to be associated with HSC expansion.

The first migration involves the colonization of the fetal liver by hematopoietic cells at E9–E10 (Fig. 2.1); this may be accomplished by migration of HSC from the yolk sac (Weissman et al., 1978; Yoder et al., 1997a, 1997b), AGM (Medvinsky and Dzierzak, 1996), or both, to the liver.

Attempts to isolate adult-type HSC from precirculation embryos have not been successful, so it is not clear whether the HSC that seed the liver arise from intra- or extraembryonic sources. For example, it could be argued that the E9 yolk sac HSC that reconstituted adults injected as newborns (Yoder et al., 1997a,b) originated in the AGM, and traveled via the newly formed circulation to the yolk sac. Conversely, the E10 AGM cells that (after 2 days of culture) fully reconstituted irradiated adults (Medvinsky and Dzierzak, 1996) might have originated in the yolk sac.

The second presumed migration is from the fetal liver to the spleen and bone marrow (Fig. 2.1) later in gestation.† Since HSC from fetal liver can repopulate irradiated adults (Micklem et al., 1972), or adults injected as unirradiated fetuses (Fleischman et al., 1982), or as neonates (Capel et al., 1989), it appears likely that fetal liver HSC are the precursors of HSC in adult bone marrow, although this has not been demonstrated. The phenotypes of fetal liver and adult bone marrow HSC differ (Jordan and Lemischka, 1990; Morrison et al., 1995a; Trevisan and Iscove, 1995).

In the case of migrations of HSC from AGM and /or yolk sac to liver, and from liver to spleen and bone marrow, cells may be mobilized in narrow windows of development. For this to be true, there must be tightly regulated changes in the adhesive and /or chemotactic properties of HSC, as well as mechanisms to direct their homing to specific microenvironments in target tissues. As will be described in the following, recent work has shown that migration of adult HSC in response to administration of cyclophosphamide and granulocyte colony-stimulating factor (G-CSF) is tightly synchronized with the cell cycle (D. E. Wright, S. H. Cheshier, I. L. Weissman, unpublished date, 2000) (submitted). It remains to be tested whether mechanisms also exist to coordinate migration of embryonic and/or fetal HSC with the cell cycle.

Some progress has been made in defining molecular interactions responsible for fetal HSC migrations. Chrimeric mice made from β_1 integrin-deficient embryonic stem (ES) cells were used to demonstrate a requirement for the common β_1 chain in the homing of hematopoietic precursor cells to the fetal liver (Hirsch et al., 1996). ($\beta_1^{-/-};^{+/+}$ chimeric mice were necessary because β_1 null embryos die in utero.) $\beta_1^{-/-}$ cells from yolk sacs of E10.5 chimeric embryos were capable of forming myeloid and erythroid colonies in vitro, and $\beta_1^{-/-}$ ES cells differentiated without impairment in vitro into mature B cells with rearranged antigen receptors. However, although the blood of E10.5 chimeric fetuses contained $\beta_1^{-/-}$ hematopoietic cells, the fetal liver (and the adult bone marrow, thymus, and spleen) did not, suggesting that β_1 integrins are required for engraftment of HSC in the liver. A β_1

---

†It has also been proposed that the spleen and bone marrow are seeded by progenitors from the P-Sp/AGM region (Delassus and Cumano, 1996).

integrin present on adult HSC with a proposed role in their attachment to bone marrow stroma and in their migration (Miyake et al., 1991b; Papayannopoulou et al., 1995; Papayannopoulou and Nakamoto, 1993) is very late antigen—4 (VLA-4; $\alpha_4\beta_1$). However, knockout studies showed that α_4 integrins are not required for transitions of HSC among sites of fetal hematopoiesis (Arroyo et al., 1996), so β_1 integrins other than VLA-4 must, at least in part, mediate colonization of the fetal liver.

Adult Hematopoietic Ontogeny

The bone marrow is the direct or indirect source of the entire daily output of hematopoietic cells in normal adult mammals. The productivity of the bone marrow is truly astounding; an estimated 1×10^{10} granulocytes are made each day in humans to replace senescing cells, along with 2×10^{11} erythrocytes and 4×10^{11} platelets (Tavassoli, 1979). Some cells, such as erythrocytes and neutrophils, mature fully in the bone marrow prior to entering the circulation, whereas other cells, such as T and B lymphocytes, mature to varying degrees in extramedullary sites like the thymus, spleen, and lymph nodes.

The bone marrow presents obstacles to in situ study, in part because it is encased in bone, so gaining access to undisturbed tissue can be difficult, and also because bone marrow cells with vastly different functions and developmental potentials are often morphologically indistinguishable. For example, HSC resemble large lymphocytes, and can only be identified at present by analyzing a sufficiently complex set of markers that in situ localization of HSC is precluded. Because of these obstacles, and because hematopoietic cells can be transplanted easily, more is known about the function of bone marrow cells in vitro, or in the setting of transplantation, than about in vivo bone marrow biology.

The Architecture of Bone Marrow

Bone marrow, because of its encasement in bone, is restricted in its ability to expand if the demand for hematopoiesis should increase. This limitation may explain why limited hematopoiesis is observed outside marrow (extramedullary hematopoiesis) in certain diseases and under conditions of hematopoietic stress.

The marrow can be divided into vascular and stromal spaces. The vascular space consists of arteries and arterioles that ramify into a network of broad (5–30) µ diameter in the mouse) continuous-type capillaries called *sinusoids* (Lichtman, 1981). In rodents, the sinusoids are bounded by a continuous single layer of vascular endothelium covered by a basement membrane.‡

‡The basement membrane on the abluminal surface of the sinusoidal endothelium is discontinuous in the rat, and may be absent in the human (Wickramasinghe, 1991).

The stromal space contains fibroblastic reticular cells, adipocytes, macrophages, and irregular strings or "cords" of developing hematopoietic cells. Reticular cells appear to be important in the structural organization of bone marrow, in that both stroma and vessels are supported by a three-dimensional meshwork that is, in part, composed of cytoplasmic projections of reticular cells as well as fibers (reticulin fibers of type III collagen) secreted by them. The stromal meshwork also contains hyaluronate, proteoglycans, and extracellular matrix (ECM) proteins such as laminin, type I collagen, and fibronectin.

The Concept of the Hematopoietic Niche

Bone marrow has the daunting task of supporting partial or complete maturation of numerous cell lineages, including erythrocytes, megakaryocytes (platelet precursors), lymphocytes (B cells, T cells, and natural killer, or NK cells), and several types of granulocytes (Fig. 2.2). The presumption that various lineages have special requirements for maturation has given rise to the concept that bone marrow is functionally divided into specialized microenvironments or "niches." In human bone marrow, for example, erythropoiesis occurs in small islands of cells that, at least superficially, appear to be zones specialized for erythropoiesis (granulopoiesis, however, is dispersed). Although myelopoiesis and erythropoiesis are sometimes observed in extramedullary locations, substantial levels of lymphomyeloid multilineage hematopoiesis cannot be sustained by tissues other than bone marrow. This is consistent with the notion that bone marrow contains specialized microenvironments. Niches have not been biochemically or ultrastructurally characterized, however.

Further support for the niche concept comes from several sources. First, despite much effort, investigators have been unable to create conditions for sustained hematopoiesis in vitro in the absence of stromal cell lines. Because of the proximity of cords of developing hematopoietic cells with cytoplasmic processes of reticular cells and with other stromal cells, it has been speculated that stromal cells maintain and/or regulate HSC development, although direct evidence supporting either of these possibilities is lacking. Cloned stromal lines are heterogeneous in their ability to maintain hematopoiesis in vitro (Williams et al., 1988; Rios and Williams, 1990; Wineman et al., 1996). Following 3 weeks of co-culture of stem cells on cloned fetal liver stromal cell lines, only 1 of 16 lines tested maintained HSC to a significant extent, although all lines promoted growth of myeloid cells (Wineman et al., 1996). The heterogeneity of cloned stromal lines in their ability to support hematopoiesis is consistent with the concept of specialized hematopoietic niches; the niche hypothesis would predict that only rare cells in bone marrow could maintain HSC. However, the study of hematopoiesis on single cloned lines in vitro surely fails to recapitulate the full complexity of bone marrow microenvironments.

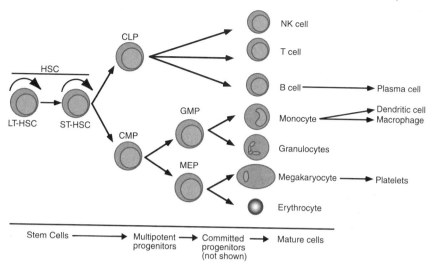

Fig. 2.2. Hematopoietic ontogeny in adults: Long-term hematopoietic stem cells (LT-HSC) can self-renew or differentiate. Differentiating LT-HSC become short-term (ST) HSC that produce multipotent progenitors. The self-renewal potential of LT-HSC exceeds the life span of the animal, whereas that of ST-HSC is much more limited. Self-renewal in multipotent progenitors, if present, is minimal. Multipotent progenitors become committed progenitors that produce all lineages of mature cells; CLP, common lymphoid progenitor; CMP, common myeloid progenitor; GMP, granulocyte/macrophage progenitor; MEP, megakaryocyte/erythroid progenitor; NK, natural killer.

Another observation used to support the niche concept is that donor-marked, transplanted HSC are unable to engraft bone marrow of syngeneic recipient animals, unless the HSC (or whole bone marrow cell preparations containing HSC) are given in extremely large numbers (Micklem et al., 1968; Takada et al., 1971; Takada and Takada, 1971; Brecher et al., 1982; Saxe et al., 1984), or unless the recipient's bone marrow is damaged by radiation and /or cytotoxic drugs. Ablation of bone marrow is necessary, by this reasoning, because normally all of the niches that support HSC are occupied. But it is also possible that normally there are excess sites in bone marrow that could support HSC development, but that most transplanted HSC cannot access these sites due to limitations in their homing ability. The fact that substantial levels of engraftment can be achieved by injecting large numbers of HSC without myeloablative treatment argues that if specialized niches exist as structural entities, they are not all continuously occupied by HSC.

No matter how bone marrow microenvironments are organized, one might expect specific factors made by stromal cells and hematopoietic cells to be important for maintenance of hematopoiesis. Although many colony-stimulating factors and synergistic factors that affect hematopoiesis have been described (for review, see Metcalf, 1993), we will focus here on three growth factors and their receptors that, directly or indirectly, influence the behavior of HSC and early hematopoietic progenitors: (a) steel factor and its receptor c-Kit; (b) thrombopoietin and its receptor c-Mpl; and (c) FLT3/FLK-2 ligand and its receptor FLT3/FLK-2.

Steel Factor and C-Kit Receptor

Steel factor (SlF, also called stem cell factor, mast cell growth factor, and c-Kit ligand), can be either secreted as a soluble molecule or expressed on the plasma membrane of some stromal cells (for review, see Williams et al., 1992). The SlF ligand is c-Kit, a receptor tyrosine kinase expressed by HSC and downstream progenitors (Williams et al., 1992). The genes encoding SlF (Copeland et al., 1990) and c-Kit (Chabot et al., 1988; Geissler et al., 1988) are mutated in two naturally occurring mouse strains called steel (Sl: Sarvella and Russell, 1956) and dominant white spotting (W; Dunn, 1937; Gruneberg, 1942; Mintz and Russell, 1957), respectively.

Homozygotes of the Sl strain die in utero, and those of the W strain die in their first postnatal week, but heterozygous Sl and W mice or homozygous strains with less severe alleles are viable and have hematopoietic and other defects that are similar.[§] This suggested that these two genes function in the same pathway. Early transplantation experiments established that the steel defect was caused by the microenvironment supporting HSC (McCulloch et al., 1965), whereas the white spotting defect was caused by a defect of HSC themselves (McCulloch et al., 1964). This led to the idea that c-Kit and SlF might be a receptor–ligand pair, which indeed they are (Huang et al., 1990; Williams et al., 1990; Zsebo et al., 1990).

About 10% of bone marrow cells express c-Kit, including most or all hematopoietic progenitors (Ogawa et al., 1991), although it has recently been claimed that rare cells, which otherwise resemble long-term repopulating HSC but lack expression of c-Kit (Randall and Weissman, 1998), are actually primitive, dormant HSC, capable of delayed but complete engraftment of all lineages (Ortiz et al., 1999). However, it should be noted that *single* c-Kit–positive HSC can provide long-term, multilineage engraftment in the long-term competitive repopulation assay (Smith et al., 1991; Osawa et al., 1996). In the study by Ortiz et al. (1999), very large numbers (2.5×10^4–1 $\times 10^5$ of c-Kit–negative bone marrow cells were transplanted in long-term competitive repopulation assays, raising the concern that the observed delayed reconstitution activity of those cells could have been due to small numbers of contaminating c-Kit–positive cells. To be definitive, such

---

[§]In addition to its role in hematopoiesis, the SlF–c-Kit interaction functions in neural, germ cell, and melanocyte development. Defective melanocyte development is responsible for the white spots of W strain mice.

experiments will need to be repeated with clonal populations of cells at limiting dilution numbers.

Two alternative splice variants of SlF are initially expressed on the cell surface. The longer of the two forms contains a proteolytic cleavage site that enables soluble SlF to be released, whereas the shorter form remains membrane-bound (Flanagan et al., 1991; Huang et al., 1992). A natural mouse mutant has arisen in which the membrane-bound (steel–Dickie, Sl^d; Brannan et al., 1991), but not the secreted, form of SlF is missing. Although viable, Sl^d mice lack pigmentation and are sterile and severely anemic (Green, 1966), underscoring the importance of membrane-bound SlF to hematopoiesis. Studies in which SlF-deficient strains of mice that overexpressed transgenes that produce the soluble or the membrane-restricted form of SlF suggest that the soluble form may be more important for myelopoiesis, and the membrane-restricted form may be more important for erythropoiesis (Kapur et al., 1998). Antibody blocking studies showed that the c-Kit–SlF interaction is required for the expansion of hematopoietic progenitors at several stages of differentiation in fetal and adult hematopoiesis (Okada et al., 1991, Ogawa et al., 1991, 1993). When E13–E15 Sl/Sl homozygous embryos were examined, however, HSC were found to be present at 30%–40% of normal numbers and expanding, which suggests that the c-Kit–SlF interaction is not required for self-renewal, at least for fetal HSC (Ikuta and Weissman, 1992).

Thrombopoietin and c-Mpl Receptor

A second interaction that appears to support hematopoiesis at the stem cell/early progenitor cell level is between thrombopoietin (TPO), a key regulator of platelet production, and its receptor c-Mpl. A vexing problem that has confronted stem cell biologists for years has been that long-term repopulating HSC could not be maintained in culture for more than a few days. Attempts to stimulate HSC proliferation resulted in their differentiation or death (van der Loo and Ploemacher, 1995; Traycoff et al., 1996; Ogawa et al., 1997). Recently, however, HSC were maintained in vitro by adding TPO to bone marrow cultures. When TPO was added to long-term Dexter-type (Dexter et al., 1984) bone marrow cultures, the long-term repopulating ability of HSC from these cultures was maintained at approximately starting levels for 2 months (Yagi et al., 1999). The issue of whether TPO acted directly on HSC, or indirectly through other cells was not addressed in this study. Although convincing evidence of significant ex vivo HSC expansion is still lacking, the maintenance of HSC in vitro is a significant step forward.

The TPO receptor is c-Mpl (Bartley et al., 1994; de Sauvage et al., 1994; Kaushansky et al., 1994; Lok et al., 1994; Wendling et al., 1994; Zeigler et al., 1994). The TPO–c-Mpl interaction appears important for supporting HSC and multiple hematopoietic progenitors in vivo as well as in vitro, as knockout studies of TPO and c-Mpl have shown (Alexander et al., 1996; Carver-

Moore et al., 1996; Kimura et al., 1998). For example, bone marrow cells from c-Mpl$^{-/-}$ mice formed about two- to ten-fold fewer colonies (in vitro) derived from several lineages, and formed about ten-fold fewer CFU–S when transferred into irradiated recipients than wild-type cells (Kimura et al., 1998). Also, c-Mpl null bone marrow cells were far inferior in giving rise to long-term reconstitution in irradiated animals than wild-type cells (Kimura et al., 1998).

FLT3/FLK-2 Ligand and FLT3/FLK-2 Receptor

A third interaction that affects early hematopoietic progenitors and HSC is that between the FLT3/FLK-2, a receptor tyrosine kinase in the same family as c-Kit and platelet-derived growth factor (PDGF), and the FLT3/FLK-2 ligand (FL). FLT3/ FLK-2 is found on hematopoietic stem and progenitor cells, but not on more mature cells (Matthews et al., 1991; Rosnet et al., 1991, 1993; Small et al., 1994). FL acts synergistically with other cytokines such as SlF, G-CSF, granulocyte macrophage colony-stimulating factor (GM-CSF), interleukin-3 (IL-3), IL-6, IL-11, and IL-12 (Tsuji et al., 1992; Hirayama et al., 1995; Jacobsen et al., 1995; Lyman and Jacobsen, 1998). Mice with a targeted disruption of the *flt3/flk-2* gene were viable, fertile, and superficially normal, but had reduced numbers of pro-B and pre-B cells (Mackarehtschian et al., 1995). Further defects were uncovered in long-term reconstitution assays, in which *flt3/flk-2* null bone marrow cells were outcompeted dramatically in B, T, and myeloid lineages by wild-type bone marrow. It is not clear whether the observed poor competitive ability of the mutant bone marrow was attributable to the lack of the FLT3/FLK-2 receptor on HSC or on other cells. In the same study, mice deficient in both c-Kit (W/W^v) and FLT3/FLK-2 had more severe hematopoietic defects than W/ W^v, suggesting that c-Kit and FLT3/FLK-2 have additive functions (Mackarehtschian et al., 1995).

One property that SlF (Molineux et al., 1991; Fleming et al., 1993b; de Revel et al., 1994; Harrison et al., 1994; Mauch et al., 1995), TPO (Torii et al., 1998), and FL (Molineux et al., 1997; Papayannopoulou et al., 1997; Sudo et al., 1997; Luens et al., 1998) have in common is that when administered to primates, humans, and/or mice, either alone or in combination with other cytokines, these factors induce HSC to migrate from the bone marrow to the blood and peripheral sites. This is termed *HSC mobilization,* and will be discussed in more detail later.

In summary, although it is plausible and perhaps likely that there are specialized lineages of stromal cells critical for the development of specific hematopoietic cells, at present there is little understanding of the structure of bone marrow microenvironments, and incomplete understanding of the molecular interactions between stromal cells and hematopoietic cells, which regulate and/or support HSC and hematopoiesis.

The Blood-Marrow Barrier

Remarkably, given the heavy minute-to-minute cellular traffic from the hematopoietic space to the vascular space of the bone marrow, immature progenitor cells are normally only infrequently found in the periphery, and, conversely, mature erythrocytes are rare in the hematopoietic space. This is due to the physical separation of the stromal and vascular compartments by the sinusoidal endothelial cells, their basement membranes, and by cells and cell processes associated with the sinusoids. Collectively, these structures are termed the *blood–marrow barrier*. Anatomically, the blood–marrow barrier would appear to be in a position to exercise great control over the hematopoietic and immune systems by regulating the entry of newly formed blood cells into the circulation at appropriate developmental stages, and by determining how many cells of each lineage are released into the periphery. However, the extent and mechanism of such control exerted by the blood–marrow barrier are unknown.

Prominent on the abluminal surface of the sinusoids are cell bodies and branching processes of reticular cells that cover up to approximately 65% of the endothelial surface in the mouse (Weiss, 1970; Chamberlain et al., 1975b). Circumstantial evidence that reticular cell processes may control cellular transit across the endothelium comes from studies in which the increase in erythrocyte production and release induced by administration of erythropoietin (EPO) to mice was associated with a reduction in the degree to which sinusoids were covered with cytoplasmic processes of adventitial reticular cells (Chamberlain et al., 1975a).

In addition to reticular cells and their processes, the abluminal surface of sinusoids is studded with macrophages and megakaryocytes that occasionally extend processes across the endothelium into the lumen. Cells entering the circulation may thus have to navigate around macrophages or megakaryocytes, and between reticular cell processes, prior to crossing the basement membrane (if present) and the endothelium itself. It has been reported in electron microscopy studies that cells do not cross the sinusoidal endothelium at endothelial cell junctions, but instead, pass across endothelial cells through transcellular pores (Muto, 1976; Tavassoli and Aoki, 1981). Such studies may be subject to fixation artifacts and interpretive biases, however.

Adult Hematopoietic Stem Cell Populations

We now know that early multipotent (lymphomyeloid) progenitors consist of at least three populations: long-term repopulating HSC (LT-HSC; Harrison and Zhong, 1992; Morrison and Weissman, 1994; Osawa et al., 1996) with a massive self-renewal capacity; short-term HSC (ST-HSC) with finite self-renewal capacity; and multipotent progenitors (MPP) that apparently have no self-renewal capacity (Morrison and Weissman, 1994; Morrison, et al.,

1997a). The three populations will be referred to collectively as HSC, although that is a semantic notation that evades a much-needed improved definition of HSC versus other clonal multipotent progenitors. Some groups have reported that all three populations are radioprotective (Morrison and Weissman, 1994), although others have reported a rare subset of LT-HSC with diminished or no radioprotective capacity (Jones et al., 1996; Osawa et al., 1996). LT-HSC have been distinguished from ST-HSC and/or MPP by flow cytometry analysis of their surface markers (Spangrude et al., 1988; Morrison and Weissman, 1994; Osawa et al., 1996), by analysis of both surface markers and the degree to which certain dyes, such as the mitochondrial supravital dye rhodamine-123, stain cells (Mulder and Visser, 1987; Spangrude and Johnson, 1990; Li and Johnson, 1992), as well as by physical separation techniques such as velocity centrifugation, combined with analysis of surface markers (Jones et al., 1990; Jones et al., 1996; Sharkis et al., 1997).

In addition to HSC, other multipotent progenitors with more restricted developmental potential are being defined. Rare bone marrow cells termed *common lymphoid precursors* (CLP; Fig. 2.2), which are capable of giving rise to T cells upon intrathymic injection and B cells and NK cells upon intravenous injection, were recently recovered from adult mouse bone marrow based on their surface phenotype (Kondo et al., 1997). Importantly, CLP were never able to give rise to erythrocytes, megakaryocytes, monocytes, or granulocytes under culture conditions favoring growth of these cells, suggesting a major branch point in hematopoiesis at which lymphoid and non-lymphoid lineages diverge.[‖] Complementing the CLP, our laboratory has also recently purified a second rare progenitor, the *common myeloid precursor* (CMP; Fig. 2.2), which is almost entirely restricted to the granulocyte, erythrocyte, megakaryocyte, and monocyte (GEMM) lineages (Akashi et al., 2000). The existence of the CMP was long expected, based on in vitro colony-forming unit (CFU) assays in which uncharacterized single cells gave rise to the GEMM lineages (the activity had been given the name CFU-GEMM). Downstream of the CMP are two bipotent progenitors, one capable of giving rise only to megakaryocytes and erythrocytes, and another restricted to granulocytes and macrophages (MEP and GMP, respectively; Akashi et al., 2000). A model showing likely relationships among LT-HSC, ST-HSC, hematopoietic progenitors, and mature effector cells is shown in Figure 2.2. Physical isolation of these cells should speed research on the genetic programs controlling lineage "choices" made by developing multipotent progenitors.

Adhesive Interactions Involving Primitive Hematopoietic Progenitor Cells

Having stressed the importance of interactions among hematopoietic progenitor cells and stromal and endothelial cells in the bone marrow, we will

---

[‖]Adult CLP are probably not the only multipotent progenitors capable of giving rise to lymphocytes (see Cumano et al., 1992, 1994).

briefly discuss some of the adhesion molecules that promote such interactions. Several classes of molecules appear to be of primary importance: integrins, selectins, isoforms of CD44, and the corresponding ligands of these molecules.

Integrins

Leukocyte integrins are heterodimeric transmembrane adhesion and signaling molecules consisting of alpha and beta chains. Short cytoplasmic tails function in signal transduction and provide links between the exterior of the cell and the actin-based cytoskeleton (for review, see Clark and Brugge, 1995). Integrins can exist on the cell surface as either adhesion-incompetent or adhesion-competent forms, the differences relating to the state of activation of the cell (Dustin and Springer, 1989; see Chapter 13 and Chapter 14 for a detailed discussion). Integrins are versatile molecules, because their avidity can be regulated not only by expression levels, but also by rapid modulation of ectodomain structure. Furthermore, the surface distribution of integrins and their interaction with the actin-based cytoskeleton can be modulated (Tamkun et al., 1986), making them well suited to participate in cell motility.

Most hematopoietic progenitors express $\alpha_4 \beta_1$ (VLA-4), $\alpha_5 \beta_1$ (VLA-5), and $\alpha_L \beta_2$ (LFA-1) integrins, although primitive progenitors with colony-forming and radioprotective capacity were reported to lack LFA-1 (Pruijt et al., 1999). VLA-4 binds, at distinct sites on its ectodomain, vascular cell adhesion molecule-1 (VCAM-1) and fibronectin (Elices et al., 1990); VLA-5 binds fibronectin; and LFA-1 binds intercellular adhesion molecule-1 (ICAM-1; Clark and Brugge, 1995). VCAM-1, in most tissues, is an endothelial adhesion molecule whose expression is induced by cytokines such as IL-1 or TNF-α. In bone marrow, however, VCAM-1 is constitutively expressed on both stromal and endothelial cells (Simmons et al., 1992; Jacobsen et al., 1996). Interactions among hematopoietic progenitors and HSC with stromal cells are mediated at least in part by VLA-4–VCAM-1 (Miyake et al., 1991a, 1991b; Teixido et al., 1992; Oostendorp et al., 1995; Oostendorp and Dormer, 1997). Papayannopoulou et al. (1995; Papayannopoulou and Nakamoto, 1993) found that in vivo administration of anti-α_4 integrin or VCAM-1 antibodies caused hematopoietic progenitors and HSC to leave the bone marrow and enter the circulation. Although the mechanism of this phenomenon is unknown, administration of anti-α_4 integrin or VCAM-1 antibodies to c-Kit–deficient (W/W^v) mice revealed that the c-Kit–SlF interaction is required for progenitor/HSC mobilization by this method (Papayannopoulou et al., 1998). It is unlikely that simple disruption of the VLA-4–VCAM-1 interaction would be sufficient to cause progenitors to "leak" from the bone marrow stromal spaces into the circulation, because the stromal and vascular spaces are separated by a continuous endothelium that must be crossed by cells entering the circulation. A possibility that has not been excluded is that there is normally a pool of marginated HSC and progenitors that are already inside the vasculature of the bone marrow or other sites. If marginated cells were attached to the luminal walls principally through VLA-4–VCAM-1, antibody-mediated disruption of the interaction might lead to release of progenitors into the circulation. This explanation does not account for the requirement for the c-Kit–SlF interaction, however.

In addition to mobilization of stem/progenitor cells by administration of anti-α_4 integrin or VCAM-1 antibodies to mice, Papayannopoulou and colleagues (1995) found that these antibodies inhibited the homing of CFU-C (an in vitro measure of hematopoietic progenitor cell activity) and CFU-S to the bone marrow by about 50%. However, administration of blocking anti–VCAM-1 antibodies by another group had no effect on CFU-C homing to bone marrow (Frenette et al., 1998), although homing was assessed after a longer time period in the latter study (14 hours vs. 3 hours).

As mentioned previously, chimeric mice containing some hematopoietic cells in which the β_1 integrin chain was deleted by gene targeting were used to demonstrate an absolute requirement for β_1 integrin(s) for colonization of the fetal liver by HSC (Hirsch et al., 1996). Because β_1 can pair with any of several α subunits, it was not clear from this study which α subunit(s) is (are) required for liver colonization. It is not the α_4 subunit, because α_4 null cells in chimeric embryos colonize fetal liver normally (Arroyo et al., 1996).

The α_4 subunit pairs with either of two β subunits, forming $\alpha_4\beta_1$ (discussed previously), or $\alpha_4\beta_7$, which binds endothelial-expressed MAdCAM-1 and facilitates migration of lymphocytes into mucosal-associated lymphoid tissue (Holzmann et al., 1989; Hamann et al., 1994). Although α_4 integrins are not required for HSC colonization of fetal liver or bone marrow, the study by Arroyo and colleagues (1996) revealed a complex role for α_4 integrins in adult life. Functionally normal α_4 null CD4 and CD8 T cells were present in the periphery of chimeric animals in the first few weeks of life, but the number of α_4 null thymic CD4/CD8 double-negative and double-positive cells gradually fell. Interestingly, primary or secondary transplantation of bone marrow cells into sublethally irradiated RAG-1$^{-/-}$ mice (RAG-1$^{-/-}$ mice are unable to produce mature lymphocytes on their own) resulted in short-term reconstitution of peripheral T cells. These data suggest that α_4 null bone marrow T-cell precursors form normally in the bone marrow and are able to colonize the adult thymus, but are unable to migrate out of the bone marrow. The fact that peripheral T-cell reconstitution occurred even when bone marrow from secondary recipients was transferred suggests that HSC are capable of entering the bone marrow and giving rise to T-cell progenitors in the absence of α_4 integrins (Arroyo et al., 1996). In addition, although α_4 null T cells were able to migrate normally to lymph nodes, they were unable to colonize the Peyer's patches. Although NK cells and monocytes developed normally in the absence of α_4 integrin expression, B-cell development in the bone marrow of adult mice was blocked at an early stage. In contrast to the adult, fetal B lymphopoiesis was reported to be α_4 integrin-independent (Arroyo et al., 1996).

Mebius et al., (1996) demonstrated that in the case of immigration of CD4$^+$ CD3$^-$ cells into developing lymph nodes, alterations in interactions between adhesion molecules and their ligands can function as "developmental switches" by facilitating a function only in a specific window of time. The dependence of B and T lymphopoiesis on α_4 integrin during adult but not fetal life appears to represent another such developmental switch mediated by adhesion molecules. Also, as evidenced by the observations that B-cell development (of α_4 integrin null cells) appeared to be blocked at an earlier stage than T-cell development, and that monocyte and NK cell development were α_4 integrin-independent, specific adhesion molecules can play both lineage- and developmental stage-specific roles.

Selectins

Another family of adhesion molecules that mediates interactions among hematopoietic cells and other cells is the selectins. Selectins allow initial attachment, or rolling of leukocytes on vascular endothelium, which is considered to be the first step of leukocyte extravasation (reviewed in Butcher, 1991; Springer, 1994). The three selectins are expressed on leukocytes and endothelial cells, and bind sugar moieties on specific glycoproteins or glycolipids through lectin domains at their N-terminals (reviewed in Lasky, 1992). L-selectin (CD62L), the first adhesion molecule described (Gallatin et al., 1983), is expressed constitutively on most leukocytes (Tedder et al., 1990) and interacts through a lectin domain (Lasky et al., 1989) with ligands that are constitutively expressed by high endothelial venules (HEV, Spertini et al., 1991), and inducibly expressed by other endothelia (Ley et al., 1993). L-selectin–deficient mice have no reported hematopoietic defects (Arbones et al., 1994; Xu et al., 1996). E-selectin (CD62E) is synthesized de novo and expressed on endothelia in humans and mice following stimulation (Bevilacqua et al., 1987; Bevilacqua et al., 1989; Picker et al., 1991), and has been reported to be expressed constitutively on endothelia of fetal and adult hematopoietic organs (Schweitzer et al., 1996). P-selectin (CD62P) is stored in α granules of platelets and Weibel–Palade bodies of endothelial cells and is translocated rapidly to the plasma membrane following exposure to inflammatory mediators (Berman et al., 1986; McEver et al., 1989). P-selectin interacts with P-selectin glycoprotein ligand-1 (PSGL-1) on hematopoietic cells (Zannettino et al., 1995; Tracey and Rinder, 1996). A recent study of human $CD34^+/CD38^-$ cells, a population enriched for primitive hematopoietic progenitors and HSC, found that PSGL-1 is the only ligand for P-selectin on these cells (Levesque et al., 1999). Intriguingly, ligation of PSGL-1 by either soluble or immobilized P-selectin, or by anti–PSGL-1 antibody, resulted in marked inhibition of growth of $CD34^+$ / $CD38^-$ cells in culture, and in apoptosis of some $CD34^+/CD38^-$ cells (Levesque et al., 1999). This study, along with recent work linking ligation of PSGL-1 to activation of an integrin (Evangelista et al., 1999), suggests that, like other adhesion molecules on hematopoietic cells, PSGL-1 may have roles in signaling as well as adhesion. Recent work in our laboratory has confirmed the surface expression of PSGL-1 by highly enriched long-term mouse HSC (A. J. Wagers and I.L.W. unpublished data, 2000).

The possibility of involvement of sugar-binding moieties in homing of hematopoietic cells was raised in a study in which bone marrow cells were transplanted into irradiated animals in the presence of various synthetic neo-glycoproteins containing galactosyl or mannosyl residues. The claim was made that hematopoietic progenitor cells expressed lectins that might be involved in their homing to hematopoietic sites (Aizawa and Tavassoli, 1988). Another study by the same group implicated lectin–carbohydrate interactions involving sulfated proteoglycans in binding of hematopoietic progenitor cell lines to stroma, but because this work was done with cell lines it is of uncertain relevance to in vivo biology (Minguell et al., 1992).

Recent evidence suggests that the endothelial P-and E-selectins may participate, along with the VLA-4–VCAM-1 interaction, in homing of hematopoietic progenitors to bone marrow (Frenette et al., 1998; Mazo et al., 1998). (Hematopoietic progenitors must, of course, home to bone marrow following clinical transplantation, but as will be discussed later, they may also be released constitutively from bone marrow of normal animals, and then home back to, and engraft at, other bone marrow sites; D.E.W., A. Pathak, I.L.W. unpublished data, 2000). Although deletion by gene targeting of either P-or E-selectin by itself resulted in a mild phenotype (Mayadas et al., 1993; Labow et al., 1994), the double mutant mice had severe hematopoietic alterations and susceptibility to infection consistent with an inability of leukocytes to exit the circulation (Bullard et al., 1996; Frenette et al., 1996). When wild-type bone marrow was transferred into lethally irradiated P-/E-selectin double-mutant mice ($P/E^{-/-}$), the recipient mice all died about 10–15 days later at doses of bone marrow sufficient to radioprotect most wild-type recipients (Frenette et al., 1998). The authors attributed this early death to a failure of homing by hematopoietic progenitors to the bone marrow. However, $P/E^{-/-}$ recipients exhibited substantially higher levels of bone marrow granulopoiesis at the time of death than did wild-type recipients. This suggests that homing of progenitors to bone marrow was not a limiting factor for hematopoiesis, and that alternate explanations for the early death are possible. Lethally irradiated $P/E^{-/-}$ mice injected 14 hours earlier with wild-type bone marrow had up to 50% fewer CFU-C in their bone marrow, with a much more pronounced reduction in bone marrow CFU-C if the $P/E^{-/-}$ recipients were pretreated with anti–VCAM-1 antibodies (Frenette et al., 1998). Taken together, these data suggested collaborative roles for endothelial P- and E-selectin and VCAM-1 in homing of progenitors to bone marrow. It should be noted, however, that selectin usage by leukocytes can change under the influence of inflammatory mediators (Ley et al., 1995).

A more direct approach taken by the same group was to study homing of fluorescently labeled cells to the marrow of the thin skull bones in situ using intravital microscopy (Mazo et al., 1998). Labeled, unfractionated E11 fetal liver cells, or FDCP-mix or M1 (progenitor cell lines) cells were injected into the carotid artery of wild-type or $P/E^{-/-}$ mice, in the presence or absence of function-blocking antibodies to all three selectins, VCAM-1, or VLA-4 (Mazo et al., 1998). Although rolling on bone marrow endothelia was L-selectin–independent, P- and E-selectin–dependent rolling was observed, as was selectin-independent rolling mediated by VLA-4 on the input cells and endothelial VCAM-1. Confirming the earlier work, P- and E-selectin, as well as VCAM-1, all contributed to rolling on bone marrow endothelia by the cells studied. Unfortunately, the relevance of the behavior in these assays of immortalized hematopoietic progenitor cell lines (the cell lines, as well as the fetal liver cells, were used because the assay required large numbers of input cells) to that of any unaltered hematopoietic progenitor population is unknown. Likewise, it is not safe to assume that the homing behavior of E11 fetal liver cells represents that of adult HSC or progenitor populations, especially in light of the clear differences in adhesion molecule usage between fetal and adult hematopoietic progenitors that have been demonstrated (Arroyo et al., 1996; Hirsch et al., 1996).

Isoforms of CD44

Hematopoietic progenitors also express isoforms of the glycoprotein CD44 (Pgp-1, H-CAM), a receptor for hyaluronic acid (HA; Turley, 1982; Turley and Moore, 1984; Turley and Torrance, 1985) and fibronectin (Jalkanen and Jalkanen, 1992). In the hematopoietic system, CD44 is expressed by adult pluripotent HSC (Antica et al., 1994; D.E.W. and I.L.W., unpublished data, 1996) and hematopoietic progenitors (Horst et al., 1990; Kansas et al., 1990; Lesley et al., 1993; Wu et al., 1993; Antica et al., 1994), but may not be expressed by fetal liver HSC (Huang and Auerbach, 1993). HA, a disaccharide polymer consisting of repeat units of N-acetyl-D-glucosamine and N-acetyl-D-glucuronic acid, is ubiquitous in extracellular matrix (ECM) and in circulation. HSC, as well as common myeloid precursor (CLP) and other bone marrow progenitors, express CD44 (Kansas et al., 1990; Lewinsohn et al., 1990; Kondo et al., 1997). Like the integrins, CD44 may also function as a signal transducer as well as an adhesion molecule with adjustable ligand affinity and cytoskeletal associations (Chiu et al., 1995; Liu et al., 1998).

Antibody blockade of CD44–HA inhibited myelopoiesis in long-term Dexter-type cultures and lymphopoiesis in Whitlock–Witte cultures (Miyake et al., 1990). However, antibody studies can be confounded by toxicity or other effects of the antibody itself, and the relevance of in vitro assays to in vivo biology must of course always be tested. Indeed, in the case of CD44, data from work done with knockout mice are not easily reconciled with the in vitro data. Mice made defective in all isoforms of CD44 by gene targeting had elevated colony-forming unit–granulocyte-macrophage (CFU-GM, an in vitro assay of myelomonocytic progenitor activity) activity in the bone marrow (Schmits et al., 1997), and reduced CFU-GM activity in the blood and spleen. If CD44 were required for myelopoiesis, as the in vitro data suggested, one would not expect elevated CFU-GM in the bone marrow of CD44 null animals. It might be that myeloid progenitors in the bone marrow have interactions with ligands not present in the in vitro cultures that relieve them of dependence on CD44. CD44 null mice also displayed impaired mobilization of progenitors from bone marrow to blood after administration of the mobilizing cytokine G-CSF (Schmits et al., 1997). Taken together, the knockout data suggested that CD44 may be involved in egress of progenitors from the bone marrow, although it was not clear whether this is a direct or indirect effect. A possible role of CD44 in mobilization of HSC was not addressed in this study.

Hematopoietic Homeostasis

The hematopoietic system must not only produce a huge array of effector cells, but must also produce all classes of cells in the right numbers to re-place senescing cells under steady-state conditions, and in elevated numbers under certain conditions of hematopoietic stress. The rather static-looking hematopoietic "tree" in Figure 2.2 should be understood as a highly dy-namic matrix of cells with various degrees of developmental flexibility. HSC can theoretically undergo symmetric (daughter cells with identical fates) or asymmetric (daughter cells with different fates) divisions, and these divisions can either lead only to self-renewal (symmetric division), only to differen-tiation (symmetric division), or to both (asymmetric division). Self-renewal by some progenitors developmentally downstream from HSC is reduced or absent (Morrison et al., 1997a), but some of these progenitors apparently retain the capacity to undergo asymmetric divisions, so that lineages can diverge.

In considering the structure and control of the hematopoietic system, it is useful to estimate how many cell divisions lie between HSC and mature cells, because each cell division represents a potential control point. The number of cell divisions between HSC and mature cells can be estimated crudely as follows: The adult C57BL mouse has roughly 8×10^4 long-term HSC (Mor-rison et al., 1997b), about 8% (6400) of which enter the cell cycle daily (Cheshier et al., 1999). We will assume that each of these 6,400 cells divides asymmetrically, producing one daughter cell that differentiates, and one that remains a stem cell. The dividing HSC pool must produce an estimated 4×10^6 nonlymphoid cells, as well as 2.4×10^8 erythrocytes daily (Metcalf, 1988). Ignoring lymphocyte production, and making the simplifying assumptions that the same number of cell divisions are required for all cells to reach maturity and that no cells die before maturity, each HSC must produce about 38,000 erythrocytes and nonlymphoid cells daily ($2.44 \times 10^8/6400 = 38,000$. This corresponds to a minimum average of about 15–16 cell divisions be-tween HSC and mature cells (this number will be slightly higher still if lym-phocyte production is added). However, the early compartment of the he-matopoietic system has been estimated to have a large excess capacity in the form of much higher numbers of primitive progenitors than are actually needed to meet daily demands (Necas et al., 1995). Many of these primitive progenitors die by apoptosis, the extent of which decreases as one moves toward more committed bone marrow precursors (Necas et al., 1998). This excess capacity implies that more than the minimum number of cell divisions lie between HSC and mature cells.

In this (oversimplified) model, HSC have the greatest capacity to produce downstream descendants and thus have the highest "proliferative potential." Accordingly, more mature progenitors have a lower proliferative potential. In vitro assays of HSC and progenitor function generally support this notion, in that immature progenitors are observed to produce colonies consisting of more cells than committed progenitors (Ogawa, 1993).

It follows, then, that regulation of hematopoietic homeostasis could be accomplished globally and more crudely at the level of HSC and primitive progenitors, or more finely at the level of progenitors with more restricted proliferative and developmental potential, or at multiple levels. Although it is not known at which levels the system is regulated on a day-to-day basis, a significantly increased proportion of LT-HSC enters the cell cycle in mice under hematopoietic stress following blood loss (S. H. Cheshier, I.L.W., unpublished data, 1999). Strikingly, HSC frequencies and absolute numbers vary considerably among mouse strains. Although there is modest variability in leukocyte counts among strains (red blood cell counts, however, are nearly identical among different strains; Green, 1966), these variations are much less than the variations in HSC numbers. In particular, AKR/J and DBA/2 mice have high HSC numbers, and C57BL/6 mice have low HSC numbers (de Haan and Van Zant, 1997; Muller-Sieburg and Riblet, 1996). Using the same 26 AKR/J × DBA/2 recombinant inbred strains in which polymorphic markers had previously been mapped, two groups mapped loci controlling HSC numbers. This was done by estimating the HSC content of bone marrow in each strain using in vitro assays and looking for associations between stem cell content and previously mapped markers. Even though both groups analyzed the same strains of mice using similar assays, they arrived at different conclusions. Linkage analysis by one group yielded an association between control of stem cell frequency and a marker on chromosome 1 (Muller-Sieburg and Riblet, 1996), whereas the other group found high concordance between this trait and a marker on chromosome 18 (de Haan and Van Zant, 1997). The reasons for this discrepancy are unclear, but may relate to differences in the way the assays were scored, or may suggest that multiple genes control this trait.

Adding complexity to the picture, at the HSC level at least four developmental "choices" are available: self-renewal, differentiation, apoptosis, and migration (Fig. 2.3). Any or all of these choices could be used to regulate hematopoiesis. Experiments in which clones of HSC were marked retrovirally suggested that only one, or a few, HSC clones contributed to hematopoiesis at any given time, with clones being replaced after they had exhausted their proliferative potential (Lemischkta et al., 1986; Snodgrass and Keller, 1987; Capel et al., 1989). This was taken as evidence in support of the "clonal succession" model (Kay, 1965). Most HSC were thought to be deeply quiescent (G_0) cells that basically sat in the bone marrow awaiting their turn to enter the cell cycle and contribute to hematopoiesis. This view was supported by the observation that, at any given time, only a small fraction of LT-HSC are in the S-, G_2-, or M-phases of the cell cycle. However, recent studies in which mice have been administered bromodeoxyuridine (BrdU), a thymidine analogue incorporated by DNA at synthesis, have shown that all LT-HSC

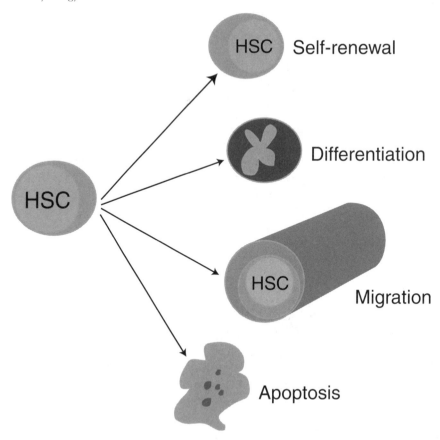

Fig. 2.3. Development choices of hematopoietic stem cells (HSC): It is likely that fate decisions of HSC are made upon cell division, at which point several choices are available. Daughter cells can self-renew, remain as HSC, or they can differentiate. LT-HSC differentiate to ST-HSC, which become multipotent progenitors. Multipotent progenitors in turn become committed progenitors that produce mature hematopoietic cells (see Fig. 2.2). A third fate is HSC migration and seeding of other sites. Migration of HSC mediates transitions among sites of hematopoiesis in fetal life, and provides for a continual, low-level supply of HSC in adult blood that can repopulate available niches. HSC migration can also be induced by drugs and is currently of great significance in clinical HSC transplantation. A fourth HSC fate is apoptosis, which is one means by which HSC numbers are maintained.

continually enter and exit the cell cycle, such that about 8% of LT-HSC enter the cell cycle per day. Individual LT-HSC were estimated to divide an average of about once a month (Bradford et al., 1997; Cheshier et al., 1999). At the population level, at least half of these monthly divisions must be partly (an asymmetric division can be partly self-renewing) or fully self-renewing divisions, because the overall number of HSC remains approximately constant.

The degree to which HSC divide symmetrically versus asymmetrically, as well as the genetic determinants of this choice are under study.

The role of apoptosis in the regulation of stem cell numbers also deserves mention. Although a review of the effects of manipulation of the many pro- and antiapoptotic genes in hematopoietic cells is beyond the scope of this chapter, recent studies suggest strongly that apoptosis has a role in regulation of HSC numbers. Transgenic mice overexpressing the human antiapoptotic proto-oncogene *BCL-2* on HSC under the control of the MHC class I promoter have markedly elevated numbers of all classes of HSC (Domen et al., 2000). HSC from H2K–*BCL-2* are more resistant than wild-type HSC to insults ranging from ionizing radiation (Domen et al., 1998) to exposure to cytotoxic drugs, and they show markedly increased survival in vitro with and without growth factors (Domen et al., 2000; J. Domen and I.L.W., unpublished data 1999). The facts that HSC from H2K–*BCL-2* mice display increased survival whether or not they are in the presence of other cells, and that they outcompete wild-type cells when injected into irradiated recipients (even though they have fewer HSC in the S/G_2-, or M-phases of the cell cycle than wild-type mice), indicate that the trait is cell intrinsic (Domen et al., 2000). The simplest explanation for these findings is that apoptosis is one of the ways in which HSC numbers are regulated, and that *BCL-2* overexpression directly blocks apoptosis of HSC.

It is likely that on a day-to-day basis, the maintenance of appropriate numbers of cells in each lineage is mostly effected at the level of progenitors more committed than HSC. In addition to apoptosis, numerous cytokines, such as IL-1, IL-3, IL-4, IL-5, IL-6, IL-11, IL-12, monocyte colony-stimulating factor (M-CSF), G-CSF, GM-CSF, erythropoietin (EPO), and leukemia inhibitory factor (LIF) have been implicated by in vitro or in vivo studies in regulation or maintenance of hematopoietic progenitors. A full review of the often-overlapping effects of these factors will not be attempted here, but is useful to try to place them in a conceptual framework. As discussed previously, some factors, such as SlF, TPO, and FL appear to affect HSC, directly or indirectly.

Other, "late-acting" factors function in a lineage-specific manner on progenitors that are already committed to a lineage (for review, see Ogawa, 1993). G-CSF, among other functions, regulates proliferation and maturation of neutrophil precursors. Mice in which the G-CSF gene was disrupted showed marked reductions in both circulating neutrophils and granulocyte and macrophage precursors in the bone marrow (Lieschke et al., 1994). Disruption of the gene for GM-CSF, which was thought to promote granulocyte and macrophage development based on its potent activity in vitro, revealed that it is dispensable, at least for hematopoiesis (Dranoff et al., 1994; Stanley et al., 1994). TPO, as well as a number of other factors, promotes megakaryopoiesis and platelet production (Alexander et al., 1996), and EPO is the key regulator of erythropoiesis; it appears to function as a survival factor (for review, see LaCombe and Mayeux, 1998). Eosinophil production is influenced by IL-5 (Sanderson, 1992), and the monocyte/macrophage lineage is regulated by M-CSF (Fixe and Praloran, 1998).

IL-3 and IL-4 have been categorized as "intermediate-acting, lineage-nonspecific" factors (Ogawa, 1993), in that they support growth of multi-potent progenitors (Fig. 2.2). GM-CSF has been included in this category of intermediate-acting factors, but it is not necessary for hematopoiesis. Perhaps the IL-3 receptor, which in humans shares its β subunit with the GM-CSF receptor (Kitamura et al., 1991), allows IL-3 to compensate for the lack of GM-CSF in GM-CSF–knockout animals.

This extremely truncated overview by no means does justice to the complexity of the regulation of hematopoiesis by cytokines, or to their often overlapping and synergistic actions. The extent to which cytokines function to actively promote development of a particular lineage, rather than acting simply as survival factors is under study. For example, Akashi et al., (1997) showed that although T and B lymphopoiesis in mice lacking the α chain of the IL-7 receptor is severely disrupted, enforced expression of the *bcl-2* gene in a T-lineage–specific manner in these mice restored thymic T lymphopoiesis to near-normal levels. This suggests that the IL-7 receptor transmits cell survival signals that can be bypassed nonspecifically. Other cytokines may function similarly (Lagasse and Weissman, 1997). Whether or not some cytokines may have a role in specification of cell fate, rather than simply supporting already-committed cells, is under investigation.

Cell Migration During Adult Hematopoiesis

Cell migration is vital to hematopoiesis. The entire output of the bone marrow (approximately 3×10^{10} leukocytes/day in the human) migrates from the stromal to the vascular space. Among these cells are thymus-seeding cells (bone marrow cells that seed the thymus are still poorly defined and may include HSC, CLP, or other cells), naïve B cells that home to the spleen or lymph nodes, and monocytes and myeloid precursors that home to various tissues to complete their maturation. Recently described c-Kit^{+} lineage^{-} T-cell progenitors (or precursors of these cells), which appear to develop in gut microcrypts called *cryptopatches*, may also be among the bone marrow emigrant populations (Saito et al., 1998).

Likewise, it is a reasonable assumption that immature hematopoietic cells must move among stromal microenvironments as they develop. Although the details of these movements are unknown, recent work in several labs has provided the conceptual framework for how some of these migrations may take place. First, a distinction should be made between cell movement within hematopoietic organs, and extravasation, which requires that cells in the bloodstream contact the endothelial wall and come to a stop prior to passing through the endothelium. Extravasation of cells in the vasculature has been extensively studied (although not in bone marrow), and a multistep model of the process has emerged from the work of several labs (Butcher, 1991, 1992; Springer, 1994). Simply stated, leukocytes, which are initially moving rapidly with respect to the vasculature, begin to roll along the endothelium through tethering interactions involving leukocyte or endothelial selectins and their ligands, and/or other molecules such as integrins (Berlin et al., 1995). Rolling leukocytes can sample the endothelial microenvironment for chemokine signals. If appropriate chemokines are present, and if the right chemokine receptors are expressed on the rolling cell, a rapid signaling cascade is initiated, starting with G-proteins linked to the chemokine receptors, and including up-regulation of affinity of integrins for their endothelial ligands. The increased ligand affinity of integrins causes the cells to stop rolling. The arrested cells can then further sample the environment, and either cross the endothelial wall or not, most likely depending on whether other chemokine signals that trigger extravasation are present. Minimal requirements for the tethering/rolling and arrest steps have been elucidated (Campbell et al., 1998).

In contrast to extravasation, few details are available about movements of cells within hematopoietic organs. The beginnings of a conceptual framework for how hematopoietic cells may navigate in complex environments containing many stimuli, such as bone marrow, have been advanced in an elegant study by Foxman et al. (1997). In that study, neutrophils were found capable of serially responding to multiple chemotactic factors, even in the presence of disorienting concentrations of chemotactic factors, which they had very recently responded to by migrating. In effect, the investigators could steer the migration of neutrophils by setting up appropriate gradients of chemotactic factors. It is appreciated that specificity of cell migration can be achieved at the levels of adhesion receptors and/or chemotactic factors such as chemokines. Prior to the study by Foxman et al. (1997), however, it was difficult to understand how cells could navigate in complex environments where they might come under the opposite influences of two gradients of chemotactic factors. Apparently, at least some cells can migrate in response to, and then ignore, a chemotactic gradient before newly responding to a second stimulus.

Hematopoietic Stem Cell Migration and Mobilization

Unlike some other leukocytes that migrate often, HSC are probably only occasionally migratory. HSC migration is observed in several settings. As described previously, the primary site of hematopoiesis changes several times during normal mammalian embryonic and fetal development, culminating in the establishment of hematopoiesis in the bone marrow of adult animals (reviewed in Morrison, et al., 1995b). In normal adult mammals, constitutive migration of small numbers of HSC from bone marrow is believed to account for the low frequency of HSC that can be found in the blood (Cavins et al., 1964; Appelbaum, 1979). Although the significance and function of these blood-borne HSC is not known, the phenomenon is currently being investigated using parabiotic mice. Within three days of being surgically joined along their sides, vascular anastamoses form, and the pairs of mice develop a shared vasculature. Adult parabiotic mice in which hematopoietic cells from each partner were genetically marked were used to show that, given several weeks of exposure, blood-borne HSC from one member of a pair engrafted the (unconditioned) bone marrow of the partner mouse (D.E.W., A. Pathak, I.L.W., unpublished data, 2000). This suggests that a fraction of HSC may be continuously redistributed, perhaps as a means of efficiently filling HSC niches as they become available.

HSC migration may also be responsible for initiation of extramedullary hematopoiesis observed in diseases such as chronic myelogenous leukemia (Tsukamoto et al., 1994), and in some genetically altered animals (Lagasse and Weissman, 1994). HSC migration has been studied extensively recently, not only because of its role in development, but also because of its importance in clinical stem cell transplantation for the treatment of malignancies and other diseases.

HSC and/or hematopoietic progenitors can be "mobilized" from bone marrow to the periphery in large numbers by administration of any of a variety of cytoreductive drugs (Richman et al., 1976; Appelbaum, 1979; Abrams et al., 1981; Juttner et al., 1985), and/or cytokines, alone or in combination. The list of mobilizing agents includes G-CSF (Molineux et al., 1990), GM-CSF (Socinski et al., 1988), SlF (Gianni et al., 1989; Siena et al., 1989; Molineux et al., 1991; Andrews et al., 1992; McNiece et al., 1993; de Revel et al., 1994), IL-1 (Fibbe et al., 1992), IL-3 (Brugger et al., 1992; Geissler et al., 1996; Huhn et al., 1996; Rosenfeld et al., 1996), IL-7 (Grzegorzewski et al., 1995), IL-11 (Mauch et al., 1995), IL-12 (Jackson et al., 1995), FL (Papayannopoulou et al., 1997; Ashihara et al., 1998), the chemokines IL-8 (Laterveer et al., 1995, 1996) and MIP-1α (Lord et al., 1995; Marshall et al., 1997), as well as antibodies to either member of the adhesion receptor–ligand pair $\alpha_4 \beta 1$ integrin/VCAM-1 (Papayannopoulou and Nakamoto, 1993; Papayannopoulou et al., 1995). Cytokine-mobilized HSC are widely used in clinical transplantation, but the biology of mobilization and homing to hematopoietic sites is poorly understood.

The kinetics of mobilization by these diverse agents varies widely. Administration of some agents, such as IL-8 (Laterveer et al., 1995, 1996) or SlF + G-CSF (Bodine et al., 1996), results in rapid (within 15–30 minutes) release of some HSC into the periphery, whereas for most agents the response takes several days (Morrison et al., 1997b). Proliferation of HSC is associated with mobilization by some, but not all, agents. When the most commonly used mobilizing agents administered to humans, cyclophosphamide (CY) and G-CSF, are given to mice, HSC expand greatly in the bone marrow prior to mobilization. After the initial expansion phase, HSC are released abruptly into the blood, apparently in substantially higher numbers than are released following IL-8 treatment (Morrison et al., 1997b). Recent BrdU studies our laboratory have shown that HSC egress from bone marrow is tightly coordinated with the cell cycle; cycling HSC enter the blood specifically after undergoing mitosis, but prior to DNA synthesis (Wright et al., submitted). This phenomenon may result from a cell cycle–dependent de-adhesion from substrate analogous to that which is observed in cultured adherent cells during M-phase (Aggeler et al., 1982). Cytokine mobilization of adult HSC may use mechanisms that evolved to regulate the subtle recirculation of HSC in adult animals, or to regulate transitions among hematopoietic organs during fetal development (Aguila et al., 1997), or both.

Down-regulation of $\alpha_4\beta_1$ integrin expression on hematopoietic progenitors after mobilizing regimens has been reported (Dercksen et al., 1995; Prosper et al., 1998), and is proposed to facilitate egress of HSC from bone marrow. Rapid IL-8–induced mobilization is blocked by pretreatment of mice with antibodies to the integrin LFA-1 ($\alpha_L\beta_2$ integrin; Pruijt et al., 1998), suggesting that interactions involving LFA-1 are required for mobilization by IL-8. It is not clear whether the observed effect of anti–LFA-1 resulted from a simple blockade of an adhesive interaction involving LFA-1, or from another cause, such as interference by the antibody with LFA-1–mediated signaling, nor is it clear which cells are involved. The G-CSF receptor (G-CSFR) is required for mobilization of progenitors by CY or interleukin-8 but not by FL (Liu et al., 1997), suggesting either that different mechanisms exist for mobilization by FL compared to CY or IL-8, or that FL acts downstream of signaling through the G-CSFR in a pathway common to all three agents. The question of which cells were required to express the G-CSF receptor was not addressed in Liu et al. (1997).

Given the importance of chemokines in leukocyte trafficking (for review, see Premack and Schall, 1996), one would predict that stem cell mobilization and homing might be regulated at least in part by chemokines, although there is no direct evidence to date that this is so. The chemokine stromal cell-derived factor (SDF-1), originally described as a growth factor for early stage B-cell precursors (Tashiro et al., 1993; Nagasawa et al., 1994), and monocyte/lymphocyte chemoattractant (Bleul et al., 1996), caused chemotaxis of human CD34$^+$ cells (in the human, CD34$^+$ cells are partially enriched for HSC) in vitro (Aiuti et al., 1997). Mice made deficient for either SDF-1 or its ligand CXCR4 die perinatally of similar severe neurological, cardiac, vascular, and hematopoietic defects, suggesting that they are a monogamous receptor–ligand pair (Nagasawa et al., 1996; Ma et al., 1998; Tachibana et al., 1998; Zou et al., 1998). Due to the lethality of homozygous null mutations of either SDF-1 or CXCR4, research into the effect of homozygous null alleles is difficult. Study of CXCR4-deficient cells was made possible, however, by production of chimeric animals in which the hematopoietic system derives wholly or partly from ES cells in which both alleles of the gene of interest (in this case CXCR4) have been disrupted (Chen et al., 1993). In addition to abnormal granulopoiesis and B lymphopoiesis in chimeric animals generated by this technique, elevated levels of CXCR4-null B lymphocyte and granulocyte precursors were found in the peripheral blood (Ma et al., 1999). Based on this observation, the authors suggested that SDF-1, acting through CXCR4, may function as a "retention factor" that holds some myeloid and B-cell progenitors in the bone marrow.

A role for CXCR4 in engraftment of transplanted progenitor cells was suggested in a recent report in which CD34$^+$CD38$^{-/low}$ cells pretreated with anti-CXCR4 antibody, engrafted NOD/SCID mice less well than control cells pretreated with anti-CD34 antibody (Peled et al., 1999). In this study, CXCR4 expression could be up-regulated by treatment with S1F and IL-6, and CXCR4 levels on CD34$^+$ cells correlated with their engraftment potential. In adoptive transfer experiments (Kawabata et al., 1999), donor fetal liver cells lacking CXCR4 contributed poorly to long-term lymphoid and myeloid reconstitution, although it was unclear whether defective homing of progenitors to bone marrow was responsible for any of the observed defects.

SDF-1 has also been suggested to function in mobilization of hematopoietic progenitor cells from bone marrow to blood. This was based on the observation that CD34$^+$ cells obtained from mobilized peripheral blood of cancer patients migrated less well in response to SDF-1 in in vitro chemotaxis assays than did CD34$^+$ cells obtained from bone marrow of normal donors (Aiuti et al., 1997). Experiments in which migration of highly purified mouse ST-HSC and LT-HSC from mobilized peripheral blood was compared with migration of the same HSC populations from bone marrow of untreated animals showed no difference in the responsiveness of the two HSC populations (D.E.W., E. P. Bowman, E. C. Butcher, and I.L.W., unpublished data, 2000. This may be attributable to species differences, or it may suggest that differences exist between the behavior of CD34$^+$ cells, only a small fraction of which are HSC, and that of purified HSC. Also, it should be noted that another group did not observe differences in migration between CD34$^+$ cells obtained from mobilized peripheral blood and CD34$^+$ cells obtained from bone marrow. (In fact, a slightly higher fraction of CD34$^+$ cells from mobilized blood migrated to SDF-1, on average; Peled et al., 1999.)

Mobilization of HSC in response to cytoreductive agents or cytokines has been observed in all mammals studied to date (Richman et al., 1976; Abrams et al., 1981; Socinski et al., 1988; Molineux et al., 1990; Andrews et al., 1992; Gratwohl et al., 1995). The fact that cytokine mobilization is evolutionarily conserved suggests that a naturally occurring version of this response may have physiological significance to many species, perhaps as a way of quickly expanding and restoring hematopoiesis, for example, after consumption of myeloablative compounds (Christopher Goodnow, personal communication, 1997) or after blood loss. Cytokine treatment may activate pathways that normally lead to mobilization of HSC during prenatal development, to constitutive migration of small numbers of HSC from bone marrow to blood in adult animals, or both.

Homing of Transplanted HSC: Effect of the Cell Cycle

As mentioned previously, HSC must home to proper microenvironments following clinical HSC transplantation. When used to support high-dose chemotherapy and/or radiotherapy in cancer treatment, the bone marrow is conditioned by lethal ablation and the patient will die if engraftment fails. It is therefore considered of primary importance to understand the molecular mechanisms of HSC homing and engraftment following transplantation.

Perhaps surprisingly, a key factor in predicting whether or not HSC can engraft successfully is position in the cell cycle at the time of transplantation. Progenitors or HSC that are in the $S/G_2/M$-phases of the cell cycle have poor engraftment potential compared to progenitors or stem cells that are in the G_0-or G_1-phases (Quesenberry et al., 1973; Monette and DeMello, 1979; Fleming et al., 1993a). In a recent study, HSC were induced by cytokines to cycle synchronously in vitro, and then removed from culture at 2- to 4-hour intervals and placed in long-term reconstitution assays (Habibian et al., 1998). Strikingly, the engraftment potential varied dramatically and reversibly, in a cell cycle-dependent manner, with an engraftment nadir at the S/G_2 boundary. It is tempting to speculate that cell cycle-dependent alterations in homing molecules may in part explain these differences in engraftment potential.

Future Directions

Prenatal and adult hematopoiesis are both rich areas for future study because so many fundamental questions remain unanswered. For example, the relationship between fetal and adult stem cells is poorly understood, as is the relationship among HSC, primitive mesenchymal cells, and stem cells of other tissues. It is reasonable to assume that some of the genetic programs and molecular mechanisms that direct the development of primitive hematopoietic cells will be shared by mature cells. In other cases, different mechanisms may be the rule.

In adult hematopoiesis, it is perhaps surprising that despite the enormous daily volume of cellular traffic across the sinusoidal endothelium, little is known about the molecular mechanisms or control of these movements. Remarkably, amotile cells, such as mature erythrocytes, as well as motile cells, like granulocytes, normally make the passage to blood successfully, and at the proper maturational stage.

Bone marrow microenvironments are poorly defined, and there is little information about how or whether developing cells move among these microenvironments, or whether the microenvironments change as cells develop. It is likely that chemokines and specific adhesion receptors will be found to play roles in the orchestration of appropriate trafficking of maturing hematopoietic cells, although few details are now available. Developing hematopoietic cells may signal their maturational state to the surrounding stromal cells that support their development, but this has yet to be demonstrated. Also, the sensing and effector mechanisms responsible for the fact that appropriate numbers of mature cells of all of the many hematopoietic lineages are normally maintained are mostly unknown. Addressing the basic biology of hematopoiesis will undoubtedly deepen our understanding of the immune system and of inflammatory processes.

We gratefully acknowledge Julie Christensen, Jos Domen, and Amy J. Wagers for careful reading of this chapter, Koichi Akashi for helpful advice, and David Traver for Figure 2.2.

References

Abrams, R. A., McCormack, K., Bowles, C., and Deisseroth, A. B. (1981) Cyclophosphamide treatment expands the circulating hematopoietic stem cell pool in dogs. *J. Clin. Invest.* 67:1392–1399.

Aggeler, J., Kapp, L. N., Tseng, S. C., and Werb, Z. (1982) Regulation of protein secretion in Chinese hamster ovary cells by cell cycle position and cell density. Plasminogen activator, procollagen fibronectin. *Exp. Cell. Res.* 139:275–283.

Aguila, H. L., Akashi, K., Domen, J., Gandy, K. L., Lagasse, E., Mebius, R. E., Morrison, S. J., Shizuru, J., Strober, S., Uchida, N., Wright, D. E., and Weissman, I. L. (1997) From stem cells to lymphocytes: biology and transplantation. *Immunol. Rev.* 157:13–40.

Aiuti, A., Webb, I. J., Bleul, C., Springer, T., and Gutierrez-Ramos, J. C. (1997) The chemokine SDF-1 is a chemoattractant for human CD34+ hematopoietic progenitor cells and provides a new mechanism to explain the mobilization of CD34+ progenitors to peripheral blood. *J. Exp. Med.* 185:111–120.

Aizawa, S., and Tavassoli, M. (1988) Molecular basis of the recognition of intravenously transplanted hemopoietic cells by bone marrow. *Proc. Natl. Acad. Sci. USA* 85:3180–3183.

Akashi, K., Kondo, M., von Freeden-Jeffry, U., Murray, R., and Weissman, I. L. (1997) Bcl-2 rescues T lymphopoiesis in interleukin-7 receptor-deficient mice. *Cell* 89:1033–1041.

Akashi, K., Traver, D., Miyamoto, T., and Weissman, I. L. (2000) A clonogenic common myeloid progenitor that gives rise to all myeloid lineages. *Nature* 404:193–197.

Alexander, W. S., Roberts, A. W., Nicola, N. A., Li, R., and Metcalf, D. (1996) Deficiencies in progenitor cells of multiple hematopoietic lineages and defective megakaryocytopoiesis in mice lacking the thrombopoietic receptor c-Mpl. *Blood* 87:2162–2170.

Andrews, R. G., Bensinger, W. I., Knitter, G. H., Bartelmez, S. H., Longin, K., Bernstein, I. D., Appelbaum, F. R., and Zsebo, K. M. (1992) The ligand for c-kit, stem cell factor, stimulates the circulation of cells that engraft lethally irradiated baboons. *Blood* 80:2715–2720.

Antica, M., Wu, L., Shortman, K., and Scollay, R. (1994) Thymic stem cells in mouse bone marrow. *Blood* 84:111–117.

Appelbaum, F. R. (1979) Hemopoietic reconstitution following autologous bone marrow and peripheral blood mononuclear cell infusions. *Exp. Hematol.* 7 (suppl. 5): 7–11.

Arbones, M. L., Ord, D. C., Ley, K., Ratech, H., Maynard-Curry, C., Otten, G., Capon, D. J., and Tedder, T. F. (1994) Lymphocyte homing and leukocyte rolling and migration are impaired in L-selectin–deficient mice. *Immun.* 1:247–260.

Arroyo, A. G., Yang, J. T., Rayburn, H., and Hynes, R. O. (1996) Differential requirements for alpha4 integrins during fetal and adult hematopoiesis. *Cell* 85:997–1008.

Ashihara, E., Shimazaki, C., Sudo, Y., Kikuta, T., Hirai, H., Sumikuma, T., Yamagata, N., Goto, H., Inaba, T., Fujita, N., and Nakagawa, M. (1998) FLT-3 ligand mobilizes hematopoietic primitive and committed progenitor cells into blood in mice. *Eur. J. Haematol.* 60:86–92.

Bartley, T. D., Bogenberger, J., Hunt, P., Li, Y. S., Lu, H. S., Martin, F., Chang, M. S., Samal, B., Nichol, J. L., Swift, S., et al. (1994) Identification and cloning of a megakaryocyte growth and development factor that is a ligand for the cytokine receptor Mpl. *Cell* 77:1117–1124.

Becker, A. J., McCulloch, E. A., and Till, J. E. (1963) Cytological demonstration of the clonal nature of spleen colonies derived from transplanted mouse marrow cells. *Nature* 197:452–454.

Berlin, C., Bargatze, R. F., Campbell, J. J., von Andrian, U. H., Szabo, M. C., Hasslen, S. R., Nelson, R. D., Berg, E. L., Erlandsen, S. L., and Butcher, E. C. (1995) Alpha 4 integrins mediate lymphocyte attachment and rolling under physiologic flow. *Cell* 80:413–422.

Berman, C. L., Yeo, E. L., Wencel-Drake, J. D., Furie, B. C., Ginsberg, M. H., and Furie, B. (1986) A platelet alpha granule membrane protein that is associated with the plasma membrane after activation: Characterization and subcellular localization of platelet activation-dependent granule-external membrane protein. *J. Clin. Invest.* 78:130–137.

Bevilacqua, M. P., Pober, J. S., Mendrick, D. L., Cotran, R. S., and Gimbrone, M. A. Jr. (1987) Identification of an inducible endothelial–leukocyte adhesion molecule. *Proc. Natl. Acad. Sci. USA* 84:9238–9242.

Bevilacqua, M. P., Stengelin, S., Gimbrone, M. A. Jr., and Seed, B. (1989) Endothelial leukocyte adhesion molecule 1: an inducible receptor for neutrophils related to complement regulatory proteins and lectins. *Science* 243:1160–1165.

Bleul, C. C., Fuhlbrigge, R. C., Casasnovas, J. M., Aiuti, A., and Springer, T. A. (1996) A highly efficacious lymphocyte chemoattractant, stromal cell-derived factor 1 (SDF-1). *J. Exp. Med.* 184:1101–1109.

Bodine, D., Seidel, N. E., and Orlic, D. (1996) Bone marrow collected 14 days after administration of granulocyte colony-stimulating factor and stem cell factor to mice has 10-fold more repopulating ability than untreated bone marrow. *Blood* 88:89–97.

Bradford, G. B., Williams, B., Rossi, R., and Bertoncello, I. (1997) Quiescence, Cycling, and turnover in the primitive hematopoietic stem cell compartment. *Exp. Hematol.* 25:445–453.

Brannan, C. I., Lyman, S. D., Williams, D. E., Eisenman, J., Anderson, D. M., Cosman, D., Bedell, M. A., Jenkins, N. A., and Copeland, N. G. (1991) Steel–Dickie mutation encodes a c-Kit ligand lacking transmembrane and cytoplasmic domains. *Proc. Natl. Acad. Sci. USA* 88:4671–4674.

Brecher, G., Ansell, J. D., Micklem, H. S., Tjio, J. H., and Cronkite, E. P. (1982) Special proliferative sites are not needed for seeding and proliferation of transfused bone marrow cells in normal syngeneic mice. *Proc. Natl. Acad. Sci. USA* 79:5085–5087.

Brugger, W., Bross, K., Frisch, J., Dern, P., Weber, B., Mertelsmann, R., and Kanz, L. (1992) Mobilization of peripheral blood progenitor cells by sequential administration of interleukin-3 and granulocyte-macrophage colony-stimulating factor following polychemotherapy with etoposide, ifosfamide, and cisplatin. *Blood* 79:1193–2000.

Bullard, D. C., Kunkel, E. J., Kubo, H., Hicks, M. J., Lorenzo, I., Doyle, N. A., Doerschuk, C. M., Ley, K., and Beaudet, A. L. (1996) Infectious susceptibility and severe deficiency of leukocyte rolling and recruitment in E-selectin and P-selectin double mutant mice. *J. Exp. Med.* 183: 2329–2336.

Butcher, E. C. (1991) Leukocyte–endothelial cell recognition: three (or more) steps to specificity and diversity. *Cell* 67:1033–1036.

Butcher, E. C. (1992) Leukocyte–endothelial cell adhesion as an active, multi-step process: a combinatorial mechanism for specificity and diversity in leukocyte targeting. *Adv. Exp. Med. Biol.* 323:181–194.

Campbell, J. J., Hedrick, J., Zlotnik, A., Siani, M. A., Thompson, D. A., and Butcher, E. C. (1998) Chemokines and the arrest of lymphocytes rolling under flow conditions. *Science* 279:381–384.

Capel, B., Hawley, R., Covarrubias, L., Hawley, T., and Mintz, B. (1989) Clonal contributions of small numbers of retrovirally marked hematopoietic stem cells engrafted in unirradiated neonatal W/Wᵛ mice. *Proc. Natl. Acad. Sci. USA* 86:4564–4568. [Published erratum appears in *Proc. Natl. Acad. Sci. USA* 1989, 86 (18): 7048]

Carpenter, K. L., and Turpen, J. B. (1979) Experimental studies on hemopoiesis in the pronephros of *Rana pipiens. Differ.* 14:167–174.

Carver-Moore, K., Broxmeyer, H. E., Luoh, S. M., Cooper, S., Peng, J., Burstein, S. A., Moore, M. W., and de Sauvage, F. J. (1996) Low levels of erythroid and myeloid progenitors in thrombopoietin- and c-Mpl–deficient mice. *Blood* 88:803–808.

Cavins, J. A., Scheer, S. C., Thomas, E. D., and Ferrebee, J. W. (1964) The recovery of lethally irradiated dogs given infusions of autologous leulocytes preserved at −80°. *Blood* 23:38–43.

Chabot, B., Stephenson, D. A., Chapman, V. M., Besmer, P., and Bernstein, A. (1988) The proto-oncogene c-Kit encoding a transmembrane tyrosine kinase receptor maps to the mouse W locus. *Nature* 335:88–89.

Chamberlain, J. K., Leblond, P. F., and Weed, R. I. (1975a) Reduction of adventitial cell cover: An early direct effect of erythropoietin on bone marrow ultrastructure. *Blood Cells* 1: 655–674.

Chamberlain, J. K., Weiss, L., and Weed, R. I. (1975b) Bone marrow sinus cell packing: a determinant of cell release. *Blood* 46:91–102.

Chen, J., Lansford, R., Stewart, V., Young, F., and Alt, F. W. (1993) RAG-2–deficient blastocyst complementation: an assay of gene function in lymphocyte development. *Proc. Natl. Acad. Sci. USA* 90:4528–4532.

Cheshier, S. H., Morrison, S. J., Liao, X., and Weissman, I. L. (1999) In vivo proliferation and cell cycle kinetics of long-term self-renewing hematopoietic stem cells. *Proc. Natl. Acad. Sci. USA* 96:3120–3125.

Chiu, R. K., Droll, A., Cooper, D. L., Dougherty, S. T., Dirks, J. F., and Dougherty, G. J. (1995) Molecular mechanisms regulating the hyaluronan binding activity of the adhesion protein CD44. *J. Neurooncol.* 26:231–239.

Clark, E. A., and Brugge, J. S. (1995) Integrins and signal transduction pathways: the road taken. *Science* 268:233–239.

Copeland, N. G., Gilbert, D. J., Cho, B. C., Donovan, P. J., Jenkins, N. A., Cosman, D., Anderson, D., Lyman, S. D., and Williams, D. E. (1990) Mast cell growth factor maps near the steel locus on mouse chromosome 10 and is deleted in a number of steel alleles. *Cell* 63:175–183.

Cumano, A., Paige, C. J., Iscove, N. N., and Brady, G. (1992) Bipotential precursors of B cells and macrophages in murine fetal liver. *Nature* 356:612–615.

Cumano, A., Kee, B. L., Ramsden, D. A., Marshall, A., Paige, C. J., and Wu, G. E. (1994) Development of B lymphocytes from lymphoid committed and uncommitted progenitors. *Immunol. Rev.* 137:5–33.

de Haan, G., and Van Zant, G. (1997) Intrinsic and extrinsic control of hemopoietic stem cell numbers: mapping of a stem cell gene. *J. Exp. Med.* 186:529–536.

Delassus, S., and Cumano, A. (1996) Circulation of hematopoietic progenitors in the mouse embryo. *Immun.* 4:97–106.

Dercksen, M. W., Gerritsen, W. R., Rodenhuis, S., Dirkson, M. K., Slaper-Cortenbach, I. C., Schaasberg, W. P., Pinedo, H. M., von dem Borne, A. E., and van der Schoot, C. E. (1995) Expression of adhesion molecules on CD34+ cells: CD34+ L-selectin+ cells predict a rapid platelet recovery after peripheral blood stem cell transplantation. *Blood* 85:3313–3319.

de Revel, T., Appelbaum, F. R., Storb, R., Schuening, F., Nash, R., Deeg, J., McNiece, I., Andrews, R., and Graham, T. (1994) Effects of granulocyte colony-stimulating factor and stem cell factor, alone and in combination, on the mobilization of peripheral blood cells that engraft lethally irradiated dogs. *Blood* 83:3795–3799.

de Sauvage, F. J., Hass, P. E., Spencer, S. D., Malloy, B. E., Gurney, A. L., Spencer, S. A., Darbonne, W. C., Henzel, W. J., Wong, S. C., Kuang, W. J., et al. (1994) Stimulation of megakaryocytopoiesis and thrombopoiesis by the c-Mpl ligand [see comments]. *Nature* 369:533–538.

Dexter, T. M., Simmons, P., Purnell, R. A., Spooncer, E., and Schofield, R. (1984) The regulation of hemopoietic cell development by the stromal cell environment and diffusible regulatory molecules. *Prog. Clin. Biol. Res.* 148:13–33.

Dieterlen-Lievre, F. (1975) On the origin of haemopoietic stem cells in the avian embryo: an experimental approach. *J. Embryol. Exp. Morphol.* 33:607–619.

Dieterlen-Lievre, F., and Martin, C. (1981) Diffuse intraembryonic hemopoiesis in normal and chimeric avian development. *Dev. Biol.* 88:180–191.

Domen, J., Gandy, K. L., and Weissman, I. L. (1998) Systemic overexpression of BCL-2 in the hematopoietic system protects transgenic mice from the consequences of lethal irradiation. *Blood* 91:2272–2282.

Domen, J., Cheshier, S. H., and Weissman, I. L. (2000) The role of apoptosis in the regulation of hematopoietic stem cells; overexpression of BCL-2 increases both their number and repopulation potential. *J. Exp. Med.* 191:253–264.

Dranoff, G., Crawford, A. D., Sadelain, M., Ream, B., Rashid, A., Bronson, R. T., Dickersin, G. R., Bachurski, C. J., Mark, E. L.; Whitsett, J. A., et al. (1994) Involvement of granulocyte-macrophage colony-stimulating factor in pulmonary homeostasis. *Science* 264:713–716.

Dunn, L. C. (1937) Studies on spotting patterns. II. Genetic analysis of variegated spotting in the house mouse. *Genetics* 22:43–64.

Dustin, M. L., and Springer, T. A. (1989) T-cell receptor cross-linking transiently stimulates adhesiveness through LFA-1. *Nature* 341:619–624.

Elices, M. J., Osborn, L., Takada, Y., Crouse, C., Luhowskyj, S., Hemler, M. E., and Lobb, R. R. (1990) VCAM-1 on activated endothelium interacts with the leukocyte integrin VLA-4 at a site distinct from the VLA-4/fibronectin binding site. *Cell* 60:577–584.

Evangelista, V., Manarini, S., Sideri, R., Rotondo, S., Martelli, N., Piccoli, A., Totani, L., Piccardoni, P., Vestweber, D., de Gaetano, G., and Cerletti, C. (1999) Platelet/polymorphonuclear leukocyte interaction: P-selectin triggers protein-tyrosine phosphorylation-dependent CD11b/CD18 adhesion: role of PSGL-1 as a signaling molecule. *Blood* 93:876–885.

Fibbe, W. E., Hamilton, M. S., Laterveer, L. L., Kibbelaar, R. E., Falkenburg, J. H., Visser, J. W., and Willemze, R. (1992) Sustained engraftment of mice transplanted with IL-1–primed blood-derived stem cells. *J. Immunol.* 148:417 21.

Fixe, P., and Praloran, V. (1998) M-CSF: haematopoietic growth factor or inflammatory cytokine? *Cytokine* 10:32–37.

Flanagan, J. G., Chan, D. C., and Leder, P. (1991) Transmembrane form of the kit ligand growth factor is determined by alternative splicing and is missing in the Sld mutant. *Cell* 64:1025–1035.

Fleischman, R. A., Custer, R. P., and Mintz, B. (1982) Totipotent hematopoietic stem cells: normal self-renewal and differentiation after transplantation between mouse fetuses. *Cell* 30:351–359.

Fleming, W. H., Alpern, E. J., Uchida, N., Ikuta, K., Spangrude, G. J., and Weissman, I. L. (1993a) Functional heterogeneity is associated with the cell cycle status of murine hematopoietic stem cells. *J. Cell. Biol.* 122:897–902.

Fleming, W. H., Alpern, E. J., Uchida, N., Ikuta, K., and Weissman, I. L. (1993b) Steel factor influences the distribution and activity of murine hematopoietic stem cells in vivo. *Proc. Natl. Acad. Sci. USA* 90:3760–3764.

Foxman, E. F., Campbell, J. J., and Butcher, E. C. (1997) Multistep navigation and the combinatorial control of leukocyte chemotaxis. *J. Cell. Biol.* 139:1349–1360.

Frenette, P. S., Mayadas, T. N., Rayburn, H., Hynes, R. O., and Wagner, D. D. (1996) Susceptibility to infection and altered hematopoiesis in mice deficient in both P- and E-selectins. *Cell* 84:563–574.

Frenette, P. S., Subbarao, S., Mazo, I. B., von Andrian, U. H., and Wagner, D. D. (1998) Endothelial selectins and vascular cell adhesion molecule-1 promote hematopoietic progenitor homing to bone marrow [see comments]. *Proc. Natl. Acad. Sci. USA* 95:14423–14428.

Gallatin, W. M., Weissman, I. L., and Butcher, E. C. (1983) A cell-surface molecule involved in organ-specific homing of lymphocytes. *Nature* 304:30–34.

Geissler, E. N., Ryan, M. A., and Housman, D. E. (1988) The dominant-white spotting (W) locus of the mouse encodes the c-Kit proto-oncogene. *Cell* 55:185–192.

Geissler, K., Peschel, C., Niederwieser, D., Strobl, H., Goldschmitt, J., Ohler, L., Bettelheim, P., Kahls, P., Huber, C., Lechner, K., Hocker, P., and Kolbe, K. (1996) Potentiation of granulocyte colony-stimulating factor-induced mobilization of circulating progenitor cells by seven-day pretreatment with interleukin-3. *Blood* 87:2732–2739.

Gianni, A. M., Siena, S., Bregni, M., Tarella, C., Stern, A. C., Pileri, A., and Bonadonna, G. (1989) Granulocyte-macrophage colony-stimulating factor to harvest circulating haemopoietic stem cells for autotransplantation. *Lancet* 2:580–585.

Godin, I., Garcia-Porrero, J. A., Dieterlen-Lievre, F., and Cumano, A. (1999) Stem cell emergence and hemopoietic activity are incompatible in mouse intraembryonic sites. *J. Exp. Med.* 190:43–52.

Gratwohl, A., Baldomero, H., John, L., Gimmi, C., Pless, M., Tichelli, A., Nissen, C., Filipowicz, A., and Speck, B. (1995) Transplantation of G-CSF mobilized allogeneic peripheral blood stem cells in rabbits. *Bone Marrow Transplant* 16:63–68.

Green, E. L. (1966) *Biology of the laboratory mouse.* New York: McGraw-Hill, p. 706.

Gruneberg, H. (1942) Inhereted macrocytic anemias in the house mouse. II. Dominance relationships. *J. Genetics* 43:285–293.

Grzegorzewski, K. J., Komschlies, K. L., Jacobsen, S. E., Ruscetti, F. W., Keller, J. R., and Wiltrout, R. H. (1995) Mobilization of long-term reconstituting hematopoietic stem cells in mice by recombinant human interleukin 7. *J. Exp. Med.* 181:369–374.

Habibian, H. K., Peters, S. O., Hsieh, C. C., Wuu, J., Vergilis, K., Grimaldi, C. I., Reilly, J., Carlson, J. E., Frimberger, A. E., Stewart, F. M., and Quesenberry, P. J. (1998) The fluctuating phenotype of the lymphohematopoietic stem cell with cell cycle transit. *J. Exp. Med.* 188:393–398.

Hamann, A., Andrew, D. P., Jablonski-Westrich, D., Holzmann, B., and Butcher, E. C. (1994) Role of alpha 4-integrins in lymphocyte homing to mucosal tissues in vivo. *J. Immunol.* 152: 3282–3293.

Harrison, D. E., and Zhong, R. K. (1992) The same exhaustible multilineage precursor produces both myeloid and lymphoid cells as early as 3–4 weeks after marrow transplantation. *Proc. Natl. Acad. Sci. USA* 89:10134–10138.

Harrison, D. E., Zsebo, K. M., and Astle, C. M. (1994) Splenic primitive hematopoietic stem cell (PHSC) activity is enhanced by steel factor because of PHSC proliferation. *Blood* 83:3146–3151.

Hirayama, F., Lyman, S. D., Clark, S. C., and Ogawa, M. (1995) The flt3 ligand supports proliferation of lymphohematopoietic progenitors and early B-lymphoid progenitors. *Blood* 85: 1762–1768.

Hirsch, E., Iglesias, A., Potocnik, A. J., Hartmann, U., and Fassler, R. (1996) Impaired migration but not differentiation of haematopoietic stem cells in the absence of beta-1 integrins. *Nature* 380:171–175.

Holzmann, B., McIntyre, B. W., and Weissman, I. L. (1989) Identification of a murine Peyer's patch-specific lymphocyte homing receptor as an integrin molecule with an alpha chain homologous to human VLA-4 alpha. *Cell* 56:37–46.

Horst, E., Meijer, C. J., Radaskiewicz, T., van Dongen, J. J., Pieters, R., Figdor, C. G., Hooftman, A., and Pals, S. T. (1990) Expression of a human homing receptor (CD44) in lymphoid malignancies and related stages of lymphoid development. *Leukemia* 4:383–389.

Huang, E., Nocka, K., Beier, D. R., Chu, T. Y., Buck, J., Lahm, H. W., Wellner, D., Leder, P., and Besmer, P. (1990) The hematopoietic growth factor KL is encoded by the Sl locus and is the ligand of the c-Kit receptor, the gene product of the W locus. *Cell* 63:225–233.

Huang, E. J., Nocka, K. H., Buck, J., and Besmer, P. (1992) Differential expression and processing of two cell associated forms of the kit-ligand: KL-1 and KL-2. *Mol. Biol. Cell.* 3:349–362.

Huang, H., and Auerbach, R. (1993) Identification and characterization of hematopoietic stem cells from the yolk sac of the early mouse embryo. *Proc. Natl. Acad. Sci. USA* 90:10110–10114.

Huhn, R. D., Yurkow, E. J., Tushinski, R., Clarke, L., Sturgill, M. G., Hoffman, R., Sheay, W., Cody, R., Philipp, C., Resta, D., and George, M. (1996) Recombinant human interleukin-3 (rhIL-3) enhances the mobilization of peripheral blood progenitor cells by recombinant human granulocyte colony-stimulating factor (rhG-CSF) in normal volunteers. *Exp. Hematol.* 24:839–847.

Ikuta, K., and Weissman, I. L. (1992) Evidence that hematopoietic stem cells express mouse c-kit but do not depend on steel factor for their generation. *Proc. Natl. Acad. Sci. USA* 89:1502–1506.

Jackson, J. D., Yan, Y., Brunda, M. J., Kelsey, L. S., and Talmadge, J. E. (1995) Interleukin-12 enhances peripheral hematopoiesis in vivo. *Blood* 85:2371–2376.

Jacobsen, K., Kravitz, J., Kincade, P. W., and Osmond, D. G. (1996) Adhesion receptors on bone marrow stromal cells: in vivo expression of vascular cell adhesion molecule-1 by reticular cells and sinusoidal endothelium in normal and gamma-irradiated mice. *Blood* 87:73–82.

Jacobsen, S. E., Okkenhaug, C., Myklebust, J., Veiby, O. P., and Lyman, S. D. (1995) The FLT3 ligand potently and directly stimulates the growth and expansion of primitive murine bone marrow progenitor cells in vitro: synergistic interactions with interleukin (IL) 11, IL-12, and other hematopoietic growth factors. *J. Exp. Med.* 181:1357–1363.

Jalkanen, S., and Jalkanen, M. (1992) Lymphocyte CD44 binds the COOH-terminal heparin-binding domain of fibronectin. *J. Cell. Biol.* 116:817–825.

Jones, R. J., Wagner, J. E., Celano, P., Zicha, M. S., and Sharkis, S. J. (1990) Separation of pluripotent haematopoietic stem cells from spleen colony-forming cells. *Nature* 347:188–189.

Jones, R., Collector, M., Barber, J., Vala, M., Fackler, M., May, W., Griffin, C., Hawkins, A., Zehnbauer, B., Hilton, J., Colvin, O., and Sharkis, S. (1996) Characterization of mouse lymphohematopoietic stem cells lacking spleen colony-forming activity. *Blood* 88:487–491.

Jordan, C. T., and Lemischka, I. R. (1990) Clonal and systemic analysis of long-term hematopoiesis in the mouse. *Genes Dev.* 4:220–232.

Juttner, C. A., To, L. B., Haylock, D. N., Branford, A., and Kimber, R. J. (1985) Circulating autologous stem cells collected in very early remission from acute non-lymphoblastic leukaemia produce prompt but incomplete haemopoietic reconstitution after high dose melphalan or supralethal chemoradiotherapy. *Br. J. Haematol.* 61:739–745.

Kansas, G. S., Muirhead, M. J., and Dailey, M. O. (1990) Expression of the CD11/CD18, leukocyte adhesion molecule 1, and CD44 adhesion molecules during normal myeloid and erythroid differentiation in humans. *Blood* 76:2483–2492.

Kapur, R., Majumdar, M., Xiao, X., McAndrews-Hill, M., Schindler, K., and Williams, D. A. (1998) Signaling through the interaction of membrane-restricted stem cell factor and c-Kit receptor tyrosine kinase: genetic evidence for a differential role in erythropoiesis. *Blood* 91:879–889.

Kaushansky, K., Lok, S., Holly, R. D., Broudy, V. C., Lin, N., Bailey, M. C., Forstrom, J. W., Buddle, M. M., Oort, P. J., Hagen, F. S., et al. (1994) Promotion of megakaryocyte progenitor expansion and differentiation by the c-Mpl ligand thrombopoietin [see comments]. *Nature* 369: 568–571.

Kawabata, K., Ujikawa, M., Egawa, T., Kawamoto, H., Tachibana, K., Iizasa, H., Katsura, Y., Kishimoto, T., and Nagasawa, T. (1999) A cell-autonomous requirement for CXCR4 in long-term lymphoid and myeloid reconstitution. *Proc. Natl. Acad. Sci. USA* 96:5663–5667.

Kay, H. E. M. (1965) How many cell generations? *Lancet* 2:418.

Kimura, S., Roberts, A. W., Metcalf, D., and Alexander, W. S. (1998) Hematopoietic stem cell deficiencies in mice lacking c-Mpl, the receptor for thrombopoietin. *Proc. Natl. Acad. Sci. USA* 95:1195–2000.

Kitamura, T., Sato, N., Arai, K., and Miyajima, A. (1991) Expression cloning of the human IL-3 receptor cDNA reveals a shared beta subunit for the human IL-3 and GM-CSF receptors. *Cell* 66:1165–1174.

Kondo, M., Weissman, I. L., and Akashi, K. (1997) Identification of clonogenic common lymphoid progenitors in mouse bone marrow. *Cell* 91:661–672.

Labow, M. A., Norton, C. R., Rumberger, J. M., Lombard-Gillooly, K. M., Shuster, D. J., Hubbard, J., Bertko, R., Knaack, P. A., Terry, R. W., Harbison, M. L., et al. (1994) Characterization of E-selectin–deficient mice: demonstration of overlapping function of the endothelial selectins. *Immun.* 1:709–720.

Lacombe, C., and Mayeux, P. (1998) Biology of erythropoietin. *Haematologica* 83:724–732.

Lagasse, E., and Weissman, I. L. (1994) Bcl-2 inhibits apoptosis of neutrophils but not their engulfment by macrophages. *J. Exp. Med.* 179:1047–1052.

Lagasse, E., and Weissman, I. (1997) Enforced expression of Bcl-2 in monocytes rescues macrophages and partially reverses osteopetrosis in op/op mice. *Cell* 89:1021–1031.

Lasky, L. A., Singer, M. S., Yednock, T. A., Dowbenko, D., Fennie, C., Rodriguez, H., Nguyen, T., Stachel, S., and Rosen, S. D. (1989) Cloning of a lymphocyte homing receptor reveals a lectin domain. *Cell* 56:1045–1055.

Lasky, L. A. (1992) Selectins: interpreters of cell-specific carbohydrate information during inflammation. *Science* 258:964–969.

Laterveer, L., Lindley, I. J., Hamilton, M. S., Willemze, R., and Fibbe, W. E. (1995) Interleukin-8 induces rapid mobilization of hematopoietic stem cells with radioprotective capacity and long-term myelolymphoid repopulating ability. *Blood* 85:2269–2275.

Laterveer, L., Lindley, I. J., Heemskerk, D. P., Camps, J. A., Pauwels, E. K., Willemze, R., and Fibbe, W. E. (1996) Rapid mobilization of hematopoietic progenitor cells in rhesus monkeys by a single intravenous injection of interleukin-8. *Blood* 87:781–788.

Lemischka, I. R., Raulet, D. H., and Mulligan, R. C. (1986) Development potential and dynamic behavior of hematopoietic stem cells. *Cell* 45:917–927.

Lesley, J., Hyman, R., and Kincade, P. W. (1993) CD44 and its interaction with extracellular matrix. *Adv. Immunol.* 54:271–335.

Levesque, J. P., Zannettino, A. C., Pudney, M., Niutta, S., Haylock, D. N., Snapp, K. R., Kansas, G. S., Berndt, M. C., and Simmons, P. J. (1999) PSGL-1–mediated adhesion of human hematopoietic progenitors to P-selectin results in suppression of hematopoiesis. *Immun.* 11:369–378.

Lewinsohn, D. M., Nagler, A., Ginzton, N., Greenberg, P., and Butcher, E. C. (1990) Hematopoietic progenitor cell expression of the H-CAM (CD44) homing-associated adhesion molecule. *Blood* 75:589–595.

Ley, K., Tedder, T. F., and Kansas, G. S. (1993) L-selectin can mediate leukocyte rolling in untreated mesenteric venules in vivo independent of E- or P-selectin. *Blood* 82; 1632–1638.

Ley, K., Bullard, D. C., Arbones, M. L., Bosse, R., Vestweber, D., Tedder, T. F., and Beaudet, A. L. (1995) Sequential contribution of L- and P-selectin to leukocyte rolling in vivo. *J. Exp. Med.* 181:669–675.

Li, C. L., and Johnson, G. R. (1992) Rhodamine-123 reveals heterogeneity within murine Lin-, Sca-1+ hemopoietic stem cells. *J. Exp. Med.* 175:1443–1447.

Lichtman, M. A. (1981) The ultrastructure of the hemopoietic environment of the marrow: a review. *Exp. Hematol.* 9:391–410.

Lieschke, G. J., Grail, D., Hodgson, G., Metcalf, D., Stanley, E., Cheers, C., Fowler, K. J., Basu, S., Zhan, Y. F., and Dunn, A. R. (1994) Mice lacking granulocyte colony-stimulating factor have chronic neutropenia, granulocyte and macrophage progenitor cell deficiency, and impaired neutrophil mobilization. *Blood* 84:1737–1746.

Liu, D., Liu, T., Li, R., and Sy, M. S. (1998) Mechanisms regulating the binding activity of CD44 to hyaluronic acid. *Front. Biosci.* 3:D631-D636.

Liu, F., Poursine-Laurent, J., and Link, D. C. (1997) The granulocyte colony-stimulating factor receptor is required for the mobilization of murine hematopoietic progenitors into peripheral blood by cyclophosphamide or interleukin-8 but not flt-3 ligand. *Blood* 90:2522–2528.

Lok, S., Kaushansky, K., Holly, R. D., Kuijper, J. L., Lofton-Day, C. E., Oort, P. J., Grant, F. J., Heipel, M. D., Burkhead, S. K., Kramer, J. M., et al. (1994) Cloning and expression of murine thrombopoietin cDNA and stimulation of platelet production in vivo. *Nature* 369:565–568.

Lord, B. I., Woolford, L. B., Wood, L. M., Czaplewski. L. G., McCourt, M., Hunter, M. G., and Edwards, R. M. (1995) Mobilization of early hematopoietic progenitor cells with BB-10010:a genetically engineered variant of human macrophage inflammatory protein-1 alpha. *Blood* 85:3412–3415.

Luens, K. M., Travis, M. A., Chen, B. P., Hill, B. L., Scollay, R., and Murray, L. J. (1998) Thrombopoietin, kit ligand, and flk2/flt3 ligand together induce increased numbers of primitive hematopoietic progenitors from human CD34+Thy-1+Lin–cells with preserved ability to engraft SCID-hu bone. *Blood* 91:1206–1215.

Lyman, S. D., and Jacobsen, S. E. (1998) C-Kit ligand and Flt3 ligand: stem/progenitor cell factors with overlapping yet distinct activities. *Blood* 91:1101–1134.

Ma, Q., Jones, D., Borghesani, P. R., Segal, R. A., Nagasawa, T., Kishimoto, T., Bronson, R. T., and Springer, T. A. (1998) Impaired B-lymphopoiesis, myelopoiesis, and derailed cerebellar neuron migration in CXCR4- and SDF-1–deficient mice. *Proc. Natl. Acad. Sci. USA* 95:9448–9453.

Ma, Q., Jones, D., and Springer, T. A. (1999) The chemokine receptor CXCR4 is required for the retention of B lineage and granulocytic precursors within the bone marrow microenvironment. *Immun.* 10:463–471.

Mackarehtschian, K., Hardin, J. D., Moore, K. A., Boast, S., Goff, S. P., and Lemischka, I. R. (1995) Targeted disruption of the *flk2/flk3* gene leads to deficiencies in primitive hematopoietic progenitors. *Immun.* 3:147–161.

Marshall, E., Woolford, L. B., and Lord, B. I. (1997). Continuous infusion of macrophage inflammatory protein MIP-1 alpha enhances leucocyte recovery and haemopoietic progenitor cell mobilization after cyclophosphamide. *Br. J. Cancer.* 75:1715–1720.

Matthews, W., Jordan, C. T., Wiegand, G. W., Pardoll, D., and Lemischka, I. R. (1991) A receptor tyrosine kinase specific to hematopoietic stem and progenitor cell-enriched populations. *Cell* 65:1143–1152.

Mauch, P., Lamont, C., Neben, T. Y., Quinto, C., Goldman, S. J., and Witsell, A. (1995) Hematopoietic stem cells in the blood after stem cells factor and interleukin-11 administration: evidence for different mechanisms of mobilization. *Blood* 86:4674–4680.

Mayadas, T. N., Johnson, R. C., Rayburn, H., Hynes, R. O., and Wagner, D. D. (1993) Leukocyte rolling and extravasation are severely compromised in P-selectin–deficient mice. *Cell* 74:541–554.

Mazo, I. B., Gutierrez-Ramos, J. C., Frenette, P. S., Hynes, R. O., Wagner, D. D., and von Andrian, U. H. (1998) Hematopoietic progenitor cell rolling in bone marrow microvessels: parallel contributions by endothelial selectins and vascular cell adhesion molecule 1. *J. Exp. Med.* 188: 465–474.

McCulloch, E. A., Siminovitch, J., and Till, J. E. (1964) Spleen-colony formation in anemic mice of genotype W/W$_v$. *Science* 144:844.

McCulloch, E. A., Siminovitch, L., Till, J. E., Russell, E. S., and Bernstein, S. E. (1965) The cellular basis of the genetically determined hemopoietic defect in anemic mice of genotype Sl-Sld. *Blood* 26:399–410.

McEver, R. P., Beckstead, J. H., Moore, K. L., Marshall-Carlson, L., and Bainton, D. F. (1989) GMP-140, a platelet alpha-granule membrane protein, is also synthesized by vascular endothelial cells and is localized in Weibel–Palade bodies. *J. Clin. Invest.* 84:92–99.

McNiece, I. K., Briddell, R. A., Hartley, C. A., Smith, K. A., and Andrews, R. G. (1993) Stem cell factor enhances in vivo effects of granulocyte colony-stimulating factor for stimulating mobilization of peripheral blood progenitor cells. *Stem Cells (Dayt)* 11 (suppl 2): 36–41.

Mebius, R. E., Streeter, P. R., Michie, S., Butcher, E. C., and Weissman, I. L. (1996) A developmental switch in lymphocyte homing receptor and endothelial vascular addressin expression regulates lymphocyte homing and permits CD4$_+$ CD3$_-$ cells to colonize lymph nodes. *Proc. Natl. Acad. Sci. USA* 93:11019–11024.

Medvinsky, A., and Dzierzak, E. (1996) Definitive hematopoiesis is autonomously initiated by the AGM region. *Cell* 86:897–906.

Metcalf, D. (1988). *The molecular control of blood cells.* Cambridge, MA: Harvard University Press.

Metcalf, D. (1993) Hematopoietic regulators: redundancy or subtlety? *Blood* 82:3515–3523.

Micklem, H. S., Clarke, C. M., Evans, E. P., and Ford, C. E. (1968) Fate of chromosome-marked mouse bone marrow cells transfused into normal syngeneic recipients. *Transplantation* 6:299–302.

Micklem, H. S., Ford, C. E., Evans, E. P., Ogden, D. A., and Papworth, D. S. (1972) Competitive in vivo proliferation of foetal and adult haematopoietic cells in lethally irradiated mice. *J. Cell. Physiol.* 79:293–298.

Minguell, J. J., Hardy, C., and Tavassoli, M. (1992) Membrane-associated chondroitin sulfate proteoglycan and fibronectin mediate the binding of hemopoietic progenitor cells to stromal cells. *Exp. Cell. Res.* 201:200–207.

Mintz, B., and Russell, E. S. (1957) Gene-induced embryological modifications of primordial germ cells in the mouse. *J. Exp. Zool.* 134:207–237.

Miyake, K., Medina, K., Hayashi, S., Ono, S., Hamaoka, T., and Kincade, P. W. (1990) Monoclonal antibodies to Pgp-1/CD44 block lympho-hemopoiesis in long-term bone marrow cultures. *J. Exp. Med.* 171:477–488.

Miyake, K., Medina, K., Ishihara, K., Kimoto, M., Auerbach, R., and Kincade, P. W. (1991a) A VCAM-like adhesion molecule on murine bone marrow stromal cells mediates binding of lymphocyte precursors in culture. *J. Cell. Biol.* 114:557–565.

Miyake, K., Weissman, I. L., Greenberger, J. S., and Kincade, P. W. (1991b) Evidence for a role of the integrin VLA-4 in lympho-hemopoiesis. *J. Exp. Med.* 173:599–607.

Molineux, G., Pojda, Z., Hampson, I. N., Lord, B. I., and Dexter, T. M. (1990) Transplantation potential of peripheral blood stem cells induced by granulocyte colony-stimulating factor. *Blood* 76:2153–2158.

Molineux, G., Migdalska, A., Szmitkowski, M., Zsebo, K., and Dexter, T. M. (1991) The effects on hematopoiesis of recombinant stem cell factor (ligand for c-kit) administered in vivo to mice either alone or in combination with granulocyte colony-stimulating factor. *Blood* 78: 961–966.

Molineux, G., McCrea, C., Yan, X. Q., Kerzic, P., and McNiece, I. (1997) Flt-3 ligand synergizes with granulocyte colony-stimulating factor to increase neutrophil numbers and to mobilize peripheral blood stem cells with long-term repopulating potential. *Blood* 89:3998–4004.

Monette, F. C., and DeMello, J. B. (1979) The relationship between stem cell seeding efficiency and position in cell cycle. *Cell Tissue Kinet.* 12:161–175.

Moore, M. A., and Metcalf, D. (1970) Ontogeny of the haemopoietic system: yolk sac origin of in vivo and in vitro colony-forming cells in the developing mouse embryo. *Br. J. Haematol.* 18:279–296.

Moore, M. A., and Owen, J. J. (1967) Chromosome marker studies in the irradiated chick embryo. *Nature* 215:1081–1082.

Morrison, S. J., and Weissman, I. L. (1994) The long-term repopulating subset of hematopoietic stem cells is deterministic and isolatable by phenotype. *Immun* 1:661–673.

Morrison, S. J., Hemmati, H. D., Wandycz, A. M., and Weissman, I. L. (1995a) The purification and characterization of fetal liver hematopoietic stem cells. *Proc. Natl. Acad. Sci. USA* 92: 10302–10306.

Morrison, S. J., Uchida, N., and Weissman, I. L. (1995b) The biology of hematopoietic stem cells. *Annu. Rev. Cell. Dev. Biol.* 11:35–71.

Morrison, S. J., Wandycz, A. M., Hemmati, H. D., Wright, D. E., and Weissman, I. L. (1997a) Identification of a lineage of multipotent hematopoietic progenitors. *Development* 124:1929–1939.

Morrison, S. J., Wright, D. E., and Weissman, I. L. (1997b) Cyclophosphamide/granulocyte colony-stimulating factor induces hematopoietic stem cells to proliferate prior to mobilization. *Proc. Natl. Acad. Sci. USA* 94:1908–1913.

Mulder, A. H., and Visser, J. W. (1987) Separation and functional analysis of bone marrow cells separated by rhodamine-123 fluorescence. *Exp. Hematol.* 15:99–104.

Muller-Sieburg, C. E., and Riblet, R. (1996) Genetic control of the frequency of hematopoietic stem cells in mice: mapping of a candidate locus to chromosome 1. *J. Exp. Med.* 183:1141–1150.

Muto, M. (1976) A scanning and transmission electron microscopic study on rat bone marrow sinuses and transmural migration of blood cells. *Arch. Histol. Jpn.* 39:51–66.

Nagasawa, T., Kikutani, H., and Kishimoto, T. (1994) Molecular cloning and structure of a pre-B-cell growth-stimulating factor. *Proc. Natl. Acad. Sci. USA* 91:2305–2309.

Nagasawa, T., Hirota, S., Tachibana, K., Takakura, N., Nishikawa, S., Kitamura, Y., Yoshida, N., Kikutani, H., and Kishimoto, T. (1996) Defects of B-cell lymphopoiesis and bone-marrow myelopoiesis in mice lacking the CXC chemokine PBSF/SDF-1. *Nature* 382:635–638.

Necas, E., Sefc, L., Brecher, G., and Bookstein, N. (1995) Hematopoietic reserve provided by spleen colony-forming units (CFU-S). *Exp. Hematol.* 23:1242–1246.

Necas, E., Sefc, L., Sulc, K., Barthel, E., and Seidel, H. J. (1998) Estimation of extent of cell death in different stages of normal murine hematopoiesis. *Stem Cells* 16:107–111.

Ogawa, M., Nishikawa, S., Ikuta, K., Yamamura, F., Naito, M., and Takahashi, K. (1988) B cell ontogeny in murine embryo studied by a culture system with the monolayer of a stromal cell clone, ST2: B cell progenitor develops first in the embryonal body rather than in the yolk sac. *Embo. J.* 1337–1343.

Ogawa, M., Matsuzaki, Y., Nishikawa, S., Hayashi, S., Kunisada, T., Sudo, T., Kina, T., and Nakauchi, H. (1991) Expression and function of c-Kit in hemopoietic progenitor cells. *J. Exp. Med.* 174:63–71.

Ogawa, M. (1993) Differentiation and proliferation of hematopoietic stem cells. *Blood* 81:2844–2853.

Ogawa, M., Nishikawa, S., Yoshinaga, K., Hayashi, S., Kunisada, T., Nakao, J., Kina, T., Sudo, T., and Kodama, H. (1993) Expression and function of c-kit in fetal hemopoietic progenitor cells: transition from the early c-kit–independent to the late c-kit–dependent wave of hemopoiesis in the murine embryo. *Dev.* 117:1089–1098.

Ogawa, M., Yonemura, Y., and Ku, H. (1997) In vitro expansion of hematopoietic stem cells. *Stem Cells* 15:7–11.

Okada, S., Nakauchi, H., Nagayoshi, K., Nishikawa, S., Miura, Y., and Suda, T. (1991) Enrichment and characterization of murine hematopoietic stem cells that express c-Kit molecule. *Blood* 78:1706–1712.

Oostendorp, R. A., Reisbach, G., Spitzer, E., Thalmeier, K., Dienemann, H., Mergenthaler, H. G., and Dormer, P. (1995) VLA-4 and VCAM-1 are the principal adhesion molecules involved in the interaction between blast colony-forming cells and bone marrow stromal cells. *Br. J. Haematol.* 91:275–284.

Oostendorp, R. A., and Dormer, P. (1997) VLA-4–mediated interactions between normal human hematopoietic progenitors and stromal cells. *Leuk. Lymphoma* 24:423–435.

Ortiz, M., Wine, J. W., Lohrey, N., Ruscetti, F. W., Spence, S. E., and Keller, J. R. (1999) Functional characterization of a novel hematopoietic stem cell and its place in the c-Kit maturation pathway in bone marrow cell development. *Immun.* 10:173–182.

Osawa, M., Hanada, K., Hamada, H., and Nakauchi, H. (1996) Long-term lymphohematopoietic reconstitution by a single CD34–low/negative hematopoietic stem cell. *Science* 273:242–245.

Palis, J., Robertson, S., Kennedy, M., Wall, C., and Keller, G. (1999) Development of erythroid and myeloid progenitors in the yolk sac and embryo proper of the mouse. *Development* 126: 5073–5084.

Papayannopoulou, T., and Nakamoto, B. (1993) Peripheralization of hemopoietic progenitors in primates treated with anti-VLA4 integrin. *Proc. Natl. Acad. Sci. USA* 90:9374–9378.

Papayannopoulou, T., Craddock, C., Nakamoto, B., Priestley, G. V., and Wolf, N. S. (1995) The VLA4/VCAM-1 adhesion pathway defines contrasting mechanisms of lodgement of transplanted murine hemopoietic progenitors between bone marrow and spleen. *Proc. Natl. Acad. Sci. USA* 92:9647–9651.

Papayannopoulou, T., Nakamoto, B., Andrews, R. G., Lyman, S. D., and Lee, M. Y. (1997) In vivo effects of Flt3/Flk2 ligand on mobilization of hematopoietic progenitors in primates and potent synergistic enhancement with granulocyte colony-stimulating factor. *Blood* 90:620–629.

Papayannopoulou, T., Priestley, G. V., and Nakamoto, B. (1998) Anti-VLA4/VCAM-1–induced mobilization requires cooperative signaling through the kit/mkit ligand pathway. *Blood* 91: 2231–2239.

Peled, A., Petit, I., Kollet, O., Magid, M., Ponomaryov, T., Byk, T., Nagler, A., Ben-Hur, H., Many, A., Shultz, L., et al. (1999) Dependence of human stem cell engraftment and repopulation of NOD/SCID mice on CXCR4. *Science* 283:845–848.

Picker, L. J., Kishimoto, T. K., Smith, C. W., Warnock, R. A., and Butcher, E. C. (1991) ELAM-1 is an adhesion molecule for skin-homing T cells [see comments]. *Nature* 349:796–799.

Premack, B. A., and Schall, T. J. (1996) Chemokine receptors: gateways to inflammation and infection. *Nat.Med.* 2:1174–1178.

Prosper, F., Stroncek, D., McCarthy, J. B., and Verfaillie, C. M. (1998) Mobilization and homing of peripheral blood progenitors is related to reversible downregulation of alpha4 beta1 integrin expression and function. *J. Clin. Invest.* 101:2456–2467.

Pruijt, J. F., van Kooyk, Y., Figdor, C. G., Lindley, I. J., Willemze, R., and Fibbe, W. E. (1998) Anti–LFA-1 blocking antibodies prevent mobilization of hematopoietic progenitor cells induced by interleukin-8. *Blood* 91:4099–4105.

Pruijt, J. F., van Kooyk, Y., Figdor, C. G., Willemze, R., and Fibbe, W. E. (1999) Murine hematopoietic progenitor cells with colony-forming or radioprotective capacity lack expression of the beta 2-integrin LFA-1. *Blood* 93:107–112.

Quesenberry, P. J., Morley, A., Miller, M., Rickard, K., Howard, D., and Stohlman, F. Jr. (1973) Effect of endotoxin on granulopoiesis and the in vitro colony-forming cell. *Blood* 41:391–398.

Randall, T. D., and Weissman, I. L. (1998) Characterization of a population of cells in the bone marrow that phenotypically mimics hematopoietic stem cells: resting stem cells or mystery population? *Stem Cells* 16:38–48.

Richman, C. M., Weiner, R. S., and Yankee, R. A. (1976) Increase in circulating stem cells following chemotherapy in man. *Blood* 47:1031–1039.

Rios, M., and Williams, D. A. (1990) Systematic analysis of the ability of stromal cell lines derived from different murine adult tissues to support maintenance of hematopoietic stem cells in vitro. *J. Cell. Physiol.* 145:434–443.

Rosenfeld, C. S., Bolwell, B., LeFever, A., Taylor, R., List, A., Fay, J., Collins, R., Andrews, F., Pallansch, P., Schuster, M. W., et al. (1996) Comparison of four cytokine regimens for mobilization of peripheral blood stem cells: IL-3 alone and combined with GM-CSF or G-CSF. *Bone Marrow Transplant* 17:179–183.

Rosnet, O., Marchetto, S., deLapeyriere, O., and Birnbaum, D. (1991) Murine Flt3, a gene encoding a novel tyrosine kinase receptor of the PDGFR/CSF1R family. *Oncogene* 6:1641–1650.

Rosnet, O., Schiff, C., Pebusque, M. J., Marchetto, S., Tonnelle, C., Toiron, Y., Birg, F., and Birnbaum, D. (1993) Human FLT3/FLK2 gene: cDNA cloning and expression in hemato-poietic cells. *Blood* 82:1110–1119.

Saito, H., Kanamori, Y., Takemori, T., Nariuchi, H., Kubota, E., Takahashi-Iwanaga, H., Iwanaga, T., and Ishikawa, H. (1998) Generation of intestinal T cells from progenitors residing in gut cryptopatches. *Science* 280:275–278.

Sanderson, C. J. (1992) Interleukin-5, eosinophils, and disease. *Blood* 79:3101–3109.

Sarvella, P. A., and Russell, L. B. (1956) Steel, a new dominant gene in the house mouse. *J. Hered.* 47:123–128.

Saxe, D. F., Boggs, S. S., and Boggs, D. R. (1984) Transplantation of chromosomally marked syngeneic marrow cells into mice not subjected to hematopoietic stem cell depletion. *Exp. Hematol.* 12:277–283.

Schmits, R., Filmus, J., Gerwin, N., Senaldi, G., Kiefer, F., Kundig, T., Wakeham, A., Shahinian, A., Catzavelos, C., Rak, J., et al. (1997) CD44 regulates hematopoietic progenitor distribution, granuloma formation, and tumorigenicity. *Blood* 90:2217–2233.

Schweitzer, K. M., Drager, A. M., van der Valk, P., Thijsen, S. F., Zevenbergen, A., Theijsmeijer, A. P., van der Schoot, C. E., and Langenhuijsen, M. M. (1996) Constitutive expression of E-selectin and vascular cell adhesion molecule-1 on endothelial cells of hematopoietic tissues. *Am. J. Pathol.* 148:165–175.

Sharkis, S. J., Collector, M. I., Barber, J. P., Vala, M. S., and Jones, R. J. (1997) Phenotypic and functional characterization of the hematopoietic stem cell *Stem Cells* 15:41–44.

Siena, S., Bregni, M., Brando, B., Ravagnani, F., Bonadonna, G., and Gianni, A. M. (1989) Cir-culation of CD34+ hematopoietic stem cells in the peripheral blood of high-dose cyclophosphamide-treated patients: enhancement by intravenous recombinant human granulocyte-macrophage colony-stimulating factor. *Blood* 74; 1905–1914.

Siminovitch, L., McCulloch, E. A., and Till, J. E. (1963) The distribution of colony-forming cells among spleen colonies. *J. Cell. Comp. Physiol.* 62:327–336.

Simmons, P. J., Masinovsky, B., Longenecker, B. M., Berenson, R., Torok-Storb, B., and Gallatin, W. M. (1992) Vascular cell adhesion molecule-1 expressed by bone marrow stromal cells mediates the binding of hematopoietic progenitor cells. *Blood* 80:388–395.

Small, D., Levenstein, M., Kim, E., Carow, C., Amin, S., Rockwell, P., Witte, L., Burrow, C., Ratajczak, M. Z., Gewirtz, A. M., et al. (1994). STK-1, the human homolog of Flk-2/Flt-3, is selectively expressed in CD34+ human bone marrow cells and is involved in the proliferation of early progenitor/stem cells. *Proc. Natl. Acad. Sci. USA* 91:459–463.

Smith, L. G., Weissman, I. L., and Heimfeld, S. (1991) Clonal analysis of hematopoietic stem-cell differentiation in vivo. *Proc. Natl. Acad. Sci. USA* 88:2788–2792.

Snodgrass, R., and Keller, G. (1987) Clonal fluctuation within the haematopoietic system of mice reconstituted with retrovirus-infected stem cells. *Embo. J.* 6:3955–3960.

Socinski, M. A., Cannistra, S. A., Elias, A., Antman, K. H., Schnipper, L., and Griffin, J. D., (1988) Granulocyte-macrophage colony stimulating factor expands the circulating haemopoietic pro-genitor cell compartment in man. *Lancet* 1:1194–1198.

Spangrude, G. J., Heimfeld, S., and Weissman, I. L. (1988) Purification and characterization of mouse hematopoietic stem cells. *Science* 241:58–62.

Spangrude, G. J., and Johnson, G. R. (1990) Resting and activated subsets of mouse multipotent hematopoietic stem cells. *Proc. Natl. Acad. Sci. USA* 87:7433–7437.

Spertini, O., Luscinskas, F. W., Kansas, G. S., Munro, J. M., Griffin, J. D., Gimbrone, M. A. Jr., and Tedder, T. F. (1991) Leukocyte adhesion molecule-1 (LAM-1, L-selectin) interacts with an inducible endothelial cell ligand to support leukocyte adhesion. *J. Immunol.* 147:2565–2573.

Springer, T. A. (1994) Traffic signals for lymphocyte recirculation and leukocyte emigration: the multistep paradigm. *Cell* 76:301–314.

Stanley, E., Lieschke, G. J., Grail, D., Metcalf, D., Hodgson, G., Gall, J. A., Maher, D. W., Cebon, J., Sinickas, V., and Dunn, A. R. (1994) Granulocyte/macrophage colony-stimulating factor–deficient mice show no major perturbation of hematopoiesis but develop a characteristic pulmonary pathology. *Proc. Natl. Acad. Sci. USA* 91:5592–5596.

Sudo, Y., Shimazaki, C., Ashihara, E., Kikuta, T., Hirai, H., Sumikuma, T., Yamagata, N., Goto, H., Inaba, T., Fujita, N., and Nakagawa, M. (1997) Synergistic effect of FLT-3 ligand on the granulocyte colony-stimulating factor–induced mobilization of hematopoietic stem cells and progenitor cells into blood in mice. *Blood* 89:3186–3191.

Tachibana, K., Hirota, S., Iizasa, H., Yoshida, H., Kawabata, K., Kataoka, Y., Kitamura, Y., Matsushima, K., Yoshida, N., Nishikawa, S., et al. (1998) The chemokine receptor CXCR4 is essential for vascularization of the gastrointestinal tract [see comments]. *Nature* 393: 591–594.

Takada, A., Takada, Y., and Ambrus, J. L. (1971) Proliferation of donor spleen and bone marrow cells in the spleens and bone marrows of unirradiated and irradiated adult mice. *Proc. Soc. Exp. Biol. Med.* 136:222–226.

Takada, Y., and Takada, A. (1971) Proliferation of donor hematopoietic cells in irradiated and unirradiated host mice. *Transplantation* 12:334–338.

Tamkun, J. W., DeSimone, D. W., Fonda, D., Patel, R. S., Buck, C., Horwitz, A. F., and Hynes, R. O. (1986) Structure of integrin, a glycoprotein involved in the transmembrane linkage between fibronectin and actin. *Cell* 46:271–282.

Tashiro, K., Tada, H., Heilker, R., Shirozu, M., Nakano, T., and Honjo, T. (1993) Signal sequence trap: a cloning strategy for secreted proteins and type I membrane proteins. *Science* 261:600–603.

Tavassoli, M. (1979) The marrow–blood barrier. *Br. J. Haematol.* 41:297–302.

Tavassoli, M., and Aoki, M. (1981) Migration of entire megakaryocytes through the marrow–blood barrier. *Br. J. Haematol.* 48:25–29.

Tedder, T. F., Penta, A. C., Levine, H. B., and Freedman, A. S. (1990) Expression of the human leukocyte adhesion molecule, LAM1. Identity with the TQ1 and Leu-8 differentiation antigens. *J. Immunol.* 144:532–540.

Teixido, J., Hemler, M. E., Greenberger, J. S., and Anklesaria, P. (1992) Role of beta 1 and beta 2 integrins in the adhesion of human CD34hi stem cells to bone marrow stroma. *J. Clin. Invest.* 90:358–367.

Till, J., and McCulloch, E. (1961) A direct measurement of the radiation sensitivity of normal mouse bone marrow cells. *Radiat. Res.* 14:213–222.

Torii, Y., Nitta, Y., Akahori, H., Tawara, T., Kuwaki, T., Ogami, K., Kato, T., and Miyazaki, H. (1998) Mobilization of primitive haemopoietic progenitor cells and stem cells with long-term repopulating ability into peripheral blood in mice by pegylated recombinant human megakaryocyte growth and development factor. *Br. J. Haematol.* 103:1172–1180.

Tracey, J. B., and Rinder, H. M. (1996) Characterization of the P-selectin ligand on human hematopoietic progenitors. *Exp. Hematol.* 24:1494–1500.

Traycoff, C. M., Cornetta, K., Yoder, M. C., Davidson, A., and Srour, E. F. (1996) Ex vivo expansion of murine hematopoietic progenitor cells generates classes of expanded cells possessing different levels of bone marrow repopulating potential. *Exp. Hematol.* 24:299–306.

Trevisan, M., and Iscove, N. N. (1995) Phenotypic analysis of murine long-term hemopoietic reconstituting cells quantitated competitively in vivo and comparison with more advanced colony-forming progeny. *J. Exp. Med.* 181:93–103.

Tsuji, K., Lyman, S. D., Sudo, T., Clark, S. C., and Ogawa, M. (1992) Enhancement of murine hematopoiesis by synergistic interactions between steel factor (ligand for c-Kit), interleukin-11, and other early acting factors in culture. *Blood* 79:2855–2860.

Tsukamoto, A. S., Reading, C., Carella, A., Frassoni, F., Gorin, C., LaPorte, J., Negrin, R., Blume, K., Cunningham, I., Deisseroth, A., et al. (1994) Biological characterization of stem cell present in mobilized peripheral blood of CML patients. *Bone Marrow Transplant* 14 (suppl. 3):S25–S32.

Turley, E., (1982) Purification of a hyaluronate-binding protein fraction that modifies cell social behavior. *Biochem. Biophys. Res. Commun.* 108:1016–1024.

Turley, E., and Moore, D. (1984) Hyaluronate binding proteins also bind to fibronectin, laminin and collagen. *Biochem. Biophys. Res. Commun.* 121:808–814.

Turley, E., and Torrance, J. (1985) Localization of hyaluronate and hyaluronate-binding protein on motile and non-motile fibroblasts. *Exp. Cell. Res.* 161:17–28.

Turpen, J. B., Knudson, C. M., and Hoefen, P. S. (1981) The early ontogeny of hematopoietic cells studied by grafting cytogenetically labeled tissue anlagen: localization of a prospective stem cell compartment. *Dev. Biol.* 85:99–112.

van der Loo, J. C., and Ploemacher, R. E. (1995) Marrow- and spleen-seeding efficiencies of all murine hematopoietic stem cell subsets are decreased by preincubation with hematopoietic growth factors. *Blood* 85:2598–2606.

Weiss, L. (1970) Transmural cellular passage in vascular sinuses of rat bone marrow. *Blood* 36: 189–208.

Weissman, I., Papaioannou, V., and Gardner, R. (1978) Fetal hematopoietic origins of the adult hematolymphoid system. In: *Cold Spring Harbor Conferences on Cell Proliferation. Vol. 5: Differentiation of Normal and Neoplastic Hematopoietic Cells,* B. Clarkson, P. Mark, and J. Till, eds. New York: Cold Spring Harbor Lab, pp. 33–47.

Wendling, F., Maraskovsky, E., Debili, N., Florindo, C., Teepe, M., Titeux, M., Methia, N., Breton-Gorius, J., Cosman, D., and Vainchenker, W. (1994) cMpl ligand is a humoral regulator of megakaryocytopoiesis. *Nature* 369:571–574.

Wickramasinghe, S. N. (1991) Observations on the ultrastructure of sinusoids and reticular cells in human bone marrow. *Clin. Lab. Haematol.* 13:263–278.

Williams, D. A., Rosenblatt, M. F., Beier, D. R., and Cone, R. D. (1988) Generation of murine stromal cell lines supporting hematopoietic stem cell proliferation by use of recombinant retrovirus vectors encoding simian virus 40 large T antigen. *Mol. Cell. Biol.* 8:3864–3871.

Williams, D. E., Eisenman, J., Baird, A., Rauch, C., Van Ness, K., March, C. J., Park, L. S., Martin, U., Mochizuki, D. Y., Boswell, H. S., et al. (1990) Identification of a ligand for the c-Kit proto-oncogene. *Cell* 63:167–174.

Williams, D. E., de Vries, P., Namen, A. E., Widmer, M. B., and Lyman, S. D. (1992) The steel factor. *Dev. Biol.* 151:368–376.

Wineman, J., Moore, K., Lemischka, I., and Muller-Sieburg, C. (1996) Functional heterogeneity of the hematopoietic microenvironment: rare stromal elements maintain long-term repopulating stem cells. *Blood* 87:4082–4090.

Wong, P. M., Chung, S. W., Chui, D. H., and Eaves, C. J. (1986) Properties of the earliest clonogenic hemopoietic precursors to appear in the developing murine yolk sac. *Proc. Natl. Acad. Sci. USA* 83:3851–3854.

Wu, A., Till, J., Siminovitch, L., and McCulloch, E. (1968) Cytological evidence for a relationship between normal hematopoietic colony-forming cells and cells of the lymphoid system. *J. Exp. Med.* 127:455–467.

Wu, A. M. (1983). Regulation of self-renewal of human T lymphocyte colony-forming units (TL-CFUs). *J. Cell. Physiol.* 117:101–108.

Wu, L., Kincade, P. W., and Shortman, K. (1993) The CD44 expressed on the earliest intrathymic precursor population functions as a thymus homing molecule but does not bind to hyaluronate. *Immunol. Lett.* 38:69–75.

Xu, J., Grewal, I. S., Geba, G. P., and Flavell, R. A. (1996) Impaired primary T-cell responses in L-selectin–deficient mice. *J. Exp. Med.* 183:589–598.

Yagi, M., Ritchie, K. A., Sitnicka, E., Storey, C., Roth, G. J., and Bartelmez, S. (1999) Sustained ex vivo expansion of hematopoietic stem cells mediated by thrombopoietin. *Proc. Natl. Acad. Sci. USA* 96:8126–8131.

Yoder, M. C., Hiatt, K., Dutt, P., Mukherjee, P., Bodine, D. M., and Orlic, D. (1997a) Characterization of definitive lymphohematopoietic stem cells in the day 9 murine yolk sac. *Immun.* 7: 335–344.

Yoder, M. C., Hiatt, K., and Mukherjee, P. (1997b) In vivo repopulating hematopoietic stem cells are present in the murine yolk sac at day 9.0 postcoitus. *Proc. Natl. Acad. Sci. USA* 94:6776–6780.

Zannettino, A. C., Berndt, M. C., Butcher, C., Butcher, E. C., Vadas, M. A., and Simmons, P. J. (1995) Primitive human hematopoietic progenitors adhere to P-selectin (CD62P). *Blood* 85: 3466–3477.

Zeigler, F. C., de Sauvage, F., Widmer, H. R., Keller, G. A., Donahue, C., Schreiber, R. D., Malloy, B., Hass, P., Eaton, D., and Matthews, W. (1994) In vitro megakaryocytopoietic and thrombopoietic activity of c-Mpl ligand (TPO) on purified murine hematopoietic stem cells. *Blood* 84:4045–4052.

Zou, Y. R., Kottmann, A. H., Kuroda, M., Taniuchi, I., and Littman, D. R. (1998) Function of the chemokine receptor CXCR4 in haematopoiesis and in cerebellar development [see comments]. *Nature* 393:595–599.

Zsebo, K. M., Williams, D. A., Geissler, E. N., Broudy, V. C., Martin, F. H., Atkins, H. L., Hsu, R. Y., Birkett, N. C., Okino, K. H., Murdock, D. C., et al. (1990) Stem cell factor is encoded at the Sl locus of the mouse and is the ligand for the c-Kit tyrosine kinase receptor. *Cell* 63: 213–224.

3

Blood Flow Regulation in Inflammation

JOEL LINDEN

Inflammation triggers the release or synthesis of a number of mediators derived from inflammatory cells, the vasculature, and nerves (see Table 3.1) Some of these compounds produce receptor-mediated effects on vascular tissues. Mast cells and macrophages are the principal cells found in tissues that release or form factors that recruit circulating leukocytes into inflamed tissues (see Chap. 23). These factors also regulate vascular tone and permeability by activating receptors found on vascular smooth muscle cells, endothelial cells, and nerve terminals. Kinins and activated products of the complement system are also increased during inflammation and produce some of their effects by direct binding to receptors on vascular tissues. This chapter reviews how the receptors that are activated by mediators released or formed during inflammation regulate vascular responses to inflammation. The main receptors involved in these responses are summarized in Table 3.2.

The major vascular events associated with acute inflammation are dilation of arterioles to increase blood flow and constriction of endothelial cells of postcapillary venules leading to the escape of plasma proteins and facilitation of diapedesis (McDonald et al., 1999). The result is tissue swelling, warmth, and redness. Inflammatory mediators derived from mast cells are present as precursors in intracellular granules. In addition to histamine, other preformed mediators include ATP and serotonin (5-HT). Inflammation stimulates the synthesis of prostaglandins, leukotrienes, and platelet-activating factor (PAF) in mast cells and other cells.

C3a and C5a

The complement peptide fragments, C3a and C5a, generated by the activation of complement during inflammation, trigger receptor-mediated increased vascular permeability due to stimulating mast cell degranulation and from direct effects on endothelium. C3a is generated in the early phase of an inflammatory reaction by proteolytic cleavage of the complement component C3. The C3a receptor is a calcium-mobilizing Gq/11 coupled receptor that, in comparison to the C5a receptor and other G-protein–coupled receptors, has a large second extracellular loop comprised of over 160 amino

Table 3.1. Some Sources of Vasoactive Inflammatory Mediators Produced During Inflammation

Mast Cells	Platelets	Macrophages	Eosinophils	Complement	Kinins	Nerves
Histamine	5-HT	TNF-α	PAF	C3a	Bradykinin	ATP
5-HT (rodent)	ADP	IL-1		C5a		SP
ATP						NKA
Prostaglandins						CGRP
Leukotrienes						
PAF						
PGD_2						
TXA_2						

Note. PAF, platelet-activating factor; PGD_2, prostaglandin D_2 TXA_2, thromboxane A_2; 5-HT, 5-hydroxytryptamine; TNF-α, tumor necrosis factor α; SP, substance P; NKA, neurokinin A; CGRP, calcitonin gene-related peptide.

acids (Ames et al., 1996). Binding of C3a to its receptor triggers chemotaxis of mast cells, neutrophils, macrophages, and eosinophils, and histamine release from mast cells (Martin et al., 1997). G-protein–coupled C5a receptors were originally described on neutrophils and monocytes but are also found on other cell types including endothelial cells and mast cells (Gasque et al., 1997).

Adenosine Triphorphate

ATP is released from autonomic nerve terminals, mast cells, platelets, endothelial cells, and other cell types. Physiological responses to extracellular nucleotides are mediated by P2X receptors that are inotropic ligand-gated channels, and by structurally distinct G-protein–coupled P2Y receptors (Fredholm et al., 1997; King et al., 1998). Seven subtypes of P2X receptors have been cloned and designated $P2X_{1-7}$. P2X receptors have intracellular amino and carboxyl terminals and span the plasma membrane twice. ATP is by far the most potent naturally occurring nucleotide ligand (Valera et al., 1994). The human P2Y receptors have variable preferences for various nucleotides: $P2Y_{12}$ receptors are selectively activated by ADP, $P2Y_2$ by ATP and UTP, $P2Y_4$ by UTP, $P2Y_6$ by UDP, and $P2Y_{11}$ by ATP. The agonist selectivity of the human $P2Y_4$ for UTP is not conserved in other species because the rat $P2Y_4$ receptor is equally activated by UTP and ATP and also is activated by ITP (Bogdanov et al., 1998b). It is not yet known how much UTP is released during inflammation, although mechanical stimulation of many different cell types has been shown, in general, to trigger the release of similar amounts of UTP and ATP (Lazarowski and Harden, 1999).

During vascular injury, nucleotides play an important role in hemostasis through activation of platelets, modulation of vascular tone, recruitment of

Table 3.2. Some Receptors Involved in Blood Flow Regulation During Inflammation (Derived in Part from the *TIPs* Receptor and Ion Channel Nomenclature Supplement 1998; Only Single Examples of Agonists and Antagonists Are Given)

Receptor	Agonist	Antagonist	Location	Effect	Coupling
A_1 adenosine	CPA	CPX	Symp. nerve terminals Myocardium	Inhibit NE release/vasodilation Decreased rate and force	Gi/o
A_{2A} adenosine	CGS21680	ZM241385	VSM Mast cells Macrophages	Dilation Inhibit degranulation Inhibit cytokine release	Gs
A_{2B} adenosine	NECA	MRS1754	VSM Endothelium Mast cells (human, canine)	Dilation NO/Dilation Degranulation	Gs–Gq/11
A_e adenosine	Cl-IB-MECA	MRS1220	Mast cells (rodent)	Degranulation	Gi/o
ATP ($P2X_1$)	2-MeSATP	PPADS	VSM	Constriction	Receptor–channel
ATP ($P2X_7$)	Bz-ATP	PPADS	Mast cells	Degranulation	Receptor–channel
ATP ($P2Y_1$)	ADP	suramin	Endothelium	NO/Dilation	Gq/11
B_2 bradykinin	[phe^8, ψ(CH2Nh)Arg^9]BK	HOE140	C-fibers Endothelium	SP, CGRP release NO/Dilation	Gq/11 Gq/11
C3a	C3a	—	Mast cells	Degranulation	Gq/11
C5a	C5a	F-[OPdChaWR]	Mast cells Endothelium	Degranulation Increased permeability	Gq/11
CGRP-1	CGRP	CGRP(8–37)	Arteriole Sympathetic nerves	Dilation NE release	Gs
H_1 histamine	TFMP-histamine	triprolidine	VSM Endothelium	Constriction Increased permeability	Gq/11

H$_2$ histamine	dimaprit	tiotidine	VSM Mast cells	Dilation Inhibit degranulation	Gs
H$_3$ histamine	R-α-methylhistamine	clobenpropit	Sympathetic nerves C-fibers	Inhibit NE release Inhibit SP, CGRP	Gs
5-HT$_{1B}$	sumatriptan	SB216441	VSM	Constriction	Gq/11
5HT$_{1D}$	sumatriptan	BRL15572	VSM	Constriction	Gq/11
5-HT$_{2A}$	α-Me-5HT	ketanserin	VSM	Constriction	Gq/11
IL-1	IL-1 beta	IL-1Ra	Fibroblast	Release VEGF-C	Tyrosine kinase
LT, cysLT$_1$	LTC$_4$	Zafurkjast	Endothelium	Increase permeability	Gq/11
NK$_1$(SP)	SP methylester	spantide	Arteriole endothelium Venule endothelium Sympathetic nerve	NO/Dilation Increased permeability NE release	Gq/11
PAF	carbamyl-PAF	WEB2086	Endothelium	Increased permeability	Gq/11
Prostanoid					
DP	BW245C	BWA868C	Veins	Relaxation	Gs
IP	cicaprost	—	Arteries and veins	Relaxation	Gs
TP	U46619	ifetroban	Arteries	Constriction	Gq/11
EP$_3$	sulprostone	—	Arteries	Constriction	Gq/11
TNF-α 1	TNF-α	etanercept	Fibroblast	Release VEGF-C, angiogenesis	Tyrosine kinase

Note. CPA, N^6-cyclopentyladenosine; CPX, 8-cyclopentyl-1,3-dipropylxanthine; CGS21680, 2-[4-(2-carboxyethyl)phenethylamino]-5'-N-ethylcarboxamidoadenosine; ZM241385, 4-(2-[7-amino-2-[2-furyl][1,2,4]triazolo[2,3-a][1,3,5]triazin-5-yl-amino]ethyl)phenol; NECA, 5'-N-ethylcarboxamidoadenosine; CI-IB-MECA, 2-chloro-N^6-(2-iodo)benzyl-5'-N-methylcarboxamidodoadenosine; PPADS, pyridoxal phosphate 6-azophenyl-2',4'-disulphonic acid; HOE140, DArg[Hyp^3, Thi^5, DTic^7, Oic^8]BK; F-[OpdChaWR], Phe-[Orn-Pro-D-cyclohexylalanine-Trp-Arg]; TFMP-histamine, 2-[3-(trifluoromethyl)phenyl]histamine; SB216441, N-[3-(2-dimethylamino)ethoxy-4-methoxyphenyl]2-methyl-4'-(5-methyl-4'(5-methyl-1,2,4oxadiazol-3-yl)-(1,1'-biphenyl)-4-carboxamide; BRL15572,3-[4-(3-chlorophenyl)piperazin-1-yl]-1,1-diphenyl-2-propanol; IL-1Ra, Interleukin-1 receptor antagonist; WEB2086, 3-(4-[2-chlorophenyl]-9-methyl-6H-thieno[3,2-f][1,2,4]triazolo[4,3-a][1,4]diazepine-2-yl)-1-(4-morpholinyl)-1-propanone; BWA868C, 3-benzyl-5-(6-carboxyhexyl)-1-(2-cyclohexyl-2-hydroxyethylamino) hydantoin; U46619, 11α,9α-epoxymethano-PGH$_2$; etanercept, soluble TNF-α receptor.

neutrophils and monocytes, and facilitation of adhesion of leukocytes to the endothelium. Activation of P2Y receptors on endothelial cells triggers the generation of nitric oxide (NO) and (PGI_2) prostacyclin. Both P2X and P2Y receptors are found on vascular smooth muscle and heart and have contractile and possibly proliferative effects (Bogdanov et al., 1998a; Murthy and Makhlouf, 1998). Activation of the $P2X_1$ receptor causes vasoconstriction that displays rapid tachyphylaxis (Malmsjo et al., 1999). The $P2X_7$ receptor (formerly called P2z) is found on mast cells and responds to ATP by triggering mast cell degranulation (Osipchuk and Cahalan, 1992; Surprenant et al., 1996). During vascular injury, nucleotides activate platelets by interacting with three nucleotide receptors on platelets, $P2Y_1$, $P2X_1$, and $P2Y_{12}$. The latter was recently cloned. $P2Y_1$ receptors mediate platelet shape change, and both the $P2Y_1$ and $P2Y_{12}$ are required for ADP-induced fibrinogen receptor activation. An endothelial P2Y receptor that is activated by UTP ($P2Y_2$ and/or $P2Y_4$) triggers the release of endothelium-derived hyperpolarizing factor, whereas NO-mediated dilation is stimulated mainly by the $P2Y_1$ receptor (Malmsjo et al., 1998).

Adenosine

The adenine nucleotides released from inflamed tissues are rapidly degraded to adenosine by ectonucleotidases including the ATP/ADPase or apyrase, CD39, and the 5'-nucleotidase, CD73. In addition, adenosine is generated intracellularly in ischemic tissues and is transported out of cells by nucleoside transport proteins. Adenosine has been shown to produce vasodilation and increase microvascular permeability in most vascular beds (Gawlowski and Duran, 1986). In vitro, the permeability of macrovascular aortic endothelial cells decreases in response to adenosine, but the permeability of microvascular endothelial cells is increased (Watanabe et al., 1992; Haselton et al., 1993). In intact vessels and in vivo adenosine increases microvascular permeability. These vascular permeability changes may result from adenosine-stimulated degranulation of perivascular mast cells (Doyle et al., 1994).

Adenosine activates four G-protein–coupled adenosine receptors (Linden and Jacobson, 1998). A_1 receptors coupled to Gi/o are found on the heart where they reduce the rate and force of contractions, and on sympathetic nerve terminals where they inhibit the release of catecholamines and indirectly reduce vascular tone (Smits et al., 1991). A_{2A} and A_{2B} adenosine receptors are coupled to Gs and are found on vascular smooth muscle where they elevate cyclic adenosine monophosphate (AMP) and produce vasodilation. A_{2B} receptors found on endothelium are dually coupled to Gs and Gq (Gao et al., 1999) and may trigger vasodilation in part by stimulating nitric oxide formation. Various vascular beds have different complements of A_2 receptor subtypes; coronary arteries are particularly enriched in A_{2A} receptors (Shryock et al., 1998). A_{2A} receptors also are found on neutrophils, macrophages, mast cells and platelets where they inhibit the release of cytokines, inhibit mast cell degranulation, and inhibit platelet aggregation (Sullivan and Linden, 1998). Activation of A_3 adenosine receptors stimulates the degranulation of perivascular mast cells in rodent species (Jin et al., 1997). However, in canine and human species, mast cell activation appears to be mediated primarily by A_{2B} receptors (Linden et al., 1999). These stimulatory effects of adenosine mediated by A_{2B} or A_3 receptors are counteracted by A_{2A} receptors that inhibit degranulation.

Histamine

Histamine is a biologically active amine that causes constriction of small blood vessels and bronchioles and increases the permeability of capillaries. It is stored in cytoplasmic granules of mast cells and basophils and is released following cross-linking of IgE antibodies by antigens or by ischemia/reperfusion (see Chapter 23). Perivascular mast cells degranulate in response to adenosine formed during ischemia or inflammation. H_1 and H_2 receptors are coupled to Gq/11 and Gs, respectively. H_3 receptors have not yet been cloned, but probably are coupled to Gs.

Histamine plays an important part in the cutaneous edematous weal and axon reflex-mediated flare responses that underlie many allergic skin conditions. Histamine directly effects vasodilation and increases microvascular permeability (Clough et al., 1998). Binding to H_1 receptors triggers vascular smooth muscle contraction and increases capillary permeability. The H_1 receptor subtype also mediates endothelium-dependent vasodilation (Adeagbo and Oriowo, 1998). H_2 and H_3 receptors produce an endothelium-independent dilation caused by the activation of small conductance Ca^{2+}-activated K^+ channels (Adeagbo and Oriowo, 1998). Binding of histamine to H_2 receptors blocks mediator release from mast cells and basophils. Histamine attracts eosinophils that produce histaminase, which degrades histamine. Prejunctional autonomic H_3 receptors and receptors on C-fiber terminals inhibit the release of autonomic transmitters and tachykinins (Imamura et al., 1996a).

Serotonin

Serotonin (5-hydroxy tryptamine) is found in rodent mast cells and human platelets. It causes contraction of smooth muscle and enhances the permeability of small blood vessels. The 5HT receptors that have been cloned include 5HT1(A/B/D) coupled to Gi/o, 5HT2(A/B/C) coupled to Gq/11, 5HT3 coupled to a cation channel, and $5HT_4$ coupled to Gs. Vasoconstriction in response to serotonin is mediated primarily by a mixture of $5HT_{1B/D}$ and $5HT_{2A}$ receptors (Cortijo et al., 1997).

Tachykinins and Calcitonin Gene-Related Peptide

Sensory nerves release neurokinins (substance P and neurokinin A) and calcitonin gene-related peptide (CGRP), neurotransmitters that mediate the process of neurogenic inflammation. An example is the weal and flare response in human skin. There are three G-protein–coupled tachykinin receptors, all coupled to Gq/11. The principal ligands and their corresponding receptors are substance P–NK_1; substance K–NK_2; and neurokinin B–NK_3. Tachykinins are subject to degradation by angiotensin-converting enzyme and neutral endopeptidase (NEP). NEP also metabolizes endothelins. Neurokinin A is a nonselective agonist of all three tachykinin receptors. CGRP receptors are members of the amylin family of G-protein–coupled receptors. CGRP acts via the Gs-coupled CGRP-1 receptor and is the principal transmitter mediating neurogenic dilation of arterioles, whereas substance P (SP) and neurokinin A (NKA) acting via NK_1 receptors mediate an increase in venular permeability (Holzer, 1998). Receptor activity-modifying proteins (RAMPs) are single transmembrane-spanning proteins that interact with the calcitonin receptor-like receptor (CRLR). The RAMP1–CRLR complex acts as a CGRP receptor (Christopoulos et al, 1999).

SP and NKA cause a marked increase in blood flow in various blood vessels (Salonen et al., 1988), and SP stimulates microvascular leak at postcapillary venules and also stimulates angiogenesis (Fan et al., 1993). NK_1 receptor antagonists block plasma exudation in response to inflammation. Neither substance P nor the NK-1 agonist, septide, increase vascular permeability in NK_1-receptor–deficient mice (Cao et al., 1999). CGRP is a vasodilator that acts directly on receptors on arterioles, but has no effect on vascular leak. CGRP and NK_1 receptors also are found on adrenergic nerve terminals and promote norepinephrine (NE) release (Seyedi et al., 1999). Capsaicin pretreatment is used to deplete neuropeptides from C-fibers. In pigs, capsaicin pretreatment inhibits the vasodilator response to allergen, which may be mediated by the release of CGRP (Alving et al., 1988). C-fiber endings are closely associated with mast cells, and CGRP is a stimulus for mast cell degranulation (Imamura et al., 1996b).

Bradykinin

Bradykinin is a 9-amino acid peptide split by plasma kallikrein from plasma kininogens in inflamed tissues. It is degraded by angiotensin-converting enzyme (ACE), and some of the effects of ACE inhibitors in man are mediated by bradykinin accumulation (Hornig et al., 1997). There are two cloned G-protein–coupled bradykinin receptors; B_1 and B_2, both coupled to Gq/11. Bradykinin is a potent activator of B_2 receptors on C-fibers and produces plasma leakage and NE release from sympathetic nerve terminals that is mediated by substance P and CGRP (Sakamoto et al., 1993; Vianna and Calixto, 1998; Seyedi et al., 1999). NE produces cardiac acceleration mediated by β1 adrenergic receptors and vasoconstriction and plasma exudation mediated by vascular and endothelial α-adrenergic receptors. B_2 receptors are found on vascular endothelium and their activation stimulates the release of nitric oxide and endothelium-dependent hyperpolarizing factor (Node et al., 1997). Inflammation induces the expression of B_1 receptors on vascular smooth muscle (Schremmerdanninger et al., 1998).

Platelet-Activating Factor

Platelet-activating factor (PAF) is a phospholipid derived from the inactive precursor, lyso-PAF, which is generated in substantial quantities by activated eosinophils and also by other cell types, including endothelial cells. The PAF receptor couples to Gq/11, and is expressed on many inflammatory cells and on vascular endothelial cells (Predescu et al., 1966 Flickinger and Olsen, 1999). PAF signaling in human umbilical vein endothelial cells (HUVECs) causes vascular cell adhesion molecule-1 (VCAM-1) expression via a pathway including mitogen-activated protein (MAP) kinase and nuclear factor κB (NF-κB) (Sultana et al., 1999), and P-selectin expression (Bunting et al., 1997). PAF also is a potent activator of angiogenesis and controls the motility and the shape of vascular endothelium by signaling through protein kinase C and tyrosine phosphorylation of focal adhesion kinase [p125(FAK)] and paxillin (Soldi et al., 1996). PAF receptor activation leads to opening of venular and capillary endothelial junctions, with the greatest receptor density on venular endothelium (Predescu et al., 1996).

Eicosanoids

Eicosanoids are arachidonic acid-derived 20 carbon cyclic fatty acids produced during inflammation from membrane phospholipids. Arachidonic acid is a precursor of prostaglandins and thromboxanes (via cyclooxygenase) and leukotrienes (via 5-lipoxygenase). Arachidonic acid production is increased in inflammatory cells as a consequence of the activation of phospholipases C or A2. Leukotrienes and thromboxanes contract smooth muscle. There are three G-protein–coupled leukotriene receptors. The leukotriene BY (BLT) receptor is dually coupled to Gq/11 and Gi/o cysteinyl-leukotriene receptors $CysLT_1$ and $CysLT_2$ are coupled to Gq/11. In addition to the well-characterized effect of leukotrienes to trigger bronchoconstriction in the lung, they also act to increase vascular permeability. Most of these effects appear to be mediated by $CysLT_1$ receptors (Devillier et al., 1999).

There are at least eight G-protein–coupled prostanoid receptors, some of which are encoded by mRNAs that can be alternatively spliced. The DP receptor is preferentially activated by prostaglandin D_2 (PGD_2); the FP receptor by $PGF_2\alpha$ the IP receptor by PGI_2; and the TP receptor by thromboxane A_2 ($TBXA_2$) and PGH_2. Four receptors, EP(1/2/3/4) preferentially bind PGE_2. Gs-coupled prostanoid receptors are DP, IP, EP_2, and EP_4; Gq/11-coupled receptors are FP, TP, and EP_1; EP_3 couples to $Gq/11$, Gi/o, and Gs. The major prostaglandin released from activated mast cells is PGD_2. In human pulmonary vessels, venous relaxation is induced by prostanoids that activate DP and IP receptors, and to a lesser extent EP receptors; however, only the IP receptor is involved in the relaxation of arterial smooth muscle (Walch et al., 1999). Prostanoids constrict pulmonary arterial vessels via TP and EP_3 receptors (Jones et al., 1997). TXA_2 is a potent inducer of vascular smooth muscle contraction and also induces platelet aggregation (Krauss et al., 1996).

Vascular Cytokine Receptors

TNF-α and IL-1 are released by many cells, including activated macrophages, and produce effects mediated by receptor tyrosine kinases (Burkegaffney and Hellewell, 1996). Two single-membrane–spanning TNF-α receptors are referred to as type I (55 kDa) and type II (75 KDa). A third related receptor, glucocorticoid-induced TNFR-related protein (GITR) has recently been identified and is expressed on vascular endothelial cells (Gurney et al., 1999). The type II TNF-α receptor appears to be confined to hematopoietic cells, whereas the type I receptor is widely distributed. TNF-α triggers the migration of cultured vascular smooth muscle cells mediated by type I receptors and mitogen-activated protein kinase (MAPK) activation (Goetze et al., 1999). Activation of TNF-α receptors in cultured human endothelial cells triggers increased expression of the intercellular adhesion molecule, ICAM-1 (Burkegaffney and Hellewell, 1996).

Vascular smooth muscle cells represent a source and a target of a number of proinflammatory cytokines, including IL-1 and its naturally occurring receptor antagonist, IL-1Ra. IL-1 induces further synthesis of itself and IL-6 by vascular endothelium. IL-1 receptors (types 1 and 2) have a single-membrane–spanning topology. IL-1 is comprised of two principal 17 kDa polypeptides: IL-1α, associated with membranes, and IL-1β, found free in the circulation. The type II receptor is identical to the type I but has a truncated intracellular carboxy-terminal region. IL-1 is a mitogen for cultured vascular smooth muscle cells. Binding of IL-1 to type 1 IL-1 receptors on vascular smooth muscle stimulates the cells to express more IL-1 (Beasley and Cooper, 1999), and stimulates the secretion of metalloproteinases that can digest vascular matrix (Lee et al., 1995). Binding of TNF-α or IL1β to receptors on fibroblasts induces the release of the proangiogenic vascular endothelial growth factor, VEGF-C. IL-1 also stimulates expression of VEGFR-2 (KDR/FLT-1) in human umbilical vein endothelial cells (Ristimaki et al., 1998).

Effects on Anti-Inflammatory Agents on Vasoactive Mediators

Steroids inhibit the conversion of fatty acids in cell membranes to arachidonic acid, the source of prostaglandins and leukotrienes. Nonsteroidal anti-inflammatory drugs inhibit the conversion of arachidonic acid to prostaglandins. Opiates have been demonstrated to inhibit the release of neuropeptides from peripheral nerve terminals in inflamed areas.

Conclusions

Inflammation leads to the release or synthesis of numerous vasoactive compounds derived from many sources including inflammatory cells, nerves, plasma precursors, and endothelium. The response of the vasculature is complex because of the number of factors that are released, and because many of these factors have physiologically antagonistic actions. It seems unlikely that inhibiting the formation or release of a single mediator, or that blocking a single receptor, will produce significant therapeutic benefits by blocking vascular changes associated with inflammation. Effective anti-inflammatory therapeutic strategies probably will require the development of interventions that simultaneously influence many signaling pathways.

References

Adeagbo, A. S., and Oriowo, M. A. (1998) Histamine receptor subtypes mediating hyperpolarization in the isolated, perfused rat mesenteric pre-arteriolar bed. *Eur. J. Pharmacol.* 347:237–244.

Alving, K., Matran, R., Lacroix, J. S., and Lundberg, J. M. (1988) Allergen challenge induces vasodilatation in pig bronchial circulation via a capsaicin-sensitive mechanism. *Acta Physiol scand.* 134:571–572.

Ames, R. S., Li, Y., Sarau, H. M., Nuthulaganti, P., Foley, J. J., Ellis, C., Zeng, Z., Su, K., Jurewicz, A. K., Hertzberg, P. P., Bergsma, D. I., and Kumar, C. (1996). Molecular cloning and characterization of the human anaphylatoxin C3a receptor. *J. Biol. Chem.* 271:20231–20234.

Beasley, D., and Cooper, A. L., (1999) Constitutive expression of interleukin-1 alpha precursor promotes human vascular smooth muscle cell proliferation. *Am. J. Physiol.* 276:H901–H912.

Bogdanov, Y., Rubino, A., and Burnstock, G. (1998a) Characterisation of subtypes of the P2X and P2Y families of ATP receptors in the foetal human heart. *Life Sci.* 62:697–703.

Bogdanov, Y. D., Wildman, S. S., Clements, M. P., King, B. F., and Burnstock, G. (1998b) Molecular cloning and characterization of rat P2Y4 nucleotide receptor. *B.J. Pharmacol.* 124:428–430.

Bunting, M., Lorant, D. E., Bryant, A. E., Zimmerman, G. A., Mcintyre, T. M., Stevens, D. I., and Prescott, S. M. (1997) Alpha toxin from clostridium perfringens induces proinflammatory changes in endothelial cells. *J. Clin. Invest.* 100:565–574.

Burkegaffney, A., and Hellewell, P. G., (1996) Tumour necrosis factor-alpha-induced ICAM-1 expression in human vascular endothelial and lung epithelial cells—modulation by tyrosine kinase inhibitors. *B.J. Pharmacol.* 119:1149–1158.

Cao, T., Gerard, N. P., and Brain, S. D. (1999) Use of NK1 knockout mice to analyze substance P-induced edema formation. *Am. J. Physiol.—Regul. Integrat. Comp. Physiol.* 46:R476–R481.

Christopoulos, G. Perry, K. I., Morfis, M. Tilakaratne, N., Gao, Y. Y., Fraser, N. J., Main, M. J., Foord, S. M., and Sexton, P. M. (1999) Multiple amylin receptors arise from receptor activity—modifying protein interaction with the calcitonin receptor gene product. *Mol. Pharmacol.* 56:235–242.

Clough, G. F., Bennett, A. R., and Church, M. K. (1998) Effects of H1 antagonists on the cutaneous vascular response to histamine and bradykinin: a study using scanning laser Doppler imaging. *Br. J., Dermatol.* 138:806–814.

Cortijo, J., Marti-Cabrera, M., Bernabeu, E., Domenech, T., Bou, J., Fernandez, A. G., Beleta, J., Palacios, J. M., and Morcillo, E. J. (1997) Characterization of 5-HT receptors on human pulmonary artery and vein: functional and binding studies. *B. J. Pharmacol.* 122:1455–1463.

Devillier, P., Baccard, N., and Advenier, C. (1999) Leukotrienes, leukotriene receptor antagonists and leukotriene synthesis inhibitors in asthma: An update. Part I: Synthesis, receptors and role of leukotrienes in asthma [Review]. *Pharmacol. Res.* 40:3–13.

Doyle, M. P., Linden, J., and Duling, B. P. (1994) Nucleoside-induced arteriolar constriction: a mast cell-dependent response. *Am. J. Physiol.* 266:H2042–H2050.

Fan, T. P., Hu, D. E., Guard, S., Gresham, G. A., and Watling, K. J. (1993) Stimulation of angiogenesis by substance P and interleukin-1 in the rat and its inhibition by NK1 or interleukin-1 receptor antagonists. *B.J. Pharmacol.* 110:43–49.

Flickinger, B. D., and Olson, M. S. (1999) Localization of the platelet-activating factor receptor to rat pancreatic microvascular endothelial cells. *Am. J. Pathol.* 254:1353–1358.

Fredholm, B. B., Abbracchio, M. P., Burnstock, G., Dubyak, G. R., Harden, T. K., Jacobson, K. A., Schwabe, U., and Williams, M. (1997) Towards a revised nomenclature for P1 and P2 receptors. *Trends in Pharmacol. Sci.* 18:79–82.

Gao, Z., Chen, T., Weber, M. J., and Linden, J. (1999) A_{2B} adenosine and $P2Y_2$ receptors stimulate mitogen-activated protein kinase in human embryonic kidney-293 cells: cross-talk between cyclic AMP and protein kinase C pathways. *J. Biol. Chem.* 274:5972–5980.

Gasque, P., Singhrao, S. K., Neal, J. W., Gotze, O., and Morgan, B. P. (1997) Expression of the receptor for complement C5a (CD88) is up-regulated on reactive astrocytes, microglia, and endothelial cells in the inflamed human central nervous system. *Am. J. Pathol.* 150:31–41.

Gawlowski, D. M., and Duran, W. N. (1986) Dose-related effects of adenosine and bradykinin on microvascular permselectivity to macromolecules in the hamster cheek pouch. *Circ. Res.* 58: 348–355.

Goetze, S., Xi, X. P., Kawano, Y., Kawano, H., Fleck, E., Hsueh, W. A., and Law, R. E. (1999) TNF–alpha-induced migration of vascular smooth muscle cells is MAPK dependent. *Hypertens.* 33:183–189.

Gurney, A. L., Marsters, S. A., Huang, R. M., Pitti, R. M., Mark, D. T., Baldwin, D. T., Gray, A. M., Dowd, AD, Brush, A. D., Heldens, A. D., et al. (1999) Identification of a new member of the tumor necrosis factor family and its receptor, a human ortholog of mouse GITR. *Curr. Biol.* 9:215–218.

Haselton, F. R., Alexander, J. S., and Mueller, S. N. (1993) Adenosine decreases permeability of in vitro endothelial monolayers. *J. Appl. Physiol.* 74:1581–1590.

Holzer, P. (1998) Neurogenic vasodilatation and plasma leakage in the skin. *Gen. Pharmacol.* 30: 5–11.

Hornig, B., Kohler, C., and Drexler, H. (1997) Role of bradykinin in mediating vascular effects of angiotensin-converting enzyme inhibitors in humans. *Circ.* 95:1115–1118.

Imamura, M., Lander, H. M., and Levi, R. (1996a) Activation of histamine H^3-receptors inhibits carrier-mediated norepinephrine release during protracted myocardial ischemia—comparison with adenosine A^1-receptors and o^2-adrenoceptors. *Circ. Res.* 78:475–481.

Imamura, M., Smith, N. C., Garbarg, M. and Levi, R. (1996b) Histamine h_3-receptors-mediated inhibition of calcitonin gene-related peptide release from cardiac C fibers—a regulatory negative-feedback loop. *Circ. Res.* 78:863–869.

Jin, X., Shepherd, R. K., Duling, B. R., and Linden, J. (1997) Inosine binds to A3 adenosine receptors and stimulates mast cell degranulation. *J. Clin. Invest.* 100:2849–2857.

Jones, R. I., Qian, Y., Wong, H. N., Chan, H., and Yim, A. P. (1997) Prostanoid action on the human pulmonary vascular system. [Review]. *Clin. Exp. Pharmacol. Physiol.* 24:969–972.

King, B. F., Townsend-Nicholson, A., and Burnstock, G. (1998) Metabotropic receptors for ATP and UTP: exploring the correspondence between native and recombinant nucleotide receptors. [Review]. *Trends Pharmacol. Sci.* 19:506–514.

Krauss, A. H., Woodward, D. F., Gibson, L. L., Protzman, C. E., Williams, L. S., Burk, R. M., Gac, T. S., Roof, M. B., Abbas, F., Marshall, K., and Senior, J. (1996) Evidence for human thromboxane receptor heterogeneity using a novel series of 9,11-cyclic carbonate derivatives of prostaglandin F2 alpha. *Br. J. pharmacol.* 117:1171–1180.

Lazarowski, E. R., and Harden, T. K. (1999) Quantitation of extracellular UTP using a sensitive enzymatic assay. *Br. J. Pharmacol.* 127:1272–1278

Lee, F., Grodzinsky, A. J., Libby, P., Clinton, S. K., Lark, M. W., and Lee, R. T. (1995) Human vascular smooth muscle cell-monocyte interactions and metalloproteinase secretion in culture. *Arterioscl. Thromb. Vasc. Biol.* 15:2284–2289.

Linden, J., and Jacobson, K. A. (1998) Molecular biology and pharmacology of recombinant human adenosine receptors. In: *Cardiovascular Biology of Purines.* G. Burnstock, J. G. Dobson Jr., B. T. Liang, and J. Linden, eds. Dordrecht: Kluwer, pp. 1–20.

Linden, J, Thai, T., Figler, H., and Robeva, A. S. (1999) Characterization of human A_{2B} adenosine receptors: radioligand binding, western blotting and coupling to Gq in HEK-293 and HMC-1 mast cells. *Mol. Pharmacol.* 56:705–713.

Malmsjo, M., Edvinsson, I., and Erlinge, D. (1998) P2U-receptor mediated endothelium—dependent but nitric oxide-independent vascular relaxation. *Br. J. Pharmacol.* 123:719–729.

Malmsjo, M., Bergdahl, A., Moller, S., Zhao, X. H., Sun, X. Y., Hedner, T., Edvinsson, L., and Erlinge, D. (1999) Congestive heart failure induces downregulation of P2X(1)-receptors in resistance arteries. *Cardiovasc. Res.* 43:219–227.

Martin, U., Bock, D., Arseniev, L. Tornetta, M. A., Ames, R. S., Bautsch, W., Kohl, J., Ganser, A., and Klos, A. (1997) The human C3a receptor is expressed on neutrophils and monocytes, but not on B or T lymphocytes. *J. Exp. Med.* 186:199–207.

McDonald, D. M., Thurston, G., and Baluk, P. (1999) Endothelial gaps as sites for plasma leakage in inflamation. *Microcirc.* 6:7–22.

Murthy, K. S., and Makhlouf, G. M. (1998) Coexpression of ligand-gated P2X and G protein-coupled P2Y receptors in smooth muscle. Preferential activation of P2Y receptors coupled to phospholipase C (PLC)-beta1 via Galphaq/11 and to PLC-beta3 via Gbetagammai3. *J. Biol. Chem.* 273:4695–4704.

Node, K. Kitakaze, M., Kosaka, H., Minamino, T., and Hori, M. (1997) Bradykinin mediation of ca2+;-activated k+ channels regulates coronary blood flow in ischemic myocardium. *Circ.* 95:1560–1567.

Osipchuk, Y., and Cahalan, M. (1992) Cell-to-cell spread of calcium signals mediated by ATP receptors in mast cells. *Nature* 359:241–244.

Predescu, D., Ihida, K., Predescu, S., and Palade, G. E. (1996) The vascular distribution of the platelet-activating factor receptor. *Eur. J. Cell. Biol.* 69:86–98.

Ristimaki, A., Narko, K., Enholm, B., Joukov, V., and Alitalo, K. (1998) Proinflammatory cytokines regulate expression of the lymphatic endothelial mitogen vascular endothelial growth factor-C. *J. Biol. Chem.* 273:8413–8418.

Sakamoto, T., Barnes, P. I., and Chung, K. F. (1993) Effect of CP-96, 345, a non-peptide NK1 receptor antagonist, against substance P-, bradykinin- and allergen-induced airway microvascular leakage and bronchoconstriction in the guinea pig. *Eur. J. Pharmacol.* 231:31–38.

Salonen, R. O., Webber, S. E., and Widdicombe, J. G. (1988) Effects of neuropeptides and capsaicin on the canine tracheal vasculature in vivo. *Br. J. Pharmacol.* 95:1262–1270.

Schremmerdanninger, E., Offner, A., Siebeck, M., and Roscher, A. A. (1998) B1 bradykinin receptors and carboxypeptidase m are both upregulated in the aorta of pigs after lps infusion. *Biochem. Biophys. Res. Commun.* 243:246–252.

Seyedi, N., Maruyama, R., and Levi, R., (1999) Bradykinin activates a cross-signaling pathway between sensory and adrenergic nerve endings in the heart: A novel mechanism of ischemic norepinephrine release? *J. Pharmacol. Exp. Ther.* 290:656–663.

Shryock, J. C., Snowdy, S., Baraldi, P. G., Cacciari, B., Spalluto, G., Monopoli, A., Ongini, E., Baker, S. P., and Belardinelli, L. (1998) A(2A)-adenosine receptor reserve for coronary vasodilation. *Circ.* 98:711–718.

Smits, P., Lenders, J. W. M., Willemsen, J. J., and Thien, T. (1991) Adenosine attenuates the response to sympathetic stimuli in humans. *Hypertens.* 18:216–223.

Soldi, R., Sanavio, F., Aglietta, M., Primo, L., Defilippi, P., Marchisio, P. C., and Bussolino, F., (1996) Platelet-activating factor (Paf) Induces the early tyrosine phosphorylation of focal adhesion kinase (P125(Fak) In human endothelial cells. *Oncogene* 13:515–525

Sullivan, G. W., and Linden, J. (1998) Role of A_{2A} adenosine receptors in inflammation. *Drug. Dev. Res.* 45:103–112.

Sultana, C., Shen, Y. M., Johnson, C., and Kalra, V. K. (1999) Cobalt chloride-induced signaling in endothelium leading to the augmented adherence of sickle red blood cells and transendothelial migration of monocyte-like HL-60 cells is blocked by PAF—receptor antagonist. *J. Cell. Physiol.* 179:67–78.

Surprenant, A., Rassendren, F., Kawashima, E., North, R. A., and Buell, G. (1996) The cytolytic P2Z receptor for extracellular ATP identified as a P2X receptor (P2X7). *Science* 272:735–738.

Valera, S., Hussy, N., Evans, R. J., Adami, N., North, R. A., Surprenant, A., and Buell, G. (1994) A new class of ligand-gated ion channel defined by P2x receptor for extracellular ATP [see comments]. *Nature* 371:516–519.

Vianna, R. M., and Calixto, J. B. (1998) Characterization of the receptor and the mechanisms underlying the inflammatory response induced by des-Arg9-BK in mouse pleurisy. *B. J. Pharmacol.* 123:281–291.

Walch, L., Labat, C., Gascard, J. P. de M, Brink, C. and Norel, X. (1999) Prostanoid receptors involved in the relaxation of human pulmonary vessels. *B. J. Pharmacol.* 126:859–866.

Watanabe, H., Kuhne, W., Schwartz, P., and Piper, H. M. (1992) A2-adenosine receptor stimulation increases macromolecule permeability of coronary endothelial cells. *Am. J. Physiol.* 262: H1174–H1181.

4

Microvascular Permeability in Inflammation

VIRGINIA H. HUXLEY and ROLANDO E. RUMBAUT

The presence of edema (tumor) was originally described by Celsus (~25 BC–AD 37; Celsus, 1938 as one of four cardinal components of the inflammatory response. Hallmarks of the inflammatory response are increases in blood flow and permeability at the site of stimulus. Inflammatory responses and the associated permeability responses are not uniform; they represent a host of reactions that appear to depend on the stimulus, the site, and the mediators. These reactions also illustrate the complex nature of the barrier separating blood from tissue. It is complex with regard to the number of components that define the barrier, and to the number of mechanisms that influence the interface between blood and tissue.

All solutes required for optimal tissue function (e.g. O_2 water, amino acids, glucose, and fatty acids carried by albumin) must traverse the walls of microvessels separating the blood and tissue compartments. The transit of metabolic byproducts (e.g., CO_2, hydrogen ions, adenosine, lactic acid), as well as hormones (e.g., steroids, growth hormones, natriuretic peptides), are also limited by the same barrier. As the nature of these components differs with regard to size, charge, and concentration gradients, the control of permeability under physiological conditions is the result of multiple mechanisms. How these mechanisms interact to control the orderly movement of molecules with diverse properties is not fully understood

Permeability is a general term used in the description of barrier properties, from cell membranes, to layers of cells such as epithelium and endothelium, to tissues. Permeability coefficients are the constants used in the description of the barrier to solute. In the context of the microcirculation, the permeability coefficient (P_d) is given by Fick's first law of diffusion where the movement of solute (solute flux, J_s) per unit surface area (S) occurs when there is a concentration gradient (ΔC) across the barrier:

$$J_s = P_d S \Delta C.$$

In biological systems, permeability to the solvent, water, is also considered. Usually water or volume flux (J_v) occurs not because of a gradient in concentration of water but in response to gradients in hydrostatic (ΔP) or osmotic $(\Delta \pi)$ pressure. The gradients of osmotic pressure arise from the partitioning of solutes (σ) across the barrier resulting in the formation of concentration gradients. The coefficient used to describe the barrier with respect to water flux is termed hydraulic conductivity (L_p). The modern form of the Starling equation summarizes the forces and coefficients describing water flux:

$$J_v = L_p S(\Delta P - \sigma \Delta \pi).$$

When solute and volume flux are measured in whole organs, where surface area for exchange is unknown, the transport coefficients are known as the permeability–surface area product (PS) and capillary filtration coefficient (CFC or K_f), respectively. Given that biological systems, especially intact microvessels, are complex, it is worth considering that the movement of water can be coupled to the movement of solutes, particularly macromolecules, and vice versa. The transport coefficient, σ, relating volume and solute flux is known as the osmotic reflection coefficient. More complete discussion of this subject can be obtained in recent reviews (Michel and Curry, 1999; Levick and Mortimer, 1999). Finally, in intact tissue preparations it is not always possible to measure solute permeability or hydraulic conductivity due to an inability to determine concentration, volume, and so forth. Under these conditions, alterations in permeability are assessed as changes in extravasation of fluorescent dye-labeled macromolecules, or the appearance of tracer materials in the interstitium or lymph.

Microvascular barrier properties can change to permit the movement of fluids and larger solutes, particularly serum proteins and inflammatory mediators, which are usually retained in the vascular compartment, into the sites of inflammation. Coupling of large molecules to fluid movement occurs as a result of the profound changes in permeability in response to inflammatory mediators, thereby accelerating the transfer of macromolecules, such as antibodies and complement, to inflamed sites.

The magnitude of the permeability responses to inflammatory stimuli provides evidence of the capacity of the barrier to change. Whether only the mechanisms involved in the control of basal permeability are responsible for inflammatory changes in permeability, or the inflammatory response involves recruitment of additional mechanisms remains to be determined.

The heterogeneity of permeability responses likely reflects the fact that inflammatory changes originate from a variety of sources, such as infection, tumor growth, ischemia–reperfusion injury, antigen challenge, neural stimuli, or tissue trauma. Inflammation generally produces conspicuous responses in the microcirculation, particularly in postcapillary venules, which represent the low-pressure end of the microvascular network. A notable response is the loss of barrier function manifest as focal increases in macromolecule leakage (leaky sites) and formation of edema. Extreme forms of the inflammatory response lead to complete loss of the microvascular barrier, evidenced by induction of ischemia due to the loss of patent vascular channels through the tissue. In contrast to the cell migration and formation of leaky sites observed in postcapillary venules, changes also occur in the capillaries, especially with regard to the movement of fluid and plasma proteins.

In view of the dramatic alterations that can occur in inflammation, it is not surprising that much research has focused on the inflammatory response with little attention given to the regulation of permeability under less conspicuous circumstances. To understand fully the myriad of processes that result in the inflammatory response, it is important to consider the notion that microvascular barrier permeability reflects the interactions of several systems. Under basal, noninflamed conditions, the microvascular barrier restricts water and solute flux at a point very different from that of inflammatory states. This basal state is analogous to that of resting arteriolar tone, where microvessels have the capacity either to dilate or to contract. Under basal conditions, exchange vessels possess the capacity either to reduce or to increase movement of substances between the vascular and tissue compartments (Huxley et al., 1993b; Rumbaut et al., 1995; Huxley and Williams, 1996; Adamson et al., 1998; Huxley, 1998). Inflammatory changes in microvessel permeability represent graded responses at one end of a spectrum of possible mechanisms. As noted earlier, under these conditions the barrier is less restrictive to macromolecules, both in capillaries and in venules.

In many cases of inflammation, vascular permeability changes develop slowly and at times well after the application of the stimulus, as in the case of photodamage (Miller et al., 1992). In other cases the inflammatory response is very rapid and of great intensity, as can happen in response to mediators such as venoms, bradykinin, or histamine. Illustrations of the temporal changes in blood flow, protein extravasation, and leukocyte adherence induced by a wide selection of inflammatory mediators can be found in the work of Raud and Lindbom (1994). In these and other states of hyperpermeability, it appears that there can be the local action of a multitude of mediators, particularly leukocytes, cytokines, and growth factors. In the intact organism the situation is complicated by the fact that the net movement of materials depends not only on changes of barrier structure, but also on blood flow to the sites of exchange, blood pressure in the microvasculature, and lymphatic function, which all serve to alter concentration and pressure gradients in the area of interest.

Structures Associated with Inflammatory Changes in Permeability

Although inflammatory changes in permeability have long been recognized and extensively studied, the mechanisms involved in the loss of barrier function remain to be fully determined. It is well known that large gaps form in endothelial cells in response to a variety of stimuli resulting in the loss of barrier integrity for macromolecules. The debate about the structure of microvascular leaks first arose in 1961 when Majno and Palade demonstrated that histamine- and serotonin-induced increases in permeability were associated with the appearance of gaps or openings in the endothelium of postcapillary venules. Whether these gaps are actually the result of cytoskeletal arrangement acting to pull apart the junctions between cells (Majno et al., 1969), the fusion of intracellular vesicles to form transcellular channels traversing the cytoplasm, or new channels, are all the foci of recent studies.

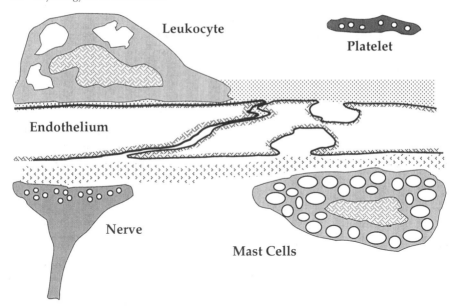

Fig. 4.1. Endothelial structures, both intracellular and extracellular, which play a role in the determination of permeability to water and solutes.

These structures and those associated with determination of basal permeability are illustrated in Figure 4.1.

In response to inflammatory stimuli, mature endothelium appears to possess the capacity to create structures not present under basal conditions. Thurston et al. (1996) used substance P to induce a neurogenic inflammatory response in tracheal postcapillary venules. This treatment resulted in the deposition of microvascular tracers as small as 5 nm (Monastral blue), which spread widely in the vessel wall and was localized to postcapillary and collecting venules. In addition, India ink particles of approximately 30 nm deposited in the regions of the endothelial perimeter. Despite traversing the endothelial cell of inflamed venules, 100 nm microspheres, remained confined to a focal region at the perimeter, as did 1000 nm microspheres. Scanning electron microscopy revealed the rapid (by 1 minute) retraction of endothelial margins and formation of gaps partitioned by fingerlike processes at the junctions. There was also evidence of a small number of transendothelial gaps by 3 minutes, but not by 1 minute following substance P application. The fingerlike structures had an average diameter of 0.7 μm. It remains to be determined how the fingerlike processes, which can be as long as 5 μm, form. It is also not known whether the same mechanisms are involved in finger formation and transendothelial gaps at the junctions, as fingers have been observed in regions devoid of gaps.

Thurston et al. (1996) also demonstrated that the glycoprotein profile at the vessel wall changes in response to inflammatory stimuli. It was suggested, from the localization of lectins, that inflammation exposed sugars resident in the basement membrane following the formation of the endothelial gaps. Furthermore, the oligosaccharide profile varied with location in the microvascular network, in that binding of specific lectins could be confined to arterioles, capillaries, and/or venules. The profile of sugars is also likely to be a component in the initiation of leukocyte interactions in selected postcapillary venules.

Alterations in the oligosaccharides of the luminal surface are consistent with a second structure, rarely examined in studies of inflammatory changes in permeability, the glycocalyx. This electron lucent layer at the endothelial surface was first demonstrated in the microcirculation by staining of the cationic dye, ruthenium red, which bound to the glycated proteins on the endothelial surface (Luft, 1965). The glycocalyx has been shown subsequently using cationic ferritin (Turner et al., 1983; Adamson and Clough, 1992) and dye-labeled lectins (Thurston et al., 1996). In the intact circulation, the glycocalyx appears to reduce contact between the surface receptors of the endothelium and the formed elements in the circulation. Under normal conditions, the glycocalyx is a barrier to water and solutes, a function that appears to require plasma proteins to maintain its optimal structure. In whole-organ preparations, absence of perfusate protein correlates with increases in capillary filtration and permeability-to-surface area (PS) product (Mann, 1981; McDonagh, 1983; Haraldsson and Rippe, 1985). In regions of the porcine aorta where Evans blue dye-labeled albumin is found to permeate, the thickness of the glycocalyx, as revealed by ruthenium red binding, was one third that of regions where Evans blue albumin failed to penetrate the endothelial layer (Gerrity et al., 1977). In capillary and postcapillary venular preparations, glycocalyx structure has been manipulated by removing protein (Mason et al., 1977; Huxley and Curry, 1985, 1991), by exposure to modified albumins and serum proteins (Haraldsson and Rippe, 1985; Huxley and Curry, 1985, 1991; Adamson and Clough, 1992; Huxley et al., 1993a), by charged probes (Turner et al., 1983; Adamson et al., 1988), and by enzyme perfusion (Adamson, 1990; Desjardins and Duling, 1990). Of interest to the mechanisms of inflammatory responses, glycocalyx structure has also been shown to change in response to electrical stimulation (Brown et al., 1996), to photodamage (Vink and Duling, 1996), or to brief heat treatment (Clough et al., 1988). The glycocalyx can restrict the movement of macromolecules on the basis of both size and charge (Adamson et al., 1988; Vink and Duling, 1996; Henry and Duling, 1999). Whether inflammatory mediators alter these properties is not known. The ability of the glycocalyx to change in thickness following inflammatory stimuli, such as heat treatment or electrical stimulus, may provide one clue about its role in inflammation and the mechanisms involved in the limitation of the inflammatory response, despite the persistence of morphological changes of the barrier (Wu and Baldwin, 1992; Neal and Michel, 1995).

Similar to the contributions of the glycocalyx to the inflammatory response, another less obvious mechanism for altering permeability involves the association of endothelial cells with the basement membrane. Disruption of focal adhesive contacts between the endothelium and the basement membrane results in increases in permeability independent of junctional or cytoplasmic structures (Kajimura et al., 1997).

In response to inflammatory stimuli, a third distinctive structural alteration, endothelial gaps arising from the fusion or coalescing of caveoli, has been observed. The clustered fused caveoli reported by Roberts and Palade (1997) appear to be equivalent to vesicular-vacuolar organelles (VVO; Dvorak et al., 1996; Feng et al., 1999). These transendothelial gap structures have been implicated in the acute inflammatory response in some vascular beds as they appear near endothelial junctions in capillaries and venules within 5 minutes of application of a variety of inflammatory mediators (Feng et al., 1999). The formation of transendothelial gaps, spatially removed from endothelial junctions, has been extensively documented in response to heat treatment, the calcium ionophore A23187, histamine, substance P, vascular endothelial growth factor (VEGF) and high intravascular hydrostatic pressure (reviewed in Michel and Neal, 1999). Whether these transendothelial gaps and VVO are separate structures is not known. It is interesting to note that all of the stimuli known to induce formation of transendothelial gaps, whether near or far from the endothelial junctions, result in transient increases in permeability. As mentioned previously, little is known about the mechanisms limiting the changes in permeability in the face of a sustained stimulus.

An additional illustration of the ability of endothelium to create structures not normally observed in the absence of inflammatory mediators is the formation of fenestrae in the small capillaries and venules of skin and skeletal muscle following exposure to VEGF (Roberts and Palade, 1997). In these studies, application of histamine while inducing increases in macromolecular leakage did not induce formation of fenestra, indicating that although the mature phenotype has the ability to make the structures, the capacity is not realized in response to inflammatory mediators universally.

It is well recognized that adhesion of leukocytes to vascular endothelium, followed by emigration from the blood to tissue is usually accompanied by enhancement of the changes in permeability mediated by the initial stimulus alone. Increases in barrier permeability usually precede the migration of white cells. Whereas leukocytes can migrate without an accompanying change in macromolecule extravasation (Gawlowski et al., 1993; Raud and Lindbom, 1994) under physiological conditions, during the inflammatory response migration is accompanied by an augmentation of macromolecular leakage. Conversely, depletion of leukocytes or inhibition of leukocyte adhesion to endothelium with specific monoclonal antibodies against adhesion molecules attenuate the increases in permeability by various inflammatory stimuli (Wedmore and Williams, 1981; Kubes et al., 1990; Harris et al., 1993; Moore et al., 1995). Whether this increase results solely from the action of mediators released by the activated white cell, by activation and release of mediators from platelets and secondary cells, particularly mast cells, from the mechanical disassociation of the endothelial cell from its basement membrane, or the enzymatic disruption of the basement membrane is an open set of questions.

The endothelium also produces mediators that appear to limit and reverse inflammatory permeability responses. Understanding these mechanisms and their time courses of action may provide some insight into the biphasic nature of the permeability response in inflammation. The best known of these is nitric oxide. The direct actions of endothelial nitric oxide on permeability are complex. At this point it appears that high concentrations of nitric oxide result in loss of barrier properties and endothelial function (Moncada et al., 1991). At lower doses, generally in the absence of the formed elements of the blood (Meyer and Huxley, 1992; Rumbaut et al., 1995; Huang and Yuan, 1997), inhibition of nitric oxide synthase induces small decreases in permeability, whereas elevation of nitric oxide induces small elevations in permeability from basal levels. In the intact circulation, or following induction of an inflammatory response, nitric oxide actually limits or attenuates the increases in protein extravasation (Kubes and Granger, 1992), possibly by its effects in inhibiting leukocyte–endothelial interactions (Kubes et al., 1991) and mast cell activation (Gaboury et al., 1996). Furthermore, endothelium produces adenosine (Smolenski et al., 1991) which can reduce permeability. Adenosine receptors of the A_2 class activate adenylyl cyclase (AC) leading to increases in cyclic adenosine monophosphate (cAMP). Direct stimulation of AC with forskolin, application of membrane-permeable analogue of cAMP, or superfusion with adenosine decrease permeability from basal or stimulated levels (Oliver, 1990; Watanabe et al., 1992; Huxley and Williams, 1996). Other "anti-inflammatory" mediators in the intact tissue that can limit the inflammatory responses include norepinephrine working through the β-receptor and the adenylyl cyclase system (Huxley et al., 1993b; Adamson et al., 1998). Adamson et al. (1998) concluded that stimulation of the AC system results in the formation of additional junctional strands between the endothelium reducing junctional width and increasing path lengths, two changes in structure that will limit the flux of water and hydrophilic solutes.

Sites of Inflammatory Responses

Although all microvessels contribute to blood-to-tissue exchange, the greatest focus in inflammatory changes in permeability has been on postcapillary venules, given the impressive responses that can occur in these vessels in response to a wide variety of mediators and stimuli (Majno and Palade, 1961; Bjork et al., 1982; Del Maestro, 1982; Bjork et al., 1985; Dillon and Dúran, 1988; Mayhan, 1993; Yuan et al., 1993; Thurston et al., 1996; Saulpaw and Joyner, 1997). Whereas the formation of focal leaky sites correlates directly with inflammatory changes in permeability, a lack of leaky sites does not mean that permeability is unchanged from basal levels (Meyer and Huxley, 1992; Michel and Curry, 1999). Capillaries, by virtue of their large number, are concluded to be the primary sites for water and small solute movement (Huxley et al., 1987; Adamson et al., 1988; Huxley and Curry, 1991; Harris et al., 1993). Study of arteriolar permeability properties has been limited (Huxley and Williams, 1996; Huxley et al., 1997; Huxley, 1998); instead, the major focus has been their role in regulating blood flow into the microvasculature.

Despite the fact that the most readily identifiable hallmarks of the inflammatory responses are observed in the postcapillary venules, it is appropriate to recognize that most of the mediators of inflammatory responses also induce alterations in the barrier properties of arterioles and capillaries. As stated previously, changes in permeability can occur without the formation of leaky sites. Chronic inflammatory increases in barrier permeability in diabetes, especially in dyslipidemia, involve the vasculature of the arterial circulation (Lever et al., 1996). Inflammatory changes in arterial vessels will influence blood flow, directly because of obstruction, and indirectly because of changes in the rate of solute flux to and from vascular smooth muscle. If the barrier properties of the endothelium change, vascular smooth muscle function (regulating blood flow) is also likely to be modified due to substrate limitation or metabolite accumulation. The same inflammatory mediator can induce differing degrees of permeability responses in different portions of the microvasculature, with regard to the magnitude of the response, the time to the peak response, and the time of recovery (Meyer and Huxley, 1992; Williams and Huxley, 1993; Raud and Lindbom, 1994). Whether the site-specific responses reflect distributions of receptors along the microvasculature, different intracellular second messenger systems, differing levels of second messenger activation, or the participation of vascular or parenchymal cells releasing additional permeability mediators, has not been determined. Although activated white cells are less likely to be observed in the arterioles and capillaries, they have been observed (most notably in the regions of atheroma, vasculitis/arteriitis, or following ischemia). Similarly, macromolecular leaks have been observed in the higher pressure vessels of the conduit circulation, albeit with much lesser frequency (Gerrity et al., 1977; Baldwin and Winlove, 1984). In fact, alterations in barrier structure resulting in increased transvascular exchange can be the very first event in the inflammatory process, well in advance of leukocyte rolling, adhesion, or emigration. Finally, the ability to study mechanisms responsible for alterations in barrier properties in these systems is providing necessary information about the capacity for change and the myriad of components that can change to both elevate and depress barrier function.

Temporal Signatures of Inflammatory Permeability Changes

Inflammatory responses can be acute and chronic. There is a well-documented transient elevation in permeability that appears to involve the mobilization of endothelial intracellular calcium stores. The response is "self-limiting" and shows a return toward baseline values in what appears to be a calcium-independent manner. Histamine, bradykinin, adenosine triphosphate (ATP), serotonin, and the calcium ionophore all elicit these kinds of responses (Svensjo et al., 1979; Wu and Baldwin, 1992; Williams and Huxley, 1993; Neal and Michel, 1995; He et al., 1997).

Vascular endothelial growth factor (VEGF) induces permeability responses over seconds and over days. The initial permeability response to VEGF (Bates and Curry, 1996) was an eight-fold rise in water conductivity immediately (23 seconds) after perfusion with 1 nm VEGF that returned to baseline by 100 seconds. On day 2 the water conductivity of vessels that had responded to VEGF was five times the basal level of day 1, and was still 40% above these levels on day 4 in the absence of any additional stimulus. In sham-treated vessels, no change in permeability or overt changes in vessel morphology were observed. Despite the ability of VEGF to induce a marked permeability response, it is notable that 30% of venules perfused with VEGF failed to respond with an increase in hydraulic conductivity. Similar non-uniformity of response with other stimuli has been provided in the literature (Meyer and Huxley, 1992). Acute hyperpermeability to VEGF in isolated coronary venules, which resulted in a transient two-to three-fold increase in permeability to albumin, was inhibited by blockade of nitric oxide synthase (Wu et al., 1996). Similarly, inhibition of guanylate cyclase with 1H-[1,2,4] oxadiazolo [4,3-a] quinoxalin-1-one (ODQ) or inhibition of protein kinase G with KT-5823 blocked the action of VEGF (Wu et al., 1996). These studies suggest that elevation of permeability can be mediated by an increase in nitric oxide, and that the permeability-elevating mechanisms are mediated by the guanylyl cyclase system and protein kinase G. It is notable that many vasodilators whose actions are mediated by guanylyl cyclase are also associated with increases in permeability (Huxley et al., 1987; Meyer and Huxley, 1992; Rumbaut et al., 1995; Huang and Yuan, 1997; He et al., 1998). In contrast, as alluded to earlier, those mechanisms mediated by adenylyl cyclase are associated with decreases in permeability (Huxley and Williams, 1996; Adamson et al., 1998).

Much of our understanding of the intracellular mechanisms controlling the barrier structures thought to be involved in the regulation of microvascular permeability has come from the extensive study of the biochemistry and cell biology of endothelial cells in culture and, most recently, co-culture with cells from the parenchyma and blood compartments (Casnocha et al., 1989; Langeler and van Hinsbergh, 1991; Oliver, 1992; Watanabe et al., 1992). To date, though, the culture systems have yet to mimic adequately the permeability responses, normal or inflammatory, observed in intact microvessel models or especially the microvascular responses of the intact circulation (van Hinsbergh, 1997). This likely reflects the absence of the physical forces, the myriad of cell types participating in the inflammatory response, or the presence of inflammatory and anti-inflammatory mediators in the interstitial tissue.

Role for More Than the Endothelium in the Control of Inflammatory Changes in Permeability

Control of permeability is a multifactorial process involving the interplay of several second messenger systems in endothelium and vascular smooth muscle, if not other closely associated vascular cells (Fig. 4.2). In intact vessels, endothelium and vascular smooth muscle are not only in close proximity, but have interconnections that can influence their electrical properties and the transfer of second messengers or other components from their cytoplasmic spaces. These systems provide substrates for mechanisms that could alter cytoskeletal structure in the cytoplasm itself, or at the points of contact between cells. Furthermore, the cytoplasmic environment regulates passage through connexins as well as attachments of the cells to the basement membrane. How all of these components result in the control of permeability remains to be determined.

Various cellular components other than endothelium can mediate increases in permeability in response to several inflammatory mediators (Table 4.1). For example, neutrophils participate in the increases in macromolecule leakage induced by agents such as leukotriene B$_4$, C5a, 1-formyl-methionyl-leucyl-phenylalanine (FMLP), and platelet-activating factor (PAF; Wedmore and Williams, 1981; Bjork et al., 1982; Hughes et al., 1990; Kubes et al., 1990). Agents such as histamine, bradykinin, serotonin, and leukotriene C$_4$ can increase extravasation independent of neutrophils (Svensjo et al., 1979; Bjork et al., 1982; Wu and Baldwin, 1992; Mayhan, 1993; Williams and Huxley, 1993; Yuan et al., 1993). In addition, activation of mast cells (which lie in close proximity to microvessels) can lead to degranulation and release of several inflammatory mediators including those listed in Table 4.1 (reviewed in Galli, 1993), which in turn can mediate increases in macromolecule extravasation from the microvasculature, especially postcapillary venules.

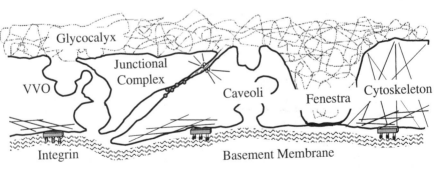

Fig. 4.2. Cell types associated closely with endothelial cells that can participate in augmenting microvascular permeability during inflammation. The four major cell types, leukocytes and platelets, circulating in the vascular compartment, in addition to nerves and mast cells, resident in the tissue compartment, all contain mediators in secretory granules that can be released during inflammation.

Table 4.1. Examples of Inflammatory Mediators Associated with Loss of Microvascular Barrier Function

Histamine

Bradykinin

Serotonin

Substance P

Leukotrienes (C_4, B_4)

Platelet-activating factor

Interleukins (IL-2, IL-8)

Tumor necrosis factor–α

C5a

FMLP (N-formyl-methionyl-leucyl-phenylalanine)

VEGF (vascular erdothelial growth factor)

Reactive oxygen species

Nitric oxide

The situation is more complex in the intact circulation. The mechanisms mediating increases in permeability are interrelated with those mediating decreases in permeability. Ample evidence exists to demonstrate cross-talk between systems within the endothelium as well as between the endothelium and the cells of the immune system, resulting in permeability responses that change in time, space, and magnitude. Furthermore, these levels of inter-action provide the means to limit, if not reverse, changes in barrier structure to forestall loss of organ function and morbidity.

Inflammatory alterations in microvascular permeability are often consid-ered as pathological and may lead to loss of circulatory function and possibly death. However, when properly regulated, the inflammatory process may be physiological. Take, for example, the processes involved in the adaptation of microvascular function in response to chronic exercise training or vascular occlusion. Both of these events can produce alterations in flow leading to ischemic or hypoxic episodes. Ischemia and hypoxia are both stimuli that can induce release of vasoactive hormones, such as atrial (ANP) and brain natriuretic peptide (BNP) and growth factors, such as VEGF from the en-dothelium and/or vascular smooth muscle. All of the substances mentioned have been shown to elevate microvascular permeability. If vascular adaptation employs inflammatory mediators and results in augmented function of the organism, then inflammation and the accompanying alterations in perme-ability represent a physiological rather than a pathological process. This view would support the picture of inflammatory changes in permeability as being a set of points on a continuum. Inflammatory processes appear to be in-volved in the process of angiogenesis and neovasculogenesis. Many of the angiogenic stimuli also induce increases in permeability; several of the in-hibitors of vascular growth also limit changes in permeability. Indeed, increases in permeability of the microvascular barrier occur in advance of basement membrane degradation or formation of microvascular buds.

Conclusion

It is evident that the mechanisms responsible for regulation of microvascular permeability during normal conditions, as well as during inflammation, are complex. Barrier alteration in response to inflammation serves to facilitate the egress of leukocytes and plasma constituents to the site of infection or tissue damage. The process involves not only the endothelium across which activated cells migrate, but can also involve platelets and leukocytes in the circulatory compartment and mast cells and other cells in the parenchyma. Each of these players participates directly and indirectly to release inflammatory and anti-inflammatory mediators over time courses that define the distinctive temporal signatures of the stimuli. Alterations in endothelial structures, those involved in the regulation of basal permeability and those unique to inflammation, provide the microvascular barrier with the capacity to elicit reversible changes in permeability that are orders of magnitude above basal levels.

References

Adamson, R. H., Huxley, V. H., and Curry, F. E. (1988). Single capillary permeability to proteins having similar size but different charge. *Am. J. Physiol.* 254:H304–H312.

Adamson, R. H. (1990). Permeability of frog mesenteric capillaries after partial pronase digestion of the endothelial glycocalyx. *J. Physiol.* 428:1–13.

Adamson, R. H., and Clough, G. (1992). Plasma proteins modify the endothelial cell glycocalyx of frog mesenteric microvessels. *J. Physiol.* 445:473–486.

Adamson, R. H., Liu, B., Fry, G. N., Rubin, L. L., and Curry, F. E. (1998). Microvascular permeability and number of tight junctions are modulated by cAMP. *Am. J. Physiol.* 274:H1885–H1894.

Baldwin, A. L., and Winlove, C. P. (1984). Effects of perfusate composition on binding of ruthenium red and gold colloid to glycocalyx of rabbit aortic endothelium. *J. Histochem. Cytochem* 32:259–266.

Bates, D. O. and Curry, F. E. (1996). Vascular endothelial growth factor increases hydraulic conductivity of isolated perfused microvessels. *Am. J. Physiol.* 271:H2520–2528.

Bjork, J., Hedqvist, P., and Arfors, K. E. (1982). Increase in vascular permeability induced by leukotriene B4 and the role of polymorphonuclear leukocytes. *Inflamm.* 6:189–200.

Bjork, J., Hugli, T. E., and Smedegard, G. (1985). Microvascular effects of anaphylatoxins C3a and C5a. *J. Immunol.* 134:1115–1119.

Brown, M. D., Egginton, S., Húdlicka, O., and Zhou, A. L. (1996) Appearance of the capillary endothelial glycocalyx in chronically stimulated rat skeletal muscles in relation to angiogenesis. *Exp. Physiol.* 81:1043–1046.

Casnocha, S. A., Eskin, S. G., Hall, E. R., and McIntire, L. V. (1989). Permeability of human endothelial monolayers: effect of vasoactive agonists and cAMP. *J. Appl. Physiol.* 67:1997–2005.

Celsus (1938). *De Medicina.* W. G. Spencer, Trans. Cambridge: Harvard University Press.

Clough, G., Michel, C. C., and Phillips, M. E. (1988). Inflammatory changes in permeability and ultrastructure of single vessels in the frog mesenteric microcirculation. *J. Physiol.* 395:99–114.

Del Maestro, R. F. (1982). Role of superoxide anion radicals in microvascular permeability and leukocyte behaviour. *Can. J. Physiol. Pharmacol.* 60:1406–1414.

Desjardins, C., and Duling, B. R. (1990). Heparinase treatment suggests a role for the endothelial cell glycocalyx in regulation of capillary hematocrit. *Am. J. Physiol.* 258:H647–H654.

Dillon, P. K., and Dúran, W. N. (1988). Effect of platelet-activating factor on microvascular perm-selectivity: dose–response relations and pathways of action in the hamster cheek pouch microcirculation. *Circ. Res.* 62:732–740.

Dvorak, A. M., Kohn, S., Morgan, E. S., Fox, P., Nagy, J. A., and Dvorak, H. F. (1996). The vesiculo-vacuolar organelle (VVO): a distinct endothelial cell structure that provides a trans-cellular pathway for macromolecular extravasation. *J. Leukocyte Biol.* 59:100–115.

Feng, D., Nagy, J. A., Pyne, K., Hammel, I., Dvorak, H. F., and Dvorak, A. M. (1999) Pathways of macromolecular extravasation across microvascular endothelium in response to VPF/VEGF and other vasoactive mediators. *Microcirc.* 6:23–44.

Gaboury, J. P., Niu, X. F., and Kubes, P. (1996) Nitric oxide inhibits numerous features of mast cell-induced inflammation. *Circ.* 93:318–326.

Galli, S. J. (1993) New concepts about the mast cell. *N. Engl. J. Med.* 328:257–265.

Gawlowski, D. M., Benoit, J. N., and Granger, H. J. (1993) Microvascular pressure and albumin extravasation after leukocyte activation in hamster cheek pouch. *Am. J. Physiol.* 264:H541–H546.

Gerrity, R. G., Richardson, M., Somer, J. B., Bell, F. P., and Schwartz, C. J. (1977) Endothelial cell morphology in areas of in vivo Evans blue uptake in the aorta of young pigs. II. Ultrastructure of the intima in areas of differing permeability to proteins. *Am. J. Pathol.* 89:313–334.

Haraldsson, B., and Rippe, B. (1985) Serum factors other than albumin are needed for the maintenance of normal capillary permselectivity in rat hindlimb muscle. *Acta Physiol. Scand.* 123:427–436.

Harris, N. R., Benoit, J. N., and Granger, D. N. (1993) Capillary filtration during acute inflammation: role of adherent neutrophils. *Am. J. Physiol.* 265:H1623–H1628.

He, P., Liu, B., and Curry, F. E. (1997) Effect of nitric oxide synthase inhibitors on endothelial [Ca2+]i and microvessel permeability. *Am. J. Physiol.* 272:H176–H185.

He, P., Zeng, M., and Curry, F. E. (1998) Cyclic-GMP modulates basal and activated microvessel permeability independently of [Ca2+]i. *Am. J. Physiol.* 274:H1865–H1874.

Henry, C. B. S., and Duling, B. R. (1999) Permeation of the luminal capillary glycocalyx is determined by hyaluronan. *Am. J. Physiol.* 277:H508–H514.

Huang, Q., and Yuan, Y. (1997) Interaction of PKC and NOS in signal transduction of microvascular hyperpermeability. *Am. J. Physiol.* 273:H2442–H2451.

Hughes, S. R., Williams, T. J., and Brain, S. D. (1990) Evidence that endogenous nitric oxide modulates oedema formation induced by substance P. *Eur. J. Pharmacol.* 191:481–484.

Huxley, V. H., and Curry, F. E. (1985) Albumin modulation of capillary permeability: test of an adsorption mechanism. *Am. J. Physiol.* 248:H264–H273.

Huxley, V. H., Tucker, V. L., Verburg, K. M., and Freeman, R. H. (1987) Increased capillary hydraulic conductivity induced by atrial natriuretic peptide. *Circ. Res.* 60:304–307.

Huxley, V. H., and Curry, F. E. (1991) Differential actions of albumin and plasma on capillary solute permeability. *Am. J. Physiol.* 260:H1645–H1654.

Huxley, V. H., Curry, F. E., Powers, M. R., and Thipakorn, B. (1993a) Differential action of plasma and albumin on transcapillary exchange of anionic solute. *Am. J. Physiol.* 264:H1428–H1437.

Huxley, V. H., McKay, M. K., Meyer, D. J. Jr, Williams, D. A., and Zhang, R. S. (1993b) Vasoactive hormones and autocrine activation of capillary exchange barrier function. *Blood Cells* 19:309–320.

Huxley, V. H., and Williams, D. A. (1996) Basal and adenosine-mediated protein flux from isolated coronary arterioles. *Am. J. Physiol.* 271:H1099–H1108.

Huxley, V. H., Williams, D. A., Meyer Jr., D. J., and Laughlin, M. H. (1997) Altered basal and adenosine-mediated protein flux from coronary arterioles isolated from exercise trained pigs. *Acta Physiol. Scand.* 160:315–325.

Huxley, V. H. (1998) What do measures of flux tell us about vascular wall biology? *Microcirc.* 5:109–116.

Kajimura, M., O'Donnell, M. E., and Curry, F. E. (1997) Effect of cell shrinkage on permeability of cultured bovine aortic endothelia and frog mesenteric capillaries. *J. Physiol.* 503: 413–425.

Kubes, P., Suzuki, M., and Granger, D.!N. (1990) Platelet-activating factor-induced microvascular dysfunction: role of adherent leukocytes. *Am. J. Physiol.* 258:G158–G163.

Kubes, P., Suzuki, M., and Granger, D. N. (1991) Nitric oxide: an endogenous modulator of leukocyte adhension. *Proc. Natl. Acad. Sci. USA* 88:4651–4655.

Kubes, P., and Granger, D.N. (1992) Nitric oxide modulates microvascular permeability. *Am. J. Physiol.* 262:H611–H615.

Langeler, E. G. and van Hinsbergh, V. W. (1991) Norepinephrine and iloprost improve barrier function of human endothelial cell monolayers: role of cAMP. *Am. J. Physiol.* 260:C1052–C1059.

Lever, M. J., Jay, M. T., and Coleman, P. J. (1996) Plasma protein entry and retention in the vascular wall: possible factors in atherogenesis. *Can. J. Physiol. Pharmacol.* 74:818–823.

Levick, J. R., and Mortimer, P. S. (1999) Fluid 'balance' between microcirculation and interstitium in skin and other tissues: Revision of the classical filtration–reabsorption scheme. In: *Microcirculation in Chronic Venous Insufficiency.* K. Messmer, ed. Basel: Krager, vol. 23, pp. 42–62.

Luft, J. H. (1965) Fine structure of capillary and endocapillary layer as revealed by ruthenium red. *Proc. FASEB* 25:1773–1783.

Majno, G., and Palade, G. E. (1961) Studies on inflammation. I. The effect of histamine and serotonin on vascular permeability: An electron microscopic study. *J. Biophys. Biochem. Cytol.* 11:571–605.

Majno, G., Shea, S. M., and Leventhal, M. (1969) Endothelial contraction induced by histamine-type mediators: an electron microscopic study. *J. Cell Biol.* 42:647–672.

Mann, G. E. 1981 Alterations of myocardial capillary permeability by albumin in the isolated, perfused rabbit heart. *J. Physiol.* 319:311–323.

Mason, J. C., Curry, F. E., and Michel, C. C. (1977) The effects of proteins upon the filtration coefficient of individually perfused frog mesenteric capillaries. *Microvasc. Res.* 13:185–202.

Mayhan, W. G. (1993) Role of nitric oxide in leukotriene C_4-induced increases in microvascular transport. *Am. J. Physiol.* 265:H409–H414.

McDonagh, P. F. (1983) Both protein and blood cells reduce coronary microvascular permeability to macromolecules. *Am. J. Physiol.* 245:H698–H706.

Meyer, D. J. Jr, and Huxley, V. H. (1992) Capillary hydraulic conductivity is elevated by cGMP-dependent vasodilators. *Circ. Res.* 70:382–391.

Michel, C. C., and Curry, F. E. (1999) Microvascular permeability. *Physiol. Rev.* 79:703–761.

Michel, C. C. and Neal, C. R. (1999) Openings through endothelial cells associated with increased microvascular permeability. *Microcirc.* 6:45–54.

Miller, F. N., Sims, D. E., Schuschke, D. A., and Abney, D. L. (1992) Differentiation of light-dye effects in the microcirculation. *Microvasc. Res.* 44:166–184.

Moncada, S., Palmer, R. M., and Higgs, E. A. (1991) Nitric oxide: physiology, pathophysiology, and pharmacology. *Pharmacol. Rev.* 43:109–142.

Moore, T. M., Khimenko, P., Adkins, W. K., Miyasaka, M., and Taylor, A. E. (1995) Adhesion molecules contribute to ischemia and reperfusion-induced injury in the isolated rat lung. *J. Appl. Physiol.* 78:2245–2252.

Neal, C. R., and Michel, C. C. (1995) Transcellular gaps in microvascular walls of frog and rat when permeability is increased by perfusion with the ionophore A23187. *J. Physiol.* 488:427–437.

Oliver, J. A. (1990) Adenylate cyclase and protein kinase C mediate opposite actions on endothelial junctions. *J. Cell. Physiol.* 145:536–542.

Oliver, J. A. (1992) Endothelium-derived relaxing factor contributes to the regulation of endothelial permeability. *J. Cell. Physiol.* 151:506–511.

Raud, J., and Lindbom, L. (1994) Studies by intravital microscopy of basic inflammatory mechanisms and acute allergic inflammation. In: *Immunopharmacology of the Microcirculation.* S. D. Brain, ed. London: Academic Press, pp. 127–170.

Roberts, W. G., and Palade, G. E. (1997) Neovasculature induced by vascular endothelial growth factor is fenestrated. *Cancer Res.* 57:765–772.

Rumbaut, R. E., McKay, M. K., and Huxley, V. H. (1995) Capillary hydraulic conductivity is decreased by nitric oxide synthase inhibition. *Am. J. Physiol.* 268:H1856–H1861.

Saulpaw, C. E., and Joyner, W. L. (1997) Bradykinin and tumor necrosis factor-alpha alter albumin transport in vivo: a comparative study. *Microvasc. Res.* 54:221–232.

Smolenski, R. T., Schrader, J., de Groot, H., and Deussen, A. (1991) Oxygen partial pressure and free intracellular adenosine of isolated cardiomyocytes. *Am. J. Physiol.* 260:C708–C714.

Celsus (1938) *De Medicina.* W. G. Spencer, Trans. Cambridge: Harvard University Press.

Svensjo, E., Arfors, K. E., Raymond, R. M., and Grega, G. J. (1979) Morphological and physiological correlation of bradykinin-induced macromolecular efflux. *Am. J. Physiol.* 236:H600–H606.

Thurston, G., Baluk, P., Hirata, A., and McDonald, D. M. (1996) Permeability-related changes revealed at endothelial cell borders in inflamed venules by lectin binding. *Am. J. Physiol.* 271:H2547–H2562.

Turner, M. R., Clough, G., and Michel, C. C. (1983) The effects of cationised ferritin and native ferritin upon the filtration coefficient of single frog capillaries. Evidence that proteins in the endothelial cell coat influence permeability. *Microvasc. Res.* 25:205–222.

van Hinsbergh, W. M. (1997) Endothelial permeability for macromolecules. Mechanistic aspects of pathophysiological modulation. *Arterioscler. Thromb. Vasc. Biol.* 17:1018–1023.

Vink, H., and Duling, B. R. (1996). Identification of distinct luminal domains for macromolecules, erythrocytes, and leukocytes within mammalian capillaries. *Circ. Res.* 79:581–589.

Watanabe, H., Kuhne, W., Schwartz, P., and Piper, H. M. (1992) A2-adenosine receptor stimulation increases macromolecule permeability of coronary endothelial cells. *Am. J. Physiol.* 262:H1174–H1181.

Wedmore, C. V., and Williams, T. J. (1981) Control of vascular permeability by polymorphonuclear leukocytes in inflammation. *Nature (Lond.)* 289:646–650.

Williams, D. A., and Huxley, V. H. (1993) Bradykinin-induced elevations of hydraulic conductivity display spatial and temporal variations in frog capillaries. *Am. J. Physiol.* 264:H1575–H1581.

Wu, H. M., Huang, Q., Yuan, Y., and Granger, H. J. (1996) VEGF induces NO-dependent hyperpermeability in coronary venules. *Am. J. Physiol.* 271:H2735–H2739.

Wu, N. Z., and Baldwin, A. L. (1992) Transient venular permeability increase and endothelial gap formation induced by histamine. *Am. J. Physiol.* 262:H1238–H1247.

Yuan, Y., Granger, H. J., Zawieja, D. C., DeFily, D. V., and Chilian, W. M. (1993). Histamine increases venular permeability via a phospholipase C-NO synthase-guanylate cyclase cascade. *Am. J. Physiol.* 264:H1734–H1739.

5

Cytokines and Endothelial Cell Activation

FRANCIS W. LUSCINSKAS

The vascular endothelium plays a critical role in regulating the blood vessel wall in normal and pathophysiological settings such as inflammation. Inflammation can be defined in the broadest terms as a host defense in response to injury of vascularized tissues (Majno and Joris, 1996). It is now well recognized that the endothelium is not just a passive barrier, rather a large multifunctional organ that actively participates in many critical processes including inflammation and response to injury, selective barrier function, regulation of vascular tone by producing vasoconstricting and vasorelaxing substances, hemostatic functions, chronic vascular remodeling, extracellular matrix production, and transduction of biomechanical forces (reviewed in Cines et al., 1998; Cotran, 1998). This chapter will touch selectively on the cytokines IL-1, IL-6, and TNF-α and their effects on endothelial cells in the context of inflammation.

In Vitro Culture of Endothelial Cells

In general, the properties of the endothelial cell in blood vessels differ depending on their location within the vasculature and from organ to organ (see Cines et al., 1998). The inflammatory response is a good example of endothelial cell specialization because recruitment of leukocytes occurs preferentially in small venules and correlates with adhesion molecule expression in a number of experimental models (see Cotran et al., 1986; Munro et al., 1989; Briscoe et al., 1992). An important milestone for study of the endothelium was the ability to isolate and then propagate primary cultures of human endothelial cells in sufficient number for detailed biochemical analyses. A reliable and well-characterized model for in vitro study has been endothelial cells derived from human umbilical veins (HUVEC; Gimbrone, 1976; Cines et al., 1998). In addition to HUVEC, researchers now have available endothelial cells derived from large arteries or veins, as well as microvessels from a number of tissues and organs. In some cases, in vitro cultured cells have recapitulated some features of that particular organ's or tissue's endothelial cell phenotype during responses to pro-inflammatory cytokines (for examples, see Petzelbauer et al., 1993; Binion et al., 1998). Limitations, however, of cultured endothelial cells exist because cultured cells require growth factors and thus have much higher rates of cell division when compared to quiescent cells in vivo. Multiple-passaged cells may lose specialized functions associated with intact perfused vessels or organs.

Other key advances have been the molecular cloning of genes implicated in inflammation, and the subsequent development of "knockout" mice that are genetically deficient in specific adhesion molecules, cytokines, and accessory molecules (see Chap. 18). In aggregate, these achievements have led to a detailed molecular definition of the mechanisms underlying the inflammatory response, and in particular, the mediators of inflammation and the mechanisms of leukocyte recruitment.

Inflammatory Mediators and Endothelial Cell Responses in Inflammation

Chemical Mediators of Inflammation

The number of acute and chronic inflammatory mediators found in the plasma and secreted by cells are legion and include lipid factors, for example, platelet-activating factor and the arachidonate-derived products, leukotrienes and lipoxins (see Chap. 7); activated complement-derived proteins (see Chap. 8); and bacterial endotoxin, pro-inflammatory cytokines, and interleukins (for a comprehensive review, see Abbas, 1996; Cines et al., 1998; Cotran, 1998). In spite of this list, the triad of IL-1, TNF-α, and LPS are considered good paradigms for pro-inflammatory mediators (Cines et al., 1998) and are responsible for much of the host's innate immune response to microbes and will be considered here along with IL-6. It is worth emphasizing two important concepts concerning cytokine biology. First, most inflammatory cytokines are not preformed molecules stored in cytosolic compartments that are released upon cell activation; rather, their production is usually transient and regulated transcriptionally. Second, IL-1 and TNF have overlapping biological actions and can act systemically (endocrine-like effect), or on the same cells that produced them (autocrine activity), or locally, on one or several cell types (paracrine activity).

Lipopolysaccharide and Cytokines and Their Receptor Signal Pathways

Lipopolysaccharide (LPS) is a complex glycolipid composed of two chemically dissimilar hydrophobic structures, polysaccharide and lipid A, and is found in the outer membrane of gram-negative bacteria. LPS is a very potent stimulus of the host's innate immune system (i.e., the physical and chemical barriers such as epithelium, the blood proteins, and the phagocytic cells), and stimulates the sequence of events that lead to the hemodynamic and hematological responses observed in patients with septic shock. LPS shed from bacteria is bound by the plasma protein LPS-binding protein (termed LBP) and is recognized by CD14, which exists as a glycoslyphosphatidylinositol (GPI)-anchored surface membrane protein expressed by myeloid lineage cells, or in plasma as a soluble form (see Ulevitch and Tobias, 1995). LPS stimulates production of cytokines IL-1, IL-6, TNF-α, and a family of low molecular mass cytokines with chemoattractant properties, termed *chemokines* (see Chap. 6) by mononuclear phagocytes and by other cells including the endothelium. The mechanism of signal transduction by the LBP-LPS–CD14 complex is less clear (Ulevitch and Tobias, 1995). Recent studies, however, have suggested that members of the Toll-like receptor family, TLR2 and/or TLR4, which share homology with the IL-1 receptor cytoplasmic tail (and in *Drosophila* induce an antifungal immune response), act as co-receptors for the LSP-LBP–CD14 complex mediated signal transduction via kinase cascades (Poltorak et al., 1998; Yang et al., 1998). These findings provide a good starting point for future experiments designed to elucidate signaling pathways for LPS. LPS also has been reported to stimulate the endothelium in in vivo and in vitro experiments (Bannerman et al., 1998) and result in reduced barrier function and programmed cell death, termed *apoptosis* (see Ashkenazi and Dixit, 1998).

The cytokines TNF-α and IL-β are considered the principal mediators of acute inflammation induced by LPS shed from gram-negative bacteria and other microbes (for review, see Abbas, 1996; Cotran, 1998). These cytokines have pleiotrophic effects because they can induce diverse responses including cell activation, proliferation, differentiation, and apoptosis, depending upon the receptor that is signaling, the cell type, and the concomitant signal(s) received; however, here the emphasis will be on their pro-inflammatory effects on endothelial cells.

TNF and IL-1 are produced by activated mononuclear phagocytes and other leukocyte types, epithelium, and endothelium. TNF encompasses two distinct species, TNF-α and TNF-β, or lymphotoxin (LT, TNF-β), which recognize the same receptors. LT/TNF-β and TNF-α have a similar profile of biological activities, but TNF-β is synthesized in much lesser quantities by activated macrophages during inflammation.

TNF circulates as a homotrimer. Two receptors have been described for TNF, a 55 kD protein TNF-RI (p55 receptor, CD120a) and a 75 kD protein, TNF-RII (p75 receptor, CD120b), and both receptors are members of the large TNF-receptor family (TNF-R) that are commonly expressed by many cell types including leukocytes and the endothelium (see Vassalli, 1992). The biological consequences of TNF-α are broad and indicate effects on cell proliferation, activation, or cell death, and thus, much work remains to be done to ferret out how these distinct or opposing outcomes are mediated by the same receptor–ligand pair (see Fig. 5.1).

In endothelium, TNF-α binding to TNF-RI appears to induce binding of TNF-R associated factors (TRAFs) to the receptor cytoplasmic domains and triggers activation of multiple transcription factors that mediate adhesion molecules expression and chemokine synthesis, as well as IL-1 and TNF production (see Fig. 5.1 and the section on transcription factors). The precise identity and nature of the interaction(s) of the adapter protein TRAFs receptor interacting protein (RIP) with the TNF-R are controversial and continue to be studied intensely. If protein synthesis is blocked transiently in

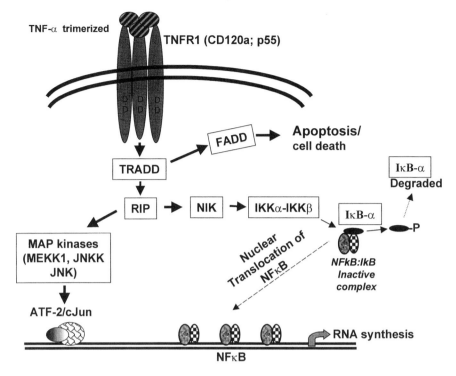

E-selectin Promotor

Fig. 5.1. Endothelial cell activation by TNF-α/TNFRI ligation via NF-kB and mitogen-activated protein (MAP) kinase systems (Abbas, 1996; Read et al., 1997; Ashkenazi and Dixit, 1998). TNFR, tumor necrosis factor receptor; TRADD, TNFR-associated death domain protein; FADD, Fas-associated death domain; I κB, Inhibitor (κB; RIP, receptor interacting protein; NIK, NF-κB-inducing kinase; IKK-α and β, Inhibitor κB kinase-α and β; ATF-2/cJUN, activating transcription factor-2/cJun heterodimer; MAP, mitogen-activating protein; MAPK, mitogen activating protein kinase; ERK, extracellular signal—regulated protein; MEK, MAPK/ERK kinase; JNK, cJun amino (N)-terminal kinase.

vitro prior to TNF-α activation, TNF-α can induce significant cell apoptosis (~50%), suggesting the presence of preexisting factors that block the TNF-α induced death signal. The interactions of other TNF-R family members, such as Fas (CD95) binding to Fas-ligand (CD95L), which is expressed on immune cells destined for elimination or by virus-infected cells, causes binding of cytosolic adapter proteins (Fas-associate death domain, FADD) that recruit and activate caspases. Caspases, which are a family of cysteine proteases that cleave certain proteins at specific sites, can initiate programmed cell death or apoptosis (for review, see Ashkenazi and Dixit, 1998).

IL-1 is composed of two different species called IL-1α and IL-1β, which share almost 25% homology, but bind to the same cell surface receptor and mediate the same effects on the endothelium. Interestingly, the nascent IL-1α and IL-1β polypeptides do not contain a hydrophobic signal sequence to target the protein for secretion, and the mechanism of secretion is less well understood. IL-1β is synthesized as a precursor and is thought to be cleaved to its mature 17 kDa form by a plasma membrane associated IL-1β–converting enzyme (ICE). Two distinct IL-1 receptors, IL-1RI and IL-1RII, and a nonbinding signaling accessory protein (IL-1 RAcP), which contain three Ig-like domains and thus belong to the immunoglobulin gene family, have been described and are responsible for signal transduction (Greenfeder et al., 1995). IL-1RI is the major receptor for IL-1–induced effects and once IL-1 is bound, the receptor–ligand complex recruits IL-1 RAcP (Cullinan et al., 1998) and its associated cytosolic kinases for downstream signal transduction via activation of transcription factors nuclear factor kappa-B (NF-κB) and mitogen-activated protein (MAP) kinases as detailed later and in Figure 5.1. IL-1RII does not transmit an activation signal and is thought to act as a decoy receptor by competitively inhibiting IL-1 binding to IL-1RI. As discussed previously, the cytoplasmic portion of IL-1RI shares homology with the Toll family of membrane receptors, which participate in the LPS-LBP and CD14 complex signal transduction. It is worth mentioning that a naturally occurring IL-1 receptor antagonist (IL-1RA) protein was identified in the early 1990s and was shown to have receptor antagonist activities in certain animal models but not in human sepsis syndromes (see Arent et al., 1998, for a recent review).

IL-6 exerts a variety of effects, which is probably reflected by the variety of names that it was originally assigned, including hepatocyte stimulating factor, B-cell differentiation factor and/or B-cell stimulatory factor 2. Several cytokines compose the IL-6 gene family based on similarities in structure and their receptor subunit composition. IL-6 functions as a homodimer. IL-1 and TNF-α stimulate IL-6 production by mononuclear phagocytes, endothelium, fibroblasts, and other cell types. The functional receptor for IL-6 consists of two transmembrane glycoproteins, the IL-6 receptor that binds the cytokine (IL-6R, CD126, gp80) and subsequently associates with a transmembrane protein gp130 (CD130), which forms multimers and transmits signals through the Janus-family kinases (JAK) and signal transducer and activator of transcription (STAT) proteins. IL-6 signals through STAT1, STAT3, and the Ras/Raf and Src-family of kinases. In the liver, these pathways are reported to induce activation of the CAAT/enhancer-binding protein family (C/EBP), and together with other transcription factor(s), lead to induction of acute-phase gene production (e.g., complement proteins, serum amyloid A, fibrinogen; see Poli, 1998). Other publications on the JAK/STAT pathways in lymphocytes used by interferons and cytokines to transduce their signal and effect gene transcription and biological responses can be found in Abbas (1996) and references therein.

It is worth mentioning briefly two other cytokines, IL-4 and IL-10, which have important biological activities (Abbas, 1996) in innate immunity. In general, IL-4, a product of T-cell subsets, basophils, and mast cells, acts on endothelium to induce surface expression of vascular cell adhesion molecule-

1 (VCAM-1) and production of monocyte chemoattractant protein-1 (MCP-1) while suppressing certain macrophage activities. IL-4 also induces isotype switching in B cells to produce immunoglobulin E, which can prime mast cells for antigen-specific degranulation. In the setting of allergic reactions, IL-4 is thought to play an important role in recruitment of leukocyte subsets (eosinophils and T helper-2 cell subsets). IL-10 is produced primarily by macrophages and also by T cells, and its primary action is to down-regulate activated macrophage production of inflammatory cytokines (IL-12, TNF, IFN-γ). This array of anti-inflammatory actions suggests an important role for IL-10 in regulation of inflammation and innate immunity.

The common denominator for IL-1, TNF-α, and IL-6 cytokines is their fundamental role in induction of the inflammatory response, including induction and release of additional cytokine cascades or waves of TNF, IL-1, and IL-6 into blood. This leads to fever, production of plasma factors produced by the liver including C-reactive protein, fibrinogen, and serum amyloid A protein, and general activation of mononuclear phagocyte and the endothelium. The activation of endothelium triggers a critical component of the inflammatory response, namely, localized recruitment of circulating blood leukocytes. This is briefly summarized in the following and examined in detail in Chapters 12–14 and 16–18.

Biological Actions of Cytokines and Lipopolysaccharide: Recruitment of Blood Leukocytes

Localized leukocyte accumulation is the cellular hallmark of inflammation (see Chap. 1). It is now well established that local tissue "activation" of normally quiescent endothelial cells is a critical event to (a) initiate and maintain the influx of leukocytes in a spatial and temporal fashion, and (b) provide leukocyte-type specific selectivity. The notion that vascular endothelial cells actively participate in the inflammatory process came from in vitro experiments that showed that inflammatory cytokines IL-1β, TNF-α, and LPS activated endothelium to become prothrombotic and proadhesive for peripheral blood leukocytes (Bevilacqua, 1993). The in situ consequences of inflammation on vessel permeability and regulation of blood flow are profound and are examined in depth in Chapters 3 and 4.

The multistep paradigm (Butcher, 1991) of cellular events involved in leukocyte extravasation are briefly listed in the following and are detailed in Chapters 12–18. Circulating leukocytes initially marginate at sites of injury and roll at low velocities on endothelium (step 1), arrest stably (step 2), and crawl to endothelial cell lateral borders. Ultimately, a significant proportion of adherent leukocytes transmigrate, or diapedese (step 3), into tissues (Bianchi et al., 1997). In general, the selectin family of adhesion molecules (endothelial cell E- and P-selectins, and leukocyte L-selectin that bind carbohydrate ligands) and the α_4 integrin mediates initial attachment and rolling, whereas other leukocyte integrins $\alpha_4\beta_1$ and β_2 integrins become activated by locally released chemokines and mediate the arrest step and motility by recognition of endothelial cell counter receptors, immunoglobulin (Ig) gene family members intercellular adhesion molecule-1 (ICAM-1) and VCAM-1 (Springer, 1994). Endothelial cell molecules at the lateral borders are thought to participate in leukocyte passage through the endothelial cell to cell borders (Allport et al., 2000) during diapedesis (see Chap. 17). It is worthwhile to restate that quiescent endothelium lining peripheral vessels, in the absence of injury or inflammation, is nonthrombogenic, does not express E-selectin, P-selectin, or VCAM-1, and does not secrete chemokines.

Regulation and Transcriptional Control of Endothelial Cell Adhesion Molecules

Treatment of endothelial cells with LPS, TNF-α, or IL-1 induces a striking and dramatic increase in leukocyte adhesion and subsequent transmigration in vivo and under static or flow conditions in vitro (Bevilacqua, 1993, Granger and Kubes, 1994). Based on experimental results, many but not all inflammatory mediators produced by activated endothelium are transcriptionally regulated, including plasma membrane expressed adhesion molecules that bind leukocytes, cytokines and chemokines. The elevated leukocyte adhesion correlates with rapid induction of mRNA transcripts (through de novo gene transcription) for E-selectin and VCAM-1, while ICAM-1, which is constitutively expressed, undergoes a dramatic up-regulation (Bevilacqua, 1993). In contrast to E-selectin and VCAM-1 genes, the human P-selectin gene is not induced by TNF-α or IL-1β, whereas the murine gene is responsive.

Transcription Factors Implicated in Cytokine-Induced Endothelial Cell Activation

Nuclear factor-κB (NF-κB/Rel) is an inducible transcription factor that performs an important function in transcriptional regulation of genes that are responsive to pro-inflammatory stimuli (Ghosh et al., 1998). The role of NF-κB in endothelial cell cytokine responsiveness has been explored in some detail. The relevant NF-κB/Rel protein for cytokine-mediated activation is the p50/p65 (NF-κB1/RelA) heterodimer (Fig. 5.1). For clarity, it will be referred to as NF-κB. The NF-κB normally resides in an inactive form in the cytosol complexed to an inhibitor IκBα (NF-κB : IκBα). In response to cytokines, IκBα is phosphorylated by at least two recently described intracellular kinases [NF-κB-inducing kinase (NIK) and inhibitor κB kinase (IKK-α–IKK-β)] and subsequently ubiquinated, targeting IκBα for degradation by the proteasome. This process releases active NF-κB to translocate to the nucleus where it binds to NF-κB recognition sites in the E-selectin (3 sites), VCAM-1 (2 sites) and ICAM-1 (1 site; Collins et. al., 1995) genes. Interestingly, the IκBα gene also has an NF-κB site, and becomes activated by nuclear NF-κB. This feedback loop serves to replenish the cytosolic pools of IκBα and thus negatively regulates cell activation. Cytokine activation also induces nuclear translocation of activator protein-1 (AP-1), which is a heterodimer composed of the c-Jun transcription factor and either a member of the Fos or activating transcription factor (ATF) family of transcription factor proteins (Read et al., 1997).

A less well understood process, but of fundamental importance, is how transcription factors such as NF-κB and associated proteins can control such a large number of genes that encode inflammatory mediators. One model suggests that specific coactivators are present in limiting quantities in the nucleus and thus foster competition among transcription factors activated by stimuli. Studies of the promotor regions of the E-selectin gene have revealed that IL-1 and TNF-α can induce synergistic interactions among a small number of transactivating factors to form specialized protein–DNA complexes, termed *enhanceosomes*, which leads to transcription of these adhesion molecules (Collins et al., 1995). The transcription factors include NF-κB and members of the MAP kinase family, JNK and p38 kinases (Read et al., 1997; Pan et al., 1998), and a family of coactivator proteins, termed cAMP [adenosine 3', 5'-cyclic monophosphate] response element binding protein (CREB-binding protein), and another related molecule, termed p300 (Wadgaonkar et al., 1999). These observations provide working models that must be further refined and extended to gain an understanding of the complex interplay between different pathways of gene activation in endothelium during response to inflammatory stimuli.

Integrative Function of Endothelium in Inflammation

In summary, the vascular endothelium plays an essential and active role in inflammation by expression of adhesion molecules and secretion of chemokines. These inducible effector functions are important factors in providing the temporal and spatial patterns of leukocyte recruitment. The underlying mechanisms appear to involve cytokine cascades, including release of IL-1, TNF-α, and IL-6, which act locally or systemically, to promote the inflammatory response and have specific effects on endothelial cells via defined receptor-mediated signaling pathways.

I wish to thank Drs. Jennifer Allport, Han Ding, Yaw-Chyn Lim, Sunil Shaw, Tucker Collins, Andrew Connolly, Andy Lichtman, and Michael Gimbrone of the Vascular Research Division, as well as numerous colleagues for helpful discussions. I also gratefully acknowledge Dr. Tucker Collins for assistance in generating Fig. 5.1 I am indebted to the support of the National Institutes of Health (NHLBI) through grants HL36028, HL53993, HL65090, and HL56985.

References

Abbas, A. K. (2000) *Cellular and Molecular Immunology*. Philadelphia: W. B. Saunders.

Allport, J. R. Ding, H., Muller, W. A., Luscinskas, F. W. (2000) Monocytes induce reversible focal changes in VE-cadherin complex during transendothelial migration under flow. *J. Cell. Biol.* 148:203–216.

Arent, W. P., Malyak, M., Guthridge, C. J., and Gabay, C. (1998) Interleukin-1 receptor antagonist: role in biology. *Ann. Rev. Immunol.* 16:27–56.

Ashkenazi, A., and Dixit, V. M. (1998) Death receptors: signaling and modulation. *Science* 281: 1305–1308.

Bannerman, D. D., Sathyamoorthy, M., and Goldblum, S. E. (1998) Bacterial lipopolysaccharide disrupts endothelial monolayer integrity and survival signaling events through caspase cleavage of adherens junction proteins. *J. Biol. Chem.* 273:35371–35380.

Bevilacqua, M. P. (1993) Endothelial–leukocyte adhesion molecules. *Annu. Rev. Immunol.* 11:767–804.

Bianchi, E., Bender, J. R., Blasi, F., and Pardi, R. (1997) Through and beyond the wall: late steps in leukocyte transendothelial migration. *Immunol. Today* 18:586–591.

Binion, D. G., West, G. A., Volk, E. E., Drazba, J. A., Ziats, N. P., Petras, R. E., and Fiocchi, C. (1998) Acquired increase in leucocyte binding by intestinal microvascular endothelium in inflammatory bowel disease. *Lancet* 352:1742–1746.

Briscoe, D. M., Cotran, R. S., and Pober, J. S. (1992) Effects of tumor necrosis factor, lipopolysaccharide, and IL-4 on the expression of vascular cell adhesion molecule-1 in vivo. *J. Immunol.* 149:2954–2960.

Butcher, E. C. (1991) Leukocyte–endothelial cell recognition: three (or more) steps to specificity and diversity. *Cell* 67:1033–1036.

Cines, D. B., Pollak, E. S., Buck, C. A., Loscalzo, J., Zimmerman, G. A., McEver, R. P., Pober, J. S., Wick, T. M., Konkle, B. A., Schwartz, B. S., et al. (1998) Endothelial cells in physiology and in the pathophysiology of vascular disorders. *Blood* 91:3527–3561.

Collins, T., Read, M. A., Neish, A. S., Whitley, M. Z., Thanos, D., and Maniatis, T. (1995) Transcriptional regulation of endothelial cell adhesion molecules: NF-kB and cytokine-inducible enhancers. *FASEB J.* 9:899–909.

Cotran, R. S., Gimbrone, M. A. Jr., Bevilacqua, M. P., Mendrick, D. L., and Pober, J. S. (1986) Induction and detection of a human endothelial activation antigen in vivo. *J. Exp. Med.* 164: 661–666.

Cotran, R. S. (1998) *Robbins Pathological Basis of Disease.* Philadelphia: W. B. Saunders.

Cullinan, E. B., Kwee, L., Nunes, P., Shuster, D. J., G. Ju, G., McIntyre, K. W., Chizzonite, R. A., and Labow, M. A. (1998) IL-1 receptor accessory protein is an essential component of the IL-1 receptor. *J. Immunol.* 161:5614–5620.

Ghosh, S., May, M. J., and Kopp, E. B. (1998) NF-kappa B and Rel proteins: evolutionarily conserved mediators of immune responses. *Annu. Rev. Immunol.* 16:225–260.

Gimbrone, M. A. Jr. (1976) Culture of vascular endothelium. *Prog. Hem. Throm.* 3:1–28.

Granger, D. N., and Kubes, P. (1994) The microcirculation and inflammation: modulation of leukocyte–endothelial cell adhesion. *J. Leuko. Biol.* 55:662–675.

Greenfeder, S. A., Nunes, P., Kwee, L., Labow, M., Chizzonite, R. A., and Ju, G. (1995) Molecular cloning and characterization of a second subunit of the interleukin-1 receptor complex. *J. Biol. Chem.* 270:13757–13765.

Majno, G., and Joris, I. (1996) Introduction to inflammation. In: *Cells, Tissues, and Disease: Principles of General Pathology.* G. Majno and I. Joris, eds. Cambridge: Blackwell, pp. 291–000.

Munro, J. M., Pober, J. S., and Cotran, R. S. (1989) Tumor necrosis factor-α and interferon-γ induce distinct patterns of endothelial activation and associated leukocyte accumulation in skin of *Papio anubis.* *Am. J. Pathol.* 135:121.

Pan, J., Xia, L., Yao, L., and McEver, R. P. (1998) Tumor necrosis factor-α or lipopolysaccharide-induced expression of the murine P-selectin gene in endothelial cells involves novel kappa-B sites and a variant activating transcription factor/cAMP response element. *J. Biol. Chem.* 273:10068–10077.

Petzelbauer, P., Bender, R. R., Wilson, J., and Pobe, J. S. (1993) Heterogeneity of dermal microvascular endothelial cell antigen expression and cytokine responsiveness in situ and in cell culture. *J. Immunol.* 151:5062–5072.

Poli, V. (1998) The Role of C/EBP isoforms in the control of inflammatory and native immunity functions. *J. Biol. Chem.* 273:29279–29282.

Poltorak, A., He, X., Smirnova, I., Liu, M. Y., Huffel, C. V., Du, X., Birdwell, D., Alejos, E., Silva, M., Galanos, C., et al., (1998) Defective LPS signaling in C3H/HeJ and C57BL/10ScCr mice: mutations in Tlr4 gene. *Science.* 282:2085–2088.

Read, M. A., Whitley, M. Z., Gupta, S., Pierce, J. W., Best J., Davis, R. J., and Collins, T. (1997)

Tumor necrosis factor α-induced E-selectin expression is activated by the nuclear factor-kB and c-JUN N-terminal kinase/p38 mitogen-activated protein kinase pathways. *J. Biol. Chem.* 272:2753–2761.

Springer, T. A. (1994) Traffic signals for lymphocyte recirculation and leukocyte emigration: the multistep paradigm. *Cell* 76:301–314.

Ulevitch, R. J., and Tobias, P. S (1995) Receptor-dependent mechanisms of cell stimulation by bacterial endotoxin. *Annu. Rev. Immunol.* 13:437–457.

Vassalli, V. (1992) The pathophysiology of tumor necrosis factors. *Ann. Rev. Immunol.* 10:411–452.

Wadgaonkar, R., Phelps, K. M., Haque, Z., Williams, A. J., Silverman, E. S., and Collins, T. (1999) CREB-binding protein is a nuclear integrator of nuclear factor-kappaB and p53 signaling. *J. Biol. Chem.* 274:1879–1882.

Yang, R. B., Mark, M. R., Gray, A., Huang, A., Xie, M. H., Zhang, M., Goddard, A., Wood, W. I., Gurney, A. L., and Godowski, P. J. (1998) Toll-like receptor-2 mediates lipopolysaccharide-induced cellular signalling. *Nature* 395:284–288.

6

Chemokines and Chemokine Receptors

ANDREW D. LUSTER and JAMES MACLEAN

The recruitment of cells to sites of inflammation is an essential component of the host inflammatory response. Cell recruitment relies on the coordinated action of cell activation, cell adhesion, chemoattraction, and transmigration across the endothelial barrier. The chemokines (chemotactic cytokines) are a newly described superfamily of secreted proteins that play an important role in cellular chemotaxis. In this chapter we will review chemokine structure, emphasizing how certain structural elements confer differential functional activity. We will also discuss chemokine receptors, their cellular expression, and their intracellular signaling mechanisms. The role of chemokines in cell trafficking will be reviewed in terms of their role in homeostasis and development and their participation in cell recruitment to sites of inflammation. Illustrative examples of chemokine action in vivo will be drawn from specific human diseases and animals models.

Chemokine Structure and Function

The chemokines are a superfamily of small, secreted proteins (8–10 kDa) that share the ability to chemoattract leukocytes. To date, close to 50 distinct chemokine molecules have been described (Fig. 6.1). The chemokines are structurally homologous and are subdivided into four families based on the position of conserved cysteine residues near the N-terminals of the molecules. CXC chemokines (also known as α-chemokines), are characterized by the presence of two cysteine residues near the N-terminus that are separated by one amino acid (CXC motif). In contrast, CC chemokines (also known as β-chemokines) have two cysteine residues that are adjacent (CC motif). The CC and CXC chemokines represent the largest of the chemokine families and contain many members. The C chemokine family contains only a single member, lymphotactin, which has one cysteine residue near the N-terminus (C motif). Likewise, the CXXXC family has only a single member, fractalkine (also called neurotactin), whose N-terminal cysteines are separated by three amino acids (CXXXC motif). Fractalkine is unique in that it contains a mucinlike stalk and has both transmembrane and cytoplasmic domains, suggesting that it is expressed on cell surfaces. The N-terminal

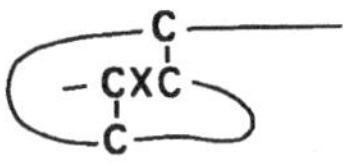

	Chemokine	Receptor

CXC(α)

CXC

Chemokine	Receptor
IL-8	CXCR1
GCP-2	CXCR1, CXCR2
GROα (MGSA)	CXCR2
GROβ (MIP-2α)	CXCR2
GROb (MIP-2β)	CXCR2
ENA-78 (LIX)	CXCR2
NAP-2	CXCR2
IP-10 (crg-2, mob-1)	CXCR3
Mig	CXCR3
I-TAC (βR1, IP-9)	CXCR3
SDF-1	CXCR4
BCA-1(BLC)	CXCR5
PF4	?
BRAK	?
Lungkine (mouse only)	?

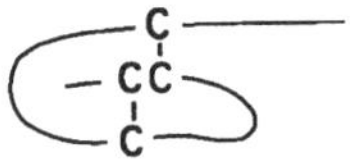

CC(β)

CC

Chemokine	Receptor
MIP-1α	CCR1, CCR5
MIP-1β	CCR5
RANTES	CCR1, CCR3, CCR5
HCC-1	CCR1
MCP-1	CCR2
MCP-2	CCR1, CCR2, CCR3, CCR5
MCP-3 (FIC, MARC)	CCR2, CCR3
MCP-4	CCR2, CCR3
MCP-5 (mouse only)	CCR2
Eotaxin	CCR3
Eotaxin-2 (MPIF2)	CCR3
Eotaxin-3	CCR3
Leukotactin-1 (HCC-2, MIP-5)	CCR1, CCR3
MDC (STCP-1, ABCD-1)	CCR4
TARC	CCR4
SLC (Exodus-2, 6CKine, TCA4)	CCR6, CCR7
MIP-3α (LARC, Exodus-1)	CCR6
ELC (MIP-3β)	CCR7
I-309 (TCA3)	CCR8
TECK	CCR9
DC-CK1 (PARC, AMAC-1, MIP-4)	?
MPIF1 (MIP-3)	?
MIP-5 (HCC-2)	?
HCC-4 (NCC-4)	?
MIP-1γ (MRP-2, CCF18)(mouse only)	?
C-10 (MRP-1)(mouse only)	?

C

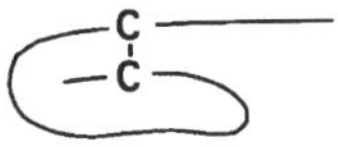

C

Chemokine	Receptor
Lymphotactin	XCR1

CXXXC

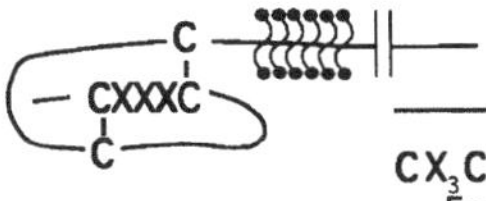

CX₃C

Chemokine	Receptor
Fractalkine (Neurotactin)	CX₃CR1

Fig. 6.1. Chemokines and their receptors: Chemokines are grouped by subfamily and listed individually (alternative names are indicated in parenthesis); receptors for each chemokine are indicated where known.

cysteines in the chemokine molecules form important intrachain disulfide bonds that determine, in part, the secondary structure of these molecules.

The CXC chemokines can be further subdivided based on the presence or absence of an ELR sequence (i.e., glutamatic acid–lysine–arginine) preceding the CXC motif, near the N-terminal of the molecule (Clark-Lewis et al., 1991). This structural difference is important because it determines separate functional activities of chemokines in this family. In general, the CXC chemokines that contain an ELR sequence (e.g., IL-8) are chemotactic for neutrophils, whereas non–ELR-containing cxc chemokines (e.g., IP-10 and SDF-1) are active on lymphocytes.

In general, the CC chemokines are chemotactic for monocytes, eosinophils, basophils, and lymphocytes, with variable selectivity, but are inactive on neutrophils. Within the CC chemokines, the monocyte chemoattractant proteins (MCPs 1–5) and the eotaxin molecules (eotaxin 1–3) share approximately 65% identity, and represent a subfamily within the β-chemokines (Luster and Rothenberg, 1997). Like the CXC chemokines, the N-terminal amino acids preceding the CC residues of the CC chemokines are critical for their biological activity and leukocyte selectivity. For example, the addition or deletion of a single amino acid residue at the N-terminus of MCP-1 reduces its biological activity on monocytes by 100- to 1000-fold (Gong and Clark-Lewis, 1995), and the deletion converts it from an activator of basophils to an eosinophil chemoattractant (Weber et al., 1996b).

Several chemokines undergo N-terminal proteolytic processing after secretion that alters their activity, and can activate, inactivate, or even create natural inhibitors. For example, the inactive platelet granule chemokine, platelet basic protein, is N-terminally processed by monocyte proteases to generate neutrophil-activating peptide-2 (NAP-2), which is a CXC chemokine active on neutrophils (Walz et al., 1989) In contrast, other chemokines, such as RANTES and stromal cell-derived factor-1 (SDF-1), are cleaved and inactivated by CD26, a leukocyte cell surface dipeptidyl exopepdiase IV (Oravecz et al., 1997; Proost et al., 1998a). CD26 cleaves the first two amino acids from peptides with penultimate proline or alanine residues, a sequence found at the N-terminals of many chemokines. Still other chemokines, such as MCP-2, can undergo posttranslation modification that removes the first 5 amino acids, resulting in a natural inhibitor of MCP-1, MCP-2, MCP-3, and RANTES (Proost et al., 1998b). Thus, posttranslational modification may be a general mechanism whereby local factors can positively or negatively regulate chemokine activity.

Chemokine Receptors

Chemokines induce cell migration and activation by binding to specific G-protein–coupled cell surface receptors on target cells (Murphy, 1994; Premack and Schall, 1996). Five human CXC chemokine receptors (CXCR1–5) and nine human CC chemokine receptors (CCR1–9) have been identified (Fig. 6.1). Most receptors recognize more than one chemokine, and several chemokines can bind to more than one receptor. However, there is receptor–ligand specificity within chemokine subfamilies, with CXC chemokines binding exclusively to CXC receptors and CC chemokines binding to CC receptors. The molecular explanation for this ligand–receptor subfamily restriction may be related to structural differences between CC and CXC chemokines. Although they share similar primary, secondary, and tertiary structures, CC and CXC chemokines have different quaternary structures (Lodi et al., 1994).

Chemokine receptors are expressed on multiple cell types, including all mature hematopoietic cells. Certain receptors have a restricted expression (e.g., CCR3 predominantly on eosinophils and basophils, and CXCR1 and CXCR2 predominantly on neutrophils), whereas other receptors are more widely expressed (e.g., CXCR4 on most cells, including all leukocytes). Expression of a given receptor on a given cell type can vary with the state of cellular differention and activation. For example, CCR1 and CCR2 are constitutively expressed on monocytes, but are expressed on lymphocytes only after stimulation by IL-2 (Loetscher et al., 1996b). Constitutive chemokine receptor expression can be down-regulated following cellular activation. For example, CCR2 is down-regulated by lipopolysaccharide, making the cells unresponsive to MCP-1. Interestingly, these cells remain responsive to chemokines that signal through other receptors, such as macrophage inflammatory protein-1α, which binds to CCR1 and CCR5 (Sica et al., 1997).

Certain chemokine receptors are only expressed on activated cells. For example, CXCR3 appears to be expressed only on activated T lymphocytes (Loetscher et al., 1996a). As such, transient up-regulation of chemokine receptors on leukocytes allows for the amplification of immune responses. The expression of chemokine receptors has been characterized most extensively on hematopoietic cells; however, chemokine receptor expression is not restricted to cells of this lineage. For example, CXCR4 is expressed on endothelial cells, epithelial cells, and neurons (Gupta et al., 1998; Klein et al., 1999; Salcedo et al., 1999), suggesting roles for the chemokine system in addition to leukocyte chemotaxis.

In addition to these receptors, the chemokines interact with two types of nonsignaling receptors. One is the promiscuous erythrocyte chemokine receptor, Duffy antigen receptor for chemokines (DARC; Horuk et al., 1993). This receptor has been known since the 1950s as the Duffy blood group determinant and is expressed on erythrocytes and on endothelial cells. Although DARC is structurally related to the chemokine receptors and both CXC and CC chemokines bind to it, chemokine binding does not induce a calcium flux. This receptor may function as a chemokine sink, clearing chemokines from the circulation.

The other type of "receptor" that the chemokines interact with are heparan sulfate proteoglycans. The chemokines are basic proteins and bind avidly to negatively charged heparin and heparan sulfate (Rot, 1992; Tanaka et al., 1993; Luster et al., 1995; Middleton et al., 1997). Heparan sulfate proteoglycans serve to capture chemokines in the extracellular matrix and on the surface of endothelial cells, which may serve to establish a local concentration gradient from the point source of chemokine secretion (Tanaka et al., 1993).

Chemokine Receptor Signaling

The signal transduction events activated by ligand binding that control leukocyte migration are not well defined and involve many different signaling pathways (Fig. 6.2) that are differentially utilized by different receptors (Bokoch, 1995; Hall et al., 1999). However, chemokine receptors are coupled to the Gi subfamily of G-proteins. Pertussis toxin (PTX), which ADP-ribosylates and irreversibly inactivates the G_α subunits of the α_i class, inhibits the majority of chemokine-induced effects on leukocytes, including chemotaxis, calcium

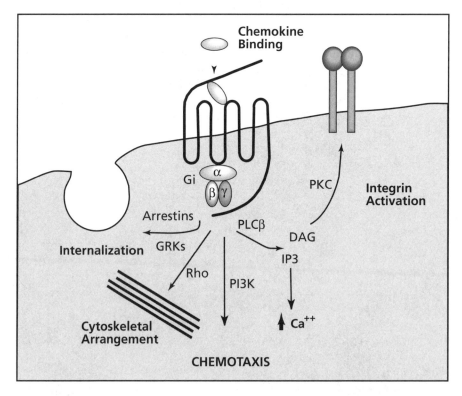

Fig. 6.2. Chemokine receptor signal transduction: Chemokine receptors are a subfamily of G-protein–coupled seven transmembrane-spanning cell surface receptors. They are coupled to heterotrimeric G-proteins of the Gi subclass, which are distinguished by their pertussis toxin (PTX) sensitivity. Chemokine receptor activation leads to the stimulation of multiple signal transduction pathways, including the activation of phosphatidylinositol 3-kinase (P13K) and phospholipase C (PLC), leading to generation of inositol triphosphates, intracellular calcium release, and protein kinase C (PKC) activation. Chemokine signaling also induces the up-regulation of integrin affinity and the activation of Rho leading to cytoskeletal reorganization. Agonist-stimulated receptors also activate G-protein–receptor kinases (GRKs), which leads to receptor phosphorylation, arrestin binding, G-protein uncoupling (desensitization), and clathrin-mediated receptor endocytosis (internalization).

flux, and integrin activation (Becknew, 1997). Other signaling events activated by the majority of chemokine receptors include the activation of phospholipase C (PLC) leading to generation of inositol triphosphates, intracellular calcium release, and protein kinase C (PKC) activation. Inhibition of chemokine-induced chemotaxis by wortmannin implicates phosphatidylinositol 3-kinase (PI3K) in chemokine receptor signal transduction. Phorbol-12-myrisate 13-acetate (PMA) activation of integrins implicates PKC as a potential mediator by which chemokines activate integrins. Chemokine signaling also leads to guanine nucleotide exchange on Rho, indicating the activation of Rho (Laudanna et al., 1996). Rac and Rho are small GTP-binding proteins involved in controlling cell locomotion through regulation of actin cytoskeletal rearrangement leading to membrane ruffling and pseudopod formation. Agonist-stimulated receptors also activate G-protein–receptor kinases (GRKs). Activated GRKs phosphorylate serine and threonine residues in the tail of G-protein–coupled receptors (GPCRs; Richmond et al., 1997). Receptor phosphorylation is followed by binding of arrestins, which bind specifically to phosphorylated receptors and uncouple the receptors from G-proteins (desensitization), and function as adaptor molecules leading to clathrin-mediated endocytosis (internalization). These internalized receptors are either dephosphorylated by phosphatases and recycled to the cell surface or targeted for degradation. Desensitization and recycling of chemokine receptors may be an important mechanism by which leukocytes maintain their ability to sense a chemoattractant gradient during an inflammatory response, whereas degradation of chemokine receptors may lead to termination of migration. Thus, chemokine receptors activate multiple intracellular signaling pathways that regulate the intracellular machinery necessary to propel the cell in its chosen direction.

Role in the Multistep Model of Leukocyte Recruitment

Leukocyte extravasation from the blood into the tissues is a regulated multistep process involving a series of coordinated leukocyte–endothelial cell interactions (Fig. 6.3; Springer, 1995; Butcher et al., 1999). Several families of molecular regulators such as the selectins, the integrins, and the chemokines, are thought to control different aspects of the process. In the multistep model, leukocyte extravasation begins with leukocyte rolling, a process dependent on selectins. Conversion of rolling to firm adherence depends on the activation of leukocyte integrins, a process dependent on cell signaling. Increasing evidence supports a role for chemokines as important activators of the leukocyte integrins.

The activation of integrins by chemokines has been shown for many leukocytes, including lymphocytes, monocytes, eosinophils, and neutrophils. The activation of leukocyte integrins by chemokines has been demonstrated experimentally by examining the expression of integrin activation epitopes and the adhesion of leukocytes to purified counterligands or endothelium under static and flow conditions. Using the more physiologically relevant

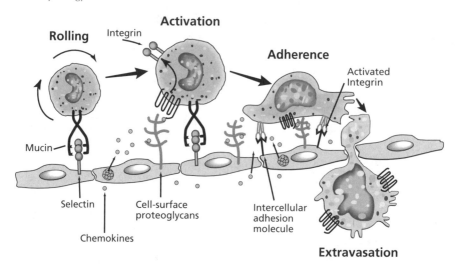

Fig. 6.3. Chemokines activate integrins and convert leukocyte rolling to firm adhesion, which ultimately leads to diapedesis. Chemokines are produced by endothelial cells or transported across endothelial cells if produced by cells in tissue and presented bound to proteoglycans, which help maintain a local concentration gradient. Leukocytes roll along endothelium in a process dependent on selections and their mucin receptors sampling the endothelial surface. Ligand activation of leukocyte chemokine receptors induces a conformational change in surface integrins that favor binding to intercelluar adhesion molecules on the surface of endothelial cells. This leads to firm adhesion and arrest of rolling leukocytes prior to extravasation through the endothelial layer.

flow-based adhesion assays, SDF-1, 6-C-kine, and MIP-3β, induced the rapid adhesion of naive lymphocytes to VCAM-1 (Campbell et al., 1998) and mucosal cell adhesion molecule-1 (MAdCAM-1; Pachynski et al., 1998). In contrast, firm adhesion of naive lymphocytes was not induced by other chemokines, including MIP-1α, MIP-1β, RANTES, GRO-α, IL-8, IP-10, or eotaxin, demonstrating the selective nature of this chemokine-induced adhesiveness. IP-10 and Mig induced firm adhesion of activated, but not resting, T cells to purified VCAM-1 and ICAM-1 (Piali et al., 1998). These chemokine-induced increases in integrin affinity and cellular adhesion were PTX sensitive, suggesting a dependence on $G\alpha_i$ linked chemokine receptor signaling.

Chemokine-induced adhesiveness to vascular endothelium has also been demonstrated for monocytes. Exposure of peripheral blood monocytes to MCP-1 or IL-8 led to rapid adhesion to vascular endothelium under flow conditions (Gerszten et al., 1999). Blocking studies with integrin-specific monoclonal antibodies suggest that this adhesion is mediated in part through β_2 integrins.

An additional complexity of chemokine-induced integrin activation is beginning to be elucidated with the demonstration that individual chemokines can differentially activate specific integrin avidity on the same cell type. For example, MCP-1 differentially activates β_1 and β_2 integrins on lymphocytes (Carr et al., 1996), whereas RANTES and MCP-3 differentially activate β_1 and β_2 integrins on eosinophils (Weber et al., 1996a), and IL-8 differentially activated β_2, β_3, and β_7 integrins in a B-lymphoblastoid line transfected with the IL-8 receptor (Sadhu et al., 1998). The exact signaling pathways downstream of PTX-senstive G-proteins, whereby chemokines induce activation of specific integrins, remains to be established and is an active area of investigation.

Taken together, these data support the concept that chemokines are important activating signals of leukocytes that convert selectin-mediated interactions into stable integrin-mediated adhesion. This ultimately leads to firm adherence of leukocytes to the vessel wall, prior to the transmigration of the endothelial barrier. As such, at least certain members of the α- and β-chemokines can function not only as leukocyte chemoattractants, but also as proadhesive agents in the recruitment of leukocytes to sites of inflammation.

Role of Chemokines in Development and Homeostasis

Chemokines provide the directional cues for the movement of leukocytes in development and homeostasis.

Development

The importance of chemokines in development can be demonstrated by analyzing the effects of targeted deletions of chemokines and chemokine receptors in mice. Such experiments heve elucidated unexpected roles for chemokines in vivo. For example, mice deficient in SDF-1 (Nagasawa et al., 1996) or its receptor CXCR4 (Tachibana et al., 1998; Zou et al., 1998) have defects in B-cell lymphopoiesis and the recruitment of hematopoietic progenitors from the fetal liver into the bone marrow, suggesting an important role for this chemokine in these processes. However, these mice also demonstrated defects in cardiac, cerebellar, and vascular morphogenesis. This dramatic phenotype underscores the possibility that, aside from directing the migration of leukocytes to sites of inflammation and infection, chemokines may play an important role in orchestrating the movement of cells during development. Dramatic developmental defects appears to be the exception rather than the rule for targeted deletions of chemokines or their receptors. For example, mice with a targeted deletion of CCR1 (Gao et al., 1997; Gerard et al., 1997), CCR2 (Boring et al., 1997), CCR5 (Zhou et al., 1998), MIP-1α (Cook et al., 1995), MCP-1 (Lu et al., 1998), eotaxin (Rothenberg et al., 1997), or IP-10 (A. D. Luster, unpublished observations) develop normally and do not manifest any significant pathologic lesions at baseline. In these circumstances, defects in immune function can sometimes be demonstrated after specific immunologic challenge. For example, deletion of MCP-1 and its receptor CCR2 result in mice that did not manifest any gross pathological defect but did manifest clear defects of macrophage/monocyte recruitment upon stimulation (Boring et al., 1997; Lu et al., 1998).

Homeostasis

Chemokines are also believed to control the baseline trafficking of leukocytes through tissues. Lymphocytes continuously recirculate through the blood, tissues, and lymphatics in an organized manner, bringing naive lymphocytes into the lymph nodes where they encounter antigen and memory lymphocytes into inflamed tissue to ensure immunity. T cells routinely patrol the body in search of foreign antigens and recirculate through the blood, tissue, and lymphatics, making over 20 round trips each day. Several recently identified chemokines are believed to participate in guiding T cells in this process. One such chemokine independently identified by several groups and given the names of SLC (secondary lymphoid-tissue chemokine), Exodus-2, 6Ckine, and TCA-4, appears to play an important role in directing T cells into peripheral lymph nodes. A role for SLC in the trafficking of T cells into lymph nodes has been suggested from studies that have examined the mutant mouse strain DDD (Nakano et al., 1998). This mutant mouse strain has a paucity of lymph node T cells because of a defect in the lymph node stroma. It has recently been shown that lymph nodes from the DDD mouse do not express the SLC chemokine (Gunn et al., 1999). Furthermore, genetic analysis has revealed that the mutant allele maps to mouse chromosome 4, the same chromosome where SLC has been mapped.

Much the same way as T cells recirculate, B cells also traffic through the body, and this process is also controlled by chemokines (Cyster et al., 1999). The B-cell specific CXC chemokine independently identified as BCA-1 (B-cell attracting chemokine-1) and BLC (B lymphocyte chemoattractant) is an important participant in this process (Legler et al., 1988; Gunn et al., 1998). BCA is a potent chemotactic factor for B cells and is expressed in the follicles of Peyer's patches, the spleen, and lymph nodes. BCA is a ligand for CXCR5, which is highly expressed on peripheral blood B cells. A role for BCA and CXCR5 in B-cell trafficking was revealed by the generation of a mouse strain deficient in CXCR5 (Forster et al., 1996). These mice have an impairment in the trafficking of peripheral blood B cells into lymph nodes.

Other leukocytes such as macrophages, neutrophils, eosinophils, and mast cells also traffic into tissue. Although these cells are produced in the bone marrow, they reside primarily in other tissues. The role of chemokines in regulating this process has begun to be elucidated from studies in mice deficient in chemokines. For example, the IL-8 receptor homologue in mice, murine CXCR2, plays an important role in drawing circulating neutrophils into tissues in unchallenged mice (Shuster et al., 1995). Likewise, eotaxin plays a critical role in normal eosinophil recruitment into tissues, especially the gastrointestinal tract where eosinophils are thought to play an important role in host defense against helminthic pathogens (Rothenberg et al., 1997).

Role in Orchestrating the Immune Response: Linking Innate and Adaptive Immunity

Chemokines provide the directional cues necessary to bring together T cells, B cells, and dendritic cells to generate an immune response and to recruit leukocytes into sites of inflammation and infection.

Generation of Effector Lymphocytes

Chemokines coordinate the movement of T cells, B cells, and dendritic cells necessary to generate an immune response (Fig. 6.4). Dendritic cells are thought to play a pivotal role in generating an immune response by capturing and presenting antigen to lymphocytes in a process that leads to the activation of T and B cells. Dendritic cells in tissue capture and process antigen and transport it to local lymph nodes for presentation to lymphocytes. Several recent studies have suggested that chemokines participate in this process (Cyster, 1999; Sozzani et al., 1999). Immature dendritic cells reside in the tissue where they are very efficient at engulfing antigen but are not very efficient at activating lymphocytes. Immature CD34+ Langerhans-like dendritic cells respond to a number of chemokines, including the CC chemokine MIP-1α (macrophage inflammatory protein-1a) and MIP-3α, which has also been called LARC (liver and activation-regulated chemokine) or Exodus. MIP-3α is a ligand for CCR6, which is highly expressed on immature dendritic cells. MIP-3α is expressed in tonsils by inflamed epithelium, a site known to be infiltrated by immature dendritic cells (Dieu et al., 1998). Moreover, MIP-3α and MIP-1α are induced by inflammatory stimuli such as LPS or TNFα. It has been hypothesized that a stimulus such as LPS induces the local tissue production of MIP-1α and MIP-3α, which attracts immature dendritic cells into the tissue. Once in the vicinity of the inflammatory stimulus, immature dendritic cells pick up antigen and then differentiate into cells more capable of activating lymphocytes. During this maturation process, dendritic cells down-modulate the expression of CCR6 and hence responsiveness to MIP-3α. At the same time, they up-regulate their expression of CCR7, allowing them to respond to SLC and ELC. This switch in chemokine receptor expression and chemokine responsiveness results in the dendritic cells leaving the tissue and being drawn into the lymphatics, and ultimately, into the T-cell–rich regions of lymph nodes.

Although the molecular details still remain to be fully elucidated, it is likely that the expression of chemokines by lymph node stroma and dendritic cells coordinate the juxtaposition of antigen-loaded dendritic cells with recirculating T and B cells. Chemokines that may play a role in this process are DC-CK1 (dendritic cell chemokine 1, which was also identified as PARC, AMAC-1, and MIP-4), MDC, TECK, and ELC (MIP-3β). DC-CK1 and ELC are expressed by activated mature dendritic cells and recruit naive T cells (Adema et al., 1997; Ngo et al., 1998). In contrast, MDC is induced in Langerhans cells migrating from contact-sensitized skin during maturation into

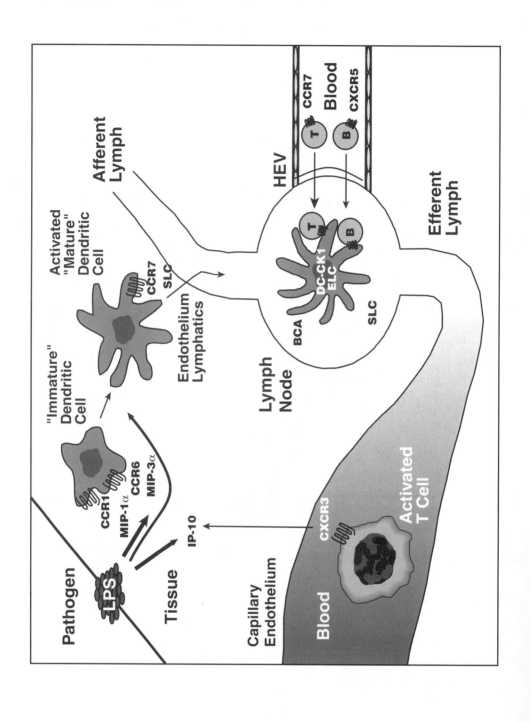

Fig. 6.4. Chemokines orchestrate the trafficking of dendritic cells, T cells, and B cells necessary to generate an immune response. In the example depicted, lipopolysaccharide (LPS) on the surface of bacterial pathogens stimulates the local release of chemokines, such as MIP-1α, MIP-3α, and IP-10. Immature dendritic cells are attracted to this site through the activation of chemokine receptors, such as CCR1 and CCR6, which they constitutively express. Immature dendritic cells are very efficient at picking up antigen, but need to mature and differentiate into cells capable of activating naive T cells. The local mileu into which the immature dendritic cell has been attracted contains factors, such as LPS and TNF, that induce dendritic cell differentiation and maturation into potent antigen-presenting cells. In this process, the dendritic cell down-regulates CCR6 and up-regulates CCR7, which leads to its migration into the afferent lymphatic. The CCR7 ligand SLC, which is expressed on the endothelium of afferent lymphatics, likely plays an important role in directing the migration of the antigen-loaded mature dendritic cells. Chemokines also play an important role in bringing naive T cells and B cells across high endothelial venules (HEV) into the lymph nodes and into contact with the activated dendritic cell. Although the molecular details remain to be elucidated, it is likely that chemokines, such as DC-CK1 and ELC, play an important role in juxtapositioning these cells in the lymph node. T cells activated in regional lymph nodes, following encounter with antigen-loaded dendritic cells, subsequently return to sites of inflammation by sensing chemokine gradients established at these local sites. Chemokines such as IP-10, a chemokine induced by LPS and IFNγ, and a ligand for CXCR3, which is highly expressed on activated T cells, are believed to play an important role in this process.

lymph node dendritic cells, and chemoattracts antigen-specific T cells but not naive T cells (Tang and Cyster, 1999).

T cells activated in regional lymph nodes, following encounter with antigen-loaded dendritic cells, subsequently return to sites of inflammation by sensing chemokine gradients established at those local sites. Chemokines such as IP-10, a chemokine induced by LPS and IFNγ, and a ligand for CXCR3, which is highly expressed on activated T cells, are believed to play an important role in this process (Farber, 1997; see Fig. 6.4).

Chemokines and Lymphocyte Effector Function: Localization of Cells to Tissue

Chemokines also participate in the effector phase of immune responses to coordinate the localization and specificity of the immune response. This is exemplified in T-cell–mediated immune responses. T-cell–mediated inflammatory responses can be segregated into distinct patterns based on the cytokine secretion pattern of CD4+ T-helper lymphocytes. T-helper (Th1) cells secrete mainly IL-2, IFN-γ, and IL-12, and mediate immune responses characterized by delayed-type hypersensitivity with activated T cells and macrophages. In contrast, Th2 cells secrete IL-4, IL-5, IL-10, and IL-13, which are involved in allergic inflammatory responses and favor the development of humoral immunity (antigen-specific IgE), and mast cell and eosinophil activation. Recent studies suggest that under certain conditions Th1 and Th2 cells can express different chemokine receptors (Sallusto et al., 1998). In these studies, Th1 cells preferentially expressed CXCR3 and CCR5 following activation, whereas activated Th2 cells expressed CCR3, CCR4, and CCR8. This differential expression of chemokine receptors may play an important role in the selective recruitment of polarized lymphocyte subsets in different disease states.

Allergic pulmonary inflammation exemplifies a specific disease state in which a polarized inflammatory response (Th2 biased) occurs (Fig. 6.5). In certain individuals, primary sensitization with an airborne allergen leads to the development of antigen-specific CD4+ T cells with a Th2 cytokine secretory phenotype. A secondary encounter with antigen leads to the elaboration of Th2 cytokines that promote the growth and maturation of eosinophils (IL-5) and mast cells (IL-3), and favor the class switch of immunoglobulin to the production of IgE (IL-4). These three developments are the hallmark of allergic inflammation. Th2 cells also secrete cytokines that promote the production of eosinophil-active chemokines, such as eotaxin and MCP-4. The production of cytokines, such as IL-13, at the site of antigen deposition (e.g., respiratory tract) leads to the localized production of eotaxin and MCP-4 from endothelial and epithelial cells resulting in eosinophilic tissue inflammation (Luster and Rothenberg, 1997).

Chemokines also play a role in the effector function of CD8+ cytotoxic T lymphocytes (CTLs). CD8+ lymphocytes play an important role in the host defense against viral infection, including HIV-1 (Yang and Walker, 1997). CD8+ T cells exert their effector functions through both cytolytic and noncytolitic mechanisms (Yang, 1997). Chemokines have been shown to be im-

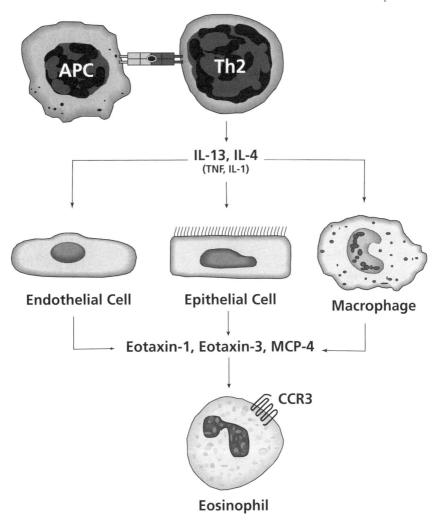

Fig. 6.5. Chemokines link Th2 lymphocyte activation and tissue eosinophilia: Antigen-activated CD4+ Th2 cells elaborate IL-4 and IL-13 that synergizes with proinflammatory cytokines, such as IL-1 and TNF, stimulating the production of eosinophil chemoattractants, such as eotaxin-1, eotaxin-3 and MCP-4 from epithelial and endothelial cells and tissue macrophages. These chemokines, in turn, attract acivated eosinophils into the tissue, resulting in the hallmark of allergic diseases.

portant effector molecules in preventing viral entry into cells by HIV (Cocchi et al., 1995). CD8+ T cells are at least one important source of these chemokines. The release of chemokines from CD8+ T cells is dependent on the activation of these cells through their T-cell receptors (Price et al., 1998; Fig. 6.6). These chemokines, which include RANTES, MIP-1α, and MIP-1β, are stored performed in cytolytic granules, co-localized with granzyme A and

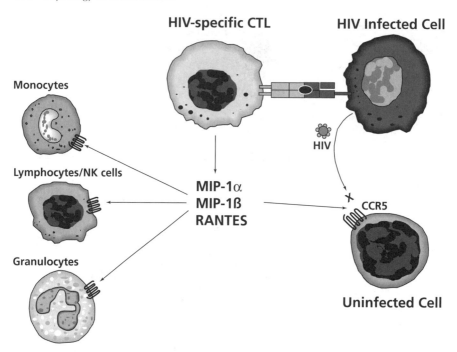

Fig. 6.6. Chemokines released from CTL localize and amplify the immune response by recruiting leukocytes to the site of viral replication and inhibit HIV-1 entry into cells. Antigen activation of CD8+ cytotoxic T cells results in the release of MIP-1α, MIP-1β, and RANTES directly onto the target cell. The release of these chemokines at the site of infection serves as a beacon to call in additional leukocytes, such as macrophages, granulocytes, and NK cells, resulting in the amplification of the local immune response. In the case of HIV-1 infection, these CCR5 ligands have the additional property of inhibiting HIV entry into nearby cells.

proteoglycans (Wagner et al., 1998). Following CTL activation, the contents of the cytolytic granules, which include chemokines complexed to proteoglycans, are coordinately released where they participate in antiviral effector functions by inhibiting viral entry into uninfected cells. This finding demonstrates the coupling of cytolytic and noncytolitic antiviral functions of CD8+ T cells, which is regulated by antigen-specific T-cell activation.

The release of chemokines from CTLs following antigen-specific activation is a general property of these cells and is not restricted to HIV-specific CTLs. CTLs specific for hepatitis B and C virus infected cells also release large amounts of chemokines when activated by antigen (Yang, 1997). The release of chemokines directly onto the infected cell recruits other inflammatory cells, including professional phagocytes to the site of viral replication, amplyfing the response to include the power of the innate immune system.

Role in Human Disease

It is likely that chemokines play a role in most disease processes that result in the accumulation and activation of leukocytes in tissues (Luster, 1998). Chemokines have been detected during inflammation in most organs, including the skin, brain, joints, meninges, lungs, blood vessels, kidneys, and gastrointestinal tract. In these organs chemokines can be detected in many types of cells, suggesting that most, if not all, cells have the capacity to secrete them given the appropriate stimulus. Major stimuli for chemokine production are early proinflammatory cytokines such as IL-1 and TNF-α, bacterial products such as LPS, and viral infections. In addition, IFNγ and IL-4, products of Th1 and Th2 lymphocytes, respectively, can induce the production of chemokines and also synergize with IL-1 and TNF-α to stimulate chemokine secretion. The capacity to control precisely the movement of inflammatory cells suggests that the various chemokines and their receptors might provide novel targets for therapeutic interventions to modify disease courses.

The nature of inflammatory infiltration that characterizes a specific disease is controlled, in part, by the subset of chemokines expressed in the disease. For example, many acute disease processes, such as bacterial pneumonia and the acute respiratory distress syndrome, are characterized by a massive influx of neutrophils into the tissue. The concentration of chemokines that are potent neutrophil chemoattractants, such as IL-8, are increased in the bronchoalveolar fluid of patients with these diseases (Chollet-Martin et al., 1993). Other acute diseases, particularly nonbacterial infectious diseases, such as viral meningitis, are characterized by the recruitment of monocytes and lymphocytes into the tissue. The cerebrospinal fluid concentrations of chemokines active on these cells, such as IP-10 and MCP-1, are increased in these patients, and the concentrations are correlated with the extent of mononuclear cell infiltration of the meninges (Lahrtz et al., 1997).

Many chronic disease processes are characterized by tissue infiltration of lymphocytes and macrophages. The delayed-type hypersensitivity granulomatous lesions of tuberculoid leprosy and sarcoidosis are characterized by the accumulation of activated lymphocytes, and high concentrations of IP-10 have been detected in these lesions (Kaplan et al., 1987; Agostini et al., 1998). In addition, levels of IP-10 in the bronchoalveolar fluid of patients with active sarcoidosis correlated with the number of T-lymphocytes in the fluid (Agostini et al., 1998).

In atherosclerosis, macrophages and lymphocytes are the major inflammatory cells found in the diseased blood vessels. These cells are thought to be central to the pathogenesis of this disease, both as progenitors of lipid-laden foam cells and a source of growth factors that mediate intimal hyperplasia. The CC chemokines MCP-1, MCP-4, RANTES, PARC, and ELC, and the CXC chemokines IL-8, SDF-1, IP-10, Mig, and I-TAC have all been detected in diseased vessels but not in normal arteries. A functional role for MCP-1 (Gu et al., 1998) and its receptor CCR2 (Boring et al., 1998), as well as the mouse IL-8 receptor CXCR2 (Boisvert et al., 1998) in the recruitment of monocytes into atherosclerotic lesions has been revealed when mice deficient in these genes were bred with mouse strains prone to develop atherosclerosis, such as the ApoE-deficient and LDL-receptor–deficient mouse strains. These mice had a decrease in the number of lesional macrophages and a decrease in atherosclerotic lesion formation, establishing a role for chemokines in the pathogenesis of this disease.

In allergic diseases, such as asthma, rhinitis, and atopic dermatitis, the inflammatory reaction is characterized by the selective accumulation and activation of eosinophils and mast cells, and their mediators are strongly associated with the pathogenesis of these diseases. Agents that induce the release of histamine from mast cells and basophils, so-called histamine-releasing factors, are also strongly associated with the pathogenesis of allergic diseases. Chemokines, in particular eotaxin and the monocyte chemoattractant proteins, are potent eosinophil chemoattractants and histamine-releasing factors, making them particularly important in the pathogenesis of allergic inflammation. In fact, the chemokines may be the major histamine-releasing factors in the absence of antigen and IgE antibody. Many chemokines have been detected in the airways of patients with asthma. In addition, several eosinophil-active chemokines are increased in the epithelial tissue of patients with atopic dermatitis, allergic rhinitis, and asthma after antigen challenge, making it likely that the chemokines are one of the molecular links between antigen-specific immune activation and tissue recruitment of eosinophils. In animals with allergic pulmonary inflammation, expression of eotaxin, MIP-1α, and MCP-1, MCP-3, and MCP-5 precede the massive airway recruitment of mononuclear cells and eosinophils. From studies using antibodies that inhibit the action of these chemokines, and studies of mice with a targeted disruption of the eotaxin gene, it is clear that all of these chemokines are participating in the recruitment of eosinophils into the airways.

Summary

Although initially identified as chemotactic factors profoundly induced by pro-inflammatory stimuli that mobilize the innate immune system and control the recruitment of leukocytes into inflammatory foci, chemokines have emerged as important regulators of cellular trafficking in development and homeostasis. In addition, they are critical for the coordinated movement of dendritic cells and lymphocytes necessary to link the acquired immune response to the innate response and generate long-lasting antigen-specific immunity. Chemokines are highly expressed in human inflammatory diseases and their specific roles in disease pathogenesis are being elucidated, revealing that these fascinating molecules offer a new class of targets for the treatment of a variety of human diseases.

References

Adema, G. J., Hartgers, F., Verstraten, R., de Vries, E., Marland, G., Menon, S., Foster, J., Xu, Y., Nooyen, P., McClanahan, T., et al. (1997) A dendritic-cell-derived C-C chemokine that preferentially attracts naive T cells. *Nature* 387:713–717.

Agostini, C., Cassatella, M., Sancetta, R., Zambello, R., Trentin, L., Gasperini, S., Perin, A., Piazza, F., Siviero, M., Facco, M., et al. (1998) Involvement of the IP-10 chemokine in sarcoid granulomatous reactions. *J. Immunol.* 161:6413–6420.

Becknew, S. (1997) G-protein activation by chemokines. In: *Methods in Enzymology, Chemokine Receptors.* R. Horuk, ed. San Diego: Academic Press, pp. 309–326.

Boisvert, W. A., Santiago, R., Curtiss, L. K., and Terkeltaub, R. A. (1998) A leukocyte homologue of the IL-8 receptor CXCR-2 mediates the accumulation of macrophages in atherosclerotic lesions of LDL receptor-deficient mice. *J. Clin. Invest.* 101:353–363.

Bokoch, G. M. (1995) Chemoattractant signaling and leukocyte activation. *Blood* 86:1649–1660.

Boring, L., Gosling, J., Chensue, S., Kunkel, S., Farese, R. J., Broxmeyer, H., and Charo, I. (1997) Impaired monocyte migration and reduced type 1 (Th1) cytokine responses in C-C chemokine receptor 2 knockout mice. *J. Clin. Invest.* 100:2552–2561.

Boring, L., Gosling, J., Cleary, M., and Charo, I. F. (1998) Decreased lesion formation in CCR2$^{-/-}$ mice reveals a role for chemokines in the initiation of atherosclerosis. *Nature* 394:894–897.

Butcher, E., Williams, M., Youngman, K., Rott, L., and Briskin, M. (1999) Lymphocyte trafficking and regional immunity. *Adv. Immunol.* 72:209–253.

Campbell, J. J., Bowman, E. P., Murphy, K., Youngman, K. R., Siani, M. A., Thompson, D. A., Wu, L., Zlotnik, A., and Butcher, E. C. (1998) 6-C-kine (SLC), a lymphocyte adhesion-tiggering chemokine expressed by high endothelium, is an agonist for the MIP-3beta receptor CCR7. *J. Cell. Biol.* 141:1053–1059.

Carr, M., Alon, R., and Springer, T. (1996) The C-C chemokine MCP-1 differentially modulates the avidity of beta 1 and beta 2 integrins on T lymphocytes. *Immun.* 4:179–187.

Chollet-Martin, S., Montravers, P., Gibert, C., Elbim, C., Desmonts, J. M., Fagon, J., Y., and Gougerot-Pocidalo, M. A. (1993) High levels of interleukin-8 in the blood and alveolar spaces of patients with pneumonia and adult respiratory distress syndrome. *Infect. Immun.* 61:4553–4559.

Clark-Lewis, I., Schumacher, C., Baggiolini, M., and Moser, B. (1991) Structure-activity relationships of interleukin-8 determined using chemically synthesized analogs. Critical role of NH2-terminal residues and evidence for uncoupling of neutrophil chemotaxis, exocytosis, and receptor binding activities. *J. Biol. Chem.* 266:23128–23134.

Cocchi, F., DeVico, A. L., Garzino-Demo, A., Arya, S. K., Gallo, R. C., and Lusso, P. (1995) Identification of RANTES, MIP-1a, and MIP-1b as the major HIV-suppressive factors produced by CD8+ T cells. *Science* 270:1811–1815.

Cook, D. N., Beck, M. A., Coffman, T. M., Kirby, S. L., Sheridan, J. F., Pragnell, I. B., and Smithies, O. (1995) Requirement of MIP-1a for an inflammatory response to viral infection. *Science* 269:1583–1585.

Cyster, J. (1999) Chemokines and the homing of dendritic cells to the T cell areas of lymphoid organs. *J. Exp. Med.* 189:447–450.

Cyster, J., Ngo, V., Ekland, E., Gunn, M., Sedgwick, J., and Anse, K. (1999) Chemokines and B-cell homing to follicles. *Curr. Top. Microbiol. Immunol.* 246:87–92.

Dieu, M. C., Vanbervliet, B., Vicari, A., Bridon, J. M., Oldham, E., Ait-Yahia, S., Briere, F., Zlotnik, A., Lebecque, S., and Caux, C. (1998) Selective recruitment of immature and mature dendritic cells by distinct chemokines expressed in different anatomic sites. *J. Exp. Med.* 188:373–383.

Farber, J. M. (1997) Mig and IP-10: CXC chemokines that target lymphocytes. *J. Leuk. Biol.* 61: 246–257.

Forster, R., Mattis, A. E., Kremmer, E., Wolf, E., Brem, G., and Lipp, M. (1996) A putative chemokine receptor, BLR1, directs B-cell migration to defined lmphoid organs and specific anatomic compartments of the spleen. *Cell* 87:1037–1047.

Gao, J., Wynn, T., Chang, Y., Lee, E., Broxmeyer, H., Cooper, S., Tiffany, H., Westphal, H., Kwon-Chung, J., and Murphy, P. (1997) Impaired host defense, hematopoiesis, granulomatous inflammation and type 1–type 2 cytokine balance in mice lacking CC chemokine receptor 1. *J. Exp. Med.* 185:1959–1969.

Gerard, C., Frossard, J. L., Bhatia, M., Saluja, A., Gerard, N. P., Lu, B., and Steer, M. (1997) Targeted disruption of the beta-chemokine receptor CCR1 protects against pancreatitis-associated lung injury. *J. Clin. Invest.* 100:2022–2027.

Gerszten, R., Garcia-Zepeda, E., Lim, Y., Yoshida, M., Ding, H., Gimbrone, M., Luster, A., Luscinskas, F., and Rosenzweig, A. (1999) MCP-1 and IL-8 trigger firm adhesion of monocytes to vascular endothelium under flow conditions. *Nature* 398:718–723.

Gong, J. H., and Clark-Lewis, I. (1995) Antagonists of monocyte chemoattractant protein 1 identified by modification of functionally critical NH2-terminal residues. *J. Exp. Med.* 181:631–640.

Gu, L., Okada, Y., Clinton, S. K., Gerard, C., Sukhova, G. K., Libby, P., and Rollins, B. J. (1998) Absence of monocyte chemoattractant protein-1 reduces atherosclerosis in low-density lipoprotein receptor-deficient mice. *Mol. Cell* 2:275–281.

Gunn, M., Kyuwa, S., Tam, C., Kakiuchi, T., Matsuzawa, A., Williams, L., and Nakano, H. (1999) Mice lacking expression of secondary lymphoid organ chemokine have defects in lymphocyte homing and dendritic cell localization. *J. Exp. Med.* 189:451–460.

Gunn, M. D., Ngo, V. N., Ansel, K. M., Ekland, E. H., Cyster, J. G., and Williams, L. T. (1998) A B-cell–homing chemokine made in lymphoid follicles activates Burkitt's lymphoma receptor-1. *Nature* 391:799–803.

Gupta, S., Lysko, P., Pillarisetti, K., Ohlstein, E., and Stadel, J. (1998) Chemokine receptors in human endothelial cells. Functional expression of CXCR4 and its transcriptional regulation by inflammatory cytokines. *J. Biol. Chem.* 273:4282–4287.

Hall, R., Premont, R., and Lefkowitz, R. (1999) Heptahelical receptor signaling: beyond the G protein paradigm. *J. Cell. Biol.* 145:927–932.

Horuk, R., Chitnis, C. E., Darbonne, W. C., Colby, T. J., Rybicki, A., Hadley, T. J., and Miller, L. H. (1993) A receptor for the malarial parasite *Plasmodium vivax*: The erythrocyte chemokine receptor. *Science* 261:1182–1184.

Kaplan, G., Luster, A. D., Hancock, G., and Cohn, Z. A. (1987) The expression of a gamma interferon-induced protein (IP-10) in delayed immune responses in human skin. *J. Exp. Med.* 166:1098–1108.

Klein, R., Williams, K., Alvarez-Hernandez, X., Westmoreland, S., Force, T., Lackner, A., and Luster, A. (1999) Chemokine receptor expression and signaling in macaque and human fetal neurons and astrocytes: implications for the neuropathogenesis of AIDS. *J. Immunol.* 163:1636–1646.

Lahrtz, F., Piali, L., Nadal, D., Pfister, H. W., Spanaus, K. S., Baggiolini, M., and Fontana, A. (1997) Chemokines in viral meningitis: Chemotactic cerebrospinal fluid factors include MCP-1 and IP-10 for monocytes and activate T lymphocytess. *Eur. J. Immunol.* 27:2484–2489.

Laudanna, C., Campbell, J. J., and Butcher, E. C. (1996) Role of rho in chemoattractant-activated leukocyte adhesion through integrins. *Science* 271:981–983.

Legler, D. F., Loetscher, M., Roos, R. S., Clark-Lewis, I., Baggiolini, M., and Moser, B. (1988) B-cell–attracting chemokine 1, a human CXC chemokine expressed in lymphoid tissues, selectively attracts B lymphocytes via BLR1/CXCR5. *J. Exp. Med.* 187:655–660.

Lodi, P. J., Garrett, D. S., Kuszewski, J., Tsang, M. L., Weatherbee, J. A., Leonard, W. J., Gronenborn, A. M., and Clore, G. M. (1994) High-resolution solution structure of the beta chemokine hMIP-1b by multidimensional NMR. *Science* 263:1762–1767.

Loetscher, M., Gerber, B., Loetscher, P., Jones, S. A., Piali, L., Clark-Lewi, I., Baggiolini, M., and Moser, B. (1996a) Chemokine receptor specific for IP10 and Mig: structure, function, and expression in activated T lymphocytes. *J. Exp. Med.* 184:963–969.

Loetscher, P., Seitz, M., Baggiolini, M., and Moser, B. (1996b) Interleukin-2 regulates CC chemokine receptor expression and chemotactic responsiveness in T lymphocytes. *J. Exp. Med.* 184:569–577.

Lu, B., Rutledge, B. J., Gu, L., Fiorillo, J., Lukas, N. W., Kunkel, S. L., North, R., Gerard, C., and Rollins, B. J. (1998) Abnormalities in monocyte recruitment and cytokine expression in monocyte chemoattractant protein 1-deficient mice. *J. Exp. Med.* 187:601–608.

Luster, A. D. (1998) Chemokines: Chemotactic cytokines that mediate inflammation. *N. Eng. J. Med.* 388:436–445.

Luster, A. D., Greenberg, S., and Leder, P. (1995) The IP-10 chemokine binds to a specific cell surface heparan sulfate site shared with platelet factor 4 and inhibits endothelial cell proliferation. *J. Exp. Med.* 182:219–231.

Luster, A. D., and Rothenberg, M. E. (1997) The role of the monocyte chemoattractant protein and eotaxin sub-family of chemokines in allergic inflammation. *J. Leuk. Biol.* 62:620–633.

Middleton, J., Neil, S., Wintle, J., Clark-Lewis, I., Moore, H., Lam, C., Auer, M., Hub, E., and Rot, A. (1997) Transcytosis and surface presentation of IL-8 by venular endothelial cells. *Cell* 91:385–395.

Murphy, P. M. (1994) The molecular biology of leukocyte chemoattractant receptors. *Annu. Rev. Immunol.* 12:593–633.

Nagasawa, T., Hirota, S., Tachibana, K., Takakura, N., Nishikawa, S., Kitamura, Y., Yoshida, N., Kikutani, H., and Kishimoto, T. (1996) Defects of B-cell lymphopoiesis and bone-marrow myelopoiesis in mice lacking the CXC chemokine PBSF/SDF-1. *Nature* 382:635–638.

Nakano, H., Shigeyuki, M., Yonekawa, H., Nariuchi, H., Matsuzawa, A., and Kakiuchi, T. (1998) A novel mutant gene involved in T-lymphocyte–specific homing into peripheral lymphoid organs on mouse chromosome 4. *Blood* 91:2886–2895.

Ngo, V. N., Tang, L., and Cyster, J. G. (1998) Epstein-Barr-virus-induced molecule 1 ligand chemokine is expressed by dendritic cells in lymphoid tissue and strongly attracts naive T cells and activated B cells. *J. Exp. Med.* 188:181–191.

Oravecz, T., Pall, M., Roderiquez, G., Gorrell, M. D., Ditto, M., Nguyen, N. Y., Boykins, R., Unsworth, E., and Norcross, M. A. (1997) Regulation of the receptor specificity and function of the chemokine RANTES (regulated on activation, normal T cell Expressed and secreted) by dipeptidyl peptidase IV (CD26)-mediated cleavage. *J. Exp. Med.* 186:1865–1872.

Pachynski, R., Wu, S., Gunn, M., and Erie, D. (1998) Secondary lymphoid-tissue chemokine (SLC) stimulates integrin $\alpha_4 \beta_7$-mediated adhesion of lymphocytes to mucosal addressin cell adhesion molecule-1 (MAdCAM-1) under flow. *J. Immunol.* 161:952–956.

Piali, L., Weber, C., LaRosa, G., Mackay, C. R., Springer, T. A., Clark-Lewis, I., and Moser, B. (1998) The chemokine receptor CXCR3 mediates rapid and shear-resistant adhesion induction of effector T lymphocytes by the chemokines IP10 and Mig. *Eur. J. Immunol.* 28:961–972.

Premack, B. A., and Schall, T. J. (1996) Chemokine receptors: Gateways to inflammation and infection. *Nat. Med.* 2:1174–1178.

Price, D. A., Sewell, A. K., Dong, T., Tan, R., Goulder, P.J.R., Rowland-Jones, S. L., and Phillips, R. E. (1998) Antigen-specific release of b-chemokines by anti-HIV-1 cytotoxic T lymphocytes. *Curr. Biol.* 8:355–358.

Proost, P., De Meester, I., Schols, D., Struyf, S., Lambeir, A., Wuyts, A., Opdenakker, G., De Clercq, E., Scharpe, S., and Van Damme, J. (1998a) Amino-terminal truncation of chemokines by CD26/dipeptidylpeptidase IV. *J. Biol. Chem.* 273:7222–7227.

Proost, P., Struyf, S., Couvreur, M., Lenaerts, J., Conings, R., Menten, P., Verhaert, P., Wuyts, A., and Van Damme, J. (1998b) Posttranslational modifications affect the activity of the human monocyte chemotactic proteins MCP-1 and MCP-2: Identification of MCP-2 (6–76) as a natural chemokine. *J. Immunol.* 160:4034–4041.

Richmond, A., Mueller, S., White, J. R., and Schraw, W. (1997) C-X-C chemokine receptor desensitization mediated through ligand-enhanced receptor phosphorylation on serine residues. In: *Methods in Enzymology, Chemokine Receptors.* R. Horuk, ed. San Diego: Academic Press, pp. 3–15.

Rot, A. (1992). Endothelial cell binding of NAP-1/IL-8: role in neutrophil emigration. *Immunol. Today* 13:291–294.

Rothenberg, M. E., MacLean, J. A., Pearlman, E., Luster, A. D., and Leder, P. (1997) Targeted disruption of the chemokine eotaxin only partially reduces antigen-induced tissue eosinophilia. *J. Exp. Med.* 185:785–790.

Sadhu, C., Masinovsky, B., and Staunton, D. (1998) Differential regulation of chemoattractant-stimulated beta 2, beta 3, and beta 7 integrin activity. *J. Immunol.* 160:5622–5628.

Salcedo, R., Wasserman, K., Young, H., Grimm, M., Howard, O., Anver, M., Kleinman, H., Murphy, W., and Oppenheim, J. (1999) Vascular endothelial growth factor and basic fibroblast growth factor induce expression of CXCR4 on human endothelial cells: In vivo neovascularization induced by stromal-derived factor-1 alpha. *Am. J. Pathol.* 154:1125–1135.

Sallusto, F., Lanzavecchia, A., and Mackay, C. R. (1998) Chemokines and chemokines receptors in T-cell priming and Th1/Th2-mediated responses. *Immunol. Today* 19:568–574.

Shuster, D. E., Kehrli, M. E. Jr., and Ackermann, M. R. (1995) Neutrophilia in mice that lacked the murine IL-8 receptor homolog. *Science* 269:1590–1591.

Sica, A., Saccani, A., Borsatti, A., Power, C. A., Wells, T. N., Luini, W., Polentarutti, N., Sozzani, S., and Mantovani, A. (1997) Bacterial lipopolysaccharide rapidly inhibits expression of C-C chemokine receptors in human monocytes. *J. Exp. Med.* 185:969–974.

Sozzani, S., Allavena, P., Vecchi, A., and Mantovani (1999) The role of chemokines in the regulation of dendritic cell trafficking. *J. Leuk. Biol.* 66:1–9.

Springer, T. (1995) Traffic signals on endothelium for leukocyte emigration. *Annu. Rev. Physiol.* 57:827–872.

Tachibana, K., Hirota, S., Iizasa, H., Yoshida, H., Kawabat, K., Kataoka, Y., Kitamura, Y., Matsushima, K., Yoshida, N., Nishikawa, S.-I., et al. (1998) The chemokine receptor CXCR4 is essential for vascularization of the gastrointestinal tract. *Nature* 393:591–594.

Tanaka, Y., Adams, D. H., Hubscher, S., Hirano, H., Siebenlist, U., and Shaw, S. (1993) T-cell adhesion induced by proteoglcan-immobilized cytokine MIP-1b. *Nature* 361:79–82.

Tang, H., and Cyster, J. (1999) Chemokine up-regulation and activated T-cell attraction by maturing dendritic cells. *Science* 284:819–822.

Wagner, L., Yang, O. O., Garcia-Zepeda, E. A., Ge, Y., Kalams, S., Walker, B. D., Pasternack, M., and Luster, A. D. (1998) b-Chemokines are released from HIV-1 specific cytolytic T-cell granules complexed to proteoglycans. *Nature* 391:908–911.

Walz, A., Dewald, B., von, T. V., and Baggiolini, M. (1989) Effects of the neutrophil-activating peptide NAP-2, platelet basic protein, connective tissue-activating peptide III and platelet factor 4 on human neutrophils. *J. Exp. Med.* 170:1745–1750.

Weber, C., Kitayama, J., and Springer, T. A. (1996a) Differential regulation of β1 and β2 integrin avidity by chemoattractants in eosinophils. *Proc. Natl. Acad. Sci. USA* 93:10939–10944.

Weber, M., Uguccioni, M. Baggiolini, M., Clark-Lewis, I., and Dahinden, C. A. (1996b) Deletion of the NH2-terminal residue converts monocyte chemotactic protein 1 from an activator of basophil mediator release to an eosinophil chemoattractant. *J. Exp. Med.* 183:681–685.

Yang, O. O., Kalams, S. A., Trocha, A., Cao, H., Luster, A. D., Johnson, R. P., Walker, B. D. (1997) Suppression of HIV replication by CD8 + cells: evidence for HLA class I–restricted triggering of cytolytic and non-cytolytic mechanisms. *J. Virol.* 71:3120–3128.

Yang, O. O., and Walker, B. D. (1997) CD8+ cells in human immunodeficiency virus type 1 pathogenesis: cytolytic and noncytolytic inhibition of viral replication. *Adv. Immunol.* 66:273–311.

Zhou, Y., Kurihara, T., Ryseck, R. P., Yang, Y., Ryan, C., Loy, J., Warr, G., and Bravo, R. (1998) Impaired macrophage function and enhanced T-cell–dependent immune response in mice lacking CCR5, the mouse homologue of the major HIV-1 coreceptor. *J. Immunol.* 160:4018–4025.

Zou, Y.-R., Kottmann, A. H., Kuroda, M., Taniuchi, I., and Littman, D. sR. (1998) Function of the chemokine receptor CXCR4 in haematopoiesis and in cerebellar development. *Nature* 393:595–599.

7

Lipid Mediators of Inflammation

PER HEDQVIST and LENNART LINDBOM

Inflammatory processes are the response of the organism to potentially harmful stimuli, such as infection, trauma, and immunological events. The inflammatory reaction is characterized by the release of a variety of inflammatory mediators and modulators that alter microvascular functions and govern leukocyte recruitment and extravasation of plasma components. Activation of phospholipase A_2 (PLA_2) induces the mobilization of fatty acids, particularly arachidonic acid (AA), from the membrane phospholipid pool. AA is the principal precursor of the eicosanoid family, which comprises the prostaglandins, prostacyclin, and thromboxanes formed along the cyclooxygenase pathway, and leukotrienes, lipoxins, and a number of hydroxy acids derived from AA via the lipoxygenase pathway. The eicosanoids are remarkably prevalent and contribute to a broad spectrum of physiological and pathological processes, such as vascular and nonvascular smooth muscle tone, thrombosis, parturition, gastric secretion, inflammation, and wound healing. Several classes of substances, most notably the nonsteroidal anti-inflammatory drugs (NSAIDs), owe their therapeutic potential to inhibition of eicosanoid biosynthesis. PLA_2 also generates a set of modified phospholipids, currently referred to as platelet-activating factor (PAF), thought to be involved in inflammatory processes.

This chapter reviews the formation and action of lipid mediators in host defense and inflammatory disorders. Special attention is paid to mechanisms of eicosanoid action and interaction in the microvascular bed, and the potential of leukotrienes as mediators of allergic and nonallergic inflammation. A schematic representation of lipid mediator actions in the microvasculature is given in Figure 7.1.

Prostaglandin Cyclooxygenases

Prostaglandins are autacoids with an impressive range of physiological and pathophysiological activities. They are formed principally from arachidonic acid (AA) by the catalytic activity of the enzyme cyclooxygenase (COX), also referred to as prostaglandin G/H synthase (Fig. 7.2). This rate-limiting committed step in the production of prostaglandins results in formation of the

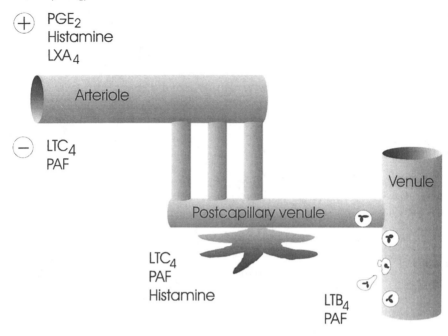

Fig. 7.1. Actions of lipid mediators and histamine in the microvasculature. Prostaglandin E_2 (PGE_2), lipoxin A_4 (LXA_4), and histamine dilate arterioles, whereas leukotriene C_4 (LTC_4) and platelet-activating factor (PAF) are potent vasoconstrictors. LTC_4 and histamine provoke increased permeability and macromolecular leakage specifically in postcapillary venules. LTB_4 and PAF cause extravasation of leukocytes and plasma components in postcapillary and larger venules. Note that none of these mediators act on capillaries.

unstable endoperoxide PGH_2 which, in turn, serves as substrate for cell-specific isomerases and synthases to produce the prostaglandins PGD_2, PGE_2, $PGF_{2\alpha}$, prostacyclin (PGI_2) and thromboxane A_2 (TXA_2) (Smith et al., 1991). Two distinct isoforms of COX have been identified and designated COX-1 and COX-2. COX-1 is widely distributed and constitutively expressed in most tissues, and is thought to catalyze formation of prostaglandins involved in maintenance of essential physiological functions, such as integrity of gastrointestinal mucosa and vascular homeostasis (Smith, 1989; O'Neill and Ford-Hutchinson, 1993). COX-2 is, with few exceptions, undetectable in normal tissue but may be induced in various cell types, including neutrophils, monocytes, and endothelial cells (Hla and Neilson, 1992; Niiro et al., 1997). The expression of COX-2 is up-regulated by stimulants of inflammation, such as tumor necrosis factor (TNF), interleukin-1 (IL-1), and bacterial lipopolysaccharides (Fu et al., 1990; Jones et al., 1993), whereas expression of this isoform is inhibited by the glucocorticoid dexamethasone and the anti-inflammatory cytokines IL-4 and IL-10 (Crofford et al., 1994; Mertz et al., 1994; Dworski and Sheller, 1997).

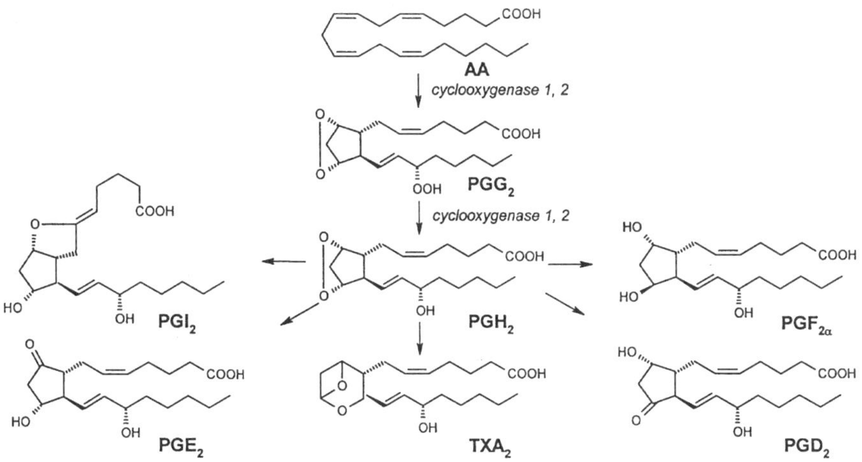

Fig. 7.2. Biosynthesis of prostaglandins (PGD_2, PGE_2 $PGF_{2\alpha}$), thromboxane A_2 (TXA_2), and prostacyclin (PGI_2) via the cyclooxygenase pathway.

Studies of recombinant enzymes in vitro and in cell lines have documented that NSAIDs, in general, inhibit both COX-1 and COX-2. The view that NSAID-induced gastrointestinal damage and renal and platelet dysfunction are the result of COX-1 inhibition, and that the beneficial effects of NSAIDs in inflammatory disorders are due to COX-2 inhibition has stimulated efforts to develop drugs that selectively inhibit either the production or function of COX-2. A number of such drugs have appeared; so far, however, none with absolute selectivity for COX-2. Numerous animal experiments indicate that these relatively selective inhibitors of COX-2 are effective anti-inflammatory, analgesic, and antipyretic agents, with little or no gastroduodenal toxicity in therapeutic dosage (Futaki et al., 1993; Masferrer et al., 1994; Seibert et al., 1994; Anderson et al., 1996). Short-term clinical trials with celecoxib, one of the new inhibitors of COX-2, have shown analgesic and anti-inflammatory efficacy in patients with rheumatoid arthritis or osteoarthritis, without causing any sign of gastric damage (Simon et al., 1998). The drug is also reported to be well tolerated by healthy individuals; however, it markedly inhibited excretion of the major urinary metabolite of prostacyclin (McAdam et al., 1999). If this effect of a COX-2 inhibitor is sustained during chronic treatment, it may have negative implications in age groups at risk for cardiovascular disease.

Another potential side effect of COX-2 inhibitors relates to wound healing. In normal gastrointestinal mucosa, COX-1 is the predominant isoform expressed. However, in situations in which the mucosa is inflamed or damaged, COX-2 may be markedly up-regulated, resulting in much higher prostaglandin production than in normal tissue (Reuter et al., 1996; Mizuno et al., 1997). There are indications that the use of selective COX-2 inhibitors in different models of rat gastric damage or colitis is associated with markedly retarded ulcer healing or such profound exacerbation that perforation occurs (Reuter et al., 1996; Mizuno et al., 1997; Schmassmann et al., 1998). Presently, no clinical data are available but it is of obvious concern, and a serious implication if selective inhibition of COX-2 expression were to delay wound healing in humans.

Prostaglandins

The discovery early in the 1970s that aspirin and other NSAIDs can inhibit prostaglandin biosynthesis (Smith and Willis, 1971; Vane, 1971) soon led to the conclusion that the antiphlogistic action of NSAIDs was due to inhibition of prostaglandin formation, a view further supported by observations that the anti-inflammatory potency of different NSAIDs apparently correlated with the degree of COX inhibition. A wealth of research has been devoted to the role of COX products in microvascular control and inflammation. Unless administered in excessive concentrations, prostaglandins per se have little or no capacity to cause plasma extravasation or overt pain (Williams and Morley, 1973; Ford-Hutchinson et al., 1978; Williams, 1979). Although these observations seemingly are at variance with the concept that the antiphlogistic effects of NSAIDs are due to COX inhibition, it has been convincingly documented that vasodilating prostaglandins potentiate the pain- and edema-producing effects of histamine and bradykinin (Ferreira, 1972; Williams and Morley, 1973; Ferreira et al., 1978; Ford-Hutchinson et al., 1978; Williams, 1979), and also potentiate leukocyte extravasation and the accompanying plasma leakage evoked by different chemotactic mediators (Bray et al., 1981; Williams, 1983; Rampart and Williams, 1986). The mechanism by which vasodilating prostaglandins enhance edema and leukocyte diapedesis is therefore considered related to their capacity to increase blood flow in inflamed tissue. As a consequence of increased flow, there is an increased intravenular hydrostatic pressure that aids outward flow of plasma through leaky venules. Increased flow also means augmented accumulation of neutrophils (Xie et al., 1999), which may stimulate additional prostaglandin production to sustain or strengthen the inflammatory reaction when they come in contact with the endothelium. This mode of action is supported by observations that vasodilators other than prostaglandins, for example, VIP, CGRP, forskolin, and nitroprusside, enhance plasma extravasation induced by different permeability-increasing mediators (Williams, 1982; Sugio and Daly, 1983; Brain and Williams 1985; Raud, 1990). Among the prostanoids formed via the COX pathway and potentially present in inflamed peripheral tissue, PGE_1, PGE_2 and PGI_2 are potent vasodilators, whereas PGD_2 displays little vasoactivity, and $PGF_{2\alpha}$ and TXA_2 are powerful vasoconstrictors (Raud, 1990).

In contrast to the stated pro-inflammatory role, numerous in vitro studies have shown that vasodilating prostaglandins also display anti-inflammatory actions. These effects include suppression of evoked release of different inflammatory mediators from neutrophils, basophils, and mast cells via cyclic adenosine monophosphate (cAMP)-dependent mechanisms (Lichtenstein and Bourne, 1971; Loeffler et al., 1971; Camussi et al., 1981), as well as enhanced release of inflammatory mediators after inhibition of prostaglandin biosynthesis (Okazaki et al., 1977; Hitchcock, 1978). Complementary to these in vitro data, NSAIDs have varyingly been reported to suppress or enhance immunologically induced edema, including IgE-mediated allergic reaction in human skin (e.g., Williams et al., 1986; Watanabe et al., 1987; Grönneberg and Dahlén, 1990).

The possibility that all these discordant data could be explained in terms of vasodilating prostaglandins actually acting in reverse at two different levels of the inflammatory process has been explored by means of intravital microscopy and animals immunized for immediate-type inflammation. Thus, in a series of experiments aimed at characterizing allergic inflammation in the hamster cheek pouch (Raud et al., 1988, 1989; Raud, 1989, 1990) it was noted that two different NSAIDs, indomethacin and diclofenac, invariably caused a marked enhancement of antigen-induced edema and leukocyte recruitment, concomitant with reduced blood flow. The two drugs also potentiated the inflammatory effects of the mast cell secretagogue compound 48/80. Furthermore, by measuring in vivo release of histamine to the interstitial fluid of the cheek pouch, it was found that indomethacin and diclofenac increased the release of histamine in response to mast cell activation by specific antigen or compound 48/80. When the cheek pouch was challenged with antigen at the same time as PGE_2 (or PGI_2) and indomethacin (or diclofenac) were present in the superfusion buffer, the NSAID-evoked potentiation of plasma leakage and leukocyte accumulation was prevented, despite marked increase in arteriolar diameter and increased blood flow. Furthermore, PGE_2, in low nanomolar concentration, completely reversed the enhanced release of histamine in indomethacin-treated hamsters challenged with antigen and in diclofenac-treated animals challenged with compound 48/80. However, PGE_2 and PGI_2 potentiated the microvascular effects of individual inflammatory mediators, including plasma leakage induced by leukotriene C_4 (LTC_4) or histamine, and leukocyte emigration and associated plasma leakage in response to local challenge with leukotriene B_4 (LTB_4). Taken together, these findings indicate that PGE_2 and PGI_2 inhibit mast cell-dependent reactions at the level of mediator release, not by reducing the actions of the mediator on the target. Thus, it may be concluded that vasodilating prostaglandins can operate through two distinct and independent mechanisms—inhibition of mediator release and enhancement of mediator actions on the target—to suppress or strengthen inflammation in vivo.

There is considerable in vitro evidence that PGE_2 and PGI_2 inhibit evoked mediator release through increased levels of cyclic adenosine monophosphate (cAMP) in the mast cells. That this mechanism is operative also in vivo is supported by the finding that forskolin, a potent vasodilator and specific activator of adenylyl cyclase, mimicked the dual activity of PGE_2 and PGI_2 in the cheek pouch (Raud, 1990). On the other hand, the vasodilator nitroprusside, which stimulates cyclic guanosine monophosphate (cGMP), potentiated the response to both antigen challenge and individual mediators, and thus displayed no inhibitory action on mediator release from the mast cells. This suggests that combined pro- and anti-inflammatory activity is confined to vasodilators that, like PGE_2, PGI_2, and forskolin, increase the cAMP level.

Heterogeneous distribution of prostaglandin receptors in different tissues, different vascular beds, and different species, and quiescent or up-regulated expression of COX-2, which governs both the rate of prostaglandin release and sites of production, are examples of factors with potential to influence vasodilating prostaglandins to exert predominantly pro- or anti-inflammatory activity. In addition, in a tissue with low basal blood flow, vasodilating prostaglandins may potentiate immunologically induced inflammation because of mediator synergism dominating suppressed mediator release, whereas the opposite result is more likely to occur in a tissue with relative high basal blood flow.

The effects of vasodilating prostaglandins also appear to vary with the route of administration. Locally applied PGE_2 and PGI_2 generally potentiate edema formation and leukocyte emigration induced by mediators, such as histamine, bradykinin, LTB_4, and C5a. However, when administered systemically PGE_2 and PGI_2 inhibit the inflammatory response to these mediators (Fantone et al., 1980; Rampart and Williams, 1986; McLeish et al., 1987). The mechanism for the anti-inflammatory effects of systemic prostaglandin treatment is not clarified, but reduced blood pressure, suppressed leukocyte function, and diminished formation of endothelial gaps have been suggested. Systemic treatment with PGE_2 and PGI_2 is commonly reported to reduce immunologically induced inflammation and tissue injury (cf. Raud and Lindbom, 1994).

Leukotrienes

Biosynthesis and Fate of Leukotrienes

Studies of the metabolism of arachidonic acid by leukocytes and parallel structural work on the slow-reacting substance of anaphylaxis (SRS-A) in the late 1970s led to the discovery of the leukotriene family and its principal members: the dihydroxy acid LTB_4 and the cysteinyl-containing LTC_4, LTD_4, and LTE_4 (Murphy et al., 1979; Samuelsson, 1983; Fig. 7.3). Leukotrienes are not stored to any appreciable extent, but are rapidly synthesized de novo on demand. Their formation from arachidonic acid can be stimulated by a variety of signals, such as antigen–antibody interactions, cytokines and growth factors, toxins, heat, and tissue trauma (cf. Denzlinger, 1996). The first step in leukotriene biosynthesis is brought about by receptor-mediated influx of Ca^{2+}, translocation of cytosolic PLA_2, and release of arachidonic acid from membrane phospholipids. The capacity to release arachidonic acid is considered to be the rate-limiting step, whereas the enzymes that catalyze subsequent transformations of arachidonic acid govern the sites where leukotrienes are synthesized. The 5-lipoxygenase (5-LO), which catalyzes formation of the leukotriene precursor LTA_4, is largely restricted to cells of the myeloic lineage, which have the greatest capacity for leukotriene generation. In addition, the cell's complement of LTA_4 hydrolase (to yield LTB_4) and/

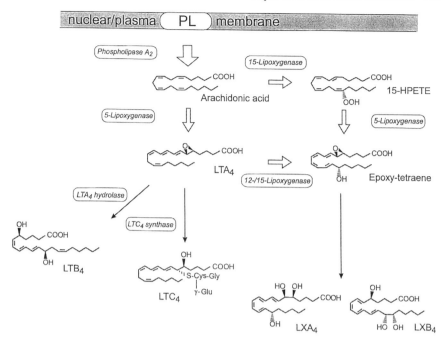

Fig. 7.3. Biosynthesis of leukotrienes (LTB₄, LTC₄, LTD₄, LTE₄) and lipoxins (LXA₄,LXB₄) via the 5 and 15-lipoxygenase pathways.

or LTC₄ synthase dictates the profile of leukotriene generation by that cell. Neutrophils make predominantly LTB₄, and mast cells and eosinophils mainly make LTC₄. Monocytes/macrophages synthesize a mixture of LTB₄ and LTC₄, with some variation between different species. In addition, LTA₄ may be released from polymorphonuclear cells and monocytes and taken up by adjacent cells devoid of 5-LO but expressing LTA₄ hydrolase and/or LTC₄ synthase. Endothelial cells, erythrocytes, lymphocytes, and platelets are examples of cell types that can complete leukotriene synthesis from LTA₄ (Keppler, 1992; Lindgren and Edenius, 1993).

LTB₄ and LTC₄ are transported out of the cell by carrier-mediated processes, which, in the case of LTC₄ has been shown to be primarily adenosine triphosphate (ATP)-dependent (Lam et al., 1990; Leier et al., 1994). Extracellular LTC₄ is converted to LTD₄ through cleavage of glutamic acid by γ-glutamyl-transferase, a glycoprotein enzyme widely distributed on cell surfaces and detectable in blood plasma. A variety of dipeptidases catalyzes the further metabolism of LTD₄ to LTE₄ by cleaving the glycine moiety. LTB₄ on the other hand, is not subject to significant extracellular modification. The half-life of leukotrienes is relatively short (4 minutes in the circulation of human beings), and they are functionally eliminated by uptake and degradation in leukocytes and hepatocytes and/or excretion in bile and urine (Keppler, 1992).

Cardiovascular Actions of Leukotrienes

The vascular response to cysteinyl-leukotrienes is, in general, vasoconstriction both in vivo and in vitro. Prominent constrictor effects have been noted in pulmonary and coronary circulation of sheep, dogs, and pigs (Michelassi et al., 1982; Woodman and Dusting, 1982; Ezra et al., 1983). In hamster microcirculation, LTC_4 and LTD_4 are as potent vasoconstrictors as angiotensin II, and LTC_4 can provoke vasoconstriction up to stasis of blood flow in gastric mucosal circulation of the rat (Dahlén et al., 1981; Whittle et al., 1985). Injection of LTC_4 into the right atrium of anesthetized monkeys causes a prompt rise of mean arterial pressure and pulmonary arterial pressure, reflecting increased resistance in both pulmonary and systemic vascular beds (Smedegård et al., 1982). The pressor response is followed by a period of hypotension and markedly diminished cardiac output. Because total peripheral resistance remains elevated, the hypotension is ascribed to impaired cardiac performance due to coronary vasoconstriction and/or negative inotropy. Intravenous or intracoronary administration of a few nanomoles of LTC_4 or LTD_4 in individuals undergoing diagnostic cardiac catheterization has been reported to provoke an increase in coronary vascular resistance and myocardial oxygen extraction (Vigorito et al., 1997).

There is little or no evidence that leukotrienes, circulating or locally formed, contribute significantly in the physiological regulation of cardiac functions, but detrimental effects may be envisaged under pathophysiological conditions. Enhanced LTE_4 excretion in urine has been documented in patients with acute myocardial ischemia, and patients undergoing cardiopulmonary bypass surgery reportedly have increased blood levels of LTB_4 (Carry et al., 1992; Gadelata et al., 1994). Enhanced cardiac production of leukotrienes has been demonstrated in rat and rabbit models of ischemia–reperfusion (global or coronary ligation-induced), and in perfused rabbit hearts with recirculating leukocytes and ionophore challenge (Hughes et al., 1991; Lee et al., 1993; Sala et al., 1993). The consequences of ischemia are accumulation of leukocytes, extravasation of macromolecules, and tissue damage. Numerous pharmacologic observations suggest that these detrimental effects are mediated, in part, by leukotrienes. Thus, inhibitors of leukotriene synthesis or action have been shown to reverse increased coronary resistance and functional impairment after global cardiac ischemia in rats, and to reduce mortality rate or myocardial damage and infarct size after coronary occlusion in rabbits, rats, and cats (Hock et al., 1992; Lee et al., 1993; Rossoni et al., 1996). Protective effects of antileukotrienes against ischemia-induced leukocyte accumulation and tissue damage have also been reported for other vascular beds, including canine intestine and hamster cheek pouch (Lehr et al., 1991; Mangino et al., 1994). The potential of leukotrienes to provoke coronary constriction and accumulation and activation of leukocytes, as well as the protective effect of antileukotrienes in a number of animal models of cardiac ischemia–reperfusion, implies a detrimental effect of endogenous leukotrienes in cardiac diseases and cardiac surgery in humans. Convincing data have yet to be presented and it may be noted that accumulating leukocytes, thought to have a pivotal role in cardiac damage, release not only leukotrienes but other potentially harmful agents, such as oxygen-derived free radicals, chemokines, proteases, and lipid mediators distinct from leukotrienes.

Leukotrienes in Host Defense and Inflammation

Acute inflammatory reactions are characterized by a series of microvascular events, including changes in vessel caliber, increased vascular permeability, and recruitment of leukocytes. Leukotrienes have been ascribed the role of inflammatory mediators because of documented increased leukotriene production during inflammation in a number of animal and human systems (Malmsten, 1984; Lewis et al., 1990; Keppler et al., 1991), and their capacity to evoke cardinal signs of inflammation. The most prominent effect of LTB_4 is recruitment of leukocytes (Smith et al., 1980; Dahlén et al., 1981; Soter et al., 1983). In addition, LTB_4 has been reported to induce degranulation and lysosomal enzyme release in neutrophils and to provoke neutrophil-dependent hyperalgesia (Palmblad et al., 1981; Sha'afi et al., 1981; Levine et al., 1984). The microvascular effects of cysteinyl-leukotrienes include vaso-constriction, endothelial contraction, and extravasation of plasma macro-molecules (Hedqvist et al., 1980; Dahlén et al., 1981; Soter et al., 1983; Joris et al., 1987).

Detailed information about the microvascular effects of leukotrienes has been obtained by intravital microscopy of the microcirculation in various tissues. The cysteinyl-leukotrienes have been shown to elicit dose-dependent extravasation of plasma, with a potency over a thousand times that of histamine. The increase in permeability is localized almost exclusively to postcapillary venules, and electron microscopic studies have documented that markers for plasma proteins leak out through gaps between adjacent contracted endothelial cells (Dahlén et al., 1981; Joris et al., 1987).

LTB_4 causes leukocytes to adhere to the endothelium in venules of all sizes, and with some latency to emigrate to the extravascular interstitium. This process is accompanied by plasma leakage, which may occur without formation of visible endothelial gaps but requires intact adhesive function of the leukocytes (Björk et al., 1982; Lindbom et al., 1982; Thureson-Klein et al., 1986; Arfors et al., 1987). It has been suggested that LTB_4-induced leakage of plasma proteins is directly coupled to the process of neutrophil chemotaxis (Rosengren et al., 1991). However, recent observations indicate that the component of plasma leakage may be separated from leukocyte transmigration (Gautam et al., 1998).

The hamster cheek pouch model has been widely used in studies of the role of endogenous leukotrienes in the inflammatory process. Some rather unspecific 5-lipoxygenase (5-LO) inhibitors slightly reduced antigen-induced plasma leakage in animals immunized for either immune complex reactions or immediate-type allergic inflammation (Björk and Smedegård, 1987; Raud, 1989). With the advent of potent and selective inhibitors of leukotriene biosynthesis and action, the issue has been readdressed in hamsters immunized to respond with allergic type 1 inflammatory reactions. Antihistamines and COX inhibitors were used to provide an experimental condition dissociated from influence of liberated histamine and prostaglandins. The results of these experiments indicate a significant role of endogenous leukotrienes as inflammatory mediators (Raud et al., 1988; Raud, 1989; Hedqvist et al., 1990, 1991, 1994). Thus, the acute microvascular events in response to antigen challenge, that is, transient arteriolar constriction, followed by plasma leakage and accumulation of leukocytes, were fully mimicked by the combined action of LTB_4 and LTC_4 in low nanomolar concentrations. Second, the microvascular components of the response to antigen challenge were profoundly inhibited by antileukotrienes, in such a way that $cysLT_1$ antagonists almost abolished vasoconstriction and plasma leakage, and 5-LO inhibitors substantially reduced leukocyte accumulation in addition to suppressing plasma leakage. Third, both LTB_4- and LTC_4-like immunoreactive substances were formed and released to the interstitial fluid of the cheek pouch in response to antigen challenge.

Experiments with antileukotrienes provide indirect evidence for endogenous leukotrienes as significant mediators of inflammatory reactions in other animal species as well, including rats, guinea pigs, and monkeys (cf. Raud and Lindbom, 1994). Antileukotrienes have been reported to accelerate healing in rat colitis models (Empey et al., 1992; Zingarelli et al., 1993).

Both 5-LO inhibitors and $cysLT_1$ receptor antagonists are in clinical practice and used in the treatment of human inflammatory disorders. Bronchial asthma is associated with increased leukotriene production, and the bronchoobstruction characteristic of this disease may be successfully treated with antileukotrienes. Furthermore, repeated administration of antileukotrienes has been reported to cause a progressive increase in the therapeutic response over time, suggesting long-term effects on the underlying inflammatory process in the airways. There are also indications that airway hyperresponsiveness, the extent of which is considered related to the degree of airway inflammation, is attenuated by treatment with antileukotrienes (cf. Dahlén, 1998).

Lipoxins

The lipoxins represent a group of arachidonic acid derivatives that may interfere with leukotriene actions in the microvasculature. Biosynthesis of lipoxins can be initiated by the 15-lipoxygenase pathway, but their formation is also linked to leukotriene generation because LTA_4 may serve as a substrate for intracellular and transcellular synthesis of lipoxins (Serhan, 1994). The lipoxins have vasoregulatory properties and stimulate generation of nitric oxide, which in turn may mediate a component of lipoxin-induced vasodilatation (Serhan, 1997). Some effects of lipoxins are antagonistic to leukotriene actions, including LTB_4-induced chemotaxis, leukocyte–endothelial cell adhesion, and plasma leakage (Hedqvist et al., 1990; Serhan, 1994). Parts of these effects may be due to down-regulation of adhesion molecules (Papayianni et al., 1996). Lipoxins may, thus, have the potential to act as feedback modulators of leukotriene action in inflammation.

Like the lipoxins, eicosanoid products of cytochrome P450 epoxygenases (epoxyeicosatrienoic acids, or EETs; Oliw et al., 1982) have vasodilatory capacity and may also have anti-inflammatory properties. Specific regioisomers of EET (i.e., [11, 12]-EET) suppress cytokine- and LPS-induced adhesion molecule expression (VCAM-1 and to a lesser extent ICAM-1 and E-selectin) in models of vascular inflammation due to an effect at the gene transcription level and distinct from the vasodilatory property (Node et al., 1999). Functionally, this mechanism may result in in reduced leukocyte adhesion to the endothelium in cytokine-driven inflammation.

Histamine and Leukotriene Interactions

Histamine is a major mediator of mast cell-dependent inflammatory reactions, and it shares with cysteinyl-leukotrienes the capacity of inducing plasma leakage selectively from postcapillary venules (Majno and Palade, 1961; Joris et al., 1987). In contrast to leukotrienes, histamine is a potent vasodilator, and as such, it potentiates target microvascular actions of leukotrienes (Raud, 1989). However, it has been documented that histamine and LTC_4 in threshold concentrations can act synergistically to cause a dramatic increase in vascular permeability by a mechanism that is unrelated to changes in vessel tone and blood flow (Raud et. al., 1992, 1994). This mutual potentiation is thus distinct and clearly separated from enhancement of leukotriene actions mediated by prostaglandins and other vasodilators. The mechanism for synergism between histamine and LTC_4 is not entirely clear, but it requires intact H_1 and $cysLT_1$ receptors, and likely relates to the capacity of histamine and cysteinyl-leukotrienes to provoke functional gaps between adjacent endothelial cells (Majno and Palade, 1961; Joris et al., 1987).

Observations that antihistamines may reduce allergen-induced leukocyte accumulation (Woodward et al., 1985; Ciprandi et al., 1992) imply that histamine, which lacks chemotactic properties per se, may act in concert with chemotactic inflammatory mediators to enhance leukocyte recruitment. This possibility has been explored in the hamster cheek pouch, using a threshold concentration of LTB_4 and low concentration of histamine (Raud et al., 1994; Hedqvist et al., 1996). Combined administration of histamine and LTB_4 strikingly potentiates the microvascular effects of LTB_4 with respect to both leukocyte accumulation and plasma leakage. However, PGE_2 also enhances the responses to LTB_4 thus indicating the presence of a blood-flow-dependent mechanism. Intravital microscopic studies of the microcirculation of the rat mesentery may shed some light on this flow dependency. Thus, it has been shown that leukocytes rolling along the venular endothelium represent the first critical step in the process of leukocyte recruitment, and that the degree of rolling apparently determines the magnitude of leukocyte firm adhesion to the endothelium (Lindbom et al., 1992; von Andrian et al., 1992). Histamine causes a significant and concentration-dependent increase in leukocyte rolling that correlates with histamine-induced vasodilatation (Raud et al., 1994; Thorlacius et al., 1995). In addition, histamine induces increased expression of P-selectin on the endothelial cells (Gaboury et al., 1995). Finally, histamine provokes formation of gaps in the endothelial lining (Majno and Palade, 1961), and may have a direct stimulating effect on the endothelial cells, promoting sustained leukocyte adhesion (Thorlacius and Xie, 1995). Considered together, these observations may also help explain why histamine appears more potent than other vasodilators for example, PGE_2 and acetylcholine, in enhancing chemotactically induced leukocyte recruitment.

Platelet-Activating Factor

Platelet-activating factor PAF (1-alkyl-2-acetyl-sn-glycero-3-phosphocholine) is a partly PLA_2-dependent phospholipid. PAF can be de novo synthesized from 1-alkyl-2-lyso-sn-glycerophosphate, an intermediate in the formation of ether-linked membrane phospholipids. Alternatively, the synthesis of PAF occurs via the remodeling pathway. This route involves conversion of 1-alkyl-2-acyl-sn-glycero-3-phosphocholine into lyso-PAF, followed by the addition of acetate, and catalyzed by a specific acetyltransferase to form PAF. The initial step in the inactivation of PAF is its deacetylation by PAF actylhydrolase to form lyso-PAF, a biologically inactive molecule (Snyder, 1994). It has been suggested that the de novo pathway is involved in the production of PAF to sustain physiological levels, and that the remodeling pathway may be responsible for high levels of PAF occurring in pathological conditions (Snyder et al., 1996). Thus, eosinophils from patients with eosinophilia have extremely high levels of lyso-PAF acetyltransferase, whereas the activity is not detectable in eosinophils from normal individuals (Lee et al., 1982). Lyso-PAF acetyltransferase activity is also higher in neutrophils from atopic patients than in those from healthy individuals (Misso et al., 1993).

The name PAF derives from early observations that a lipid factor released from IgE-stimulated basophils provoked aggregation of rabbit platelets (Benveniste et al., 1972). This designation has been retained in spite of the fact that the biological activity of PAF extends far beyond the activation of platelets to include a number of events that are relevant for inflammatory reactions. Thus, PAF promotes aggregation, chemotaxis, granule secretion, and oxygen radical generation in isolated neutrophils, eosinophils, and monocytes (O'Flaherty et al., 1981; Yasaka et al., 1982; Wardlaw et al., 1986). Application of PAF to the microcirculation of the hamster cheek pouch results in dose-dependent vasoconstriction, increase in macromolecular permeability in postcapillary and larger venules, and adhesion and transmigration of polymorphonuclear leukocytes (Björk and Smedegård, 1983). Similarly, PAF injected intradermally in rats and rabbits elicits increased vascular permeability, infiltration of neutrophils, and hyperalgesia (Bonnet et al., 1981; Humphrey et al., 1982a, 1982b). Intratracheal instillation of PAF in rabbits reportedly is associated with accumulation of alveolar macrophages and polymorphonuclear leukocytes, and degenerative changes of alveolar epithelium and microvascular endothelium (Camussi et al., 1983). PAF has also been reported to cause pulmonary vasoconstriction and edema in perfused lungs. Because LTC_4 and LTD_4 were identified in the lung effluent, it was suggested that the observed effects were partly mediated by liberated leukotrienes (Voelkel et al., 1982).

PAF can be formed by various inflammatory cells, including neutrophils, eosinophils, monocytes/macrophages, platelets, and endothelial cells, and are often targets themselves for PAF-induced bioactivities (cf. Braquet et al., 1987). PAF synthesized in endothelial cells is of particular significance because of the key position of these cells in inflammatory reactions. Examples of inflammation-associated molecules that induce PAF synthesis in endothelial cells are histamine and cysteinyl-leukotrienes, and cytokines such as TNF-α and Il-1 (McIntyre et al., 1985, 1986; Bussolino et al., 1988). Synthesized PAF is retained by the endothelial cells, and is thought to stimulate rolling neutrophils to express their β_2 integrins CD11/CD18. P-selectin, a mediator of leukocyte rolling and coexpressed with PAF on the endothelial cells, and the β_2 integrins then act in concert to support firm adhesion of the neutrophils to the endothelium. Thus, PAF and P-selectin on the surface of stimulated endothelial cells, together with their counterstructures on the neutrophils (the PAF receptor and the P-selectin glycoprotein ligand-1), may form a juxtacrine system of importance for the recruitment of leukocytes (Zimmerman et al., 1996).

Summary

It is well established that leukotrienes may be released from both blood-borne and tissue-residing cells, and that minute concentrations of these mediators provoke local tissue edema and accumulation of phagocytizing cells. Observations that selective inhibitors of leukotriene biosynthesis and action attenuate important events in immunologically induced inflammation indicate that endogenous leukotrienes may be significant mediators of inflammatory reactions. In a complex reaction, such as inflammation, a number of inflammatory mediators and modulators with different targets are likely to be active. The biological response to an external or internal stimulus is therefore not mediated by leukotrienes alone, but rather represents the composite result of mediator interactions with the ultimate goal of maintaining homeostatic control in the intact organism. Vasodilating prostaglandins, lipoxins, PAF, and histamine are some examples of endogenous substances that interact with leukotrienes in the inflammatory process.

The vasodilating prostaglandins, often referred to as pro-inflammatory, have the potential both to enhance and to inhibit different events in inflammation. The identification of the inducible isoform of prostaglandin cyclooxygenase (COX-2), specifically expressed in inflammatory lesions, has led to the design of drugs that reduce inappropriate inflammation without removing the protective prostaglandins made by the constitutive COX-1 in the stomach and kidneys.

Lipoxins apparently lack the ability to stimulate inflammation. Rather, a prime effect of lipoxins may be inhibition of neutrophil recruitment and switching the cellular response toward monocytes, thus promoting wound healing and tissue repair. The remarkable synergism between histamine and leukotrienes in causing extravasation of macromolecules and recruitment of phagocytizing cells reflects a distinct type of interaction. This synergism may be regarded as a rapid and efficient up-regulation of the host defense, but also represents a potential risk in cases of misdirected inflammation.

The phospholipid autacoid PAF displays an impressive range of biological activities, several of which have the vascular endothelium as specific target. Like the leukotrienes, PAF elicits local edema and recruitment of leukocytes, but the effect of PAF antagonists in allergic inflammation is not convincing. However, there is some evidence that PAF manufactured in endothelial cells has a signaling (juxtacrine) function in P-selectin–mediated leukocyte interaction with the endothelium.

This work was supported by grants from the Swedish Medical Research Council (04X-4342, 04P-10738), the Swedish Foundation for Health Care Science and Allergy Research (A98110), and the Karolinska Institutet. Figures 7.2 and 7.3 were kindly provided by Drs. M. Kumlin and J. Haeggström.

References

Anderson, G. D., Hauser, S. D., McGarity, K. L., Bremer, M. E., Isakson, P. C., and Gregory, S. A. (1996) Selective inhibition of cyclooxygenas (COX)-2 reverses inflammation and expression of COX-2 and interleukin 6 in rat adjuvant arthritis. *J. Clin. Invest.* 97:2672–2679.

Arfors, K. E., Lundberg, C., Lindbom, L., Lundberg, P. K., Beatty, P. G., and Harlan, J. M. (1987) A monoclonal antibody to the membrane glycoprotein complex CD18 inhibits polymorphonuclear leukocyte accumulation and plasma leakage in vivo. *Blood* 69:338–340.

Benveniste, J., Henson, P. M., and Cochrane, C. G. (1972) Leukocyte-dependent histamine release from rabbit platelets. The role of IgE, basophils, and platelet-activating factor. *J. Exp. Med.* 136:1356–1377.

Björk, J., Hedqvist P., and Arfors, K. E. (1982) Increase in vascular permeability induced by leukotriene B$_4$ and the role of polymorphonuclear leukocytes. *Inflamm.* 6:189–200.

Björk, J., and Smedegård G. (1983) Acute microvascular effects of PAF-acether, as studied by intravital microscopy *Eur. J. Pharmacol.* 96(1–2):87–94.

Björk, J., and Smedegård G. (1987) Immune-complex-induced inflammatory reaction studied by intravital microscopy: role of histamine and arachidonic acid metabolites. *Inflamm.* 11:47–58.

Bonnet, J., Loiseau, A. M., Orvoen, M., and Bessin, P. (1981) Platelet-activating factor acether (PAF-acether) involvement in acute inflammatory and pain processes. *Agents Actions* 11:559–562.

Brain S. D., and Williams, T. J., (1985) Inflammatory oedema induced by synergism between calcitonin gene-related peptide (CGRP) and mediators of increased vascular permeability. *Br. J. Pharmacol.* 86:855–860.

Braquet, P., Touqui, L., Shen, T. Y., and Vargaftig, B. B. (1987) Perspectives in platelet-activating factor research. *Pharmacol. Rev.* 39:97–145.

Bray, M. A., Cunningham, F. M., Ford-Hutchinson, A. W., and Smith, M. J. (1981) Leukotriene B$_4$; a mediator of vascular permeability. *Br. J. Pharmacol.* 72:483–486.

Bussolino, F., Camusso, G., and Baglioni, C. (1988) Synthesis and release of platelet-activating factor by human vascular endothelial cells treated with tumor necrosis factor or interleukin 1α. *J. Biol. Chem.* 263:11856–11861.

Camussi, G., Tetta, C., Segoloni, G., Chiara Deregibu, M., and Bussolino, F. (1981) Neutropenia induced by platelet-activating factor (PAF-acether) released from neutrophils: the inhibitory effect of prostacyclin (PGI₂). *Agents Actions* 11:550–553.

Camussi, G., Pawlowski, I., Tetta, C., Roffinello, C., Alberton, M., Brentjens, J., and Andres, G. (1983) Acute lung inflammation induced in the rabbit by local instillation of 1-0-octadecyl-2-acetyl-sn-glycerol-3-phosphorylcholine or of native platelet-activating factor. *Am. J. Pathol.* 112:78–88.

Carry, M., Korley, V., Willerson, J. T., Weigelt, L., Ford-Hutchinson, A. W., and Tagari, P. (1992) Increased urinary leukotriene excretion in patients with cardiac ischemia. In vivo evidence for 5-lipoxygenase activation. *Circ.* 85:230–236.

Ciprandi, G., Buscaglia, S., Iudice, A., and Canonica, G. W. (1992) Protective effect of different doses of terfenadine on the conjunctival provocation test. *Allergy* 47:309–312.

Crofford, L. J., Wilder, R. L., Ristimaki, A. P., Sano, H., Remmers, E. F., Epps, H. R., and Hla, T. (1994) Cyclooxygenase-1 and- 2 expression in rheumatoid synovial tissues. Effects of interleukin-1 beta, phorbol ester, and corticosteroids. *J. Clin. Invest.* 93:1095–1101.

Dahlén, S. E., Björk, J., Hedqvist, P., Arfors, K. E., Hammarstrom, S., Lindgren, J. A., and Samuelsson, B. (1981) Leukotrienes promote plasma leakage and leukocyte adhesion in postcapillary venules: In vivo effects with relevance to the acute inflammatory response. *Proc. Natl. Acad. Sci. USA* 78:3887–3891.

Dahlén, S. E. (1998) Leukotrienes. Inflammatory mechanisms in asthma. In: *Lung Biology in Health and Disease*, vol. 117. S. T. Holgate and W. W. Busse, eds. New York: Marcel Dekker, pp. 679–733.

Denzlinger, C. (1996) Biology and pathophysiology of leukotrienes. *Crit. Rev. Oncol. Hematol.* 23(3):167–223.

Dworski, R., and Sheller, J. R. (1997) Differential sensitivities of human blood monocytes and alveolar macrophages to the inhibition of prostaglandin endoperoxide synthase-2 by interleukin-4. *Prostaglandins* 53(4)237–251.

Empey, L. R., Walker, K., and Fedorak, R. N. (1992) Indomethacin worsens and a leukotriene biosynthesis inhibitor accelerates mucosal healing in rat colitis. *Can. J. Physiol. Pharmacol.* 70: 660–668.

Ezra, D., Boyd, L. M., Feuerstein, G., and Goldstein, R. E. (1983) Coronary constriction by leukotriene C₄, D₄, and E₄, in the intact pig heart. *Am. J. Cardiol.* 51:1451–1454.

Fantone, J. C., Kunkel, S. L., Ward, P. A., and Zurier, R. B. (1980) Suppression by prostaglandin E₁ of vascular permeability induced by vasoactive inflammatory mediators. *J. Immunol.* 125: 2591–2596.

Ferreira, S. H. (1972) Prostaglandins, aspirin-like drugs and analgesia. *Nature—New Biol.* 240(102):200–203.

Ferreira, S. H., Nakamura, M., and de Abreu Castro, M. S. (1978) The hyperalgesic effects of prostacyclin and prostaglandin E₂. *Prostaglandins* 16(1):31–37.

Ford-Hutchinson, A. W., Walker, J. R., Davidson, E. M., and Smith, M. J. (1978) PGI₂: a potential mediator of inflammation. *Prostaglandins* 16(2):253–258.

Fu, J. Y., Masferres, J. L., Seiberg, K., Raz, A., and Needleman, P. (1990) The induction and suppression of prostaglandin H₂ synthase (cyclooxygenase) in human monocytes. *J. Biol. Chem.* 265:16737–16740.

Futaki, N., Yoshikawa, K., Hamasaka, Y., Arai, I., Higuchi, J., Iizuka, H., and Otomo, S. (1993) NS-398, a novel non-steroidal anti-inflammatory drug with potent analgesic and antipyretic effects, which causes minimal stomach lesions. *Gen. Pharmacol.* 13:105–110.

Gaboury, J. P., Johnston, B., Niu, X. F., and Kubes, P. (1995) Mechanisms underlying acute mast cell-induced leukocyte rolling and adhesion in vivo. *J. Immunol.* 154:804–813.

Gadaleta, D., Fahey, A. L., Verma, M., Ko, W., Kreiger, K. H., Isom, O. W., and Davis, J. M. (1994) Neutrophil leukotriene generation increases after cardiopulmonary bypass. *J. Thorac. Cardiov. Surg.* 108:642–647.

Gautam, N., Hedqvist, P., and Lindbom, L. (1998) Kinetics of leukocyte-induced changes in endothelial barrier function. *Br. J. Pharmacol.* 125:1109–1115.

Grönneberg, R., and Dahlén, S. E. (1990) Interactions between histamine and prostanoids in IgE-dependent, late cutaneous reactions in man. *J. Allergy Clin. Immunol.* 85:843–852.

Hedqvist, P., Dahlén, S. E., Gustafsson, S. E., Hammarstrom, S., and Samuelsson, B. (1980) Biological profile of leukotrienes C_4 and D_4 *Acta Physiol. Scand.* 110:331–333.

Hedqvist, P., Raud, J., and Dahlén, S. E. (1990) Microvascular actions of eicosanoids in the hamster cheek pouch. *Adv. Prostaglandin Thromboxane Leukotriene Res.* 20:153–160.

Hedqvist, P., Raud, J., Palmertz, U., Kumlin, M., and Dahlén, S. E. (1991) Eicosanoids as mediators and modulators of inflammation. *Adv. Prostaglandin Thromboxane Leukotriene Res.* 21B: 537–543.

Hedqvist, P., Lindbom, L., Palmertz, U., and Raud, J. (1994) Microvascular mechanisms in inflammation. *Adv. Prostaglandin Thromboxane Leukotriene Res.* 22:91–99.

Hedqvist, P., Lindbom, L., Thorlacius, H., and Raud, J. (1996) Microvascular actions and interactions of eicosanoids and histamine in inflammation. In: *Eicosanoids: From Biotechnology to Therapeutic Applications*, G. C. Folco, B. Samuelsson, J. Maclouf, and G. P. Velo, eds. *NATO ASI Series A: Life Sci*, New York: Plenum Press, 283:155–163.

Hitchcock, M. (1978) Effect of inhibitors of prostaglandin synthesis and prostaglandins E_2 and $F_{2\alpha}$ on the immunologic release of mediators of inflammation from actively sensitized guinea-pig lung. *J. Pharmacol. Exp. Ther.* 20:630–640.

Hla, T., and Neilson, K. (1992) Human cyclooxygenase-2 cDNA. *Proc. Natl. Acad. Sci. USA* 89: 7384–7388.

Hock, C. E., Beck, L. D., Papa L. A. (1992) Peptide leukotriene receptor antagonism in myocardial ischaemia and reperfusion. *Cardiovasc. Res.* 26:1206–1211.

Hughes, H., Gentry, D. L., McGuire, G. M., and Taylor, A. A. (1991) Gas chromatographic–mass spectrometric analysis of lipoxygenase products in post-ischemic rabbit myocardium. *Prostaglandin Leukotriene Essays* 42(4):225–231.

Humphrey, D. M., Hanahan, D. J., and Pinckard, R. N. (1982a) Induction of leukocytic infiltrates in rabbit skin by acetyl glycerol ether phosphorylcholine. *Lab. Invest.* 47:227–234.

Humphrey, D. M., McManus, L. M., Satouchi, K., Hanahan, D. J., and Pinckard, R. N. (1982b) Vasoactive properties of acetyl glycerol ether phosphorylcholine and analogues. *Lab. Invest.* 46:422–427.

Jones, D. A., Carlton, D. P., McIntyre, T. M., Zimmerman, G. A., and Prescott, S. M. (1993) Molecular cloning of human prostaglandin endoperoxide synthase type II and demonstration of expression in response to cytokines. *J. Biol. Chem.* 268:9049–9054.

Joris, I., Majno, G., Corey, E. J., and Lewis, R. A. (1987) The mechanism of vascular leakage induced by leukotriene E_4. Endothelial contraction. *Am. J. Pathol.* 126:19–24.

Keppler, D. (1992) Leukotrienes: biosynthesis transport, inactivation, and analysis. *Rev. Physiol. Biochem. Pharmacol.* 121:1–30.

Keppler, D., Guhlmann, A., Oberdorfer, F., Krauss, K., Muller, J., Ostertag, H., and Huber, M. (1991) Generation and metabolism of cysteinyl leukotrienes in vivo. *Ann. N.Y. Acad. Sci.* 629: 100–104.

Lam, B. K., Gagnon, L., Austen, K. F., and Soberman, R. J. (1990) The mechanism of leukotriene B_4 export from human polymorphonuclear leukocytes. *J. Biol. Chem.* 265:13438–13441.

Lee, C. C., Appleyard, R. F., Byrne, J. G., and Cohn, L. H. (1993) Leukotrienes D_4 and E_4 produced in myocardium impair coronary flow and ventricular function after two hours of global ischaemia in rat heart. *Cardiovasc. Res.* 27:770–773.

Lee, T. C., Malone, B., Wasserman, S. I., Fitzgerald, V., and Snyder, F. (1982) Activities of enzymes that metabolize platelet-activating factor (1-alkyl-2-acetyl-sn-glycero-3-phosphocholine) in neutrophils and eosinophils from humans and the effect of a calcium ionophore. *Biochem. Biophys. Res. Commun.* 105:1303–1308.

Lehr, H. A., Guhlmann, A., Nolte, D., Keppler, D., and Messmer, K. (1991) Leukotrienes as mediators in ischemia-reperfusion injury in a microcirculation model in the hamster. *J. Clin. Invest.* 87:2036–2041.

Leier, I., Jedlitschky, G., Buchholz, U., and Keppler, D. (1994) Characterization of the ATP-dependent leukotriene C_4 export carrier in mastocytoma cells. *Eur. J. Biochem.* 220:599–606.

Levine, J. D., Lau, W., Kwiat, G., and Goetz, E. J. (1984) Leukotriene B_4 produces hyperalgesia that is dependent on polymorphonuclear leukocytes. *Science* 225:743–745.

Lewis, R. A., Austen, K. F., and Soberman, R. J. (1990) Leukotrienes and other products of the 5-lipoxygenase pathway. Biochemistry and relation to pathobiology in human diseases. *New. Engl. J. Med.* 323:645–655.

Liechtenstein, L. M., and Bourne, H. R. (1971) Inhibition of allergic histamine release by histamine and other agents which stimulate adenyl cyclase. In: *Biochemistry of Acute Allergic Reactions.* K. F. Austen and E. L. Becker, eds., Oxford: Blackwell, pp. 161–174.

Lindbom, L., Hedqvist, P., Dahlén, S. E., Lindgren, J. A., and Arfors, K. E. (1982) Leukotriene B$_4$ induces extravasation and migration of polymorphonuclear leukocytes in vivo. *Acta Physiol. Scand.* 116:105–108.

Lindbom, L., Xie, X., Raud, J., and Hedqvist, P. (1992) Chemoattractant-induced leukocyte adhesion to vascular endothelium in vivo is critically dependent on initial leukocyte rolling. *Acta Physiol. Scand.* 146:415–421.

Lindgren, J. A., and Edenius, C. (1993) Transcellular biosynthesis of leukotrienes and lipoxins via leukotriene A$_4$ transfer. *Trends Pharmacol. Sci.* 14:351–354.

Loeffler, L. J., Lovenberg, W., and Sjoerdsma, A. (1971) Effects of dibutyryl-3',5'-cyclic adenosine monophosphate, phosphodiesterase inhibitors and prostaglandin E$_1$ on compound 48–80-induced histamine release from rat peritoneal mast cells in vitro. *Biochem. Pharmacol.* 20:2287–2297.

Majno, G., and Palade, G. E. (1961) Studies on inflammation. I. The effect of histamine and serotonin on vascular permeability. An electron microscopic study. *J. Biophys. Biochem. Cytol.* 11:571–605.

Malmsten, C. L. (1984) Leukotrienes: mediators of inflammation and immediate hypersensitivity reactions. *Crit. Rev. Immunol.* 4:307–334.

Mangino, M. J., Murphy, M. K., and Anderson, C. B. (1994) Effects of the arachidonate 5-lipoxygenase synthesis inhibitor A-64077 in intestinal ischemia-reperfusion injury. *J. Pharmacol. Exp. Ther.* 269:75–81.

Masferrer, J. L., Zweifel, B. S., Manning P. T., Hauser, S. D., Leahy, K. M., Smith, W. G., Isakson, P. C., and Seibert, K. (1994) Selective inhibition of inducible cyclooxygenase 2 in vivo is antiinflammatory and nonulcerogenic. *Proc. Natl. Acad. Sci. USA* 91:3228–3232.

McAdam, B. F., Catella-Lawson, F., Mardini, I. A., Kapoor, S., Lawson, J. A., and FitzGerald, G. A. (1999) Systemic biosynthesis of prostacyclin by cyclooxygenase (COX)-2: The human pharmacology of a selective inhibitor of COX-2. *Proc. Natl. Acad. Sci. USA* 96:272–277.

McIntyre, T. M., Zimmerman, G. A., Satoh, K., and Prescott, S. M. (1985) Cultured endothelial cells synthesize both platelet-activating factor and prostacyclin in response to histamine, bradykinin, and adenosine triphosphate. *J. Clin. Invest.* 76:271–280.

McIntyre, T. M., Zimmerman, G. A., and Prescott, S. M. (1986) Leukotrienes C4 and D4 stimulate human endothelial cells to synthesize platelet-activating factor and bind neutrophils. *Proc. Natl. Acad. Sci. USA* 83:2204–2208.

McLeish, K. R., Wellhausen, S. R., and Stelzer, G. T. (1987) Mechanism of prostaglandin E2 inhibition of acute changes in vascular permeability. *Inflamm.* 11(3):279–288.

Mertz, P. M., De Witt, D. L., Stetler-Stevenson, W. G., and Wahl, L. M. (1994) Interleukin 10 suppression of monocyte prostaglandin H synthase-2. Mechanism of inhibition of prostaglandin-dependent matrix metalloproteinase production. *J. Biol. Chem.* 269:21322–21329.

Michelassi, F., Landa, L., Hill, R. D., Lowenstein, E., Watkins, W. D., Petkau, A. J., and Zapol, W. M. (1982) Leukotriene D$_4$ a potent coronary artery vasoconstrictor associated with impaired ventricular contraction. *Science* 217:841–843.

Misso, N. L., Gillon, R. L., Taylor, M. L., Stewart, G. A., and Thompson, P. J. (1993) Acetyl-CoA: lyso-platelet-activating factor acetyltransferase activity in neutrophils from asthmatic patients and normal subjects. *Clin. Sci.* 85:455–463.

Mizuno H., Sakamoto, C., Matsuda, K., Wada, K., Uchida, T., Noguchi, H., Akamatsu, T., and Kasuga, M. (1997) Induction of cyclooxygenase 2 in gastric mucosal lesions and its inhibition by the specific antagonist delays healing in mice. *Gastroenterol.* 112:387–397.

Murphy, R. C., Hammarstrom, S., and Samuelsson, B. (1979) Leukotriene C: a slow-reacting substance from murine mastocytoma cells. *Proc. Natl. Acad. Sci. USA* 76:4275–4279.

Niiro, H. Otsuka, T., Izuhara, K., Yamaoka, K., Ohshima, K., Tanabe, T., Hara, S., Nemoto, Y.,

Tanaka, Y., Nakashima, H., and Niho Y. (1997) Regulation by interleukin-10 and interleukin-4 of cyclooxygenase-2 expression in human neutrophils. *Blood* 89:1621–1628.

Node, K., Huo, Y., Ruan, X., Yang, B., Specker, M., Ley, K., Zeldin, D. C., and Liao, J. K. (1999) Anti-inflammatory properties of cytochrome P450 epoxygenase-derived eicosanoids. *Science* 285:1276–1279.

O'Flaherty, J. T., Wykle, R. L., Miller, C. H., Lewis, J. C., Waite, M., Bass, D. A., McCall, C. E., and DeChatelet, L. R. (1981) 1-O-Alkyl-sn-glycerol-3-phosphorylcholines: a novel class of neutrophil stimulants. *Am. J. Pathol.* 103:70–79.

Okazaki, T., Ilea, V. S., Rosario, N. A., Reisman, R. E., Arbesman, C. E., Lee, J. B., and Middleton, E. Jr. (1977) Regulatory role of prostaglandin E in allergic histamine release with observations on the responsiveness of basophil leukocytes and the effect of acetylsalicylic acid. *J. Allergy Clin. Immunol.* 60(6):360–366.

Oliw, E. H., Guengerich, F. P., and Oates, J. A. (1982) Oxygenation of arachidonic acid by hepatic monooxygenases. Isolation and metabolism of four epoxide intermediates. *J. Biol. Chem.* 257:3771–3781.

O'Neill, G. P., and Ford-Hutchinson, A. W. (1993) Expression of mRNA for cyclooxygenase-1 and cycloxygenase-2 in human tissues. *FEBS Lett.* 330(2):156–160.

Palmblad, J., Malmsten, C. L., Uden, A. M., Radmark, O., Engstedt, L., and Samuelsson, B. (1981) Leukotriene B_4 is a potent and stereospecific stimulator of neutrophil chemotaxis and adherence. *Blood* 58:658–661.

Papayianni, A., Serhan, C. N., and Brady, H. R. (1996) Lipoxin A_4 and B_4 inhibit leukotriene-stimulated interactions of human neutrophils and endothelial cells. *J. Immunol.* 156:2264–2272.

Rampart M. and Williams, T. J., (1986) Polymorphonuclear leukocyte-dependent plasma leakage in the rabbit skin is enhanced or inhibited by prostacyclin, depending on the route of administration. *Am. J. Pathol.* 124:66–73.

Raud, J., Dahlén, S. E., Sydbom, A., Lindbom, L., and Hedqvist, P. (1988) Enhancement of acute allergic inflammation by indomethacin is reversed by prostaglandin E_2: apparent correlation with in vivo modulation of mediator release. *Proc. Natl. Acad. Sci. USA* 85:2315–2319.

Raud, J. (1989) Intravital microscopic studies on acute mast cell-dependent inflammation. *Acta Physiol. Scand. (suppl.)* 578:1–58.

Raud, J., Dahlén, S. E., Sydbom, A., Lindbom, L., and Hedqvist, P. (1989) Prostaglandin modulation of mast cell-dependent inflammation. *Agents Actions* 26(1–2):42, 44.

Raud, J. (1990) Vasodilatation and inhibition of mediator release represent two distinct mechanisms for prostaglandin modulation of acute mast cell-dependent inflammation. *Br. J. Pharmacol.* 99(3):449–454.

Raud, J., Lindbom, L., and Hedqvist, P. (1992) Histamine and leukotriene C_4 act synergistically via a blood flow-independent mechanism to enhance microvascular plasma leakage. *Acta Physiol. Scand.* 146:545–546.

Raud, J., and Lindbom, L. (1994) Studies by intravital microscopy of basic inflammatory mechanisms and acute allergic inflammation. In: *Immunopharmacology of the Microcirculation*, S. D. Brain, ed. *The Handbook of Immunopharmacology.* San Diego Academic Press, pp. 127–170.

Raud, J., Thorlacius, H., Xie, X., Lindbom, L., and Hedqvist, P. (1994) Interactions between histamine and leukotrienes in the microcirculation: Aspects of relevance to acute allergic inflammation. *Ann. N.Y. Acad. Sci.* 744:191–198.

Reuter, B. K., Asfaha, S., Buret, A., Sharkey, K. A., and Wallace, J. L. (1996) Exacerbation of inflammation-associated colonic injury in rat through inhibition of cyclooxygenase-2. *J. Clin. Invest.* 98:2076–2085.

Rosengren, S., Olofsson, A. M., von Andrian, U. H., Lundgren-Akerlund, E., and Arfors, K. E. (1991) Leukotriene B4-induced neutrophil-mediated endothelial leakage in vitro and in vivo. *J. Appl. Physiol.* 71:1322–1330.

Rossoni, G., Sala, A., Berti, F., Testa, T., Buccellati, C., Molta, C., Muller-Peddinghaus, R., Maclouf, J., and Folco, G. C. (1996) Myocardial protection by the leukotriene synthesis inhibitor BAY X 1005: importance of transcellular biosynthesis of cysteinyl-leukotrienes. *J. Pharmacol. Exp. Ther.* 276:335–341.

Sala, A., Rossoni, G., Buccellati, C., Berti, F., Folco, G., and Maclouf, J. (1993) Formation of sulphidopeptide-leukotrienes by cell-cell interaction causes coronary vasoconstriction in isolated, cell-perfused heart of rabbit. *Br. J. Pharmacol.* 110:1206–1212.

Samuelsson, B. (1983) Leukotrienes: mediators of immediate hypersensitivity reactions and inflammation. *Science* 220:568–575.

Schmassmann, A., Peskar, B. M., Stettler, C., Netzer, P., Stroff, T., Flogerzi, B., and Halter, F. (1998) Effects of inhibition of prostaglandin endoperoxide synthase-2 in chronic gastrointestinal ulcer models in rats. *Br. J. Pharmacol.* 123:795–804.

Seibert, K, Zhang, Y., Leahy, K., Hauser, S., Masferrer, J., Perkins, W., Lee, L., and Isakson, P. (1994) Pharmacological and biochemical demonstration of the role of cyclooxygenase 2 in inflammation and pain. *Proc. Natl. Acad. Sci. USA* 91:12013–12017.

Serhan, C. N. (1994) Lipoxin biosynthesis and its impact in inflammatory and vascular events. *Biochim. Biophys. Acta* 1212:1–25.

Serhan, C. N. (1997) Lipoxins and novel aspirin-triggered 15-epi-lipoxins (ATL): a jungle of cell–cell interactions or a therapeutic opportunity? *Prostaglandins* 53(2):107–137.

Sha'afi, R. I., Naccache, P. H., Molski, T. F., Borgeat, P., and Goetzl, E. J. (1981) Cellular regulatory role of leukotriene B$_4$: its effects on cation homeostasis in rabbit neutrophils. *J. Cell Physiol.* 108:401–408.

Simon, L. S., Lanza, F. L., Lipsky, P. E., Hubbard, R. C., Talwalker, S., Schwartz, B. D., Isakson, P. C., and Geis, G. S. (1998) Preliminary study of the safety and efficacy of SC-58635, a novel cyclooxygenase 2 inhibitor. *Arthritis Rheum.* 41:1591–1602.

Smedegård, G., Hedqvist, P., Dahlen, S. E., Revenas, B., Hammarstrom, S., and Samuelsson, B. (1982) Leukotriene C$_4$ affects pulmonary and cardiovascular dynamics in monkey. *Nature* 295:327–329.

Smith, J. B., and Willis, A. L. (1971) Aspirin selectively inhibits prostaglandin production in human platelets. *Nature–New Biol.* 231(25):235–237.

Smith, M. J., Ford-Hutchinson, A. W., and Bray, M. A. (1980) Leukotriene B: a potential mediator of inflammation. *J. Pharm. Pharmacol.* 32:517–518.

Smith, W. L. (1989) The eicosanoids and their biochemical mechanisms of action. *Biochem. J.* 159:315–324.

Smith, W. L., Marnett, L. J., and DeWitt, D. L. (1991) Prostaglandin and thromboxane biosynthesis. *Pharmacol. Therpeut.* 49(3):153–179.

Snyder, F. (1994) Metabolic processing of PAF. *Clin. Rev. Allergy* 12:309–327.

Snyder, F., Fitzgerald, V., and Blank, M. L. (1996) Biosynthesis of platelet-activating factor and enzyme inhibitors. *Adv. Exp. Med. Biol.* 416:5–10.

Soter, N. A., Lewis, R. A., Corey, E. J., and Austen, K. F. (1983) Local effects of synthetic leukotrienes (LTC$_4$, LTD$_4$, LTE$_4$, LTB$_4$) in human skin. *J. Invest. Dermatol.* 80(2):115–119.

Sugio, K., and Daly, J. W. (1983) Effect of forskolin on alterations of vascular permeability induced with bradykinin, prostaglandin E$_1$, adenosine, histamine and carrageenin in rats. *Life Sci.* 33(1):65–73.

Thorlacius, H., Raud, J., Xie, X., Hedqvist, P., and Lindbom, L. (1995) Microvascular mechanisms of histamine-induced potentiation of leukocyte adhesion evoked by chemoattractants. *Br. J. Pharmacol.* 116:3175–3180.

Thorlacius, H., and Xie, X. (1995) Histamine modulates the nature of fMLP-induced leukocyte adhesion. *Acta Physiol. Scand.* 155:475–476.

Thureson-Klein, A., Hedqvist, P., and Lindbom, L. (1986) Leukocyte diapedesis and plasma extravasation after leukotriene B$_4$: lack of structural injury to the endothelium. *Tissue Cell* 18(1):1–12.

Vane, J. R. (1971) Inhibition of prostaglandin synthesis as a mechanism of action for aspirin-like drugs. *Nature–New Biol.* 231(25):232–235.

Vigorito, C., Giordani, A., Cirillo, R., Genovese, A., Rengo, F., and Marone, G. (1997) Metabolic and hemodynamic effects of peptide leukotriene C$_4$ and D$_4$ in man. *Int. J. Clin. Lab. Res.* 27(3):178–184.

Voelkel, N. F., Worthen, S., Reeves, J. T., Henson, P. M., and Murphy, R. C. (1982) Nonimmunological production of leukotrienes induced by platelet-activating factor. *Science* 218:286–289.

von Andrian U. H., Hansell, P., Chambers, J. D., Berger, E. M., Torres Filho, I., Butcher, E. C., and Arfors, K. E. (1992) L-selectin function is required for beta 2-integrin-mediated neutrophil adhesion at physiological shear rates in vivo. *Am. J. Physiol.* 263:H1034–1044.

Wardlaw, A. J., Moqbel, R., Cromwell, O., and Kay, A. B. (1986) Platelet-activating factor. A potent chemotactic and chemokinetic factor for human eosinophils. *J. Clin. Invest.* 78:1701–1706.

Watanabe, M., Ohuchi, K., and Tsurufuji, S. (1987) Recurrence of an allergic inflammation of air-pouch type in rats and possible participation of prostaglandin E_2. *Int. Arch. Allergy Immunol.* 83(4):390–397.

Whittle, B. J., Oren-Wolman, N., and Guth, P. H. (1985) Gastric vasoconstrictor actions of leukotriene C_4 $PGF_{2\alpha}$ an thromboxane mimetic U-46619 on rat submucosal microcirculation in vivo. *Am. J. Physiol.* 248:G580–G586.

Williams, T. J., and Morley J. (1973) Prostaglandins as potentiators of increased vascular permeability in inflammation. *Nature* 246:215–217.

Williams, T. J. (1979) Prostaglandin E_2, prostaglandin I_2 and the vascular changes of inflammation. *Br. J. Pharmacol.* 65:517–524.

Williams, T. J. (1982) Vasoactive intestinal polypeptide is more potent than prostaglandin E_2 as a vasodilator and oedema potentiator in rabbit skin. *Br. J. Pharmacol.* 77:505–509.

Williams, T. J. (1983) Interactions between prostaglandins, leukotrienes and other mediators of inflammation. *Br. Med. Bull.* 39:239–242.

Williams, T. J., Hellewell, P. G., and Jose, P. J. (1986) Inflammatory mechanisms in the Arthus reaction. *Agents Actions* 19(1–2):66–72.

Woodman, O. L., and Dusting, G. J. (1982) Coronary vasoconstriction induced by leukotrienes in the anaesthetized dog. *Eur. J. Pharmacol.* 86:125–128.

Woodward, D. F., Spada, C. S., Hawley, S. B., and Nieves, A. L. (1985) Histamine H_1- and H_2-receptor involvement in eosinophil infiltration and the microvascular changes associated with cutaneous anaphylaxis. *Agents Actions* 17:121–125.

Xie, X., Hedqvist, P. and Lindbom, L. (1999) Influence of local haemodynamics on leukocyte rolling and chemoattractant-induced firm adhesion in microvessels of the rat mesentery. *Acta Physiol Scand* 165:251–258.

Yasaka, T., Boxer, L. A., and Baehner, R. L. (1982) Monocyte aggregation and superoxide anion release in response to formyl-methionyl-leucyl-phenylalanine (FMLP) and platelet-activating factor (PAF). *J. Immunol.* 128:1939–1944.

Zimmerman, G. A., Elstad, M. R., Lorant, D. E., McIntyre, T. M., Prescott, S. M., Topham, M. K., Weyrich, A. S., and Whatley, R. E. (1996) Platelet-activating factor (PAF): signalling and adhesion in cell–cell interactions. *Adv. Exp. Med. Biol.* 416:297–304.

Zingarelli, B., Squadrito, F., Graziani, P., Camerini, P., and Capute, A. P. (1993) Effects of zileuton, a new 5-lipoxygenase inhibitor, in experimentally induced colitis in rats. *Agents Actions* 39(3–4):150–156.

8

Complement in Inflammation

B. PAUL MORGAN

Complement (C) has been linked with inflammation almost since the discovery of the C system more than a century ago. In 1909 Friedberger showed that incubation of serum with immune complexes caused the generation of anaphylaxis-inducing activity that he termed *anaphylatoxin*. The capacity of serum to generate anaphylatoxin was lost upon heating, leading Friedberger and others to consider complement as the source of this activity (Friedberger and Ito, 1911). More than half a century passed before the C-derived factors responsible for the anaphylaxis observed by Friedberger were properly characterized and shown to be fragments of the major C-proteins released during activation of the system (Dias da Silva and Lepow, 1967; Bokisch et al., 1969). It is not possible in this brief chapter to discuss in detail the fascinating history of discovery and characterization of the C-derived anaphylatoxins and other pro-inflammatory products (for excellent earlier reviews, see Hugli, 1981; Bitter-Suermann, 1982).

The Complement System

The C system is composed of a group of 12 soluble plasma proteins that interact with one another in three distinct enzymatic activation cascades (the classical, alternative, and lectin pathways) and result in the nonenzymatic assembly of a cytolytic complex (the membrane attack pathway; Fig. 8.1). Complement plays a central role in innate immune defense, providing a system for the rapid destruction of a wide range of invading microorganisms. Activation of complement on immune complexes is essential for the efficient clearance of immune complexes. These roles of complement in homeostasis and defense are well illustrated in individuals deficient in components of the C pathways who present with immune complex disease and/or multiple bacterial infections (Morgan and Walport, 1991).

The classical activation pathway (CP), so called because it was the first pathway to be described, is triggered by antibody bound to particulate antigen. Many other substances, including components of damaged cells, bacterial lipopolysaccharide, and nucleic acids, can also initiate the classical activation pathway in an antibody-independent manner. Binding of C1 to

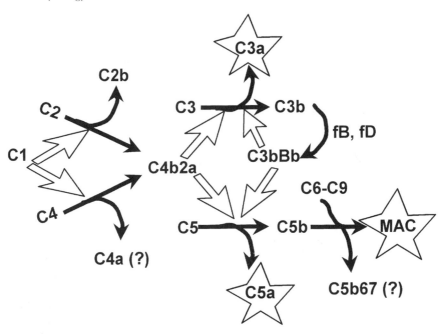

Fig. 8.1. The complement system generates multiple pro-inflammatory products. The constituent pathways of the complement system and the component proteins are shown. The lectin pathway differs from the classical activation pathway only in that the mannan-binding protein—mannan-associated serine protease (MBP-MASP) complex replaces the C1 complex. Enzymatic cleavages are represented by open arrows; pro-inflammatory products of complement activation are in "stars."

aggregated or immune complex-bound immunoglobin G (IgG) or IgM antibody is the initiating step that marks a target for C activation (Loos, 1988). Conformational changes occur upon binding of multiple heads of the C1q component of the C1 molecule by aggregates of IgG that trigger activation of an enzymatic activity in C1s within the C1 complex (Reid, 1986, Reid and Day, 1989) C1s in the activated C1 complex will enzymatically cleave and activate the next component of the classical activation pathway C4. C4 is a large abundant plasma protein (~0.6 g/1) composed of three disulphide-bonded chains (α, β and γ; Schreiber and Muller-Eberhard, 1974; Janatova and Tack, 1981). C1s cleaves plasma C4 at a single site near the amino-terminal of the α chain, releasing a small fragment, C4a, and exposing a reactive thioester group in the α chain of the large fragment, C4b. Once exposed in C4b, the thioester can form covalent amide or ester bonds with exposed amino or hydroxyl groups, respectively, on the activating surface, locking the molecule to the activating surface. The thioester group is extremely labile due to its propensity to inactivation by hydrolysis, restricting C4b binding to the immediate vicinity of the activating C1 complex and providing a receptor for the next component of the classical activation pathway, C2.

C2 is a single-chain protein present in relatively low amounts in plasma (0.1 g/l). In the presence of Mg^{2+} ions, C2 binds to C4b on the membrane and is presented for cleavage by C1s in an adjacent C1 complex. The larger fragment, C2a, remains attached to C4b to form the C4b2a complex, an enzyme that cleaves C3. C3 is a large molecule composed of two disulphide-bonded chains (α and β; Lambris, 1988). It is the most abundant of the C components (1–2 g/l). C3 binds the C4b2a complex and is then cleaved by the C2a enzyme at a single site in the α chain, releasing the small fragment, C3a, from the amino-terminal and exposing in the large fragment, C3b, a labile thioester. C3b binds either to the activating C4b2a enzyme or to the adjacent membrane (Kozono et al., 1990; Ebanks et al., 1992). C3b bound to the activating C4b2a complex yields a new enzyme, C4b2a3b, the C5 cleaving enzyme of the classical activation pathway.

C5 is a two-chain (α and β, disulphide-bonded) plasma protein ($\sim$ 0.2 g/l; 190 kDa molecular weight). C5 is structurally related to C3 and C4 but has no thioester group. C5 binds the C4b2a3b convertase and is cleaved by C2a at a single site in the α chain, releasing a small amino-terminal fragment, C5a, and exposing in the larger fragment, C5b, a labile hydrophobic surface-binding site and a site for binding C6.

The alternative pathway (AP) has many features in common with the classical activation pathway but does not require antibody for initiation. It provides a rapid system for C activation and amplification on foreign surfaces. As in the classical activation pathway, C3 is the key component, but three other proteins, factor B, factor D and properdin, are also required. Factor B, a single-chain protein closely related to C2, binds C3b in a Mg^{2+}-dependent manner and is then cleaved at a single site by factor D, a serine protease present in plasma in its active form. The large cleavage fragment, Bb, contains a serine protease domain enabling the C3bBb complex to cleave more C3 (Gotze, 1986). Properdin binds and stabilizes the C3bBb complex, extending the lifetime of the active convertase three to four-fold (Fearon et al., 1976; Weiler et al., 1976). Initiation of the alternative pathway on an "activator" surface occurs spontaneously, the phenomenon of *tickover*. C3 in plasma is hydrolyzed to form a metastable $C3(H_2.O)$ molecule that has many of the characteristics of C3b, binds factor B in solution, and renders it susceptible to cleavage by factor D to form a fluid phase C3 convertase [$C3(H_2.O)Bb$; Lachmann and Hughes-Jones, 1984; Law and Dodds, 1990].

The alternative pathway C5 convertase is composed of two molecules of C3b, one binding Bb in the C3bBb complex and an adjacent (or attached) C3b acting as receptor for C5. The site of cleavage in C5 is identical to that utilized by C2a in the classical activation pathway.

The lectin pathway provides a second antibody-independent route for activation of C on bacteria and other microorganisms. The key component of this novel pathway is mannan-binding lectin (MBL), a high molecular weight serum lectin (Holmskov et al., 1994, Reid and Turner, 1994). MBL, which resembles C1q in structure, binds mannose and N-acetyl glucosamine residues in bacterial cell walls, MBL is associated with a serine protease (MBL-associated serine protease, or MASP), which can cleave C4 and C2 in the same sites used by C1s (Matsuhita and Fujita, 1992).

The membrane attack pathway involves the noncovalent association of C5b with the four terminal C components to form an amphipathic membrane-inserted complex. Each of the terminal components is present in plasma at concentrations of about 0.1 g/l

C5b binds C6, a large single-chain plasma protein. The C5b6 complex in turn binds C7, a single-chain plasma protein that is homologous to C6. The trimolecular C5b67 complex is released to the fluid phase and then binds directly to membrane via its hydrophobic membrane-binding site.

C8, a complex molecule made up of three chains, α, β, and γ, binds the C5b67 complex and the resulting complex, C5b-8, becomes more deeply buried in the membrane (Tamura et al., 1972). C9, a single-chain plasma protein, binds the C5b-8 complex and undergoes a major conformational change from a globular, hydrophilic form to an elongated, amphipathic form that traverses the membrane and exacerbates membrane leakiness. Additional C9 molecules are recruited into the complex to form a large trans-membrane pore (the membrane attack complex, MAC) that can cause lysis of the target cell.

The C system is tightly controlled by regulatory proteins present in the plasma and on cell membranes. The details of regulation are beyond the scope of this chapter (for a comprehensive review, see Morgan and Harris, 1999).

Active Products of Complement

During C activation, numerous active products are generated that act on surrounding cells either through interaction with specific receptors, or through direct binding to the membrane (Table 8.1). Although these active products have many different effects on many different cell types, a common consequence is the amplification of inflammation.

In the activation pathways, the fragments of C4, C3, and C5 generated by their respective convertases are the most important active products. The large fragments, C4b and C3b, bind to the activating surface through the nascent thioester group and are essential components of the convertases. Surface-bound C4b and C3b and products generated during degradation of these molecules also play important roles in marking the C-activating surface for phagocytosis. Phagocytic cells express surface receptors specific for C3b, C4b, and fragments of these molecules, enabling them to bind surfaces coated (opsonized) with these C fragments. Binding and uptake of opsonized targets by phagocytes results in the clearance of the activating stimulus. Although the process of opsonization mediated by these large fragments is anti-inflammatory in that it aids removal of the C-activating surface, uptake of opsonized particles can trigger release from the phagocytes of proteolytic

Table 8.1. Pro-inflammatory Products of C Activation

Product	Target Cell	Effect Mediated	Receptor Characteristics
C3a	eosinophil	chemotaxis, degranulation	7-TM G-protein–linked; broad tissue distribution.
C5a	neutrophil eosinophil macrophage mast cell platelet others	chemotaxis, degranulation, oxidase response, adhesion, etc.	7-TM G-protein–linked; broad tissue distribution.
C5b67	neutrophil	chemotaxis, down-regulates oxidase response, etc.	not characterized
MAC	many (ubiquitous?)	varies with cell type (see Table 8.2)	direct membrane binding

Note. MAC, membrane attack complex; 7-TM, seven transmembrane.

enzymes, reactive oxygen species, and other inflammatory agents. In this way, opsonization can, in some circumstances, be pro-inflammatory.

Of more relevance to inflammation are the small fragments of C4, C3, and C5 generated upon cleavage by the convertases. All have been implicated as chemotactic and anaphylactic agents. Each of the fragments, C4a, C3a, and C5a, are generated by cleavage in the α chain of the corresponding protein to release a small N-terminal peptide. All three are of similar length (74–77 amino acids); C3a and C4a have an apparent Mr of about 8.5 kDa, whereas C5a is glycosylated, yielding an apparent molecular mass (Mr) of about 11 kDa (Hugli, 1981). A much clearer picture of the functions of these three peptides has emerged in recent years, largely as a consequence of cloning their receptors (Gerard and Gerard, 1991; Gerard and Gerard, 1994; Ames et al., 1996).

Complement-Derived Anaphylatoxins/Chemotaxins

C5a is a 74 amino acid glycopolypeptide derived from the amino-terminal end of the α chain of C5, with a molecular mass of about 11 kDa. C5a is by far the most active of the three anaphylactic/chemotactic peptides. It is a potent leukocyte chemoattractant with chemotactic activity for neutrophils, eosinophils, basophils, monocyte/macrophages, platelets, and probably several other cell types. It also exerts powerful anaphylactic actions on phagocytic cells, mast cells, and basophils. Binding of C5a triggers activation of each of these cell types, the precise effect depending on the cell. In neutrophils, the major effects of C5a include degranulation with release of proteolytic enzymes, production of reactive oxygen species, and generation of prostanoids. C5a acts not only on myeloid cells, but also on many other cell types, although the precise nature of the effects mediated are much less clear in these other cells (Wetsel, 1995).

The presence of specific receptors for C5a was first demonstrated on neutrophils and macrophages using labeled ligands (Chenoweth and Goodman, 1983; van Epps and Chenoweth, 1984). The C5a receptor (C5aR, CD88) has been cloned and shown to be a member of the 7-transmembrane-spanning receptor family that also includes the adrenergic receptor and numerous chemokine/cytokine receptors (Gerard and Gerard, 1991). All members of this family share homology and all are G-protein coupled, signaling cell activation upon binding of ligand. The process of cell activation following ligation of the C5aR and other members of this receptor family is discussed in detail in Chapter 9. Although the precise distribution of the receptor for C5a is still the subject of debate, it is now becoming clear that C5aR is present and functional on a very wide range of cells and tissues (Table 8.1; Gasque et al., 1995; Lacy et al., 1995; McCoy et al., 1995). From the viewpoint of inflammation, the most intriguing of these is the reported effect of C5a on hepatic cells, which has been implicated in triggering the acute phase response (McCoy et al., 1995). The gene encoding the C5aR has been deleted in the mouse with resultant impairment of inflammation in the reversed Arthus reaction (Hopken et al., 1997; see also Chapter 18).

C3a is a 77 amino acid unglycosylated peptide derived from the amino-terminal end of the α chain of C3 and with a molecular mass of about 9 kDa. Although there are numerous reports in the literature indicating that C3a activates all myeloid cells (Grossklaus et al., 1976; Hartung and Hadding, 1983), recent data indicate that C3a is much more restricted in its actions. When highly purified cell populations are examined, it becomes clear that eosinophils are the primary target for C3a. C3a directly triggers chemotaxis and activation of eosinophils with degranulation and release of reactive oxygen species (Daffern et al., 1995). The apparent effects of C3a on other myeloid cells are not directly attributable to C3a but occur secondary to activation of eosinophils.

As for C5aR, the presence of specific receptors for C3a (C3aR) was first demonstrated in ligand-binding studies (Fukuoka and Hugli, 1988). The C3aR was cloned in 1996 (Ames et al., 1996). It, too, is a member of the 7-transmembrane-spanning G-protein–linked receptor family but differs from the C5aR and other members of this family in that the second extracellular loop is very large (160 amino acids). Northern blotting and antibody binding studies indicate that the C3aR is widely distributed, and is expressed on the majority of cells of myeloid origin and on many other cell types. The presence of C3aR on neutrophils is surprising in light of the finding that these cells do not directly respond to C3aR (Daffern et al., 1995). The roles of C3aR expressed in nonmyeloid cells remain undefined.

C4a is a 77 amino acid (8.7 kDa) unglycosylated peptide derived from the amino-terminal end of the α chain of C4. Early studies claim weak anaphylactic and chemotactic activity for C4a, acting on a similar range of cells, albeit with much reduced activity compared to C5a (Moon et al., 1981 Hugli, 1984;) However, despite the best efforts of many researchers, no receptor for C4a has yet been identified Furthermore, in "clean" assay systems using recombinant proteins, no C4a-mediated chemotactic or anaphylactic activities have been demonstrated (Lienenklaus et al, 1998). It is likely that the activities ascribed to C4a in earlier studies were due to trace contamination of preparations with C5a.

Both C5a and C3a are regulated by a serum carboxypeptidase N, which cleaves the carboxy-terminal Arg residue from each peptide (Bokisch and Muller-Eberhard, 1970, Plummer and Hurwitz, 1978). The desArg molecules generated are either completely inactive (C3adesArg) or of much diminished activity (C5adesArg). C5adesArg has no anaphylactic activity; however, it retains weak chemotactic activity and is stable in vivo, enabling it to attract phagocytic cells at a distance from the site of C activation. For this reason, C5adesArg is an important chemotactic agent, recruiting neutrophils remote from the site of C activation.

A role for the C5b67 complex as a neutrophil chemotactic factor was first proposed 30 years ago (Lachmann et al., 1970, Ward and Becker, 1977). Interest in this phenomenon has reemerged in the last few years. Nicholson-Weller and colleagues have confirmed that hemolytically inactive C5b67 is chemotactic for neutrophils and have shown that chemotaxis is dependent on activation of G-proteins and calcium fluxes in the cell (Wang et al., 1995, 1996). The receptor responsible for these effects has yet to be identified. Interestingly, C5b67 inhibited neutrophil oxidase responses and degranulation. C5b67 would thus be predicted to attract neutrophils to the site of C activation and act to inhibit neutrophil activation by C5a and other anaphylactic agents. The biological purpose of this unique set of properties is hard to envisage. Given the abundance of C5b67-binding proteins present in plasma (S-protein, clusterin, C8), the biological relevance of C5b67-mediated chemotaxis must, in any case, be in doubt.

The Membrane Attack Complex as a Pro-inflammatory Agent

Dogma dictates that the MAC forms pores in membranes and brings about lysis of target cells (Mayer, 1977). This lytic activity of the MAC is most easily demonstrated in vitro when the targets chosen are inert and easily lysed. Lytic killing, which causes the release of cell contents, is a potentially inflammatory event and is rare in vivo. Most nucleated cell types are very resistant to the lytic effects of MAC in vitro and in vivo. Resistance is attributable in part to the abundant expression of C-regulatory molecules on the cell membrane, but active processes in the cell also aid resistance to lytic killing and recovery from attack (Morgan, 1989a). MACs formed in the membranes of metabolically active nucleated cells (and some enucleate cells such as platelets) are rapidly eliminated, either by internalization or shedding on vesicles. Escape from lysis does not mean that the target cell is unaffected by attack. MAC can cause activation of cells in the absence of lysis and this activation may be an important drive to inflammation. Nonlethal cell activation induced by MAC has been demonstrated in numerous cell types and is dis-

Table 8.2. Activation of Cells in Vitro by the Membrane Attack Complex (MAC)

Cell Type	Effect	Reference
Neutrophil	vesiculation; cell swelling; oxidase response; eicosanoid secretion	Morgan et al., 1987 Morgan, 1988 Morgan, 1989
Platelet	vesiculation; degranulation; shape changes; eicosanoid secretion; acquisition of procoagulant properties	Wiedmer and Sims, 1985 Wiedmer et al., 1986b Sims et al., 1988 Wiedmer, et al., 1986a
Endothelial	vesiculation; degranulation; loss of barrier function; eicosanoid secretion; secretion of von Willebrand factor; IL-1α synthesis and secretion; tissue factor synthesis; increased E-selectin expression; shedding of heparan sulfate prothrombinase binding; release of growth factors	Geller et al., 1992 Ando et al., 1988 Saadi and Platt, 1995 Hattori et al., 1989 Saadi et al., 1995 Ihrcke and Platt, 1996

cussed in several recent reviews (Shin and Carney, 1988; Morgan, 1988, 1989b; Morgan et al., 1989). End responses are dependent on the target cell but have included vesiculation, degranulation, release of inflammatory mediators, secretion of cytokines, proliferation, and numerous other responses, many of which can be considered pro-inflammatory. Some examples from the three most studied primary cell types are given in Table 8.2. The precise signaling pathway(s) by which MAC triggers cell activation remain(s) unclear. Even in the absence of lysis, formation of pores in the membrane disrupts ion gradients; intracellular Ca^{2+} levels may increase 100-fold, which may be an important trigger in some cell types. Numerous other signaling pathways have also been implicated in various cell types but a consistent pattern has yet to emerge. In platelets, activation of protein kinases has been implicated in signaling MAC removal (Wiedmer et al., 1987). In other cell types, activation of phospholipase C with generation of diacylglycerol and activation of adenylate cyclase with production of cyclic adenosine monophosphate (cAMP) appear to be involved (Cybulsky et al., 1989 Carney et al., 1990). In B cells, MAC attack is associated with the activation of multiple components of the mitogen-activated protein kinase (MAPK) cascade (Rus et al., 1997, Niculescu et al., 1999), a response also observed following exposure to physical stress stimuli. A recent publication has implicated the pro-inflammatory transcription factor NF-κB as a central factor in MAC-induced activation of endothelial cells (Kilgore et al., 1997); whether this holds true for other cell types is untested. Regardless of the signaling pathway involved, and in almost all tissues, the in vitro evidence indicates that MAC assembly on metabolically active nucleated host cells at the inflammatory site in vivo is likely to trigger the release of pro-inflammatory molecules and enhance the inflammatory response.

Complement in Inflammatory Disease

The complement system contributes to tissue damage in a large number of diseases of diverse etiology (Dalmasso, 1986; Morgan, 1994, 1995). An involvement of complement in pathology is perhaps clearest in those iatrogenic diseases triggered by exposure of a bioincompatible surface to the plasma (Mellbye et al., 1988, Mollnes, 1991). In cardiopulmonary bypass complement is activated in the ex vivo circuit, and complement activation products accumulate in plasma causing activation of circulating cells and endothelia. These activation events, particularly involving activation of neutrophils and platelets, are responsible for the post-bypass syndrome that causes considerable morbidity and occasional mortality.

The hallmarks of autoimmune diseases are autoantibodies and immune complexes that deposit in the affected organs where they trigger activation of complement and exacerbate inflammation. In many autoimmune diseases, from the organ specific (e.g., autoimmune thyroid disease) to the disseminated (e.g., systemic lupus erythematosus), complement deposition can be detected in the affected tissues, and products of complement activation are found in the plasma (Koffler et al., 1982). In systemic lupus erythematosus, autoantibodies are present that recognize DNA and other components of normal cells. Following any stimulus to cell death, these components are released and immune complexes form. Immune complexes deposit in capillary beds, particularly in the skin and kidney, where they activate complement to cause inflammation and further tissue destruction. A vicious cycle is triggered in which more cell killing drives the production of more immune complexes that in turn exacerbates complement activation and tissue destruction. Myasthenia gravis, an autoimmune disease in which the autoantibodies target the acetylcholine receptor at the neuromuscular junction, provides a particularly good example of the importance of complement. Local activation of complement causes destruction of the junction and is directly responsible for the muscle weakness that characterizes the disease (Engel, 1980, Engel and Arahata, 1987). In animal models of the disease, removal of C6 prevents assembly of MAC and abrogates induction of the disease (Biesecker and Gomez, 1989).

Anti-Complement Agents as Anti-inflammatories

From the preceding account of the pro-inflammatory properties of many of the products of activation, it is clear that complement activation is a powerful drive to inflammation and tissue destruction in many diseases. Therapies that inhibit complement activation or specific activation products might therefore be of broad therapeutic benefit. Numerous agents have been developed, acting at various points in the complement system (Table 8.3). To date, most success has been achieved with modified forms of the naturally occurring regulators. A recombinant soluble form of the membrane complement regulator CR1 (sCR1) has been shown to block complement activation effectively and to inhibit the progress of inflammatory disease in numerous animal models. Therapy with sCR1 blocks complement by inhibiting the convertases of the activation pathways, preventing generation of C5a and MAC. This agent and further modifications of this agent are now being tested for therapy in inflammatory disease in man (Ryan, 1995; Candinas et al., 1996; Mulligan et al., 1999).

A second strategy for complement inhibition, which has made enormous strides toward the clinic, is the use of anti-complement antibodies to block at specific stages of the pathway. A humanized single-chain antibody against C5 has been developed that blocks the cleavage of C5, preventing the generation of C5a and MAC (Kroshus et al., 1995; Thomas et al., 1996). This agent proved effective in a mouse model of lupus nephritis (Wang et al., 1996). Anti-C5 is now in clinical trials for therapy of myocardial infarction and to inhibit the negative sequelae of cardiopulmonary bypass.

An alternative approach to inhibit the pro-inflammatory effects of complement activation is to specifically block the receptor for the major anaphylactic and chemotactic product, C5a. The C5aR represents an attractive target for pharmaceutical companies in that there is a real prospect of developing small-molecule antagonists. Numerous such agents have already been developed and shown to be effective in vitro, but none have yet been developed as therapeutics (Konteatis et al., 1994). C5aR-blocking antibodies have also been developed and might prove useful as therapeutics (Morgan et al., 1993).

Table 8.3. Anti-Complement Therapeutics

Agent	Target	Stage of Development	Comments
sCR1	C3/C5 convertases	In clinical trials, transplantation, ARDS	large, expensive, limited utility
sMCP, sDAF, sDAF/MCF hybrid	C3/C5 convertase	preclinical	large, expensive, limited utility
Anti-C5 scFv	C5 cleavage	In clinical trials, MI, CPB	promising agent, systemic only
C5aR antagonist	C5a	preclinical	potential for small molecule, orally active
Anti-C5aR	C5a	in vitro	little progress

Note. CR1, C receptor 1; MCP, membrane cofactor protein; DAF, decay accelerating factor, ARDS, adult respiratory distress syndrome; MI, myocardial infarction; CPB, cardiopulmonary bypass.

Conclusion

Complement activation generates multiple pro-inflammatory activities and represents a major drive to inflammation in vivo. The relative contributions to inflammation made by the different active products will vary for different sites of activation, and there is growing evidence that the active products may synergize to exacerbate inflammation further (Czermak et al., 1999). Agents that inhibit complement activation or prevent the actions of specific active products may prove to be highly effective anti-inflammatory therapies in numerous diseases. Of note, evidence is already accumulating that anti-complement agents may be of therapeutic benefit in Alzheimer's disease where low-grade inflammation is now considered to be an important component of the pathology (McGeer and McGeer, 1992; McGeer and Rogers, 1992).

The author acknowledges the financial support of the Wellcome Trust through the award of a Senior Clinical Research Fellowship.

References

Ames, R. S., Li, Y., Sarau, H. M., Nuthulaganti, P., Foley, J. J., Ellis, C., Zeng, Z., Su, K., Jurewicz, A. J., Hertzberg, R. P. et al. (1996) Molecular cloning and characterization of the human anaphylatoxin C3a receptor J. Biol. Chem 271:20231–20234.

Ando, B., Wiedmer, T., Hamilton, K. K., and Sims, P. J. (1988) Complement proteins C5b-9 initiate secretion of platelet storage granules without increased binding of fibrinogen or von Willebrand factor to newly expressed cell surface GPIIb–IIIa. *J. Biol. Chem.* 263:11907–11914.

Biesecker, G., and Gomez, C. M. (1989) Inhibition of acute passive transfer experimental autoimmune myasthenia gravis with Fab antibody to complement C6. *J. Immunol.* 142:2654–2659.

Bitter-Suermann, D. (1982) Contribution of complement factors and reaction pathways to inflammation *Agents Actions Suppl.* 11:159–178.

Bokisch, V. A., and Muller-Eberhard, H. J., (1970) Anaphylatoxin inactivator of human plasma its isolation and characterization as a carboxypeptidase. *J. Clin. Invest.* 49:2427–2436.

Bokisch, V. A., Muller-Eberhard, H. J., and Cochrane, C. G. (1969) Isolation of a fragment (C3a) of the third component of human complement containing anaphylatoxin and chemotactic activity and description of an anaphylatoxin inactivator of human serum. *J. Exp. Med.* 129:1109–1130.

Candinas, D., Lesnikoski, B. A., Robson, S. C., Scesney, S. M., Otsu, I., Myiatake, T., Marsh, H. C. Jr., Ryan, U. S., Hancock, W. W., and Bach, F. H. (1996) Soluble complement receptor type 1 and cobra venom factor in discordant xenotransplantation *Transplant. Proc.* 28:581–582.

Carney, D. F., Lang, T. J., and Shin, M. L. (1990) Multiple signal messengers generated by terminal complement complexes and their role in terminal complement complex elimination. *J. Immunol.* 145:623–629.

Chenoweth, D. E., and Goodman, M. G. (1983). The C5a receptor of neutrophils and macrophages *Agents Actions Suppl.* 12:252–273.

Cybulsky, A. V., Salant, D. J., Quigg, R. J., Badalamenti, J., and Bonventre, J. V. (1989) Complement C5b-9 complex activates phospholipases in glomerular epithelial cells *Am. J. Physiol.* 257:F826–F836.

Czermak, B. J., Lentsch, A. B., Bless, N. M., Schmal, H., Friedl, H. P., and Ward, P. A. (1999) Synergistic enhancement of chemokine generation and lung injury by C5a or the membrane attack complex of complement. *Am. J. Pathol.* 154:1513–1524.

Daffern, P. J., Pfeifer, P. H., Ember, J. A, and Hugli, T. E. (1995) C3a is a chemotaxin for human eosinophils but not neutrophils I. C3a stimulation of neutrophil activation is secondary to eosinophil activation *J. Exp. Med.* 181:2119–2127.

Dalmasso, A. P. (1986) Complement in the pathophysiology and diagnosis of human diseases. *Crit. Rev. Clin. Lab. Sci.* 24:123–183.

Dias da Silva, W, and Lepow, I. H. (1967) Complement as a mediator of inflammation. II. Biological properties of anaphylatoxin prepared with purified components of human complement *J. Exp. Med.* 125:921–946.

Ebanks, R. O., Jaikaran, A. S., Carroll, M. C., Anderson, M. J., Campbell, R. D., and Isenman, D. E. (1992) A single arginine to tryptophan interchange at beta-chain residue 458 of human complement component C4 accounts for the defect in classical pathway C5 convertase activity of allotype C4A6. Implications for the location of a C5 binding site in C4. *J. Immunol.* 148: 2803–2811.

Engel, A. G. (1980) Morphologic and immunopathologic findings in myasthenia gravis and in congenital myasthenic syndromes *J. Neurol. Neurosurg. & Psych.* 43:577–589.

Engel, A. G., and Arahata, K (1987) The membrane attack complex of complement at the endplate in myasthenia gravis *Ann. N.Y. Acad. Sci.* 505:326–332.

Fearon, D. T., Daha, M. R., Weiler, J. M., and Austen, K. F. (1976) The natural modulation of the amplification phase of complement activation *Transplant. Rev.* 32:12–25.

Friedberger, E. (1909) Kritik der Theorien über die Anaphylaxie *Z. Immunitatsforsch.* 2:208–224.

Friedberger, E., and Ito, T. (1911) Uber anaphylaxie. XXI Mitteilung Naheres uber den mechanismus der komplementwikung bei der anaphylatoxinbildung in vitro. *Z. Immunitatsforsch.* 11:471–486.

Fukuoka, Y., and Hugli, T. E. (1988) Demonstration of a specific receptor for C3a on guinea pig platelets. *J. Immunol.* 140:3496–3501.

Gasque, P., Chan, P., Fontaine, M., Ischenko, A., Lamacz, M., Gotze, O., and Morgan, B. P. (1995) Identification and characterization of the complement C5a anaphylatoxin receptor on human astrocytes. *J. Immunol.* 155:4882–4889.

Geller, R. L., Bach, F. H., Vercellotti, G. M., Nistler, R. S, Bolman, R. M. d., Fischel, R. J., Leventhal, J., and Platt, J. L. (1992) Activation of endothelial cells in hyperacute xenograft rejection. *Transplant. Proc.* 24:592–593.

Gerard, C., and Gerard, N. P. (1994) C5a anaphylatoxin and its seven transmembrane-segment receptor. *Ann. Rev. Immunol.* 12:775–808.

Gerard, N. P., and Gerard, C. (1991) The chemotactic receptor for human C5a anaphylatoxin. *Nature* 349:614–617.

Gotze, O. (1986) The alternative pathway of activation In: *The Complement System*. K. Rother, and G. O., Till, Eds. Berlin: Springer, pp. 154–168.

Grossklaus, C., Damerau, B., Lemgo, E., and Vogt, W. (1976) Induction of platelet aggregation by the complement-derived peptides C3a and C5a *Naunyn-Schmiedebergs Arch. Pharmacol.* 295: 71–76.

Hartung, H. P., and Hadding, U. (1983) Synthesis of complement by macrophages and modulation of their functions through complement activation *Springer Seminars Immunopathol.* 6: 283–326.

Hattori, R., Hamilton, K. K., McEver, R. P, and Sims, P. J. (1989) Complement proteins C5b-9 induce secretion of high molecular weight multimers of endothelial von Willebrand factor and translocation of granule membrane protein GMP-140 to the cell surface. *J. Biol. Chem.* 264:9053–9060.

Holmskov, U., Malhotra, R, Sim, R. B., and Jensenius, J. C. (1994) Collectins: collagenous C-type lectins of the innate immune defense system *Immunol. Today* 67:74.

Hopken, U. E., Lu, B., Gerard, N. P., and Gerard, C. (1997) Impaired inflammatory responses in the reverse arthus reaction through genetic deletion of the C5a receptor *J. Exp. Med.* 186: 749–756.

Hugli, T. E. (1981) The structural basis for anaphylatoxic and chemotactic functions of C3a, C4a and C5a. *Crit. Rev. Immunol.* 1:321–366.

Hugli, T. E. (1984) Structure and function of the anaphylatoxins. *Springer Sem. Immunopathol.* 7: 193–219.

Ihrcke, N. S., and Platt, J. L. (1996) Shedding of heparan sulfate proteoglycan by stimulated endothelial cells: evidence for proteolysis of cell-surface molecules. *J. Cell. Physiol.* 168:625–637.

Janatova, J., and Tack, B. F. (1981) Fourth component of human complement studies of an amine-sensitive site comprised of a thiol component. *Biochem.* 20:2394–2402.

Kilgore, K. S., Schmid, E, Shanley, T. P., Flory, C. M., Maheswari, V., Tramontini, N. L., Cohen, H., Ward, P. A., Friedl, H. P., and Warren, J. S (1997) Sublytic concentrations of the membrane attack complex of complement induce endothelial interleukin-8 and monocyte chemoattractant protein-1 through nuclear factor-kappaB activation. *Am. J. Pathol.* 150:2019–2031.

Koffler, D., Biesecker, G., and Katz, S. M. (1982) Immunopathogenesis of systemic lupus erythematosus. *Arthritis Rheum.* 25:858–861.

Konteatis, Z. D., Siciliano, S. J., Van Riper, G., Molineaux, C. J., Pandya, S, Fischer, P., Rosen, H., Mumford, R. A., and Springer, M. S (1994) Development of C5a receptor antagonists: Differential loss of functional responses. *J. Immunol.* 153:4200–4205.

Kozono, H., Kinoshita, T., Kim, Y. U., Takata-Kozono, Y., Tsunasawa, S., Sakiyama, F., Takeda, J., Hong, K., and Inoue, K. (1990) Localization of the covalent C3b-binding site on C4b within the complement classical pathway C5 convertase, C4b2a3b. *J. Biol. Chem.* 265:14444–14449.

Kroshus, T. J., Rollins, S. A., Dalmasso, A. P., Elliott, E. A., Matis, L. A., Squinto, S. P., and Bolman, R. M. (1995) Complement inhibition with an anti-C5 monoclonal antibody prevents acute cardiac tissue injury in an ex vivo model of pig-to-human xenotransplantation *Transplant.* 60:1194–1202.

Lachmann, P. J., Kay, A. B., and Thompson, R. A. (1970) The chemotactic activity for neutrophil and eosinophil leukocytes of the trimolocular complex of the fifth, sixth and seventh components of human complement (C567) prepared in free solution by the "reactive lysis" procedure *Immunol.* 19:895–899.

Lachmann, P. J., and Hughes-Jones, N. C. (1984) Initiation of complement activation. *Springer Sem. Immunopathol.* 7:143–162.

Lacy, M., Jones, J., Whittemore, S. R., Haviland, D. L., Wetsel, R. A., and Barnum, S. R. (1995) Expression of the receptors for the C5a anaphylatoxin, interleukin-8 and FMLP by human astrocytes and microglia. *J. Neuroimmunol.* 61:71–78.

Lambris, J. D. (1988) The multifunctional role of C3, the third component of complement *Immunol. Today* 9:387–393.

Law, S. K., and Dodds, A. W. (1990) C3, C4 and C5: the thioester site. *Biochem. Soc. Transac.* 18:1155–1159.

Lienenklaus, S., Ames, R. S., Tornetta, M. A., Sarau, H. M., Foley, J. J., Crass, T., Sohns, B., Raffestseder, U., Grove, M., Holzer, A., et al. (1998) Human C4a anaphylatoxin elicits C3a-receptor mediated effects in guinea pigs but not in man *Mol. Immunol.* 35:366–367.

Loos, M. (1988) "Classical" pathway of activation. In *The Complement System.* (K Rother and G. O., Till, eds. Berlin: Springer pp. 136–153.

Matsuhita, M., and Fujita, T. (1992) Activation of the classical complement pathway by mannose-binding protein in association with a novel C1s-like serine protease *J. Exp. Med.* 176:1497–1502.

Mayer, M. M. (1977) The cytolytic attack mechanism of complement. *Monogr. Allergy* 12:1–12.

McCoy, R., Haviland, D. L., Molmenti, E. P., Ziambaras, T., Wetsel, R. A., and Perlmutter, D. H. (1995) N-formylpeptide and complement C5a receptors are expressed in liver cells and mediate hepatic acute phase gene regulation *J. Exp. Med.* 182:207–217.

McGeer, P. L., and McGeer, E. G. (1992) Complement proteins and complement inhibitors in Alzheimer's disease *Res. Immunol.* 143:621–624.

McGeer, P. L., and Rogers, J (1992) Anti-inflammatory agents as a therapeutic approach to Alzheimer's disease. *Neurol.* 42:447–449.

Mellbye, O. J, Froland, S. S., Lilleaasen, P., Svennevig, J. L., and Mollnes, T. E. (1988) Complement activation during cardiopulmonary bypass comparison between the use of large volumes of plasma and dextran 70. *Eur. Surg. Res.* 20:101–109.

Mollnes, T. E., Videm, V., Riesenfeld, J., Garred, P., Svennevig, J. L., and Fosse, E, Hogasen, K., and Harboe, M. (1991) Complement activation and bioincompatibility *Clin. exp. Immunol.* (suppl. 1) 86:21–26.

Moon, K. E., Gorski, J. P., and Hugli, T. E. (1981) Complete primary structure of human C4a anaphylatoxin *J. Biol. Chem.* 256:8685–8692.

Morgan, B. P. (1988). Non-lethal complement-membrane attack on human neutrophils: transient cell swelling and metabolic depletion *Immunol.* 63:71–77.

Morgan, B. P., Dankert, J. R., and Esser, A. F. (1987) Recovery of human neutrophils from complement attack: removal of the membrane attack complex by endocytosis and exocytosis *J. Immunol.* 138:246–253.

Morgan, B. P. (1989a) Complement membrane attack on nucleated cells resistance, recovery and non-lethal effects *Biochem. J.* 264:1–14.

Morgan, B. P. (1989b) Mechanisms of tissue damage by the membrane attack complex of complement. *Complement Inflamm.* 6:104–111.

Morgan, B. P., Vora, J. P., Bennett, A. J, Thomas, J. P., and Matthews, N (1989) A case of hereditary combined deficiency of complement components C6 and C7 in man. *Clin. Exp. Immunol.* 75:396–401.

Morgan, B. P., and Walport, M. J. (1991) Complement deficiency and disease. *Immunol. Today* 12:301–306.

Morgan, B. P. (1994) Clinical complementology recent progress and future trends. *Eur. J. Clin. Invest.* 24:219–228.

Morgan, B. P. (1995) Physiology and pathophysiology of complement progress and trends. *Crit. Rev. Clin. Lab. Sci.* 32:265–298.

Morgan, B. P., and Harris, C. L. (1999) *Complement Regulatory Proteins.* London: Academic Press.

Morgan, E. L., Ember, J. A., Sanderson, S. D, Scholz, W., Buchner, R., Ye, R. D., and Hugli, T. E. (1993) Anti-C5a receptor antibodies. Characterization of neutralizing antibodies specific for a peptide, C5aR-(9-29), derived from the predicted amino-terminal sequence of the human C5a receptor *J. Immunol.* 151:377–388.

Mulligan, M. S, Warner, R. L., Rittershaus, C. W., Thomas, L. J., Ryan, U S, Foreman, K. E, Crouch, L. D, Till, G. O., and Ward, P. A (1999) Endothelial targeting and enhanced anti-inflammatory effects of complement inhibitors possessing sialyl Lewis(x) moieties. *J. Immunol.* 162:4952–4959.

Niculescu, F., Soane, L., Badea, T, Shin, M, and Rus, H. (1999) Tyrosine phosphorylation and activation of Janus kinase 1 and STAT3 by sublytic C5b-9 complement complex in aortic endothelial cells *Immunopharmacol.* 42:187–193.

Plummer, T. H. Jr., and Hurwitz, M. Y. (1978) Human plasma carboxypeptidase N. isolation and characterization *J. Biol. Chem.* 253:3907–3912.

Reid, K. B. (1986) Activation and control of the complement system *Essays Biochem.* 22:27–68.

Reid, K. B., and Day, A. J (1989) Structure–function relationships of the complement components *Immunol. Today* 10:177–180.

Reid, K. B., and Turner, M. W (1994) Mammalian lectins in activation and clearance mechanisms involving the complement system. *Springer Sem. Immunopathol.* 15:307–326.

Rus, H., Niculescu, F., Badea, T., and Shin, M. L., (1997) Terminal complement complexes induce cell cycle entry in oligodendrocytes through mitogen activated protein kinase pathway *Immunopharmacol.* 38:177–187.

Ryan, U S. (1995) Complement inhibitory therapeutics and xenotransplantation. *Nature Med.* 1: 967–968.

Saadi, S, Holzknecht, R. A, Patte, C. P, Stern, D. M, and Platt, J. L (1995) Complement-mediated regulation of tissue factor activity in endothelium *J. Exp. Med.* 182:1807–1814.

Saadi, S., and Platt, J. L (1995) Transient perturbation of endothelial integrity induced by natural antibodies and complement *J. Exp. Med.* 181:21–31.

Schreiber, R. D., and Muller-Eberhard, H. J. (1974) Fourth component of human complement description of a three polypeptide chain structure. *J. Exp. Med.* 140:1324–1335.

Shin, M. L, and Carney, D. F. (1988) Cytotoxic action and other metabolic consequences of terminal complement proteins. *Prog. Allergy* 40:44–81.

Sims, P. J., Faioni, E. M, Wiedmer, T., and Shattil, S. J. (1988) Complement proteins C5b-9 cause release of membrane vesicles from the platelet surface that are enriched in the membrane receptor for coagulation factor Va and express prothrombinase activity. *J. Biol. Chem.* 263: 18205–18212.

Tamura, N, Shimada, A., and Chang, S. (1972) Further evidence for immune cytolysis by antibody and the first eight components of complement. *Immunol.* 22:131–140.

Thomas, T. C., Rollins, S. A., Rother, R. P., Giannoni, M. A., Hartman, S. L, Elliott, E. A., Nye, S. H., Matis, L. A., Squinto, S. P., and Evans, M. J. (1996) Inhibition of complement activity by humanized anti-C5 antibody and single-chain Fv *Mol. Immunol.* 33:1389–1401.

van Epps, D. E., and Chenoweth, D. E. (1984) Analysis of the binding of fluorescent C5a and C3a to human peripheral blood leukocytes *J. Immunol.* 132:2862–2867.

Wang, C., Barbashov, S, Jack, R. M., Barrett, T., Weller, P. F., and Nicholson-Weller, A. (1995) Hemolytically inactive C5b67 complex an agonist of polymorphonuclear leukocytes *Blood* 85: 2570–2578.

Wang, C., Gerard, N. P, and Nicholson-Weller, A (1996) Signaling by hemolytically inactive C5b67, an agonist of polymorphonuclear leukocytes. *J. Immunol.* 156:786–792.

Wang, Y., Hu, Q, Madri, J. A., Rollins, S. A., Chodera, A., and Matis, L. A (1996) Amelioration of lupus-like autoimmune disease in NZB/WF1 mice after treatment with a blocking mono-clonal antibody specific for complement component C5 *Proc. Nat. Acad. Sci. USA* 93:8563–8568.

Ward, P. A, and Becker, E L. (1977) Biology of leukotaxis. *Rev. Physiol. Biochem. & Pharmacol.* 77: 125–148.

Weiler, J. M., Daha, M. R., Austen, K. F., and Fearon, D. T. (1976). Control of the amplification convertase of complement by the plasma protein beta1H. *Proceedings of the National Academy of Sciences of the United States of America* 73, 3268–3272.

Wetsel, R. A. (1995) Expression of the complement C5a anaphylatoxin-receptor (C5aR) on non-myeloid cells. *Immunol. Lett.* 44:183–187.

Wiedmer, T, Ando, B, and Sims, P. J. (1987) Complement C5b-9-stimulated platelet secretion is associated with a Ca2+-initiated activation of cellular protein kinases. *J. Biol. Chem.* 262: 13674–13681.

Wiedmer, T., Esmon, C. T., and Sims, P. J (1986a) Complement proteins C5b-9 stimulate pro-coagulant activity through platelet prothrombinase. *Blood* 68:875–880.

Wiedmer, T., Esmon, C. T., and Sims, P. J. (1986b) On the mechanism by which complement proteins C5b-9 increase platelet prothrombinase activity. *J. Biol. Chem.* 261:14587–14592.

Wiedmer, T., and Sims, P. J. (1985) Effect of complement proteins C5b-9 on blood platelets. Evidence for reversible depolarization of membrane potential *J. Biol. Chem.* 260:8014–8019.

9

Chemoattractant Receptor–G-Protein Coupling

KATHARINA WENZEL-SEIFERT and ROLAND SEIFERT

General Principles of Chemoattractant-Mediated Signal Transduction

Chemoattractants and Chemoattractant Receptors

The "professional phagocytes", that is, neutrophils, basophils, eosinophils, monocytes, and macrophages, play key roles in host defense against invading bacteria (Rossi, 1986; Seifert and Schultz, 1991). The importance of phagocytes in host defense is highlighted by chronic granulomatous disease in which certain components of the superoxide anion (O_2^-)-generating ("respiratory burst") NADPH oxidase are defective (Seifert and Schultz, 1991; Malech et al., 1997). Patients with chronic granulomatous disease suffer from increased susceptibility to bacterial infections and develop chronic granulomas which are name-giving for the disease. Moreover, the activity of phagocytes has been implicated in the pathogenesis of nonbacterial diseases such as myocardial infarction, emphysema, rheumatoid arthritis, and psoriasis (Malech and Callin, 1987; Weiss, 1989).

Phagocytes are activated by numerous particulate and soluble stimuli. Classic soluble phagocyte activators are the chemoattractants *N*-formyl-*L*-methionyl-*L*-leucyl-*L*-phenylalanine (fMLP), complement C5a, interleukin 8 (IL-8), platelet-activating factor (PAF), and leukotriene B_4 (LTB_4). The term *chemoattractant* derives from the fact that phagocytes migrate along a concentration gradient of fMLP, complement C5a, IL-8, PAF, or LTB_4 (Dillon et al., 1988). When chemoattractants are present at high concentrations, they activate cytotoxic functions of phagocytes (Rossi, 1986; Dillon et al., 1988; Seifert et al., 1991; Klinker et al., 1996b). Specifically, phagocytes generate oxygen radicals and release lysosomal enzymes such as elastase, lysozyme, and acid hydrolases. In conjunction, these cytotoxic products destroy invading microorganisms and can also damage host tissue.

Complement C5a, IL-8, PAF, and LTB_4 are endogenous chemoattractants (Seifert et al., 1991), whereas fMLP and structurally related formyl peptides are produced in bacteria such as *Escherichia coli* and *Staphylococcus aureus* (Marasco et al., 1984; Marasco and Ward, 1988). Based on these findings, one might assume a crucial role for the formyl peptide receptor (FPR) in the clearance of bacterial infections. In phagocytes, the FPR may be expressed at levels as high as ~ 5 pmol/mg of membrane protein (Wenzel-Seifert et al., 1999). This number implies that the FPR is a receptor with one of the highest physiological expression levels reported so far. However, relatively little is known about the role of formyl peptides and the FPR in vivo. Only recently has it been demonstrated conclusively that the FPR does play a crucial role in host defense against bacterial infections. Specifically, mice lacking the *FPR* gene (*FPR* knockout mice) show increased susceptibility to infection with *Listeria monocytogenes* (Gao et al., 1999). Future studies will have to determine whether the lack of the FPR generally increases susceptibility to bacterial infections. Some reports suggest that formyl peptides are also released from damaged mitochondria (Carp, 1982; Shawar et al., 1995), but the pathophysiological role of endogenous formyl peptides is unknown.

Although the FPR is a classic phagocyte receptor, it is now recognized that the FPR is expressed more broadly, that is, in parenchymal cells of the liver, medial tissue cells of the human coronary artery, interstitial cells of the rabbit right atrium, astrocytes, microglia cells, endocrine cells, smooth muscle cells, endothelial cells, and colonic cells (Rotrosen et al., 1987; Dunkel et al., 1989; LeDuc et al., 1994; Lacy et al., 1995; McCoy et al., 1995; Keitoku et al., 1997; Becker et al., 1998). The expression of FPRs is increased in multiple sclerosis lesions (Müller-Ladner et al., 1996), and formyl peptides can induce contraction of smooth muscle cells (Marasco et al., 1982; Keitoku et al., 1997). These data point to a rather general role of the FPR in the regulation of various physiological and pathological processes. However, little is known about the G-protein coupling of, and signal transduction induced by, FPRs expressed in nonphagocytic cells. The expression of the complement C5a receptor (C5aR), IL-8 receptors, PAF receptor (PAFR) and LTB_4 receptor (BLTR) is also not confined to phagocytes (Gerard and Gerard, 1991; Murphy, 1994).

Figure 9.1 presents a scheme of some of the initial events of chemoattracant-mediated signal transduction exemplified for the FPR. The FPR, C5aR, IL-8 receptors, PAFR, and BLTR share a high degree of homology with each other and belong to the family 1b of G-protein–coupled receptors (GPCRs; Boulay et al., 1990a, 1990b, 1991; Gerard and Gerard, 1991; Murphy, 1994; Yokomizo et al., 1997; Bockaert and Pin, 1999). GPCRs possess seven transmembrane domains (TM-I through TM-VII), three extracellular loops (e1, e2, and e3), and three intracellular loops (i1, i2, and i3; Murphy, 1994; Wess, 1997; Bockaert and Pin, 1999). The receptor N-terminal faces toward the extracellular space and is, for most chemoattractant receptors, glycosylated, whereas the C-terminal is localized intracellularly. Upon binding of the appropriate agonist, chemoattractant receptors undergo a conformational change that enables them to interact with pertussis toxin (PTX)-sensitive G-proteins of the G_i-family (Seifert and Schultz, 1991; Klinker et al., 1996b). PTX blocks the interaction of chemoattractant receptors with G_i-proteins (Dillon et al., 1988; Seifert and Schultz, 1991; Klinker et al., 1996b). The fact that PTX inhibits most of the stimulatory effects of chemoattractants in intact phagocytes and phagocyte membranes (Dillon et al., 1988; Seifert

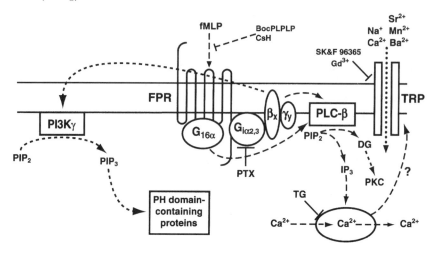

Fig. 9.1. Overview on some of the initial events of FPR-mediated signal transduction in phagocytes: The signal transduction pathways activated by fMLP, IL-8, complement C5a, LTB$_4$, and PAF are similar. The precise roles of defined G-protein βγ-complexes (β$_x$γ$_y$) in chemoattractant-mediated signal transduction are not yet well defined. A physiological role of G$_{16α}$ in chemoattractant-mediated signal transduction is not yet established. G$_{16α}$ is only included in this scheme because in transfection systems, chemoattractant receptors have been shown to couple to G$_{16α}$. *Abbreviations:* BocPLPLP, *N-t*-butoxycarbonyl-*L*-phenylalanyl-*L*-leucyl-*L*-phenylalanyl-*L*-leucyl-*L*-phenylalanine; CsH, cyclosporin H; DG, 1,2-diacylglycerol; fMLP, *N*-formyl-*L*-methionyl-*L*-leucyl-*L*-phenylalanine; FPR, formyl peptide receptor; IP$_3$, inositol-1,4,5-trisphosphate; PH domain, pleckstrin homology domain; PI3Kγ, phosphoinositide 3-kinase-γ; PIP$_2$, phosphatidylinositol-4,5-bisphosphate; PIP$_3$ phosphatidylinositol-3,4,5-trisphosphate; PKC, protein kinase C; PLC-β, β-isoenzymes of the phospholipase C family; TG, thapsigargin; TRP, mammalian homologues of the *Drosophila* transient receptor potential channels.

and Schultz, 1991; Klinker et al., 1996b) highlights the eminent importance of G$_i$-proteins in chemoattractant receptor-mediated signaling.

In expression systems, chemoattractant receptors have also been shown to couple efficiently to the G-protein G$_{16α}$. G$_{16α}$ mediates PTX-insensitive phospholipase C (PLC) activation, but the physiological importance of G$_{16α}$ in phagocytes is elusive.

During the past decade, a number of antagonists for chemoattractant receptors has been identified or specifically engineered. These antagonists compete with chemoattractants for binding to the respective receptors, thereby preventing chemoattractant-mediated cell activation. Selective antagonists are available for the FPR (Wenzel-Seifert and Seifert, 1993; De Paulis et al., 1996; Wenzel-Seifert et al., 1998a), C5aR (Konteatis et al., 1994; Pellas et al., 1998; Wong et al., 1998), IL-8 receptors (Jones et al., 1997; White et al., 1998), PAFR (Liao et al., 1997; Tavet et al., 1997), and BLTR (Daines et al., 1996; Showell et al., 1998). Given the importance of chemoattractants as phagocyte activators and the importance of phagocytes in the pathogenesis of numerous nonbacterial diseases (Malech and Gallin, 1987; Weiss, 1989), one could envisage several therapeutic applications of chemoattractant receptor antagonists. Some chemoattractant receptor antagonists are already under clinical investigation, specifically, BLTR antagonists (Liston et al., 1998; Showell et al., 1998). The neuropeptide spinorphin and a retrovirus-derived hexapeptide are formyl peptide receptor (FPR) antagonists (Oostendorp et al., 1992; Yamamoto et al., 1997). These findings suggest that efficient natural mechanisms exist to prevent excessive activation of FPRs.

G_i-Proteins and Phospholipase C Activation

All G-proteins consist of an α-subunit and a $\beta\gamma$-complex (Gilman, 1987; Birnbaumer et al., 1990; Gudermann et al., 1997). G-proteins are classified according to their α-subunits; phagocytes express G-proteins of the G_s-, G_i- and G_q-families.

G_i-proteins are the most abundant and important G-proteins in phagocytes because they mediate most, if not all, of the stimulatory effects of chemoattractants. There are three $G_{i\alpha}$ genes ($G_{i\alpha1}$, $G_{i\alpha2}$, and $G_{i\alpha3}$). Myeloid cells express only $G_{i\alpha2}$ and $G_{i\alpha3}$, with $G_{i\alpha2}$ being much more abundant than $G_{i\alpha3}$ (Didsbury et al., 1987; Murphy et al., 1987; Gierschik et al., 1989a; Klinker et al., 1994). $G_{i\alpha2}$ has a lower guanosine 5'-diphosphate (GDP)-affinity than $G_{i\alpha1}$ and $G_{i\alpha3}$ (Carty et al., 1990; Linder et al., 1990). The differential expression of $G_{i\alpha}$ subunits in phagocytes (Didsbury et al., 1987; Murphy et al., 1987; Gierschik et al., 1989a; Klinker et al., 1994), the known biochemical properties of $G_{i\alpha}$ isoforms (Carty et al., 1990; Linder et al., 1990), and the fact that the $G_{i\alpha2}$ knockout mouse shows a specific phenotype i.e., an ulcerative colitis (Rudolph et al., 1995), point to different functions of $G_{i\alpha2}$ and $G_{i\alpha3}$ in the regulation of phagocyte functions. Using fusion proteins of the FPR and $G_{i\alpha1}$, $G_{i\alpha2}$, and $G_{i\alpha3}$, respectively, a system that ensures defined GPCR/G-protein ratio and efficient coupling (Seifert et al., 1999c), we failed to detect differences in the interaction of the FPR with the three $G_{i\alpha}$ subunits (Wenzel-Seifert, 1999). However, this result should not be generalized to conclude that there is no specificity in the coupling of chemoattractant receptors to $G_{i\alpha}$ proteins (see section on differential coupling of chemoattractant receptors to G_i-proteins). To elucidate the precise roles of $G_{i\alpha1}$, $G_{i\alpha2}$, and $G_{i\alpha3}$ in signal transduction, it will be necessary to study the coupling of all permutations of chemoattractant receptors with the three $G_{i\alpha}$-proteins in appropriate expression systems such as Sf9 cells (see section on model systems for the analysis of chemoattractant receptor/G-protein coupling).

There are 5 different G-protein β-subunits and 11 G-protein γ-subunits that, in principle, allow for the formation of a vast number of G_i-protein heterotrimers (Simon et al., 1991; Gudermann et al., 1997). Human neutrophils express $G_{\beta3}$ (Virchow et al., 1998). $G_{\beta3}$ exists as a long splice variant ($G_{\beta3-l}$, the normal wild-type protein) and a short splice variant ($G_{\beta3-s}$, Siffert et al., 1998). $G_{\beta3-s}$ has been linked to the pathogenesis of hypertension and is more efficient than $G_{\beta3-1}$ at promoting binding of the hydrolysis-resistant guanosine 5'-triphosphate (GTP) analogue guanosine 5'-O-(3-thiotriphosphate) (GTPγS) to $G_{i\alpha2-s}$ expressed in Sf9 insect cells (Siffert et al., 1998). Neutrophils expressing $G_{\beta3-s}$ show enhanced fMLP-stimulated chemotaxis, whereas fMLP-stimulated increases in cytosolic Ca^{2+} concentration ($[Ca^{2+}]_i$) are diminished (Virchow et al., 1998). In contrast to neutrophils, HL-60 cells differentiated with dimethyl sulfoxide or with dimethyl sulfoxide plus retinoic acid do not express $G_{\beta3}$, but do express $G_{\beta1}$, $G_{\beta2}$, and $G_{\beta4}$ (Iiri et al., 1995; Nürnberg et al., 1996). Dimethyl sulfoxide-differentiated HL-60 cells express $G_{\gamma5}$, and $G_{\gamma7}$ but not $G_{\gamma2}$ (Iiri et al., 1995). Retinoic acid specifically induces the expression of $G_{\gamma2}$ (Iiri et al., 1995). $\beta\gamma$-Complex derived from dimethyl sulfoxide-plus retinoic acid-differentiated HL-60 cells is more efficient than $\beta\gamma$-complex from dimethyl sulfoxide-differentiated HL-60 cells at supporting high-affinity [^{3}H]fMLP binding and phospholipase C (PLC) activation (Iiri et al., 1995). Taken together, these data demonstrate differential expression of G-protein β- and γ-subunits in various myeloid cell types and point to specific roles of individual $\beta_x\gamma_y$-complexes in chemoattractant receptor-mediated signal transduction.

Upon activation by a receptor agonist, G-proteins dissociate into the α-subunit and the $\beta\gamma$-complex (Gilman, 1987; Birnbaumer et al., 1990). (The G-protein activation/deactivation cycle is explained in detail later.) In human myeloid cells, G-protein $\beta\gamma$-complexes released from G_i-protein heterotrimers activate PLC-$\beta2$ and, to a lesser extent, PLC-$\beta3$ (Camps et al., 1992; Jiang et al., 1996). (see Figure 9.1) PLC cleaves phosphatidylinositol-4,5-bisphosphate (PIP$_2$) into 1,2-diacylglycerol (DG) and inositol-1,4,5-trisphosphate (IP$_3$; Dillon et al., 1988). IP$_3$ mobilizes Ca^{2+} from nonmitochondrial stores, and DG activates Ca^{2+}-dependent and Ca^{2+}-independent protein kinase C isoenzymes. Protein kinase C isoenzymes play important and differential roles in the activation of cytotoxic effector functions of neutrophils, that is, exocytosis and O_2^- formation (Seifert and Schultz, 1991; Wenzel-Seifert et al., 1994; Mayer et al., 1996). The importance of the PLC pathway in the activation of O_2^- formation is highlighted by results obtained with the knockout mouse lacking both PLC-$\beta2$ and PLC-$\beta3$. In particular, neutrophils of these mice show a complete deficiency of fMLP-stimulated O_2^- formation (Li et al., 2000).

Activation of chemotaxis by chemoattractant receptors via G_i-proteins is dependent on the release of $\beta\gamma$-subunits, but there is no known specific role of $G_{i\alpha}$-subunits per se in the activation of chemotaxis (Neptune and Bourne, 1997; Neptune et al., 1999). Only $\beta\gamma$-subunits released from G_i-proteins but not $\beta\gamma$-subunits released from G-proteins of other families can mediate chemotaxis (Neptune et al., 1999). An explanation for this observation could be that chemoattractant receptors and G_i-proteins are in very close contact to each other and segregated from other G-proteins in specific membrane compartments (see section on localization of signaling components). Alternatively, or in addition, $G_{i\alpha}$ may interact with unique $\beta_x\gamma_y$-complexes that specifically mediate activation of chemotaxis.

Although chemotaxis is clearly $\beta\gamma$-dependent, migration is not impaired in the PLC-β2- and PLC-β3 knockout mouse (Li et al., 2000). These data point to the importance of other signaling pathways in the activation of chemotaxis. In fact, βγ-subunits also activate phosphoinositide 3-kinase-γ (PI3Kγ) (Toker and Cantley, 1997; Condliffe et al., 2000; Dekker and Segal, 2000) (see Fig. 9.1.). PI3Kγ catalyzes the phosphorylation of PIP_2 to phosphatidylinositol-3,4,5-trisphosphate (PIP_3). PIP_3 binds to proteins containing pleckstrin homology (PH) domains, resulting in down-stream signaling. As an example, protein kinase B (PKB) is a well-known effector of PI3Kγ, and upon exposure to chemoattractants, PKB is translocated to the leading edge of neutrophils (Servant et al., 2000). Other effectors regulated by PI3Kγ include low-molecular mass GTP binding proteins of the *rho* family (Servant et al., 2000; Condliffe et al., 2000; Dekker and Segal, 2000). Recently, three groups have convincingly demonstrated that PI3Kγ plays a central role in the regulation of both neutrophil chemotaxis and O_2^- formation. Specifically, PI3Kγ-knockout mice show severely impaired chemotaxis and O_2^- formation upon exposure to chemoattractants (Sasaki et al., 2000; Li et al., 2000; Hirsch et al., 2000).

Regulation of Cation Entry Pathways

As indicated previously, IP_3 mobilizes Ca^{2+} from nonmitochondrial Ca^{2+} stores, thereby inducing a transient increase in $[Ca^{2+}]_i$. Subsequent to chemoattractant-induced Ca^{2+} mobilization from intracellular stores, a sustained influx of cations through the plasma membrane takes place (see Fig. 9.1). The cations that cross the plasma membrane of phagocytes upon chemoattractant activation are Ca^{2+} and Na^+ (physiological cations) as well as Mn^{2+}, Ba^{2+} and Sr^{2+} (cations used as experimental tools; Merritt et al., 1989, 1990; Demaurex et al., 1992, 1994; Krautwurst et al., 1992; Wenzel-Seifert et al., 1996a, 1996b, 1997a). Cation entry can be blocked by lanthanides, specifically Gd^{3+}, and imidazoles, specifically SK&F 96363 (1-[β-[3-(4-methoxyphenyl)propoxy]4-methoxyphenylethyl]-1*H*-imidazole hydrochloride) and antimycotics such as econazole (Merritt et al., 1990; Krautwurst et al., 1992; Wenzel-Seifert et al., 1996a, 1996b, 1997a).

By analyzing the effects of the removal of Ca^{2+} and Na^+ alone or in combination from the extracellular medium and by studying the effects of cation-entry inhibitors, it has been clearly shown that both Ca^{2+} and Na^+ influx play crucial roles in the activation of NADPH oxidase and lysosomal enzyme release by chemoattractants (Krautwurst et al., 1992; Wenzel-Seifert et al., 1996a, 1996b). Although the mechanisms by which Ca^{2+} acts as intracellular signal molecule are well defined, for example, by activating calmodulin or Ca^{2+}-dependent protein kinase C isoenzymes (Dillon et al., 1988; Seifert et al., 1991), the mechanism of action of Na^+ remains poorly defined. Possibly, Na^+ alters GPCR-G-protein coupling by stabilizing receptors in an inactive (R) state.

There is considerable interest in the mechanisms by which chemoattractant-induced cation entry is accomplished. A commonly accepted hypothesis assumes that cation entry is regulated by Ca^{2+} store depletion. This cation entry pathway is, therefore, also referred to as *capacitative* Ca^{2+} entry or *calcium release-activated calcium entry* (CRAC) (Fasolato et al., 1994). Experimental support for this model comes from the fact that thapsigargin (TG) and cyclopiazonic acid, which both deplete intracellular Ca^{2+} stores by inhibiting the re-uptake of Ca^{2+} through the Ca^{2+} ATPase, are efficient activators of cation entry in phagocytes (Demaurex et al., 1992, 1994; Wenzel-Seifert et al., 1996b). The precise molecular mechanism by which TG activates cation entry is, however, still unknown. It has been suggested that Ca^{2+} store depletion generates a diffusible signal molecule (calcium influx factor, or CIF) that ultimately activates cation entry across the plasma membrane (Csutora et al., 1999). Recent results indicate that a direct physical interaction of intracellular Ca^{2+} stores with the cation channels in the plasma membrane is essential for activation of cation entry from the extracellular space (Ma et al., 2000).

It was postulated that chemoattractants and Ca^{2+}-ATPase inhibitors activate cation entry through a common mechanism (Demaurex et al., 1992, 1994). However, the detailed comparison of the effects of fMLP and TG on cation entry in phagocytes revealed several differences between the two stimuli. Most importantly, various cation entry blockers have different effects on fMLP- and TG-stimulated cation entry (Wenzel-Seifert et al., 1996b, 1997a), and GPCR-mediated cation entry can occur independently of Ca^{2+} mobilization from intracellular stores (Seifert et al., 1994; Burde and Seifert, 1996). These findings suggest that TG and fMLP activate cation entry through different mechanisms, and that phagocytes possess multiple types of cation channels (Wenzel-Seifert et al., 1996a, 1996b, 1997a). Most likely, the cation channels in phagocytes are mammalian homologues of the *Drosophila* transient receptor potential (TRP) channels (Birnbaumer et al., 1996; Montell, 1997).

The question whether phagocyte cation channels are under the direct control of G-proteins is unanswered, too. The fact that PTX inhibits chemoattractant-induced cation entry (Krautwurst et al., 1992; Wenzel-Seifert et al., 1996b) clearly points to the involvement of G_i-proteins in the signaling cascade, but evidence for a direct interaction of either $G_{i\alpha}$-subunits or $\beta\gamma$-subunits with cation channels has not been obtained. It is noteworthy that even cation entry activated by stimuli that bypass chemoattractant receptors, that is, TG and the *Aeromonas hydrophila* toxin aerolysin, is at least partially PTX-sensitive (Wenzel-Seifert et al., 1996b; Krause et al., 1998). These data could point to the involvement of constitutively active chemoattractant receptors and agonist-independent G_i-protein activation as tonic signals for cation channel stimulation in general (see section on constitutive activity of chemoattractant receptors). Finally, there is a feedback regulation between the activation of cation entry and NADPH oxidase stimulation. Specifically, the membrane depolarization accompanying O_2^- formation inhibits cation entry (Geiszt et al., 1997). This mechanism explains the inhibitory effect of fMLP and other activators of O_2^- formation on TG-induced cation entry (Wenzel-Seifert et al., 1996a; Geiszt et al., 1997). Because neutrophils from patients with chronic granulomatous disease cannot generate O_2^-, these cells also lack the chemoattractant-induced inhibition of cation entry (Geiszt et al., 1997).

G_i-Protein Regulation of Adenylyl Cyclase and NADPH Oxidase

Historically, G_i-proteins had been named because of their ability to *inhibit* adenylyl cyclase (AC; Gilman, 1987; Birnbaumer et al., 1990). Although chemoattractants all efficiently activate G_i-proteins, and although $G_{i\alpha}$-subunits can inhibit the activity of certain AC isoforms (Sunahara et al., 1996), there is no convincing evidence that fMLP, complement C5a, IL-8, LTB_4, or PAF can inhibit AC in intact human myeloid cells or cell membranes (Seifert and Schultz, 1991). In view of these data and the importance of G_i-protein $\beta\gamma$-subunits in PLC activation (Camps et al., 1992; Jiang et al., 1996), the term G_i-proteins in the context of phagocyte physiology is certainly misleading. As indicated previously, $G_{i\alpha}$-subunits inhibit only some, but not all, AC isoforms (Sunahara et al., 1996). Thus, the lack of inhibitory effect of chemoattractants on AC activity in phagocytes could be explained by the absence of appropriate AC isoenzyme in phagocytes. This view is supported by the fact that the FPR has the potential to mediate AC inhibition in certain mammalian expression systems (Uhing et al., 1992; Lang et al., 1993). However, to our knowledge, the expression pattern of AC isoforms in phagocytes has not yet been studied. This is quite amazing in view of the fact that neutrophils are a classic system for studying AC activation by G_s-protein-coupled receptors such as the β_2-adrenergic receptor (β_2AR) prostaglandin I- and E-type receptors and histamine H_2-receptors (Seifert and Schultz, 1991).

The role of $G_{i\alpha}$-subunits in the regulation of NADPH oxidase is still an unresolved issue. The fact that in cell-free systems, stable GTP analogues potentiate fatty acid-stimulated O_2^- formation (Seifert and Schultz, 1991), that GTP analogues are efficient activators of G-proteins (Gilman, 1987; Birnbaumer et al., 1990), and that chemoattractant-stimulated O_2^- formation is PTX-sensitive, gave rise to the hypothesis that the phagocyte NADPH oxidase is under the direct control of G_i-proteins (Seifert et al., 1986). However, it has been convincingly shown that the low-molecular mass GTP-binding proteins *rac1* and *rac2* directly regulate NADPH oxidase (see Seifert and Schultz, 1991, for a historical perspective). Nonetheless, it has never been specifically addressed whether in addition to *rac* proteins, $G_{i\alpha}$-proteins are also involved in NADPH oxidase activation. Recent support for a possible direct role of $G_{i\alpha}$-subunits in NADPH oxidase activation comes from studies on the H_2O_2-generating NADPH oxidase of human adipocytes. This NADPH oxidase can be directly activated by $G_{i\alpha2}$ (Krieger-Brauer et al., 1997). Considering that there is still no defined role of $G_{i\alpha}$-subunits in the regulation of effector systems in phagocytes, it is certainly worthwhile to study the effects of purified $G_{i\alpha}$-proteins on the phagocyte NADPH oxidase in cell-free systems.

Chemoattractant Receptor–G-Protein Coupling

Model Systems for the Analysis of Chemoattractant Receptor–G-Protein Coupling

During the past 15 years, chemoattractant-mediated signal transduction has been studied in considerable detail using native phagocytes, cultured phagocyte cell lines, and recombinant systems. Human, rabbit, and guinea pig neutrophils are classic native models for studying chemoattractant receptors, and accordingly, many studies have been performed with those cells, both at the intact cell level and the membrane level (Showell et al., 1976; Okajima et al., 1985; Feltner et al., 1986; Wilde et al., 1989; Kanaho et al., 1990; Wenzel-Seifert et al., 1991). An advantage of neutrophils is that they represent physiologically relevant cells, but a drawback of experiments with neutrophils is that they cannot be used to specifically express defined signaling proteins, and there can be substantial batch-to-batch variability in the responsiveness of cells (Seifert et al., 1991). Studies with monocytes, eosinophils, and basophils, which all express different chemoattractant receptors, are limited by the availability of cells in sufficient purity and quantity (Seifert and Schultz, 1991).

To overcome the difficulties associated with experiments using native blood cells, numerous studies were performed with cultured cell lines, specifically U937 leukemia cells and HL-60 leukemia cells. HL-60 leukemia cells are promyelocytes that can be differentiated toward neutrophils and monocytes (Klinker et al., 1996b). U937 leukemia cells can be differentiated only toward monocytes (Seifert et al., 1992b; Kew et al., 1997; Wenzel-Seifert et al., 1997b). HL-60 and U937 cells can be grown in large quantities using suspension culture techniques. HL-60 and U937 cells have been successfully used to clone the cDNAs of several chemoattractant receptors (Boulay et al., 1990a, 1991; Gerard and Gerard, 1991; Murphy and Tiffany, 1991; Yokomizo et al., 1997), to study differentiation-dependent signaling (Klinker et al., 1996b) and to analyze chemoattractant receptor–G-protein coupling both on the cellular and membrane level (Gierschik et al., 1989a, 1989b, 1989c, 1991; McLeish et al., 1989b; Klinker et al., 1996b). However, it should be emphasized that there are several functional differences between differentiated HL-60 cells and mature neutrophils, and that HL-60 cells differentiated with retinoic acid, dimethyl sulfoxide, and dibutyryl cAMP all have different phenotypes (Iiri et al., 1995; Klinker et al., 1996b).

With the cloning of cDNAs of various chemoattractant receptors, these GPCRs became available for functional analysis in mammalian expression systems (Boulay et al., 1990a, 1991; Gerard and Gerard, 1991; Prossnitz et al., 1991; Lang et al., 1993; Ali et al., 1998) and insect cells (Quehenberger et al., 1992; Wenzel-Seifert et al., 1998a). When expressed in RINm5F insulinoma cells, mouse 2071 fibroblasts and human embryonic cells (HEK293 cells), the expressed FPR mediates PTX-sensitive PLC activation as it does in native phagocytes, HL-60 cells, and U937 cells (Prossnitz et al., 1991; Didsbury et al., 1992; Lang et al., 1993). Despite the fact that COS-7 cells endogenously express G_i-proteins, the FPR and C5aR do not induce PTX-sensitive

PLC activation in these cells (Jiang et al., 1996). The failure of the FPR and C5aR to mediate PTX-sensitive PLC activation in COS-7 cells can be explained by the fact that these cells express only PLC-β3, but not PLC-β2 and that PLC-β3 is less sensitive to activation by G-protein–βγ-complexes than PLC-β2 (Jiang et al., 1996). In fact, the FPR and C5aR induce a PTX-sensitive PLC activation in COS-7 cells when co-expressed with PLC-β2. FPR- and C5aR-mediated PLC activation in COS-7 cells can also be reconstituted by coexpression of the receptors with $G_{16\alpha}$ (Amatruda et al., 1993; Offermanns and Simon, 1995). This PLC activation is PTX-insensitive. In contrast to the FPR and C5aR, the PAFR can mediate PLC activation also via the endogenous G_q-proteins of COS-7 cells (Amatruda et al., 1993). In Chinese hamster ovary (CHO) cells, the BLTR mediates a largely PTX-insensitive PLC activation without coexpression of $G_{16\alpha}$ being required (Yokomizo et al., 1997). The identity of the G-protein mediating this BLTR response is not known, but the results of cotransfection studies suggest that the BLTR does not couple to $G_{q\alpha}/G_{11\alpha}$ (Gaudreau et al., 1998). Collectively, these data show that the reconstitution of chemoattractant receptor-mediated PLC activation in commonly employed mammalian expression systems is strongly dependent on the specific complement of G-proteins and PLC-β isoforms of the host cells.

The functional reconstitution of chemoattractant receptors is even species-dependent. In particular, the rabbit FPR can be readily reconstituted in *Xenopus laevis* oocytes (Thomas et al., 1990), a commonly used system for expression cloning of GPCRs, whereas the human and murine FPR cannot be reconstituted in this system without an additional cofactor encoded by mRNA from undifferentiated HL-60 cells (Murphy and McDermott, 1991; Schultz et al., 1992; Gao and Murphy, 1993). A subsequent study identified the cofactor from HL-60 cells as the G-protein $G_{16\alpha}$ (Burg et al., 1995). Thus, the rabbit FPR can couple to the endogenous G-proteins of the *Xenopus laevis* oocytes, whereas the human and murine FPR cannot. In this context it should be noted that the FPRs from humans, rabbits, and mice are structurally quite divergent (Thomas et al., 1990; Murphy and McDermott, 1991; Gao and Murphy, 1993). Moreover, the affinity of the murine FPR for fMLP is much lower than the fMLP affinity of the human FPR (Gao and Murphy, 1993). These results point to species-specific adaptations of FPR function in host defense.

To circumvent problems associated with the availability of specific G-proteins and effectors, chemoattractant receptors have also been expressed in myeloid cells that provide a more natural complement of endogenous signaling proteins than the previously discussed expression systems. In fact, chemoattractant receptors could be reconstituted with the endogenous G_i-proteins of rat basophilic leukemia cells (RBL-2H3 cells; Hall et al., 1997; Ali et al., 1998), undifferentiated HL-60 cells (Prossnitz et al., 1993), and undifferentiated U937 cells (Kew et al., 1997). In the undifferentiated HL-60 cells and U937 cells, the transfected chemoattractant receptors did not only reconstitute, as expected, PTX-sensitive PLC activation, but also cell-type-specific responses, that is, differentiation and chemotaxis, respectively (Prossnitz et al., 1993; Kew et al., 1997). The reconstitution of cellular responses in HL-60 and U937 cells clearly documents the usefulness of these cells as expression systems for chemoattractant receptors.

A powerful approach to analyze chemoattractant receptor–G-protein coupling is to express both receptor and G-protein in a cell line of nonmammalian origin where there is no coupling of the receptor to the endogenous G-proteins of the host cell. Such a system has the evident advantage that the composition of the G-protein heterotrimer can be precisely controlled and questions regarding the specific functions of individual G-protein subunits can be addressed. The Sf9 insect cells provide a system that is devoid of mammalian-type G_i-proteins, and where the human FPR does not couple to the endogenous G_s- and G_q-like insect G-proteins (Quehenberger et al., 1992; Leopoldt et al., 1997; Wenzel-Seifert et al., 1998a, 1999). The human FPR expressed in Sf9 cells efficiently couples to the coexpressed mammalian G-protein heterotrimer $G_{i\alpha2}\beta_1\gamma_2$ (Wenzel-Seifert et al., 1998a). Additionally, there is efficient coupling between fusion proteins of the human FPR and the $G_{i\alpha}$-proteins $G_{i\alpha1}$, $G_{i\alpha2}$, and $G_{i\alpha3}$, respectively, expressed in Sf9 cells (Wenzel-Seifert et al., 1999). Thus, the Sf9 system is particularly useful to analyze systematically coupling of chemoattractant receptors to defined G-protein heterotrimers at the G-protein level, but complete reconstitution of the signaling cascade, including effectors, has not yet been accomplished. Because Sf9 cells have a low background of endogenous GPCR activity, nucleotidases, and G-proteins, these cells are also useful for the analysis of constitutive receptor activity (Seifert et al., 1998a, 1998b; Wenzel-Seifert et al., 1998a, 1999) (see section on constitutive activity of chemoattractant receptors).

By homologous recombination, mice deficient in the expression of defined chemoattractant receptors have been generated. Specifically, FPR-deficient mice are more susceptible to bacterial infection with *Listeria monocytogenes* than the wild-type animals, and neutrophils from FPR-deficient mice are not activated by fMLP (Gao et al., 1999). C5aR-deficient mice are very susceptible to pulmonary infection with *Pseudomonas aeruginosa* (Höpken et al., 1997). Surprisingly, mice deficient in the IL-8 receptor show an accumulation of mature and immature neutrophils in the spleen, pointing to an important role of the IL-8 receptor in myeloid differentiation processes (Cacalano et al., 1994). BLTR knockout mice show reduced eosinophil recruitment in thioglycollate-induced peritonitis (Tager et al., 2000). Thus, the quite different phenotypes of chemoattractant receptor-deficient mice indicate that the individual chemoattractant receptors play nonredundant roles in signal transduction. To our knowledge, PAFR knockout mice have not yet been reported, and we are not aware of studies in which chemoattractant receptors have been overexpressed in specific tissues by transgenic techniques. The BLTR has recently been implicated as a co-receptor for HIV-1 entry in CD4-positive cells (Owman et al., 1998). It remains to be determined whether BLTR antagonists are of any therapeutic value in the treatment of HIV-1 infection and whether other chemoattractant receptors have a similar function in HIV-1 entry as the BLTR.

G-Protein Activation/Deactivation Cycle

The mechanisms underlying receptor–G-protein coupling are principally the same for all GPCRs and G-proteins. The FPR, in addition to the βARs, is one of the best-studied receptors in this respect. The binding of an agonist to a GPCR induces a conformational change in the receptor that unmasks G-protein–interacting domains in the receptor (Gether et al., 1997). Generally, intracellular domains (specifically i2 and i3 and in some cases, the C-terminal) of a receptor are important for its coupling to G-proteins (Kobilka, 1992; Wess, 1997). The FPR possesses an exceptionally broad contact area for G-protein coupling, comprising i1–i3 and the C-terminal (Bommakanti et al., 1995). There is ample evidence that C-terminal regions of $G_{i\alpha}$-subunits are crucial for G-protein coupling to receptors (Gudermann et al., 1997; Iiri et al., 1998). This is highlighted by the mechanism of action of PTX. Specifically, PTX transfers a bulky ADP-ribose residue from NAD^+ to a cysteine residue at the extreme C-terminal of $G_{i\alpha}$-subunits (Gilman, 1987; Birnbaumer et al., 1990), thereby blocking the coupling of the FPR to G_i-proteins (Dillon et al., 1988; Seifert and Schultz, 1991).

Figure 9.2 illustrates the G-protein activation/deactivation cycle exemplified for the FPR. In step 1, the agonist-occupied FPR promotes the release of GDP from $G_{i\alpha}$-subunits. The release of GDP is believed to be the rate-limiting step of G-protein activation and generates guanine nucleotide-free G_α (Cassel and Selinger, 1978; Brandt and Ross, 1986; Wieland et al., 1992b). The agonist-occupied FPR, together with the guanine nucleotide-free G-protein heterotrimer, forms a *ternary complex*, which is characterized by a high agonist affinity (step 2); (Gierschik et al., 1989b, 1989c, 1991; Posner et al., 1994; Seifert et al., 1998a, 1999b; Wenzel-Seifert et al., 1998a). The receptor then catalyzes the binding of GTP to G_α (step 3a; Brandt and Ross, 1986; Gierschik et al., 1991; Iiri et al., 1998). Experimentally, the GTPase-resistant GTP analogue GTPγS (Gierschik et al., 1991; Wenzel-Seifert et al., 1998a) or the photoreactive GTP analogue GTP-azidoanlide (AA-GTP) (Offermanns et al., 1990; Klinker et al., 1994) are used instead of the natural and cleavable nucleotide to monitor GTP binding to G_α. A consequence of the binding of GTP or its analogue to G_α is the disruption of the ternary complex. Thereby, the agonist affinity of the receptor is reduced and the probability of agonist dissociation from the FPR increases (step 3b; Gierschik et al., 1989b, 1989c, 1991; Posner et al., 1994; Seifert et al., 1998a, 1999b; Wenzel-Seifert et al., 1998a). It is generally assumed that GTP/GTPγS binding to G_α impairs the interaction between the GPCR and the G-protein (Gilman, 1987; Birnbaumer et al., 1990), but this may not mean separation of the proteins. Specifically, discrepancies between the K_d values for high affinity [³H]fMLP binding and potencies of fMLP for activation of guanine nucleotide exchange suggest that even the FPR in a state of low agonist affinity can efficiently couple to G_i-proteins (Gierschik et al., 1989c; Offermanns et al., 1990; Wenzel-Seifert et al., 1998a, 1999). Similar conclusions were reached for the nociceptin receptor (Albrecht and Petty, 1998). In addition, there is circumstantial evidence that GPCRs can directly regulate the GTP

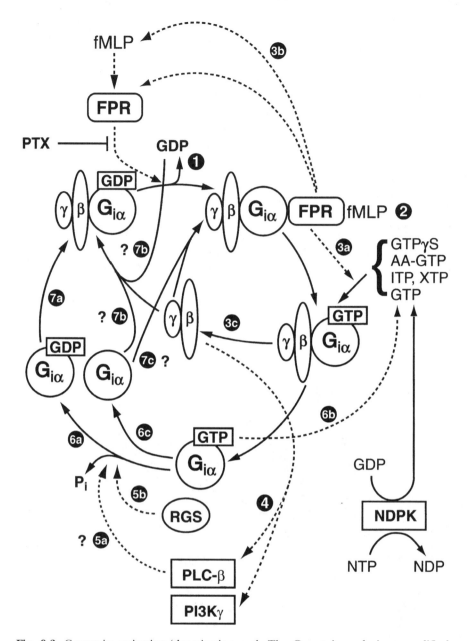

Fig. 9.2. G-protein activation/deactivation cycle: The G-protein cycle is exemplified for the FPR and G_i-proteins. The white numbers on black background define the individual steps of the cycle and are explained in detail in the text. Question marks indicate unresolved issues. Under physiological conditions, the FPR catalyzes the binding of GTP to $G_{i\alpha}$. However, several other natural nucleotides (XTP and ITP) and synthetic nucleotides (AA-GTP and GTPγS) can be used as experimental tools to analyze various aspects of the G-protein cycle and chemoattractant receptor-G-protein coupling. Abbreviations: AA-GTP, GTP-azidoanilide; fMLP, *N*-formyl-*L*-methionyl-*L*-leucyl-*L*-phenylalanine; FPR, formyl peptide receptor; GTPγS, guanosine 5'-O-(3-thiotriphosphate); NDP, nucleoside 5'-diphosphate; NDPK, nucleoside diphosphate kinase; NTP, nucleoside 5'-triphosphate; PI3Kγ, phosphoinositide 3-kinase-γ; PLC-β, β-isoenzymes of the phospholipase C family; PTX, pertussis toxin; RGS, regulators of G-protein signaling.

hydrolytic step of the G-protein cycle (step 6a; Wenzel-Seifert et al., 1998b; Seifert et al., 1999a). Such a regulation would imply that GPCRs have some physical contact with the G-protein through the entire G-protein cycle. Thus, it appears that guanine nucleotide binding to G_α modifies, but does not abrogate, G-protein interaction with GPCRs.

The binding of GTP or GTP analogue to G_α destabilizes the interaction between G_α and the $\beta\gamma$-complex, resulting in the generation of free, or at least functionally mobile, $\beta\gamma$-complex and GTP/GTP analogue-liganded G_α (step 3c; Birnbaumer et al., 1990). As discussed previously, $\beta\gamma$-complexes released from G_i-proteins activate PLC-β isoenzymes and PI3Kg (Camps et al., 1992; Jiang et al., 1996; Dekker and Segal 2000; Condliffe et al., 2000) (step 4), but an effector function for $G_{i\alpha}$ in phagocytes is yet unknown. Termination of G-protein activation is achieved by the GTPase of G_α, which cleaves GTP into GDP and inorganic phosphate (P_i) (step 6a; Gilman, 1987; Birnbaumer et al., 1990). GDP-liganded G_α and the $\beta\gamma$-complex reassociate, completing a G-protein activation/deactivation cycle (step 7a).

PLC and a novel class of proteins (Regulators of G-protein Signaling, RGS proteins) increase the intrinsic GTPase activity of G-protein α-subunits, thereby accelerating effector system shutdown (steps 5a and 5b; Berman et al., 1996a, 1996b; Biddlecome et al., 1996). Thus, RGS proteins and PLC can be considered GAP proteins (GTPase-Activating Proteins). The RGS proteins RGS1, RGS3, and RGS4 efficiently interact with G_i-proteins and block effector pathway activation by these G-proteins (Berman et al., 1996a, 1996b; Huang et al., 1997). Although the effects of RGS proteins on purified G_i-proteins in vitro have been well characterized, the role of RGS proteins in chemoattractant-mediated signal transduction is not yet completely understood. In lymphoid cells transiently expressing the FPR, RGS1, RGS3, and RGS4 efficiently inhibit fMLP-induced chemotaxis (Bowman et al., 1998). In addition, it has been shown that various human monocytic cell lines express RGS1 and that RGS1 added to membranes from monocytic cells greatly enhances steady-state GTP hydrolysis activated by several chemoattractant receptors (Denecke et al., 1999). These data are compatible with the concept that RGS proteins are negative regulators of chemoattractant receptor-coupled G_i-proteins. It should be noted that a GAP function of PLC has thus far only been documented for PLC-β1 and G_q, but not for PLC-β2 and PLC-β3 and G_i-proteins (Biddlecome et al., 1996).

Although it is generally recognized that the classic G-protein activation/deactivation cycle involves a GTPase step, the G-protein cycle can also proceed without a GTPase step as an association/dissociation cycle. The evidence for such an alternative G-protein cycle can be summarized as follows. Several GPCRs, including the FPR, not only stimulate the binding of GTPγS/guanosine 5'-[β,γ-imido]triphosphate (GppNHp) to G-proteins, but also stimulate the dissociation of GTPγS/GppNHp (step 6b; Cassel and Selinger, 1977; Hilf et al., 1992; Kupprion et al., 1993; Breivogel et al., 1998). Because GTPγS and GppNHp have high affinities for G_α (Gilman, 1987; Birnbaumer et al., 1990), it is conceivable that nucleotides with lower affinities for G_α than GTPγS, and GppNHp, such as GDP, GTP, inosine 5'-diphosphate (IDP), inosine 5'-triphosphate (ITP), and xanthosine 5'-triphosphate (XTP), dissociate from G-proteins even more rapidly (Florio and Sternweis, 1989; Seifert et al., 1999a). Unfortunately, because of their low affinity, it is technically very difficult, if not impossible, to monitor directly receptor-agonist–regulated dissociation of GDP, IDP, GTP, ITP, and XTP from G_i-proteins. Indirect evidence that nucleotide dissociation is an important G-protein deactivation mechanism comes from the observation that XTP can efficiently support activation of effector systems, but is not, or only slowly, hydrolyzed by G-proteins (Bilezikian and Aurbach, 1974; Howell et al., 1987; Stutchfield and Cockcroft, 1988; Klinker and Seifert, 1997; Seifert et al., 1999a).

An evident consequence of nucleotide dissociation from G_α as a deactivation step is the generation of nucleotide-free G_α (step 6c). It is an intriguing and yet unresolved question whether nucleotide-free G_α needs first to rebind GDP in order to be able to undergo another G-protein activation/deactivation cycle (step 7b) or whether nucleotide-free G_α is immediately available for another cycle without prior binding of GDP (step 7c). Should rebinding of GDP not be necessary, this would imply that GDP release (step 1) can not longer be the rate-limiting step of the G-protein activation/deactivation cycle. This would then point to the crucial importance of active GTP binding by GPCRs to G_α as the regulatory mechanism of G-protein activation (Brandt and Ross, 1986; Iiri et al., 1998). To explore GTPase-independent mechanisms of G_i-protein activation by chemoattractant receptors further, it will be necessary to study the GPCR-regulation of GTPase-deficient G_α-mutants (Wong et al., 1991).

It has been proposed that the FPR activates G_i-proteins catalytically, that is, one FPR molecule activates up to 20 G_i-proteins and, thereby, induces substantial signal amplification (Gierschik et al., 1991; Wieland et al., 1992a; Jacobs et al., 1995; Wenzel-Seifert et al., 1998a). This conclusion is based on the analysis of the maximum values (B_{max} values) of [³H]fMLP saturation binding and fMLP-stimulated GTPγS saturation binding. However, a recent study revealed that the [³H]fMLP binding assay grossly underestimates the true FPR expression level because a large fraction of the FPRs exists in a low-affinity state that cannot be detected in the binding assay, but functionally couples to G_i-proteins (Wenzel-Seifert et al., 1999). Therefore, one FPR molecule may not activate more than one G_i-protein. Signal transfer in phagocytes is rather linear than catalytical. Linear signal transfer could explain the different cellular responses of phagocytes over a broad range of agonist concentrations. Particularly, at low concentrations of fMLP, phagocytes migrate along the chemoattractant gradient to bacteria (Dillon et al., 1988). Once the phagocyte has reached the bacteria, the fMLP concentration increases, and cytotoxic functions including O_2^- formation and lysosomal enzyme release are activated, leading to the destruction of bacteria (Dillon et al., 1988; Seifert and Schultz, 1991). Linear signal transfer in phagocytes may prevent premature stimulation of cytotoxic cell functions and destruction of host tissue.

Constitutive Activity of Chemoattractant Receptors

Presently, the most widely accepted model of GPCR activation is the extended ternary complex model, also referred to as the *two-state model* (Lefkowitz et al., 1993; Leff, 1995). The two-state model assumes that GPCRs exist in equilibrium between an inactive state (R) and an active state (R*; Fig. 9.3A). In the R* state, GPCRs activate G-proteins and effectors. Receptor agonists stabilize the R* state and increase basal G-protein and effector activity, whereas inverse agonists and monovalent cations, specifically Na^+, stabilize the R state and decrease basal G-protein and effector activity (Costa et al., 1990; Tian et al., 1994).

The isomerization of a GPCR from R to R* does not only occur in the presence of an agonist, but also, to some extent, in the absence of an agonist. The agonist-independent (spontaneous) isomerization of a GPCR from R to R* is referred to as *constitutive activity* and results in the activation of a certain number of G-proteins and effectors. Thus, constitutive receptor activity substantially contributes to the basal G-protein and effector activity. Constitutive activity has been proven for numerous wild-type receptors, including the $\beta_2 AR$ (Chidiac et al., 1994; Gether et al., 1995; Seifert et al., 1998a), the histamine H_2-receptor (Smit et al., 1996) and δ-opioid receptor (Costa and Herz, 1989). In certain engineered and naturally occurring and disease-causing receptor mutants, the constitutive activity is much higher than in the corresponding wild-type receptors (Lefkowitz et al., 1993; Scheer and Cotecchia, 1997). Accordingly, such receptor mutants give rise to a very high basal G-protein and effector system activity that is otherwise only achieved with agonist stimulation.

It has long been assumed that the FPR is a constitutively active GPCR (Fig. 9.3B). This hypothesis is supported by the observation that PTX strongly suppresses various G-protein–dependent activities in intact phagocytes and phagocyte membranes (Brandt et al., 1983; Krause et al., 1985; Volpi et al., 1985; Gierschik et al., 1989b, 1991; Cowen et al., 1990; Sokoloski et al., 1991; Klinker et al., 1994). Since PTX selectively prevents the interaction of receptors with G_i-proteins (see Fig. 9.2), these data indicate efficient coupling of agonist-free FPRs (and/or other chemoattractant receptors) to G_i-proteins. Additionally, Na^+ efficiently reduces the basal G-protein activity in membranes expressing FPRs (Gierschik et al., 1989b, 1991), compatible with the assumption that Na^+ stabilizes the R state of the FPR.

Definitive proof for the constitutive activity of the FPR was obtained when an inverse agonist and a sensitive reconstitution system became available. By serendipity, cyclosporin H (CsH), a stereoisomer of the immunosuppressant cyclic undecapeptide cyclosporin A, was identified as highly efficient inverse agonist at the FPR coexpressed with $G_{i\alpha2}\beta_1\gamma_2$ in Sf9 insect cells. In contrast, the formyl peptide derivative *N-t*-butoxycarbonyl-*L*-phenylalanyl-*L*-leucyl-*L*-phenylalanyl-L-leucyl-L-phenylalanine (BocPLPLP) is a neutral FPR antagonist, and blocks the effects of both the agonist fMLP and the inverse agonist CsH without having an effect of its own on basal G_i-protein activity (Fig. 9.3B); Wenzel-Seifert et al., 1998a, 1999).

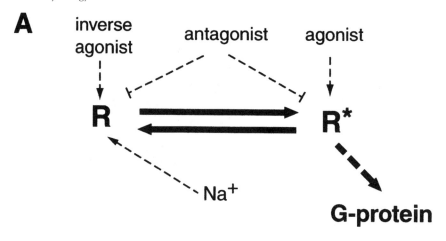

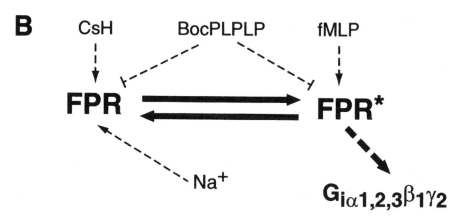

Fig. 9.3. The two-state model of GPCR activation:Panel A illustrates the general principles of the two-state model; panel B applies these principles specifically to the FPR. It is likely that other chemoattractant receptors than the FPR, specifically the C5aR, are also constitutively active. *Abbreviations*: BocPLPLP, *N-t*-butoxycarbonyl-*L*-phenylalanyl-*L*-leucyl-*L*-phenylalanyl-*L*-leucyl-*L*-phenylalanine; CsH, cyclosporin H; fMLP, *N*-formyl-*L*-methionyl-*L*-leucyl-*L*-phenyalalanine; FPR, formyl peptide receptor.

Na^+ is highly efficient at reducing basal GTPγS binding in Sf9 membranes, and in the presence of a maximally effective concentration of Na^+, CsH does not have a further inhibitory effect. These data support the assumption that CsH and Na^+ act through mechanisms that they have in common to stabilize the R state. By analogy to other GPCRs (Neve et al., 1991; Ceresa and Limbird, 1994), Na^+ presumably interacts with a highly conserved aspartate residue in TM-II (Asp71 in the FPR; Prossnitz et al., 1995b). It is noteworthy that the inhibitory effect of Na^+ on constitutive activity of the FPR is half-maximal at a concentration of 5 mmol/l and is almost maximal at 20 mmol/l. These Na^+ concentrations correspond to the intracellular free Na^+ concentrations observed in resting and fMLP-stimulated phagocytes, respectively (Wenzel-Seifert et al., 1996b). Thus, these data could provide a link between fMLP-induced Na^+ entry in phagocytes and the target of action of Na^+ as intracellular signal molecules. However, it should be emphasized that it is unknown whether Na^+ reaches its target in the receptor protein from the extracellular or intracellular side of the membrane, and how the access of Na^+ to the membrane-buried Asp71 is regulated.

The molecular basis for the high constitutive activity of the FPR is also unknown. The FPR exists in two isoforms (*i.e.*, FPR26 and FPR92; Boulay et al., 1990a), and so far, only FPR26 has been studied with regard to constitutive activity (Wenzel-Seifert et al., 1998a). FPR26 and FPR92 differ from each other in two amino acids, one localized in TM-III and the other localized in the receptor C-terminal. Changes in amino acid sequence in both locations can alter constitutive activity of GPCRs (Scheer and Cotecchia, 1997). It is now recognized that several GPCRs are polymorphic and that naturally occurring GPCR isoforms, although differing from each other only in one or two amino acids, may nonetheless show important differences in their ligand-binding and/or G-protein coupling properties (Büscher et al., 1999). Thus, it will be important to compare the constitutive activity of FPR26 to that of FPR92. These studies could provide valuable information about the structure–function relationship of the FPR.

It has been proposed that G-protein α-subunits have an impact on the constitutive activity of GPCRs (Seifert et al., 1998b). This hypothesis is based on the observation that the β_2AR coupled to the long splice variant of $G_{s\alpha}(G_{s\alpha L})$ but not the β_2AR coupled to the short splice variant of $G_{s\alpha}$ ($G_{s\alpha S}$) possesses the properties of a constitutively active GPCR (Seifert et al., 1998b). Differences in GDP-affinity of the two $G_{s\alpha}$-proteins provide the molecular basis for the differences in constitutive activity of the β_2AR. Particularly, $G_{s\alpha L}$ has a lower GDP-affinity than $G_{s\alpha S}$ (Seifert et al., 1998b). Thus, the GPCR activation energy required for dissociating GDP from $G_{s\alpha L}$ is lower than the corresponding energy required for dissociating GDP from $G_{s\alpha S}$. Experimentally, this results in an increased efficacy and potency of partial agonists and an increase in efficacy of inverse agonists at the $G_{s\alpha L}$-coupled β_2AR as compared to the corresponding ligand properties of the $G_{s\alpha S}$-coupled β_2AR.

$G_{i\alpha 2}$ has a lower GDP-affinity than $G_{i\alpha 1}$ and $G_{i\alpha 3}$ (Carty et al., 1990; Linder et al., 1990). By analogy to the observations made for G_s-proteins, one might have expected that the FPR coupled to $G_{i\alpha 2}$, but not the FPR coupled to $G_{i\alpha 1}$ or $G_{i\alpha 3}$ possesses the properties of a constitutively active GPCR. However, the FPR displays similarly high constitutive activity when coupled to all three G_i-proteins as assessed by partial agonist potencies and efficacies and inverse agonist efficacy (Wenzel-Seifert et al., 1999). These data show that with respect to $G_{i\alpha}$-proteins, G-protein GDP-affinity does not have an impact on constitutive activity of the FPR. Possibly, the intrinsic constitutive activity of the FPR is so high that modulation of constitutive activity of the FPR by GDP-affinity of G_i-proteins is too subtle to become effective.

Nevertheless, a C-terminally truncated FPR is constitutively active only with respect to a PTX-insensitive signaling pathway, but not with regard to G_i-protein–mediated signaling pathways. It is possible that defined G-protein βγ-complexes have an impact on the constitutive activity of the FPR. So far, the FPR has been reconstituted only with the $β_1γ_2$-complex (Wenzel-Seifert et al., 1998a). The $β_1γ_2$-complex increases the constitutive activity of the $β_2AR$ coupled to the long splice variant of $G_{sα}$ (Seifert et al., 1998a), and βγ-complexes containing $G_{γ2}$ are more efficient at promoting high-affinity [^{3}H]fMLP binding than βγ-complexes devoid of $G_{γ2}$ (Iiri et al., 1995). Thus, it will be very informative to analyze the impact of various βγ-dimers on constitutive activity of the FPR.

Among the chemoattractant receptors, constitutive activity does not seem to be restricted to the FPR. Specifically, a chimeric FPR, in which i1 of the FPR was replaced by i1 of the C5aR, gave rise to a higher basal PLC activity than wild-type FPR when the coupling to $G_{16α}$ was analyzed (Amatruda et al., 1995). These data suggest that the C5aR exhibits high constitutive activity and that i1 of chemoattractant receptors plays a crucial role in R to R* isomerization of the GPCRs. However, it is unknown whether the FPR chimera with i1 of the C5aR or native C5aR also display high constitutive activity when coupled to G_i-proteins. Given the fact that only two FPR antagonists had to be studied to identify an inverse agonist (Wenzel-Seifert et al., 1998a), it is likely that among the rather large number of available C5aR antagonists (Konteatis et al., 1994; Pellas et al., 1998; Wong et al., 1998), at least one compound will be identified as an inverse agonist at the C5aR.

The possible physiological relevance of the constitutive activity of chemoattractant receptors is still incompletely understood. The fact that PTX can reduce several G-protein–dependent basal activities in intact phagocytes points to the relevance of constitutive activity of chemoattractant receptors in vivo (Brandt et al., 1985; Krause et al., 1985; Volpi et al., 1985; Naccache et al., 1991; Sokoloski et al., 1991). Additional evidence for the physiological relevance of constitutive activity of chemoattractant receptors comes from studies dealing with the regulation of the expression of FPRs and G_i-proteins. Specifically, lipopolysaccharide and certain cytokines (i.e., interferon-γ, granulocyte-macrophage colony-stimulating factor, and tumor necrosis factor-α) increase the responsiveness of phagocytes to fMLP (Seifert and Schultz, 1991). This process is referred to as *priming*. The fact that cytokines also increase the expression level of FPRs and G_i-proteins in the plasma membrane (McLeish et al., 1991; Klein et al., 1992; Durstin et al., 1993; Klein et al., 1995) could provide a link to the observed cytokine-induced priming. In particular, a given cellular response requires a certain number of receptors in the R* state and active G-proteins. To achieve this, a specific concentration of fMLP is needed. An increase in the expression level of FPRs increases the absolute number of FPRs in the R* state as compared to the normal situation. As a result of the increased number of receptors in the R* state in the absence of an agonist, the threshold for achieving the required number of receptors in the R* state for effector activation is decreased; fMLP induces the biological response already at lower concentrations. In addition, when the expression level of G_i-proteins is increased, this facilitates stabilization of the R* state and pulls the equilibrium toward R*. Again, the result is that fMLP acts at a lower concentration than normally.

Both FPRs and G_i-proteins may be translocated to the plasma membrane from specific granules (Rotrosen et al., 1988; Sengelov et al., 1994), and G_i-proteins may additionally be recruited to the plasma membrane from the cytosol (Rudolph et al., 1989a, 1989b; see section on differential coupling). Finally, it should be noted that the increased expression of FPRs is not only observed under in vitro or cell culture conditions, but also in human disease (i.e., sepsis; Tschaikowsky et al., 1993).

Desensitization of Chemoattractant Receptors

It is well established that the responsiveness of GPCRs, following repeated exposure to the appropriate agonists, is diminished. This process is referred to as homologous desensitization and involves phosphorylation of the GPCRs by specific G-protein–coupled receptor kinases (GRKs). The mechanisms of GPCR desensitization in general (Lohse, 1993; Pitcher et al., 1998), and of chemoattractant receptor desensitization in particular (Ali et al., 1999), have been reviewed and will, therefore, not be dealt with in detail here.

Human phagocytes express several types of GRKs (GRK1, GRK2, GRK5, GRK6, and GRK7; Chuang et al., 1992; Haribabu et al., 1997). The C-terminal of the FPR is phosphorylated by GRK2 and GRK3, but not by GRK5 and GRK6 (Prossnitz et al., 1995a). *Homologous desensitization* is mediated by GRKs and impairs the coupling of the FPR to G_i-proteins and effectors (McLeish et al., 1989a; Seifert et al., 1989; Prossnitz, 1997). *Heterologous desensitization* involves phosphorylation of receptors by second messenger-activated protein kinases such as protein kinase C and protein kinase A (Lohse, 1993; Pitcher et al., 1998). Indeed, both protein kinases A and C exhibit inhibitory effects on chemoattractant phagocyte activation (Ervens et al., 1991; Seifert and Schultz, 1991). Within the class of chemoattractant receptors, a third type of desensitization has been defined, which is referred to as *receptor class desensitization* (Didsbury et al., 1991). Specifically, chemoattractant peptides desensitize the responses toward the lipid mediators PAF and LTB_4 whereas the lipid mediators do not desensitize the responses toward peptide chemoattractants. There is convincing evidence that desensitization of chemoattractant receptors is phosphorylation-dependent (Prossnitz, 1997), but in addition to that, there may also be phosphorylation-independent desensitization mechanisms (Richardson et al., 1998).

Methods to Study Chemoattractant Receptor–G-Protein Coupling

Because GDP release is assumed to be the rate-limiting step of G-protein activation (step 1 in Fig. 9.2), measuring GDP release provides the most proximal assay to monitor receptor–G-protein coupling at a molecular level. However, experimentally, it has been difficult to assess chemoattractant receptor-mediated GDP release from G_i-protein α-subunits directly. The reason for this difficulty is that GDP dissociates from G_i-proteins very rapidly under basal conditions (i.e., in the absence of agonist; Weiland et al., 1992b). The rapid basal GDP release is attributable both to the high endogenous GDP/GTP exchange rate of G_i-proteins (Carty et al., 1990; Linder et al., 1990) and the fact that at least one member of the chemoattractant receptors (the FPR) possesses high constitutive activity (Wenzel-Seifert et al., 1998a, 1999; see previous discussion about constitutive activity).

In contrast to GDP release, ternary complex formation (step 2 in Fig. 9.2) can be readily monitored for chemoattractant receptors (Schepers et al., 1992; Wieland et al., 1992a; Jacobs et al., 1995; Wenzel-Seifert et al., 1998a, 1999). It should be noted that not only GTP and GTPase-resistant GTP analogues reduce the high-affinity agonist binding to GPCRs in general and to the FPR in particular, but also GDP and even GMP (Gierschik et al., 1989c; Seifert et al., 1998a). These data are consistent with the concept that the guanine nucleotide-free G-protein forms the ternary complex with the agonist-occupied receptor.

Another feasible approach to analyze chemoattractant receptor–G-protein coupling is to monitor noncovalent binding of GTPγS and covalent binding of AA-GTP to $G_{i\alpha}$-subunits (step 3 in Fig. 9.2) in membranes (Offermanns et al., 1990; Gierschik et al., 1991; Wenzel-Seifert et al., 1999). A crucial prerequisite for detecting efficient agonist-stimulated GTPγS/AA-GTP binding to G_i-proteins is the presence of GDP. A straightforward explanation for the striking GDP dependence of receptor agonist-stimulated GTPγS/AA-GTP binding to G_i-proteins is the high basal GDP release from G_i-proteins, resulting in high basal binding of GTPγS/AA-GTP and blunting of the agonist response. A large molar excess of GDP relative to GTPγS/AA-GTP, by competition, forces the majority of the $G_{i\alpha}$-subunits into the GDP-liganded state in which G-proteins are then able to bind GTPγS/AA-GTP following agonist exposure.

The GTPγS binding assay is a kinetic assay that can be used to analyze the time course of G-protein activation and the stoichiometry of receptor–G-protein coupling (Gierschik et al., 1991; Schepers et al., 1992; Jacobs et al., 1995; Wenzel-Seifert et al., 1998a, 1999). The GTPγS binding assay can also be applied to permeabilized phagocytes, which provide an interesting intermediate between an intact cell system and a membrane system (Wieland et al., 1995). However, the presence of endogenous nucleotides in the permeabilized cells renders detailed analyses of nucleotide affinities of G-proteins more difficult than in carefully washed and nucleotide-depleted membranes. The GTPγS binding assay is suitable to monitor the interaction between chemoattractant receptors and G_i-proteins as a family (Gierschik et al., 1991; Klinker et al., 1994), but when used in membranes from native phagocytes or cultured cell lines, the GTPγS binding assay cannot be used to analyze the interaction of a GPCR with a given $G_{i\alpha}$ isoform. For such studies, recombinant systems such as the Sf9 cells must be employed (Wenzel-Seifert et al.,

1998a, 1999). We are not aware of reports in which the GTPγS binding assay has been successfully used to monitor the interaction of chemoattractant receptors with $G_{16\alpha}$. Possibly, the expression levels of $G_{16\alpha}$ in native phagocytes, cell lines, or recombinant systems are too low and/or the guanine nucleotide exchange rates of $G_{16\alpha}$ are too slow to allow detection of receptor–G-protein coupling in the GTPγS binding assay. In addition, GTPγS can dissociate from G_q-proteins (Biddlecome et al., 1996), a factor that could also contribute to potential difficulties monitoring chemoattractant $G_{16\alpha}$ coupling by means of GTPγS binding.

In contrast to the GTPγS binding assay, the AA-GTP photolabeling assay can be used to discriminate between various G-protein α-subunits activated by a given chemoattractant receptor in membranes from native phagocytes or cultured cell lines (Offermanns et al., 1990; Klinker et al., 1994). This is achieved because AA-GTP is covalently attached to G_α following ultraviolet irradiation of the membranes. The identification of AA-GTP–labeled G-protein α-subunits is accomplished by analyzing the comigration of the labeled G-proteins with immunologically detected G-proteins in sodium dodecyl sulfate (SDS) polyacrylamide gel electrophoresis or, more accurately, by immunoprecipitating labeled G-protein α-subunits with specific antisera. The photolabeling technique has been successfully applied to study the coupling of chemoattractant receptors to $G_{i\alpha2}$ and $G_{i\alpha3}$ but again, coupling of chemoattractant receptors to $G_{16\alpha}$ has not yet been demonstrated with this technique.

Another approach for analyzing the coupling of chemoattractant receptors to specific G_i-proteins takes advantage of the ADP-ribosylation of $G_{i\alpha}$-subunits by cholera toxin (CTX). CTX ADP-ribosylates a highly conserved arginine residue in the center of the polypeptide chain of $G_{i\alpha}$ proteins (Simon et al., 1991). In the absence of guanine nucleotides (i.e., under conditions that allow for the efficient formation of the ternary complex; see Fig. 9.2), certain chemoattractants, particularly fMLP, stimulate CTX-mediated ADP-ribosylation (Gierschik et al., 1989a; Iiri et al., 1989; McLeish et al., 1989b; Iiri et al., 1992; Klinker et al., 1994). The ADP-ribosylated $G_{i\alpha}$-subunits are then analyzed by SDS polyacrylamide electrophoresis and autoradiography. Thus, like the photolabeling technique, the ADP-ribosylation assay permits the study of the interaction of chemoattractant receptors with specific $G_{i\alpha}$ isoforms in membranes from native phagocytes and cultured cell lines. The CTX ADP-ribosylation assay is particularly powerful at dissecting different conformational states of $G_{i\alpha}$ stabilized by different chemoattractant receptors.

Because the GTPγS binding assay is a kinetic assay, the actual magnitude of the effect of an agonist or inverse agonist can vary largely, depending on which specific time point is chosen for the measurement (Gierschik et al., 1991; Wenzel-Seifert et al., 1998a, 1999). This bias in data interpretation is avoided by using the high-affinity GTPase assay. The GTPase assay is a steady-state method and measures the outcome of multiple G-protein activation/deactivation cycles (Klinker et al., 1993; Gierschik et al., 1994; Seifert et al., 1998b; Wenzel-Seifert et al., 1999). Thus, the GTPase assay is particularly useful to assess the pharmacological profile of a receptor under defined conditions (Seifert et al., 1998b; Wenzel-Seifert et al., 1999). Like the GTPγS binding assay, the GTPase assay is feasible for G_i-proteins but not G_q-proteins, and cannot discriminate between differential activation of $G_{i\alpha}$ isoforms in membranes from native phagocytes or cultured cell lines. Receptor agonists increase the maximum velocity of high-affinity GTP hydrolysis without affecting the Michaelis constant K_m ($\sim$ to 0.1–0.3 µmol/l, Feltner et al., 1986; Klinker et al., 1993; Gierschik et al., 1994). Unlike the GTPγS binding assay, conclusions about the stoichiometry of receptor–G-protein coupling (expressed as moles of activated G-proteins per mol of receptor) cannot be made with the GTPase assay. In addition, the sensitivity of the GTPase assay in terms of the relative stimulatory effects of receptor agonists is considerably lower than the sensitivity of the GTPγS binding assay (Feltner et al., 1986; Gierschik et al., 1994; Wieland and Jakobs, 1994; Seifert et al., 1998a). Fortunately, the background of low-affinity nucleotidase activity in neutrophil membranes, and particularly in HL-60 and Sf9 cell membranes, is low enough to allow for the conduction of meaningful GTPase studies (Okajima et al., 1985; Feltner et al., 1986; Wilde et al., 1989; Kupper et al., 1992; Klinker et al., 1993; Gierschik et al., 1994; Seifert et al., 1998a, 1998b; Wenzel-Seifert et al., 1999).

Several methods are available to investigate effector system activation. The direct assessment of PLC activity provides a sensitive method to monitor chemoattractant receptor–G-protein coupling in native phagocytes, cultured cell lines, and mammalian expression systems (Dillon et al., 1988; Cowen et al., 1990; Seifert et al., 1992a; Jiang et al., 1996). Unlike the GTPγS binding assay, AA-GTP–labeling assay and GTPase assay, the PLC assay can be readily used to study the interaction of chemoattractant receptors with PTX-insensitive G-proteins, particularly $G_{16\alpha}$ (Amatruda et al., 1993; Offermanns and Simon, 1995). The PLC assay requires labeling of the cells with *myo*-[2-³H]inositol.

In addition to monitoring PLC activation, chemoattractant-mediated effector system activation can be assessed by measuring PLC-triggered Ca^{2+} mobilization (and subsequent Ca^{2+} entry) by using Ca^{2+}-sensitive fluorescent dyes such as Fura-2. Again, this method can be applied to native phagocytes, cultured cell lines, and mammalian expression systems (Prossnitz et al., 1991; Didsbury et al., 1992; Seifert et al., 1992a; Wenzel-Seifert et al., 1996b; Yokomizo et al., 1997). An advantage of the Fura-2 assay, as compared to the PLC assay, is that it readily allows for high-temporal resolution of signals, avoids the use of radioisotopes, and is inexpensive. The sensitivity of the fluorescent dye-based assays is high. Like the PLC assay, the Fura-2 assay is sensitive enough to monitor coupling of receptors to PTX-insensitive G-proteins (Wenzel-Seifert and Seifert, 1990; Seifert et al., 1992a, 1992b; Yokomizo et al., 1997).

The assessment of phagocyte functions in terms of chemotaxis, O_2^- formation, and lysosomal enzyme release are also classic and widely employed methods to monitor effector system activation (Rossi, 1986; Dillon et al., 1988; Seifert and Schultz, 1991). These methods provide information about the actual biological outcome of the signal transduction process. Another advantage of these assays is that they are sensitive, inexpensive, and relatively easy to perform. A disadvantage of these cell function-based assays is that they represent a very distal readout of receptor–G-protein coupling. Specifically, multiple signaling steps, particularly phosphorylation cascades, are involved between PLC activation and actual cell functions (Rossi, 1986; Dillon et al., 1988; Seifert and Schultz, 1991). Thus, there may not necessarily be a linear relation between the extent of receptor–G-protein coupling and cell functions. However, the cell function-based assays complement the PLC and Fura 2 assays and are useful for differentiating the effects of various chemoattractants (see section on differential coupling of chemoattractant receptors to G-proteins.

Role of Transphosphorylation Reactions in Chemoattractant Receptor–G-Protein Coupling

GPCRs actively catalyze the binding of GTP/GTPγS to G-protein α-subunits (Fig. 9.2, step 3a), Brandt and Ross, 1986; Iiri et al., 1998). Thus, the availability of GTP and GTPγS in the vicinity of G_α provides an obvious mechanism by which G-protein activation can be regulated. For such a mechanism to be relevant, there must be functional and/or structural barriers between the guanine nucleotide binding cleft of G_α and the cytosol that limit the access of GTP to the G-protein. Specifically, the bulk cellular GTP concentration is ~ 50 μmol/l, whereas the affinity of G-protein α-subunits for GTP is ~ 0.3–0.1 μmol/l (Otero, 1990; Kupper et al., 1992; Klinker et al., 1993; Piacentini and Niroomand, 1996).

A mechanism by which the local supply of GTP for G-proteins is regulated is nucleoside diphosphate kinase (NDPK)-mediated transphosphorylation of GDP to GTP by a nucleoside 5'-triphosphate (NTP; see Fig. 9.2, Otero, 1990; Klinker et al., 1996a; Piacentini and Niroomand, 1996). NDPK can also use phosphorthioate analogues of NTPs as substrates, resulting in the formation of GTPγS (Seifert, et al., 1988; Wieland and Jakobs, 1989; Wieland et al., 1991a; Klinker and Seifert, 1999). NDPKs catalyze transphosphorylation via an energy-rich phosphohistidine intermediate (Otero, 1990; Piacentini and Niroomand, 1996). NDPs at high concentrations block transphosphorylation by formation of an abortive NDPK–NDP complex (Seifert et al., 1988; Klinker and Seifert, 1999).

Adenosine 5'-O-(3-thiotriphosphate) inhibits high-affinity agonist binding in HL-60 membranes in the presence of GDP, and the effect of adenosine 5'-O-(3-thiotriphosphate) is blocked by UDP at high concentrations (Wieland et al., 1991a). In addition, NDPK-generated GTPγS is more potent than exogenously added GTPγS at inhibiting ternary complex formation of chemoattractant receptors with G_i-proteins (Wieland and Jakobs, 1992). These data point to a close association of NDPKs with chemoattractant receptors and G-proteins, and to a regulatory role of NDPKs in providing GTP to G-protein α-subunits.

Although there is convincing evidence that transphosphorylation reactions are involved in G_i-protein activation by chemoattractant receptors, the question about the identity of the NDPK is still unresolved. The NDPKs cloned so far are highly conserved and form oligomers of 17–23 kDa subunits (Piacentini and Niroomand, 1996). Phagocytes express two types of NDPK (NDPK-A, 21 kDa and NDPK-B, 18 kDa) which are predominantly localized in the cytosol (Guignard and Markert, 1966). Upon exposure to fMLP, NDPKs are translocated from the cytosol to the membrane, a finding that is consistent with the role of NDPK-A and/or NDPK-B in G-protein activation (Guignard and Market, 1996).

In addition, or alternatively, to NDPK-A and NDPK-B, G-protein β-subunits may play a part in NDPK reactions. Support in favor of this model stems from the fact that G-protein β-subunits in HL-60 membranes can be transiently (thio)phosphorylated; that the (thio)phosphorylation shows the characteristics of histidine(thio)phosphorylation; and that the (thio)phosphate group attached to G_β can be retransferred to GDP (Wieland et al., 1991b, 1993; Kaldenberg-Stasch et al., 1994; Nürnberg et al., 1996). However, neither G-protein βγ-subunits alone, nor G-protein βγ-subunits in combination with G_α can reconstitute a functional NDPK, pointing to the involvement of additional regulatory and/or catalytical proteins (Kowluru et al., 1996; Klinker and Seifert, 1999).

Localization of Signaling Components

Illustrations of GPCR-mediated signal transduction, including Figure 9.1, generally suggest that the individual signaling components are freely mobile in the plasma membrane and can interact with each other in an unconstrained manner. However, this is not the case. Rather, signaling components cluster in specific microdomains or segregate from each other, thereby preventing their effective interaction (Neubig, 1994). Membrane domains that are enriched in signaling proteins are referred to as *transducisomes* (Tsunoda et al., 1997; Körschen et al., 1999). The relation of transducisomes to membrane domains, such as coated pits, and the general importance of the transducisome concept in mammalian cells remain to be established.

The FPR copurifies with G_i-proteins when isolated from HL-60 membranes (Polakis et al., 1988). The C5aR and IL-8 receptors are also in tight contact with G_i-proteins with human neutrophil membranes being the source of material (Siciliano et al., 1990; Rollins et al., 1991; Damaj et al., 1996). Tight physical association of receptors with G_i-proteins can be considered *precoupling* (Seifert et al., 1999b), may ensure rapid initiation of downstream signaling, and prevent chemoattractant receptors from interacting with G-proteins other than G_i-proteins (Neptune et al., 1999). Indeed, the formation of the ternary complex (step 2 in Fig. 9.2, Posner et al., 1994; Domalewski et al., 1996) and the onset of chemoattractant-stimulated O_2^- formation are fast (Wymann et al., 1987). These data support the concept of chemoattractant receptor–G_i-protein precoupling. The fact that only G_i-protein–derived βγ-subunits, but not βγ-subunits derived from other G-proteins, can mediate chemoattractant-induced chemotaxis points to compartmentalization of chemoattractant receptors and G_i-proteins in the same plasma membrane compartment, whereas other G-proteins are excluded (Neptune and Bourne, 1997; Neptune et al., 1999).

The translocation of chemoattractant receptors and G_i-protein α-subunits from specific granules to the plasma membrane upon stimulation may provide a mechanism by which priming is accomplished (Rotrosen et al., 1988; Sengelov et al., 1994). Whereas agonist stimulation of FPRs leads to rapid association of the receptors with actin filaments (Jesaitis et al., 1993; Särndahl et al., 1996), agonist stimulation may lead either to association of $G_{i\alpha}$ with (Wieland et al., 1996), or dissociation of $G_{i\alpha}$ from, the cytoskeleton (Särndahl et al., 1996). In addition, myeloid cells contain large amounts of cytosolic $G_{i\alpha}$, which changes its hydrodynamic properties upon binding of Mg^{2+} and GTPγS (Rudolph et al., 1989b). Thus, although the cellular trafficking and localization of chemoattractant receptors and particularly of $G_{i\alpha}$ is not yet completely understood, the available data demonstrate that myeloid cells possess mechanisms that regulate the concentration of receptors and $G_{i\alpha}$ in the plasma membrane, thus regulating the efficiency of signal transduction.

Differential Coupling of Chemoattractant Receptors to G_i-Proteins

In human phagocytes, the FPR, C5aR, IL-8 receptors, BLTR, and PAFR all couple to G_i-proteins to mediate activation of PLC, chemotaxis, and cytotoxic cell functions (Rossi, 1986; Dillon et al., 1988; Seifert and Schultz, 1991; Baggiolini et al., 1993). However, there are marked differences in the efficacies of chemoattractants at inducing O_2^- formation and lysosomal enzyme release. Specifically, in human neutrophils, fMLP, complement C5a and IL-8 are far more efficient activators of enzyme release and O_2^- formation than LTB$_4$ and PAF; that is, the former three chemoattractants can be considered *full secretagogues,* whereas the latter two chemoattractants can be considered *partial* or *incomplete secretagogues* (Rossi, 1986; Wymann et al., 1987; Dillon et al., 1988; Seifert and Schultz, 1991; Baggiolini et al., 1993). Differences in GPCR expression levels cannot explain the differences in efficacy of various chemoattractants at activating cytotoxic phagoyte functions (Schepers et al., 1992; Jacobs et al., 1995). Thus, the question arose whether the individual chemoattractant receptors stabilize different conformational states in G_i-proteins. The AA-GTP labeling technique demonstrated that the FPR, C5aR, and BLTR activate $G_{i\alpha2}$ and $G_{i\alpha3}$ with similar efficiency (Offermanns et al., 1990; Klinker et al., 1994). In addition, we could not detect differences in the coupling of the FPR of $G_{i\alpha1}$, $G_{i\alpha2}$, and $G_{i\alpha3}$ using fusion proteins which provide a defined and sensitive system for detecting differences in the coupling of a given GPCR to different G-proteins (Seifert et al., 1999c; Wenzel-Seifert et al., 1999). However, it is possible that the appropriate experimental conditions to dissect differences in the coupling of the individual chemoattractant receptors to $G_{i\alpha}$ isoforms (e.g., concentrations of GDP, NaCl, and MgCl$_2$, varied alone or in combination) have yet to be identified.

The analysis of the kinetics of GTPγS binding unmasked important differences between fMLP, complement C5a, and LTB$_4$ with respect to G_i-protein activation. First, the initial rate of GTPγS binding stimulated by the FPR is higher than the BLTR-stimulated GTPγS binding rate (Schepers et al., 1992). Second, GDP inhibits LTB$_4$-stimulated GTPγS binding more potently than fMLP-stimulated GTPγS binding (Schepers et al., 1992). These results indicate that the FPR reduces the affinity of G$_i$-proteins for GDP more efficiently than the BLTR; that is, the FPR is more efficient at catalyzing GDP release (step 1 in Fig. 9.2) than the BLTR. Finally, the GTPγS affinity of G$_i$-proteins activated by the BLTR, indicating that the FPR is more efficient than the BLTR at promoting GTPγS binding (step 3a in Fig. 9.2, Schepers et al., 1992; Jacobs et al., 1995).

The GTPγS binding data point to chemoattractant receptor-specific G$_i$-protein activation. This concept was further corroborated by analyzing the effects of chemoattractants on G$_i$-protein–mediated ITP hydrolysis. Under physiological conditions, ITP most likely does not play a significant role as G-protein activating nucleotides, but it serves an important role as an experimental tool, as do AA-GTP and GTPγS. G-proteins bind ITP with lower affinity than GTP (Northup et al., 1982; Seifert et al., 1999a). fMLP is highly potent and efficient at stimulating ITP hydrolysis in HL-60 membranes, whereas complement C5a is both less potent and efficient in this respect (Klinker and Seifert, 1997). These data suggest that the FPR is very efficient at inducing a conformational change in G$_{i\alpha}$ that promotes IDP/ITP exchange, whereas the C5aR cannot efficiently promote this conformational change.

The most striking differences between various chemoattractants were observed when CTX-catalyzed ADP-ribosylation of G$_{i\alpha}$-proteins was studied: particularly, chemoattractants stimulate the ADP-ribosylation in the order of efficacy: fMLP> complement C5a > LTB$_4$ = PAF (ineffective) (McLeish et al., 1989b; Levistre et al., 1993; Schepers and McLeish, 1993; Klinker et al., 1994). These data indicate that the various chemoattractant receptors differ dramatically in their efficacy at inducing the conformational change in G$_{i\alpha}$-proteins required for G$_{i\alpha}$ to become a substrate for CTX.

Taken together, the differential effects of chemoattractants on ITP hydrolysis by, and CTX-catalyzed ADP-ribosylation of, G$_{i\alpha}$-proteins point to receptor-specific conformational states of G$_i$-proteins. In other words, chemoattractant receptors may confer a "receptor memory" to G$_i$-proteins. An important molecular manifestation of this receptor-specific G$_i$-protein activation could be the receptor-specific changes in GDP-affinity of G$_i$-proteins. The cellular outcome of the chemoattractant receptor-specific G$_i$-protein activation is differential stimulation of O$_2^-$ formation and lysosomal enzyme release.

Role of G$_{16\alpha}$ in Chemoattractant Receptor-Mediated Signal Transduction in Phagocytes

The majority of the stimulatory effects of chemoattractants in intact phagocytes and phagocyte membranes are PTX-sensitive, indicative for the central role of G$_i$-proteins in chemoattractant receptor-mediated signal transduction

(Dillon et. al., 1988; Gierschik et al., 1991; Seifert and Schultz, 1991; Klinker et al., 1994). However, it has been repeatedly observed that some of the stimulatory effects of chemoattractants cannot be blocked by PTX (Cowen et al., 1990; Kanaho et al., 1990; Klinker et al., 1994). These findings, together with the fact that the PTX-insensitive G-protein $G_{16\alpha}$ can efficiently reconstitute chemoattractant receptor-mediated PLC activation in various expression systems gave rise to the hypothesis that the FPR, C5aR, and BLTR may couple to $G_{16\alpha}$ also in vivo (Buhl et al., 1993; Wu et al., 1993; Amatruda et al., 1995; Offermanns and Simon, 1995; Gaudreau et al., 1998).

However, despite the extensive documentation of chemoattractant receptor coupling to $G_{16\alpha}$ in cotransfection systems, evidence for coupling of chemoattractant receptors to $G_{16\alpha}$ in native neutrophils and monocytes, HL-60 cells, and U937 cells, is still missing. For example, it has not been demonstrated that chemoattractants can increase the incorporation of AA-GTP into $G_{16\alpha}$ in membranes from native phagocytes or cultured cell lines. In addition, an important paradox remains to be clarified. Although $G_{16\alpha}$ is expressed at high levels in undifferentiated HL-60 cells (Amatruda et al., 1991), chemoattractant receptors are expressed only at very low levels, if at all, in undifferentiated HL-60 cells (Klinker et al., 1996b). In contrast, differentiated HL-60 cells do not express $G_{16\alpha}$ but do express high levels of chemoattractant receptors (Amatruda et al., 1991; Klinker et al., 1996b). The opposite regulation of chemoattractant receptor and $G_{16\alpha}$ expression argues against a central role of $G_{16\alpha}$ in chemoattractant-mediated signal transduction in phagocytes in vivo. Moreover, U937 cells respond to chemoattractants in a PTX-sensitive manner and do not express $G_{16\alpha}$ at all (Vanek et al., 1994). Unlike the FPR, C5aR, IL-8 receptors, and BLTR, the PAFR can also couple to $G_{q\alpha}$ (Amatruda et al., 1993; Wu et al., 1993; Offermanns and Simon, 1995; Gaudreau et al., 1998), but the relevance of PAFR/$G_{q\alpha}$ coupling for activation of neutropils and monocytes is not known.

When discussing apparently PTX-insensitive effects in phagocytes, one must also keep in mind that G_i-proteins are highly abundant in phagocytes i.e., they account for $\sim$ 2%–3% of the total membrane protein (Murphy et al., 1987; Uhing et al., 1987; Gierschik et al., 1989a; Rudolph et al., 1989a). Second, although this fact is poorly documented in the literature, the quality of PTX preparations can vary substantially. We have experienced substantial problems with some PTX preparations from various commercial suppliers. High abundance of G_i-proteins and/or poor PTX quality can lead to incomplete ADP-ribosylation of G_i-proteins. It is, indeed, very difficult to ADP-ribosylate *all* $G_{i\alpha}$-proteins in intact cells, even when high toxin concentrations and long incubation times are used (Cowen et al., 1990; Wenzel-Seifert and Seifert, 1990). Thus, a minute fraction of the G_i-proteins may still be functional and sufficient to mediate residual chemoattractant receptor–G_i-protein coupling, although the chemoattractant effect is interpreted as being PTX-insensitive. Taken together, it is very well documented that chemoattractant receptors have the potential to couple to $G_{16\alpha}$, but the physiological importance of this coupling is unknown.

Summary

1. The professional phagocytes express receptors for the chemoattractants *N*-formyl-*L*-methionyl-*L*-leucyl-*L*-phenylalanine, complement C5a, interleukin 8, platelet-activating factor, and leukotriene B$_4$. Chemoattractant receptors couple to pertussis toxin (PTX)-sensitive G-proteins of the G$_i$-family to mediate activation of phospholipase C (PLC) with subsequent Ca^{2+} mobilization from intracellular stores and Ca^{2+} influx through the plasma membrane. Chemoattractant receptors also mediate activation of phosphoinositide 3-kinase-γ (PI3Kγ) with subsequent activation of pleckstrin domain-containing proteins. PLC and PI3Kγ activation and is mediated by βγ-complexes released from G$_i$-proteins, but there is no known role of G$_{i\alpha}$-subunits in effector system activation. The precise mechanism by which chemoattractants activate Ca^{2+} influx is unknown. Cellular responses of phagocytes following chemoattractant exposure are chemotaxis, lysosomal enzyme release, and oxygen radical formation. Activation of chemotaxis is dependent on PI3Kγ activation, whereas activation of O$_2^-$ formation is both PLC- and PI3Kγ-dependent.

2. Chemoattractant receptors are in close physical contact with G$_i$-proteins (precoupling). Individual chemoattractant receptors stabilize different conformations of G$_i$-proteins thereby inducing chemoattractant-specific phagocyte activation. Phagocytes express G$_{i\alpha 2}$ and G$_{i\alpha 3}$ and various G-protein β- and γ-subunits. However, little is known about specific functions of individual G$_{i\alpha}$-, β-, and γ-subunits in signal transduction. Cotransfection studies showed that chemoattractant receptors can also couple to the G-protein G$_{16\alpha}$ to mediate PTX-insensitive PLC activation, but the physiological relevance of the interaction of chemoattractant receptors with G$_{16\alpha}$ is unknown.

3. It is generally accepted that the G-protein activation/deactivation cycle involves GTP-hydrolysis, but it is less well known that the cycle can also proceed as a nucleotide association/dissociation cycle. Chemoattractant receptors regulate both GDP release from, and GTP binding to, G$_i$-proteins. The supply of GTP for G$_i$-proteins is controlled by an incompletely understood transphosphorylation mechanism.

4. Reconstitution of the formyl peptide receptor with G$_i$-proteins in *Spodoptera frugiperda* (Sf9) cells has shown that this receptor possesses high constitutive activity. Constitutive activity of the formyl peptide receptor is prevented by the inverse agonist cyclosporin H and Na$^+$ which both stabilize the receptor in an inactive (R) state and reduce the high basal activity of G$_i$-proteins induced by the agonist-free formyl peptide receptor.

5. Important future areas of research are the definition of the role of individual G-protein subunits (G$_{i\alpha 2, 3}$ β$_x$γ$_y$) in chemoattractant-mediated signal transduction, the molecular analysis of cation entry mechanisms, the analysis of the coupling of chemoattractant receptors to G$_{16\alpha}$ in native phagocytes and HL-60 and U937 cells, the analysis of the molecular basis and physiological role of constitutive activity of chemoattractant receptors, and the elucidation of the mechanism by which transphosphorylation reactions regulate G$_i$-protein activation by chemoattractant receptors.

References

Albrecht, E., and Petty, H. R. (1998) Cellular memory: neutrophil orientation reverses during temporally decreasing chemoattractant concentrations. *Proc. Natl. Acad. Sci. USA* 95:5039–5044.

Ali, H., Richardson, R. M., Haribabu, B., and Snyderman, R. (1999) Chemoattractant receptor cross-desensitization. *J. Biol. Chem.* 274:6027–6030.

Ali, H., Sozzani, S., Fisher, I., Barr, A. J., Richardson, R. M., Haribabu, B., and Snyderman, R. (1998) Differential regulation of formyl peptide and platelet-activating factor receptors. Role of phospholipase $C\beta_3$ phosphorylation by protein kinase A. *J. Biol. Chem.* 273:11012–11016.

Amatruda, T. T., Steele, D. A., Slepak, V. Z., and Simon, M. I. (1991) $G_{\alpha16}$, a G protein α subunit specifically expressed in hematopoietic cells. *Proc. Natl. Acad. Sci. USA* 88:5587–5591.

Amatruda, T. T., Gerard, N. P., Gerard, C., and Simon, M. I. (1993) Specific interactions of chemoattractant factor receptors with G-proteins. *J. Biol. Chem.* 268:10139–10144.

Amatruda, T. T., Dragas-Graonic, S., Holmes, R., and Perez, H. D. (1995) Signal transduction by the formly peptide receptor. Studies using chimeric receptors and site-directed mutagenesis define a novel domain for interaction with G-proteins. *J. Biol. Chem.* 270:28010–28013.

Baggiolini, M., Boulay, F., Badwey, J. A., and Curnutte, J. T. (1993) Activation of neutrophil leukocytes: chemoattractant receptors and respiratory burst. *FASEB J.* 7:1004–1010.

Becker, E. L., Forouhar, F. A., Grunnet, M. L., Boulay, F., Tardif, M., Bormann, B. J., Sodja, D., Ye, R. D., Woska, J. R. Jr., and Murphy, P. M. (1998) Broad immunocytochemical localization of the formylpeptide receptor in human organs, tissues, and cells. *Cell Tissue Res.* 292:129–135.

Berman, D. M., Kozasa, T., and Gilman, A. G. (1996a) The GTPase-activating protein RGS4 stabilizes the transition state for nucleotide hydrolysis. *J. Biol. Chem.* 271:27209–27212.

Berman, D. M., Wilkie, T. M., and Gilman, A. G. (1996b) GAIP and RGS4 are GTPase-activating proteins for the G_i subfamily of G protein α subunits. *Cell* 86:445–452.

Biddlecome, G. H., Berstein, G., and Ross, E. M. (1996) Regulation of phospholipase C-$\beta 1$ by G_q and m_1 muscarinic cholinergic receptor. Steady-state balance of receptor-mediated activation and GTPase-activating protein-promoted deactivation. *J. Biol. Chem.* 271:7999–8007.

Bilezikian, J. P., and Aurbach, G. D. (1974) The effects of nucleotides on the expression of β-adrenergic adenylate cyclase activity in membranes from turkey erythrocytes. *J. Biol. Chem.* 249:157–161.

Birnbaumer, L., Abramowitz, J., and Brown, A. M. (1990) Receptor–effector coupling by G proteins. *Biochem. Biophys. Acta* 1031:163–224.

Birnbaumer, L., Zhu, X., Jiang, M., Boulay, G., Peyton, M., Vannier, B., Brown, D., Platano, D., Sadeghi, H., Stefani, E., and Birnbaumer, M. (1996) On the molecular basis and regulation of cellular capacitative calcium entry: roles for Trp proteins. *Proc. Natl. Acad. Sci. USA* 93:15195–15202.

Bockaert, J., and Pin, J. P. (1999) Molecular tinkering of G-protein–coupled receptors: an evolutionary success. *EMBO J.* 18:1723–1729.

Bommakanti, R. K., Dratz, E. A., Siemsen, D. W., and Jesaitis, A. J. (1995) Extensive contact between G_{i2} and N-formyl peptide receptor of human neutrophils: mapping of binding sites using receptor-mimetic peptides. *Biochem.* 34:6720–6728.

Boulay, F., Tardif, M., Brouchon, L., and Vignais, P. (1990a) The human N-formypeptide receptor. Characterization of two cDNA isolates and evidence for a new subfamily of G-protein-coupled receptors. *Biochem.* 29:11123–11133.

Boulay, F., Tardif, M., Brouchon, L., and Vignais, P. (1990b) Synthesis and use of a novel N-formyl peptide derivative to isolate a human N-formyl peptide receptor cDNA. *Biochem. Biophys. Res. Commun.* 168:1103–1109.

Boulay, F., Mery, L., Tardif, M., Brouchon, L., and Vignais, P. (1991) Expression cloning of a receptor for C5a anaphylatoxin on differentiated HL-60 cells. *Biochem.* 30:2993–2999.

Bowman, E. P., Campbell, J. J., Druey, K. M., Scheschonka, A., Kehrl, J. H., and Butcher, E. C. (1998) Regulation of chemotactic and proadhesive responses to chemoattractant receptors by RGS (regulator of G-protein signaling) family members. *J. Biol. Chem.* 273:28040–28048.

Brandt, D. R., Asano, T., Pedersen, S. E., and Ross, E. M. (1983) Reconstitution of catecholamine-stimulated guanosinetriphosphatase activity. *Biochem.* 22:4357–4362.

Brandt, D. R., and Ross, E. M. (1986) Catecholamine-stimulated GTPase cycle. Multiple sites of regulation by β-adrenergic receptor and Mg^{2+} studied in reconstituted receptor-G_s vesicles. *J. Biol. Chem.* 261:1656–1664.

Brandt, S. J., Dougherty, R. W., Lapetina, E. G., and Niedel, J. E. (1985) Pertussis toxin inhibits chemotactic peptide-stimulated generation of inositol phosphates and lysosomal enzyme secretion in human leukemic (HL-60) cells. *Proc. Natl. Acad. Sci. USA* 82:3277–3280.

Breivogel, C. S., Selley, D. E., and Childers, S. R. (1998) Cannabinoid receptor agonist efficacy for stimulating [^{35}S]GTPγS binding to rat cerebellar membranes correlates with agonist-induced decreases in GDP affinity. *J. Biol. Chem.* 273:16865–16873.

Buhl, A. M., Eisfelder, B. J., Worthen, G. S., Johnson, G. L., and Russell, M. (1993) Selective coupling of the human anaphylatoxin C5a receptor and $α_{16}$ in human kidney 293 cells. *FEBS Lett.* 323:132–134.

Burde, R., and Seifert, R. (1996) Stimulation of histamine H_2- (and H_1-)receptors activates Ca^{2+} influx in *all-trans*-retinoic acid-differentiated HL-60 cells independently of phospholipase C or adenylyl cyclase. *Naunyn-Schmiedeberg's Arch. Pharmacol.* 353:123–129.

Burg, M., Raffetseder, U., Grove, M., Klos, A., Kohl, J., and Bautsch, W. (1995) $G_{α16}$ complements the signal transduction cascade of chemotactic receptors for complement factor C5a (C5a-R) and N-formylated peptides (fMLF-R) in *Xenopus laevis* oocytes: $G_{α16}$ couples to chemotactic receptors in *Xenopus* oocytes. *FEBS Lett.* 377:426–428.

Büscher, R., Herrmann, V., and Insel, P. A. (1999) Human adrenoceptor polymorphisms: evolving recognition of clinical importance. *Trends Pharmacol. Sci.* 20:94–99.

Cacalano, G., Lee, J., Kikly, K., Ryan, A. M., Pitts-Meek, S., Hultgren, B., Wood, W. I., and Moore, M. W. (1994) Neutrophil and B cell expansion in mice that lack the murine IL-8 receptor homolog. *Science* 265:682–684.

Camps, M., Carozzi, A., Schnabel, P., Scheer, A., Parker, P. J., and Gierschik, P. (1992) Isozyme-selective stimulation of phospholipase C-$β_2$ by G protein βγ-subunits. *Nature* 360:684–686.

Carp, H. (1982) Mitochondrial N-formylmethionyl proteins as chemoattractants for neutrophils. *J. Exp. Med.* 155:264–275.

Carty, D. J., Padrell, E., Codina, J., Birnbaumer, L., Hildebrandt, J. D., and Iyengar, R. (1990) Distinct guanine nucleotide binding and release properties of the three G_i-proteins. *J. Biol. Chem.* 265:6268–6273.

Cassel, D., and Selinger, Z. (1977) Catecholamine-induced release of [^{3}H]-Gpp(NH)p from turkey erythrocyte adenylate cyclase. *J. Cyclic Nucleotide Res.* 3:11–22.

Cassel, D., and Selinger, Z. (1978) Mechanism of adenylate cyclase activation through the β-adrenergic receptor: catecholamine-induced displacement of bound GDP by GTP. *Proc. Natl. Acad. Sci. USA* 75:4155–4159.

Ceresa, B. P., and Limbird, L. E. (1994) Mutation of an aspartate residue highly conserved among G-protein–coupled receptors results in nonreciprocal disruption of $α_2$-adrenergic receptor–G-protein interactions. A negative charge at amino acid residue 79 forecasts $α_{2A}$-adrenergic receptor sensitivity to allosteric modulation by monovalent cations and fully effective receptor/G-protein coupling. *J. Biol. Chem.* 269:29557–29564.

Chidiac, P., Hebert, T. E., Valiquette, M., Dennis, M., and Bouvier, M. (1994) Inverse agonist activity of β-adrenergic antagonists. *Mol. Pharmacol.* 45:490–499.

Chuang, T. T., Sallese, M., Ambrosini, G., Parruti, G., and De Blasi, A. (1992) High expression of β-adrenergic receptor kinase in human peripheral blood leukocytes. Isoproterenol and platelet activating factor can induce kinase translocation. *J. Biol. Chem.* 267:6886–6892.

Condliffe, A. M., and Hawkins, P. T. (2000) Moving in mysterious ways. *Nature* 404:135–137.

Costa, T., and Herz, A. (1989) Antagonists with negative intrinsic activity at δ opioid receptors coupled to GTP-binding proteins. *Proc. Natl. Acad. Sci. USA* 86:7321–7325.

Costa, T., Lang, J., Gless, C., and Herz, A. (1990) Spontaneous association between opioid receptors and GTP-binding regulatory proteins in native membranes: specific regulation by antagonists and sodium ions. *Mol. Pharmacol.* 37:383–394.

Cowen, D. S., Baker, B., and Dubyak, G. R. (1990) Pertussis toxin produces differential inhibitory effects on basal, P_2-purinergic, and chemotactic peptide-stimulated inositol phospholipid breakdown in HL-60 cells and HL-60 cells membranes. *J. Biol. Chem.* 265:16181–16189.

Csutora, P., Su, Z., Kim, H. Y., Bugrim, A., Cunningham, K. W., Nuccitelli, R., Keizer, J. E., Hanley, M. R., Blalock, J. E., and Marchase, R. B. (1999) Calcium influx factor is synthesized by yeast and mammalian cells depleted of organellar calcium stores. *Proc. Natl. Acad. Sci. USA* 96:121–126.

Daines, R. A., Chambers, P. A., Foley, J. J., Griswold, D. E., Kingsbury, W. D., Martin, L. D., Schmidt, D. B., Sham, K. K., and Sarau, H. M. (1996) (E)-3-[6-[[(2,6-dichlorophenyl)thio]methyl]-3-(2-phenylethoxy)-2-pyridinyl]-2-propenoic acid: a high-affinity leukotriene B_4 receptor antagonist with oral antiinflammatory activity. *J. Med. Chem.* 39:3837–3841.

Damaj, B. B., McColl, S. R., Mahana, W., Crouch, M. F., and Naccache, P. H. (1996) Physical association of $G_{i2\alpha}$ with interleukin-8 receptors. *J. Biol. Chem.* 271:12783–12789.

Dekker, L. V., and Segal, A. W. (2000) Signals to move cells. *Science* 287:982–985.

Demaurex, N., Lew, D. P., and Krause, K. H. (1992) Cyclopiazonic acid depletes intracellular Ca^{2+} stores and activates an influx pathway for divalent cations in HL-60 cells. *J. Biol. Chem.* 267:2318–2324.

Demaurex, N., Monod, A., Lew, D. P., and Krause, K. H. (1994) Characterization of receptor-mediated and store-regulated Ca^{2+} influx in human neutrophils. *Biochem. J.* 297:595–601.

Denecke, B., Meyerdierks, A., and Böttger, E. C. (1999) RGS1 is expressed in monocytes and acts as a GTPase-activating protein for G-protein-coupled chemoattractant receptors. *J. Biol. Chem.* 274:26860–26868.

De Paulis, A., Ciccarelli, A., de Crescenzo, G., Cirillo, R., Patella, V., and Marone, G. (1996) Cyclosporin H is a potent and selective competitive antagonist of human basophil activation by N-formyl-methionyl-leucyl-phenylalanine. *J. Allergy Clin. Immunol.* 98:152–164.

Didsbury, J. R., Ho, Y. S., and Snyderman, R. (1987) Human G_i protein α-subunit: deduction of amino acid structure from a cloned cDNA. *FEBS Lett.* 211:160–164.

Didsbury, J. R., Uhing, R. J., Tomhave, E., Gerard, C., Gerard, N., and Snyderman, R. (1991) Receptor class desensitization of leukocyte chemoattractant receptors. *Proc. Natl. Acad. Sci. USA* 88:11564–11568.

Didsbury, J. R., Uhing, R. J., Tomhave, E., Gerard, C., Gerard, N., and Snyderman, R. (1992) Functional high efficiency expression of cloned leukocyte chemoattractant receptor cDNAs. *FEBS Lett.* 297:275–279.

Dillon, S. B., Verghese, M. W., and Synderman, R. (1988) Signal transduction in cells following binding of chemoattractants to membrane receptors. *Virchows Arch. B Cell. Pathol. Mol. Pathol.* 55:65–80.

Domalewski, M. D., Guyer, D. A., Freer, R. J., Muthukumaraswamy, N., and Sklar, L. A. (1996) Fixation traps formyl peptide receptors in high and low affinity forms that can be regulated by GTP[S] in the absence of ligand. *J. Recept. Signal Transduct. Res.* 16:59–75.

Dunkel, C. G., Saffitz, J. E., and Evers, A. S. (1989) fMet-Leu-Phe receptor expression by an interstitial cell in rabbit right atrium following left ventricular myocardial infarction. *Cir. Res.* 65:215–223.

Durstin, M., McColl, S. R., Gomez-Cambronero, J., Naccache, P. H., and Sha'afi, R. I. (1993) Up-regulation of the amount of $G_{i\alpha2}$ associated with the plasma membrane in human neutrophils stimulated by granulocyte-macrophage colony-stimulating factor. *Biochem. J.* 292:183–187.

Ervens, J., Schultz, G., and Seifert, R. (1991) Differential inhibition and potentiation of chemoattractant-induced superoxide formation in human neutrophils by the cell-permeant analogue of cyclic GMP, N^2, 2'-O-dibutyryl guanosine 3':5'-cyclic monophosphate. *Naunyn-Schmiedeberg's Arch. Pharmacol.* 343:370–376.

Fasolato, C., Innocenti, B., and Pozzan, T. (1994) Receptor-activated Ca^{2+} influx: how many mechanisms for how many channels? *Trends Pharmacol. Sci.* 15:77–83.

Feltner, D. E., Smith, R. H., and Marasco, W. A. (1986) Characterization of the plasma membrane bound GTPase from rabbit neutrophils. I. Evidence for an N_i-like protein coupled to the formyl peptide, C5a, and leukotriene B_4 chemotaxis receptors. *J. Immunol.* 137:1961–1970.

Florio, V. A., and Sternweis, P. C. (1989) Mechanisms of muscarinic receptor action on G_o in reconstituted phospholipid vesicles. *J. Biol. Chem.* 264:3909–3915.

Gao, J. L., and Murphy, P. M. (1993) Species and subtype variants of the *N*-formyl peptide chemotactic receptor reveal multiple important functional domains. *J. Biol. Chem.* 268:25395–25401.

Gao, J. L., Lee, E. J., and Murphy, P. M. (1999) Impaired antibacterial host defense in mice lacking the *N*-formylpeptide receptor. *J. Exp. Med.* 189:657–662.

Gaudreau, R., Le Gouill, C., Metaoui, S., Lemire, S., Stankova, J., and Rola-Pleszczynski, M. (1998) Signalling through the leukotriene B_4 receptor involves both α_i and α_{16} but not α_q or α_{11} G-protein subunits. *Biochem. J.* 335:15–18.

Geiszt, M., Kapus, A., Nemet, K., Farkas, L., and Ligeti, E. (1997) Regulation of capacitative Ca^{2+} influx in human neutrophil granulocytes. Alterations in chronic granulomatous disease. *J. Biol. Chem.* 272:26471–26478.

Gerard, N. P., and Gerard, C. (1991) The chemotactic receptor for human C5a anaphylatoxin. *Nature* 349:614–617.

Gether, U., Lin, S., and Kobilka, B. K. (1995) Fluorescent labeling of purified β_2 adrenergic receptor. Evidence for ligand-specific conformational changes. *J. Biol. Chem.* 270:28268–28275.

Gether, U., Lin, S., Ghanouni, P., Ballesteros, J. A., Weinstein, H., and Kobilka, B. K. (1997) Agonists induce conformational changes in transmembrane domains III and IV of the β_2 adrenoceptor. *EMBO J.* 16:6737–6747.

Gierschik, P., Sidiropoulos, D., and Jakobs, K. H. (1989a) Two distinct G_i-proteins mediate formyl peptide receptor signal transduction in human leukemia (HL-60) cells. *J. Biol. Chem.* 264:21470–21473.

Gierschik, P., Sidiropoulos, D., Steisslinger, M., and Jakobs, K. H. (1989b) Na^+ regulation of formyl peptide receptor-mediated signal transduction in HL 60 cells. Evidence that the caution prevents activation of the G-protein by unoccupied receptors. *Eur. J. Pharmacol.* 172:481–492.

Gierschik, P., Steisslinger, M., Sidiropoulos, D., Herrmann, E., and Jakobs, K. H. (1989c) Dual Mg^{2+} control of formyl-peptide-receptor-G-protein interaction in HL 60 cells. Evidence that the low-agonist-affinity receptor interacts with and activates the G-protein. *Eur. J. Biochem.* 183:97–105.

Gierschik, P., Moghtader, R., Straub, C., Dieterich, K., and Jakobs, K. H. (1991) Signal amplification in HL-60 granulocytes. Evidence that the chemotactic peptide receptor catalytically activates guanine-nucleotide-binding regulatory proteins in native plasma membranes. *Eur. J. Biochem.* 197:725–732.

Gierschik, P., Bouillon, T., and Jakobs, K. H. (1994) Receptor-stimulated hydrolysis of guanosine 5'-triphosphate in membrane preparations. *Methods Enzymol.* 237:13–26.

Gilman, A. G. (1987) G proteins: transducers of receptor-generated signals. *Annu. Rev. Biochem.* 56:615–649.

Gudermann, T., Schöneberg, T., and Schultz, G. (1997) Functional and structural complexity of signal transduction via G-protein-coupled receptors. *Annu. Rev. Neurosci.* 20:399–427.

Guignard, F., and Markert, M. (1996) The nucleoside diphosphate kinase of human neutrophils. *Biochem. J.* 316:233–238.

Hall, A. L., Wilson, B. S., Pfeiffer, J. R., Oliver, J. M., and Sklar, L. A. (1997) Relationship of ligand–receptor dynamics to actin polymerization in RBL-2H3 cells transfected with the human formyl peptide receptor. *J. Leukoc. Biol.* 62:535–546.

Haribabu, B., Richardson, R. M., Fisher, I., Sozzani, S., Peiper, S. C., Horuk, R., Ali, H., and Snyderman, R. (1997) Regulation of human chemokine receptors CXCR4. Role of phosphorylation in desensitization and internalization. *J. Biol. Chem.* 272:28726–28731.

Hilf, G., Kupprion, C., Wieland, T., and Jakobs, K. H. (1992) Dissociation of guanosine 5'-[γ-thio] triphosphate from guanine-nucleotide-binding regulatory proteins in native cardiac membranes. Regulation by nucleotides and muscarinic acetylcholine receptors. *Eur. J. Biochem.* 204:725–731.

Hirsch, E., Katanaev, V. L., Garlanda, C., Azzolino, O., Pirola, L., Silengo, L., Sozzani, S., Mantovani, A., Altruda, F., and Wymann, M. P. (2000) Central role for G protein-coupled phosphoinositide 3-kinase γ in inflammation. *Science* 287:1049–1053.

Höpken, U. E., Lu, B., Gerard, N. P., and Gerard, C. (1997) Impaired inflammatory responses in the reverse arthus reaction through genetic deletion of the C5a receptor. *J. Exp. Med.* 186: 749–756.

Howell, T. W., Cockcroft, S., and Gomperts, B. D. (1987) Essential synergy between Ca^{2+} and guanine nucleotides in exocytotic secretion from form permeabilized rat mast cells. *J. Cell. Biol.* 105:191–197.

Huang, C., Helper, J. R., Gilman, A. G., and Mumby, S. M. (1997) Attenuation of G_i and G_q-mediated signaling by expression of RGS4 or GAIP in mammalian cells. *Proc. Natl. Acad. Sci. USA* 94:6159–6163.

Iiri, T., Tohkin, M., Morishima, N., Ohoka, Y., Ui, M., and Katada, T. (1989) Chemotactic peptide receptor-supported ADP-ribosylation of a pertussis toxin substrate GTP-binding protein by cholera toxin in neutrophil-type HL-60 cells. *J. Biol. Chem.* 264:21394–21400.

Iiri, T., Ohoka, Y., Ui, M., and Katada, T. (1992) Modification of the function of pertussis toxin substrate GTP-binding protein by cholera toxin-catalyzed ADP-ribosylation. *J. Biol. Chem.* 267; 1020–1026.

Iiri, T., Homma, Y., Ohoka, Y., Robishaw, J. D., Katada, T., and Bourne, H. R. (1995) Potentiation of G_i-mediated phospholipase C activation by retinoic acid in HL-60 cells. Possible role of $G_{\gamma2}$. *J. Biol. Chem.* 270:5901–5908.

Iiri, T., Farfel, Z., and Bourne, H. R. (1998) G-protein diseases furnish a model for the turn-on switch. *Nature* 394:35–38.

Jacobs, A. A., Huber, J. L., Ward, R. A., Klein, J. B., and McLeish, K. R. (1995) Chemoattractant receptor-specific differences in G protein activation rates regulate effector enzyme and functional responses. *J. Leukoc. Biol.* 57:679–686.

Jesaitis, A. J., Erickson, R. W., Klotz, K. N., Bommakanti, R. K., and Siemsen, D. W. (1993) Functional molecular complexes of human N-formyl chemoattractant receptors and actin. *J. Immunol.* 151:5653–5665.

Jiang, H., Kuang, Y., Wu, Y., Smrcka, A., Simon, M. I., and Wu, D. (1996) Pertussis toxin-sensitive activation of phospholipase C by the C5a and fMet-Leu-Phe receptors. *J. Biol. Chem.* 271: 13430–13434.

Jones, S. A., Dewald, B., Clark-Lewis, I., and Baggiolini, M. (1997) Chemokine antagonists that discriminate between interleukin-8 receptors. Selective blockers of CXCR2. *J. Biol. Chem.* 272: 16166–16169.

Kaldenberg-Stasch, S., Baden, M., Fesseler, B., Jakobs, K. H., and Wieland, T. (1994) Receptor-stimulated guanine-nucleotide-triphosphate binding to guanine-nucleotide-binding regulatory proteins. Nucleotide exchange and β-subunit-mediated phosphotransfer reactions. *Eur. J. Biochem.* 221:25–33.

Kanaho, Y., Kermode, J. C., and Becker, E. L. (1990) Comparison of stimulation by chemotactic formyl peptide analogs between GTPase activity in neutrophil plasma membranes and granule enzyme release from intact neutrophils. *J. Leukoc. Biol.* 47:420–428.

Keitoku, M., Kohzuki, M., Katoh, H., Funakoshi, M., Suzuki, S., Takeuchi, M., Karibe, A., Horiguchi, S., Watanabe, J., Satoh, S., et al. (1997) FMLP actions and its binding sites in isolated human coronary arteries. *J. Mol. Cell. Cardiol.* 29:881–894.

Kew, R. R., Peng, T., DiMartino, S. J., Madhavan, D., Weinman, S. J., Cheng, D., and Prossnitz, E. R. (1997) Undifferentiated U937 cells transfected with chemoattractant receptors: a model system to investigate chemotactic mechanisms and receptor structure/function relationships. *J. Leukoc. Biol.* 61:329–337.

Klein, J. B., Scherzer, J. A., and McLeish, K. R. (1992) IFN-γ enhances expression of formyl peptide receptors and guanine nucleotide-binding proteins by HL-60 granulocytes. *J. Immunol.* 148:2483–2488.

Klein, J. B., Scherzer, J. A., Harding, G., Jacobs, A. A., and McLeish, K. R. (1995) TNF-α stimulates increased plasma membrane guanine nucleotide binding protein activity in polymorphonuclear leukocytes *J. Leukoc. Biol.* 57:500–506.

Klinker, J. F., Höer, A., Schwaner, I., Offermanns, S., Wenzel-Seifert, K., and Seifert, R. (1993)

Lipopeptides activate G$_i$-proteins in dibutyryl cyclic AMP-differentiated HL-60 cells. *Biochem. J.* 296:245–251.

Klinker, J. F., Schwaner, I., Offermanns, S., Hagelüken, A., and Seifert, R. (1994) Differential activation of dibutyryl cAMP-differentiated HL-60 human leukemia cells by chemoattractants. *Biochem. Pharmacol.* 48:1857–1864.

Klinker, J. F., Laugwitz, K. L., Hagelüken, A., and Seifert, R. (1996) Activation of GTP formation and high-affinity GTP hydrolysis by mastoparan in various cell membranes. G-protein activation via nucleoside diphosphate kinase, a possible general mechanism of mastoparan action. *Biochem. Pharmacol.* 51:217–223.

Klinker, J. F., Wenzel-Seifert, K., and Seifert, R. (1996b) G-protein-coupled receptors in HL-60 human leukemia cells. *Gen. Pharmacol.* 27:33–54.

Klinker, J. F., and Seifert, R. (1997) Functionally nonequivalent interactions of guanosine 5'-triphosphate, inosine 5'-triphosphate, and xanthosine 5'-triphosphate with the retinal G-protein, transducin, and with G$_i$-proteins in HL-60 leukemia cell membranes. *Biochem. Pharmacol.* 54:551–562.

Klinker, J. F., and Seifert, R. (1999) Nucleoside diphosphate kinase activity in soluble transducin preparations biochemical properties and possible role of transducin-β as phosphorylated enzyme intermediate. *Eur. J. Biochem,* 261:72–80.

Kobilka, B. K. (1992) Adrenergic receptors as models for G protein-coupled receptors. *Annu. Rev. Neurosci.* 15:87–114.

Konteatis, Z. D., Siciliano, S. J., Van Riper, G., Molineaux, C. J., Pandya, S., Fischer, P., Rosen, H., Mumford, R. A., and Springer, M. S. (1994) Development of C5a receptor antagonists. Differential loss of functional responses. *J. Immunol.* 153:4200–4205.

Körschen, H. G., Beyermann, M., Müller, F., Heck, M., Vantler, M., Koch, K. W., Kellner, R., Wolfrum, U., Bode, C., Hofmann, K. P., and Kaupp, U. B. (1999) Interaction of glutamic-acid-rich proteins with the cGMP signalling pathway in rod photoreceptors. *Nature* 400:761–766.

Kowluru, A., Seavey, S. E., Rhodes, C. J., and Metz, S. A. (1996) A novel regulatory mechanism for trimeric GTP-binding proteins in the membrane and secretory granule fractions of human and rodent beta cells. *Biochem. J.* 313:97–107.

Krause, K. H., Schlegel, W., Wollheim, C. B., Andersson, T., Waldvogel, F. A., and Lew, P. D. (1985) Chemotactic peptide activation of human neutrophils and HL-60 cells. Pertussis toxin reveals correlation between inositol trisphosphate generation, calcium ion transients, and cellular activation. *J. Clin. Invest.* 76:1348–1354.

Krause, K. H., Fivaz, M., Monod, A., and van der Goot, F. G. (1998) Aerolysin induces G-protein activation and Ca^{2+} release from intracellular stores in human granulocytes. *J. Biol. Chem.* 273:18122–18129.

Krautwurst, D., Seifert, R., Hescheler, J., and Schultz, G. (1992) Formyl peptides and ATP stimulate Ca^{2+} and Na$^+$ inward currents through non-selective cation channels via G-proteins in dibutyryl cyclic AMP-differentiated HL-60 cells. Involvement of Ca^{2+} and Na$^+$ in the activation of β-glucuronidase release and superoxide production. *Biochem. J.* 288:1025–1035.

Krieger-Brauer, H. I., Medda, P. K., and Kather, H. (1997) Insulin-induced activation of NADPH-dependent H$_2$O$_2$ generation in human adipocyte plasma membranes is mediated by Gα$_{i2}$ *J. Biol. Chem.* 272:10135–10143.

Kupper, R. W., Dewald, B., Jakobs, K. H., Baggiolini, M., and Gierschik, P. (1992) G-protein activation by interleukin 8 and related cytokines in human neutrophil plasma membranes. *Biochem. J.* 282:429–434.

Kupprion, C., Wieland, T., and Jakobs, K. H. (1993) Receptor-stimulated dissociation of GTP[S] from G$_i$-proteins in membranes of HL-60 cells. *Cell. Signal.* 5:425–433.

Lacy, M., Jones, J., Whittemore, S. R., Haviland, D. L., Wetsel, R. A., and Barnum, S. R. (1995) Expression of the receptors for the C5a anaphylatoxin, interleukin-8 and FMLP by human astrocytes and microglia. *J. Neuroimmunol.* 61:71–78.

Lang, J., Boulay, F., Li, G., and Wollheim, C. B. (1993) Conserved transducer coupling but different effector linkage upon expression of the myeloid fMet-Leu-Phe receptor in insulin secreting cells. *EMBO J.* 12:2671–2679.

LeDuc, L. E., Brown, L., and Vidrich, A. (1994) Bradykinin and FMLP stimulate prostanoid production by adult rabbit colonocytes in culture. *Am. J. Physiol.* 267:G778–G785.

Leff, P. (1995) The two-state model of receptor activation. *Trends Pharmacol. Sci.* 16:89–97.

Lefkowitz, R. J., Cotecchia, S., Samama, P., and Costa, T. (1993) Constitutive activity of receptors coupled to guanine nucleotide regulatory proteins. *Trends Pharmacol. Sci.* 14:303–307.

Leopoldt, D., Harteneck, C., and Nürnberg, B. (1997) G proteins endogenously expressed in Sf9 cells: interactions with mammalian histamine receptors. *Naunyn-Schmiedeberg's Arch. Pharmacol.* 356:216–224.

Levistre, R., Masliah, J., and Bereziat, G. (1993) Stimulatory and inhibitory guanine-nucleotide-binding regulatory protein involvement in stimulation of arachidonic-acid release by *N*-formyl-methionyl-leucyl-phenylalanine and platelet-activating factor from guinea-pig alveolar macrophages. Differential receptor/G-protein interaction assessed by pertussis and cholera toxins. *Eur. J. Biochem.* 213:295–303.

Li, Z., Jiang, H. Xie, W., Zhang, Z., Smrcka, A. V., and Wu, D. (2000) Roles of PLC-β2 and- β3 and PI3Kγ in chemoattractant-mediated signal transduction. *Science* 287:1046–1049.

Liao, C. H., Ko, F. N., Wu, T. S., and Teng, C. M. (1997) Bakkenolide G, a natural PAF—receptor antagonist. *J. Pharm. Pharmacol.* 49:1248–1253.

Linder, M. E., Ewald, D. A., Miller, R. J., and Gilman, A. G. (1990) Purification and characterization of $G_{o\alpha}$ and three types of $G_{i\alpha}$ after expression in *Escherichia coli*. *J. Biol. Chem.* 265:8243–8251.

Liston, T. E., Conklyn, M. J., Houser, J., Wilner, K. D., Johnson, A., Apseloff, G., Whitacre, C., and Showell, H. J. (1998) Pharmacokinetics and pharmacodynamics of the leukotriene B$_4$ receptor antagonist CP-105, 696 in man following single oral administration. *Br. J. Clin. Pharmacol.* 45:115–121.

Lohse, M. J. (1993) Molecular mechanisms of membrane receptor desensitization. *Biochim. Biophys. Acta* 1179:171–188.

Ma, H.-T., Patterson, R. L., van Rossum, D. B., Birnbaumer, L., Mikoshiba, K., and Gill, D. L. (2000) Requirement of the inositol trisphosphate receptor for activation of store-operated Ca^{2+} channels. *Science* 287:1647–1651.

Malech, H. L., and Gallin, M. D. (1987) Neutrophils in human diseases. *N. Engl. J. Med.* 317:687–694.

Malech, H. L., Maples, P. B., Whiting-Theobald, N., Linton, G. F., Sekhsaria, S., Vowells, S. J., Li, F., Miller, J. A., DeCarlo, E., Holland, S. M., et al. (1997) Prolonged production of NADPH oxidase-corrected granulocytes after gene therapy of chronic granulomatous disease. *Proc. Natl. Acad. Sci. USA* 94:12133–12138.

Marasco, W. A., Fantone, J. C., and Ward, P. A. (1982) Spasmogenic activity of chemotactic *N*-formylated oligopeptides: identity of structure–function relationships for chemotactic and spasmogenic activities. *Proc. Natl. Acad. Sci. USA* 79:7470–7473.

Marasco, W. A., Phan, S. H., Krutzsch, H., Showell, H. J., Feltner, D. E., Nairn, R., Becker, E. L., and Ward, P. A. (1984) Purification and identification of formyl-methionyl-leucyl-phenylalanine as the major peptide neutrophil chemotactic factor produced by *Escherichia coli*. *J. Biol. Chem.* 259:5430–5439.

Marasco, W. A., and Ward, P. A. (1988) Chemotactic factors of bacterial origin. *Methods Enzymol.* 162:198–214.

Mayer, A. M., Brenic, S., and Glaser, K. B. (1996) Pharmacological targeting of signaling pathways in protein kinase C-stimulated superoxide generation in neutrophil-like HL-60 cells: effect of phorbol ester, arachidonic acid and inhibitors of kinase(s), phosphatase(s) and phospholipase A$_2$. *J. Pharmacol. Exp. Ther.* 279:633–644.

McCoy, R., Haviland, D. L., Molmenti, E. P., Ziambaras, T., Wetsel, R. A., and Perlmutter, D. H. (1995) *N*-formylpeptide and complement C5a receptors are expressed in liver cells and mediate hepatic acute phase gene regulation. *J. Exp. Med.* 182:207–217.

McLeish, K. R., Gierschik, P., and Jakobs, K. H. (1989a) Desensitization uncouples the formyl peptide receptor-guanine nucleotide-binding protein interaction in HL60 cells. *Mol. Pharmacol.* 36:384–390.

McLeish, K. R., Gierschik, P., Schepers, T., Sidiropoulos, D., and Jakobs, K. H. (1989b) Evi-

dence that activation of a common G-protein by receptors for leukotriene B_4 and
N-formylmethionyl-leucyl-phenylalanine in HL-60 cells occurs by different mechanisms.
Biochem. J. 260:427–434.

McLeish, K. R., Klein, J. B., Schepers, T., and Sonnenfeld, G. (1991) Modulation of transmembrane signalling in HL-60 granulocytes by tumour necrosis factor-α. *Biochem. J.* 279:455–
460.

Merritt, J. E., Jacob, R., and Hallam, T. J. (1989) Use of manganese to discriminate between
calcium influx and mobilization from internal stores in stimulated human neutrophils. *J. Biol.
Chem.* 264:1522–1527.

Merritt, J. E., Armstrong, W. P., Benham, C. D., Hallam, T. J., Jacob, R., Jaxa-Chamiec, A., Leigh,
B. K., McCarthy, S. A., Moores, K. E., and Rink, T. J. (1990) SK&F 96365, a novel inhibitor
of receptor-mediated calcium entry. *Biochem. J.* 271:515–522.

Montell, C. (1997) New light on TRP and TRPL. *Mol. Pharmacol.* 52:755–763.

Müller-Ladner, U., Jones, J. L., Wetsel, R. A., Gay, S., Raine, C. S., and Barnum, S. R. (1996)
Enhanced expression of chemotactic receptors in multiple sclerosis lesions. *J. Neurol. Sci.* 144:
135–141.

Murphy, P. M., Eide, B., Goldsmith, P., Brann, M., Gierschik, P., Spiegel, A., and Malech, H. L.
(1987) Detection of multiple forms of $G_{i\alpha}$ in HL60 cells. *FEBS Lett.* 221:81–86.

Murphy, P. M., and McDermott, D. (1991) Functional expression of the human formyl peptide
receptor in *Xenopus* oocytes requires a complementary human factor. *J. Biol. Chem.* 266:
12560–12567.

Murphy, P. M., and Tiffany, H. L. (1991) Cloning of complementary DNA encoding a functional
human interleukin-8 receptor. *Science* 253:1280–1283.

Murphy, P. M. (1994) The molecular biology of leukocyte chemoattractant receptors. *Annu. Rev.
Immunol.* 12:593–633.

Naccache, P. H., Caon, A. C., Gilbert, C., Chouinard, G., and McColl, S. R. (1991) Pertussis toxin
selectively interferes with the responses of the HL-60 human promyelocytic cell line to di-
methylsulfoxide. *Blood* 78:2534–2541.

Neptune, E. R., and Bourne, H. R. (1997) Receptors induce chemotaxis by releasing the βγ subunit of G_i, not by activating G_q or G_s. *Proc. Natl. Acad. Sci. USA* 94:14489–14494.

Neptune, E. R., Iiri, T., and Bourne, H. R. (1999) $G\alpha_i$ is not required for chemotaxis mediated
by G_i-coupled receptors. *J. Biol. Chem.* 274:2824–2828.

Neubig, R. R. (1994) Membrane organization in G-protein mechanisms. *FASEB J.* 8:939–946.

Neve, K. A., Cox, B. A., Henningsen, R. A., Spanoyannis, A., and Neve, R. L. (1991) Pivotal role
for aspartate-80 in the regulation of dopamine D_2 receptor affinity for drugs and inhibition
of adenylyl cyclase. *Mol. Pharmacol.* 39:733–739.

Northup, J. K., Smigel, M. D., and Gilman, A. G. (1982) The guanine nucleotide activating site
of the regulatory component of adenylate cyclase. Identification by ligand binding. *J. Biol.
Chem.* 257:11416–11423.

Nürnberg, B., Harhammer, R., Exner, T., Schulze, R. A., and Wieland, T. (1996) Species- and
tissue-dependent diversity of G-protein β subunit phosphorylation: evidence for a cofactor.
Biochem. J. 318:717–722.

Offermanns, S., Schäfer, R., Hoffmann, B., Bombien, E., Spicher, K., Hinsch, K.-D., Schultz, G.,
and Rosenthal, W. (1990) Agonist-sensitive binding of a photoreactive GTP analog to a
G-protein α-subunit in membranes of HL-60 cells. *FEBS Lett.* 260:14–18.

Offermanns, S., and Simon, M. I. (1995) $G\alpha_{15}$ and $G\alpha_{16}$ couple a wide variety of receptors to
phospholipase C. *J. Biol. Chem.* 270:15175–15180.

Okajima, F., Katada, T., and Ui, M. (1985) Coupling of the guanine nucleotide regulatory protein to chemotactic peptide receptors in neutrophil membranes and its uncoupling by islet-
activating protein, pertussis toxin. A possible role of the toxin substrate in Ca^{2+}-mobilizing
receptor-mediated signal transduction. *J. Biol. Chem.* 260:6761–6768.

Oostendorp, R. A., Knol, E. F., Verhoeven, A. J., and Scheper, R. J. (1992) An immunosuppressive
retrovirus-derived hexapeptide interferes with intracellular signaling in monocytes and granulocytes through N-formylpeptide receptors. *J. Immunol.* 149:1010–1015.

Otero, A. D. (1990) Transphosphorylation and G protein activation. *Biochem. Pharmacol.* 39:1399–
1404.

Owman, C., Garzino-Demo, A., Cocchi, F., Popovic, M., Sabirsh, A., and Gallo, R. C. (1998) The leukotriene B$_4$ receptor functions as a novel type of coreceptor mediating entry of primary HIV-1 isolates into CD4-positive cells. *Proc. Natl. Acad. Sci. USA* 95:9530–9534.

Pellas, T. C., Boyar, W., van Oostrum, J., Wasvary, J., Fryer, L. R., Pastor, G., Sills, M., Braunwalder, A., Yarwood, D. R., Kramer, R. (1998) Novel C5a receptor antagonists regulate neutrophil functions in vitro and in vivo. *J. Immunol.* 160:5616–5621.

Piacentini, L., and Niroomand, F. (1996) Phosphotransfer reactions as a means of G protein activation. *Mol. Cell. Biochem.* 157:59–63.

Pitcher, J. A., Freedman, N. J., and Lefkowitz, R. J. (1998) G protein-coupled receptor kinases. *Annu. Rev. Biochem.* 67:653–692.

Polakis, P. G., Uhing, R. J., and Snyderman, R. (1988) The formylpeptide chemoattractant receptor copurifies with a GTP-binding protein containing a distinct 40-kDa pertussis toxin substrate. *J. Biol. Chem.* 263:4969–4976.

Posner, R. G., Fay, S. P., Domalewski, M. D., and Sklar, L. A. (1994) Continuous spectrofluorometric analysis of formyl peptide receptor ternary complex interactions. *Mol. Pharmacol.* 45: 65–73.

Prossnitz, E. R., Quehenberger, O., Cochrane, C. G., and Ye, R. D. (1991) Transmembrane signalling by the N-formyl peptide receptor in stably transfected fibroblasts. *Biochem. Biophys. Res. Commun.* 179:471–476.

Prossnitz, E. R., Quehenberger, O., Cochrane, C. G., and Ye, R. D. (1993) Signal transducing properties of the N-formyl peptide receptor expressed in undifferentiated HL60 cells. *J. Immunol.* 151:5704–5715.

Prossnitz, E. R., Kim, C. M., Benovic, J. L., and Ye, R. D. (1995a) Phosphorylation of the N-formyl peptide receptor carboxyl terminus by the G protein-coupled receptor kinase, GRK2. *J. Biol. Chem.* 270:1130–1137.

Prossnitz, E. R., Schreiber, R. E., Bokoch, G. M., and Ye, R. D. (1995b) Binding of low affinity N-formyl peptide receptors to G protein. Characterization of a novel inactive receptor intermediate. *J. Biol. Chem.* 270:10686–10694.

Prossnitz, E. R. (1997) Desensitization of N-formylpeptide receptor-mediated activation is dependent upon receptor phosphorylation. *J. Biol. Chem.* 272:15213–15219.

Quehenberger, O., Prossnitz, E. R., Cochrane, C. G., and Ye, R. D. (1992) Absence of G$_i$ proteins in the Sf9 insect cell. Characterization of the uncoupled recombinant N-formyl peptide receptor. *J. Biol. Chem.* 267:19757–19760.

Rane, M. J., Arthur, J. M., Prossnitz, E. R., and McLeish, K. R. (1998) Activation of mitogen-activated protein kinases by formyl peptide receptors is regulated by the cytoplasmic tail. *J. Biol. Chem.* 273:20916–20923.

Richardson, R. M., Ali, H., Pridgen, B. C., Haribabu, B., and Snyderman, R. (1998) Multiple signaling pathways of human interleukin-8 receptor A. Independent regulation by phosphorylation. *J. Biol. Chem.* 273:10690–10695.

Rollins, T. E., Siciliano, S., Kobayashi, S., Cianciarulo, D. N., Bonilla-Argudo, V., Collier, K., and Springer, M. S. (1991) Purification of the active C5a receptor from human polymorphonuclear leukocytes as a receptor-G$_i$ complex. *Proc. Natl. Acad. Sci. USA* 88:971–975.

Rossi, F. (1986) The O$_2^-$-forming NADPH oxidase of the phagocytes: nature, mechanisms of activation and function. *Biochim. Biophys. Acta* 853:65–89.

Rotrosen, D., Malech, H. L., and Gallin, J. I. (1987) Formyl peptide leukocyte chemoattractant uptake and release by cultured human umbilical vein endothelial cells. *J. Immunol.* 139:3034–3040.

Rotrosen, D., Gallin, J. I., Spiegel, A. M., and Malech, H. L. (1988) Subcellular localization of G$_i\alpha$ in human neutrophils. *J. Biol. Chem.* 263:10958–10964.

Rudolph, U., Koesling, D., Hinsch, K. D., Seifert, R., Bigalke, M., Schultz, G., and Rosenthal, W. (1989a) G-protein α-subunits in cytosolic and membranous fractions of human neutrophils. *Mol. Cell. Endocrinol.* 63:143–153.

Rudolph, U., Schultz, G., and Rosenthal, W. (1989b) The cytosolic G-protein α-subunit in human neutrophils responds to treatment with guanine nucleotides and magnesium. *FEBS Lett.* 251: 137–142.

Rudolph, U., Finegold, M. J., Rich, S. S., Harriman, G. R., Srinivasan, Y., Brabet, P., Boulay, G.,

Bradley, A., and Birnbaumer, L. (1995) Ulcerative colitis and adenocarcinoma of the colon in $G\alpha_{12}$-deficient mice. *Nature Genetics* 10:143–150.

Särndahl, E., Bokoch, G. M., Boulay, F., Stendahl, O., and Andersson, T. (1996) Direct or C5a-induced activation of heterotrimeric G_{12} proteins in human neutrophils is associated with interaction between formyl peptide receptors and the cytoskeleton. *J. Biol. Chem.* 271:15267–15271.

Sasaki, T., Irie-Sasaki, J., Jones, R. G., Oliveira-dos-Santos, A., Stanford, W. L., Bolon, B., Wakeham, A., Itie, A., Bouchard, D., Kozieradzki, I. et al. (2000) Function of PI3Kγ in thymocyte development, T cell activation, and neutrophil migration. *Science* 287:1040–1046.

Scheer, A., and Cotecchia, S. (1997) Constitutively active G protein-coupled receptor: potential mechanisms of receptor activation. *J. Receptor Signal Transduct. Res.* 17:57–73.

Schepers, T. M., Brier, M. E., and McLeish, K. R. (1992) Quantitative and qualitative differences in guanine nucleotide binding protein activation by formyl peptide and leukotriene B_4 receptors. *J. Biol. Chem.* 267:159–165.

Schepers, T. M., and McLeish, K. R. (1993) Differential cholera-toxin-and pertussis-toxin-catalysed ADP-ribosylation of G-proteins coupled to formyl-peptide and leukotriene B_4 receptors. *Biochem. J.* 289:469–473.

Schultz, P., Stannek, P., Voigt, M., Jakobs, K. H., and Gierschik, P. (1992) Complementation of formyl peptide receptor-mediated signal transduction in *Xenopus laevis* oocytes. *Biochem. J.* 284:207–212.

Seifert, R., Rosenthal, W., and Schultz, G. (1986) Guanine nucleotides stimulate NADPH oxidase in membranes of human neutrophils. *FEBS Lett.* 205:161–165.

Seifert, R., Rosenthal, W., Schultz, G., Wieland, T., Gierschik, P., and Jakobs, K. H. (1988) The role of nucleoside-diphosphate kinase reactions in G protein activation of NADPH oxidase by guanine and adenine nucleotides. *Eur. J. Biochem.* 175:51–55.

Seifert, R., Burde, R., and Schultz, G. (1989) Activation of NADPH oxidase by purine and pyrimidine nucleotides involves G proteins and is potentiated by chemotactic peptides. *Biochem. J.* 259:813–819.

Seifert, R., Hilgenstock, G., Fassbender, M., and Distler, A. (1991) Regulation of the superoxide-forming NADPH oxidase of human neutrophils is not altered in essential hypertension. *J. Hypertens.* 9:147–153.

Seifert, R., and Schultz, G. (1991) The superoxide-forming NADPH oxidase of phagocytes. An enzyme system regulated by multiple mechanisms. *Rev. Physiol. Biochem. Pharmacol.* 117:1–338.

Seifert, R., Höer, A., Offermanns, S., Buschauer, A., and Schunack, W. (1992a) Histamine increases cytosolic Ca^{2+} in dibutyryl-cAMP-differentiated HL-60 cells via H_1 receptors and is an incomplete secretagogue. *Mol. Pharmacol.* 42:227–234.

Seifert, R., Höer, A., Schwaner, I., and Buschauer, A. (1992b) Histamine increases cytosolic Ca^{2+} in HL-60 promyelocytes predominantly via H_2 receptors with an unique agonist/antogonist profile and induces functional differentiation. *Mol. Pharmacol.* 42:235–241.

Seifert, R., Grünbaum, L., and Schultz, G. (1994) Histamine H_1-receptors in HL-60 monocytes are coupled to G_i-proteins and pertussis toxin-insensitive G-proteins and mediate activation of Ca^{2+} influx without concomitant Ca^{2+} mobilization from intracellular stores. *Naunyn-Schmiedeberg's Arch. Pharmacol.* 349:355–361.

Seifert, R., Lee, T. W., Lam, V. T., and Kobilka, B. K. (1998a) Reconstitution of β_2-adrenoceptor—GTP-binding-protein interaction in Sf9 cells: High coupling efficiency in a β_2-adrenoceptor–$G_{s\alpha}$ fusion protein. *Eur. J. Biochem.* 255:369–382.

Seifert, R., Wenzel-Seifert, K., Lee, T. W., Gether, U., Sanders-Bush, E., and Kobilka, B. K. (1998b) Different effects of $G_s\alpha$ slice variants of β_2-adrenoreceptor-mediated signaling. The β_2-adrenoreceptor coupled to the long splice variant of $G_s\alpha$ has properties of a constitutively active receptor. *J. Biol. Chem.* 273:5109–5116.

Seifert, R., Gether, U., Wenzel-Seifert, K., and Kobilka, B. K. (1999a) The effect of guanine-, inosine-and xanthine nucleotides on β_2-adrenoceptor/G_s interactions: Evidence for multiple receptor conformations. *Mol. Pharmacol.* 56:348–358.

Seifert, R., Wenzel-Seifert, Gether, U., Lam, V. T., and Kobilka, B. K. (1999b) Examining the efficiency of receptor/G-protein coupling with a cleavable β_2-adrenoceptor-$G_{s\alpha}$ fusion protein. *Eur. J. Biochem.* 260:661–666.

Seifert, R., Wenzel-Seifert, K., and Kobilka, B. K. (1999c) GPCR-Gα fusion proteins: molecular analysis of receptor-G-protein coupling. *Trends Pharmacol. Sci.* 20:383–389.

Sengelov. H., Boulay. F., Kjeldsen, L., and Borregaard, N. (1994) Subcellular localization and translocation of the receptor for N-formylmethionyl-leucyl-phenylalanine in human neutrophils. *Biochem. J.* 299:473–479.

Senogles, S. E., Spiegel, A. M., Padrell, E., Iyengar, R., and Caron, M. G. (1990) Specificity of receptor-G protein interactions. Discrimination of G_i subtypes by the D_2 dopamine receptor in a reconstituted system. *J. Biol. Chem.* 265:4507–4514.

Servant, G., Weiner, O. D., Herzmark, P., Balla, T., Sedat, J. W., and Bourne, H. R. (2000) Polarization of chemoattractant receptor signaling during neutrophil chemotaxis. *Science* 287: 1037–1040.

Shawar, S. M., Rich. R. R., and Becker, E. L. (1995) Peptides from the amino-terminus of mouse mitochondrially encoded NADH dehydrogenase subunit 1 are potent chemoattractants. *Biochem. Biophys. Res. Commun.* 211:812–818.

Showell, H. J., Freer, R. J., Zigmond, S. H., Schiffmann, E., Aswanikumar, S., Corcoran, B., and Becker, E. L. (1976) The structure–activity relations of synthetic peptides as chemotactic factors and inducers of lysosomal secretion for neutrophils. *J. Exp. Med.* 143:1154–1169.

Showell, H. J., Conklyn, M. J., Alpert, R., Hingorani, G. P., Wright, K. F., Smith, M. A., Stam, E., Salter, E. D., Scampoli, D. N., Meltzer, S., et al. (1998) The preclinical pharmacological profile of the potent and selective leukotriene B_4 antagonist CP-195543. *J. Pharmacol. Exp. Ther.* 285:946–954.

Siciliano, S. J., Rollins, T. E., and Springer, M. S. (1990) Interaction between the C5a receptor and G_i in both the membrane-bound and detergent-solubilized states. *J. Biol. Chem.* 265: 19568–19574.

Siffert, W., Rosskopf, D., Siffert, G., Busch, S., Moritz, A., Erbel, R., Sharma, A. M., Ritz, E., Wichmann, H. E., Jakobs, K. H., and Horsthemke, B. (1998) Association of a human G-protein β_3 subunit variant with hypertension. *Nature Genetics* 18:45–48.

Simon, M. I., Strathmann, M. P., and Gautam, N. (1991) Diversity of G proteins in signal transduction. *Science* 252:802–808.

Smit, M. J., Leurs, R., Alewijnse, A. E., Blauw, J., Van Nieuw Amerongen, G. P., Van De Vrede, Y., Roovers, E., and Timmerman, H. (1996) Inverse agonism of histamine H_2 antagonist accounts for upregulation of spontaneously active histamine H_2 receptors. *Proc. Natl. Acad. Sci. USA* 93:6802–6807.

Sokoloski, J. A., Sartorelli, A. C., Handschumacher, R. E., and Lee, C. W. (1991) Inhibition by pertussis toxin of the activation of Na^+-dependent uridine transport in dimethyl-sulphoxide-induced HL-60 leukaemia cells. *Biochem. J.* 280:515–519.

Stutchfield, J., and Cockcroft, S. (1988) Guanine nucleotides stimulate polyphosphoinositide phosphodiesterase and exocytotic secretion from HL60 cells permeabilized with streptolysim O. *Biochem. J.* 250:375–382.

Sunahara, R. K., Dessauer, C. W., and Gilman, A. G. (1996) Complexity and diversity of mammalian adenylyl cyclases. *Annu. Rev. Pharmacol. Toxicol.* 36:461–480.

Tager, A. M., Dufour, J. H., Goodarzi, K., Bercury, S. D., von Andrian, U. H., Luster, A. D. (2000). BLTR mediates leukotriene B4-induced chemotaxis and adhesion and plays a dominant role in eosinophil accumulation in a murine model of peritonitis. *J. Exp. Med.*, in press.

Tavet, F., Lamouri, A., Heymans, F., Dive, G., Touboul, E., Blavet, N., and Godfroid, J. J. (1997) Design and modeling of new platelet-activating factor antagonists. 2. Synthesis and biological activity of 1, 4-bis-(3',4',5'-trimethoxybenzoyl)-2-alkyl and 2-alkyloxymethylpiperazines. *J. Lipid Mediator Cell. Signal.* 15:145–159.

Thomas, K. M., Pyun, H. Y., and Navarro, J, (1990) Molecular cloning of the fMet-Leu-Phe receptor from neutrophils. *J. Biol. Chem.* 265:20061–20064.

Tian, W. N., Duzic, E., Lanier, S. M., and Deth, R. C. (1994) Determinants of α_2-adrenergic receptor activation of G proteins; evidence for a precoupled receptor/G protein state. *Mol. Pharmacol.* 45:524–531.

Toker, A., and Cantley, L. C. (1997) Signalling through the lipid products of phosphoinositide-3-OH kinase. *Nature* 387:673–676.

Tschaikowsky, K., Sittl, R., Braun, G. G., Hering, W., and Rugheimer, E. (1993) Increased fMet-Leu-Phe receptor expression and altered superoxide production of neutrophil granulocytes in septic and posttraumatic patients. *Clin. Invest.* 72:18–25.

Tsunoda, S., Sierralta, J., Sun, Y., Bodner, R., Suzuki, E., Becker, A., Socolich, M., and Zuker, C. S. (1997) A multivalent PDZ-domain protein assembles signalling complexes in a G-protein-coupled cascade. *Nature* 388:243–249.

Uhing, R. J., Polakis, P. G., and Snyderman, R. (1987) Isolation of GTP-binding proteins from myeloid HL-60 cells. Identification of two pertussis toxin substrates. *J. Biol. Chem.* 262:15575–15579.

Uhing, R. J., Gettys, T. W., Tomhave, E., Snyderman, R., and Didsbury, J. R. (1992) Differential regulation of cAMP by endogenous versus transfected formylpeptide chemoattractant receptors:implications for G_i-coupled receptor signaling. *Biochem. Biophys. Res. Commun.* 183:1033–1039.

Vanek, M., Hawkins, L. D., and Gusovsky, F. (1994) Coupling of the C5a receptor to G_i in U-937 cells and in cells transfected with C5a receptor cDNA. *Mol. Pharmacol.* 46:832–839.

Virchow, S., Ansorge, N., Rubben, H., Siffert, G., and Siffert, W. (1998) Enhanced fMLP-stimulated chemotaxis in human neutrophils from individuals carrying the G protein β_3 subunit 825 T-allele. *FEBS Lett.* 436:155–158.

Volpi, M., Naccache, P. H., Molski, T. F., Shefcyk, J., Huang, C. K., Marsh, M. L., Munoz, J., Becker, E. L., and Sha'afi, R. I. (1985) Pertussis toxin inhibits fMet-Leu-Phe but not phorbol ester-stimulated changes in rabbit neutrophils:role of G proteins in excitation response coupling. *Pro. Nalt. Acad. Sci. USA* 82:2708–2712.

Weiss, S. J. (1989) Tissue destruction by human neutrophils. *N. Engl. J. Med.* 320:365–375.

Wenzel-Seifert, K., and Seifert, R. (1990) Nucleotide-, chemotactic peptide-and phorbol ester-induced exocytosis in HL-60 leukemic cells. *Immunobiol.* 181:298–316.

Wenzel-Seifert, K., Grünbaum, L., and Seifert, R. (1991) Differential inhibition of human neutrophil activation by cyclosporins A, D, and H. Cyclosporin H is a potent and effective inhibitor of formyl peptide-induced superoxide formation. *J. Immunol.* 147:1940–1946.

Wenzel-Seifert, K., and Seifert, R. (1993) Cyclosporin H is a potent and selective formyl peptide receptor antagonist. Comparison with *N*-t-butoxycarbonyl-*L*-phenylalanyl-*L*-leucyl-*L*phenylalanyl-*L*-leucyl-*L*-phenylalanine and cyclosporins A, B, C, D, and E. *J. Immunol.* 150: 4591–4599.

Wenzel-Seifert, K., Schächtele, C., and Seifert, R. (1994) N-protein kinase C isoenzymes may be involved in the regulation of various neutrophil functions. *Biochem. Biophys. Res. Commun.* 200: 1536–1543.

Wenzel-Seifert, K., Krautwurst, D., Lentzen, H., and Seifert, R. (1996a) Concanavalin A and mistletoe lectin I differentially activate cation entry and exocytosis in human neutrophils: lectins may activate multiple subtypes of cation channels. *J. Leukoc. Biol.* 60:345–355.

Wenzel-Seifert, K., Krautwurst, D., Musgrave, I., and Seifert, R. (1996b) Thapsigargin activates univalent-and bivalent-cation entry in human neutrophils by a SK&F 96365- and Gd^{3+}-sensitive pathway and is a partial secretagogue:involvement of pertussis-toxin-sensitive G-proteins and protein phosphatases 1/2A and 2B in the signal–transduction pathway. *Biochem. J.* 314:679–686.

Wenzel-Seifert, K., Lentzen, H., Aktories, K., and Seifert, R. (1997a) Complex regulation of human neutrophil activation by actin filaments:dihydrocytochalasin B and botulinum C2 toxin uncover the existence of multiple cation entry pathways. *J. Leukoc. Biol.* 61:703–711.

Wenzel-Seifert, K., Lentzen, H., and Seifert, R. (1997b) In U-937 promonocytes, mistletoe lectin I increases basal $[Ca^{2+}]_i$, enhances histamine H_1 and complement C5a-receptor-mediated rises in $[Ca^{2+}]_i$, and induces cell death. *Naunyn Schmiedeberg's Arch. Pharmacol.* 355: 190–197.

Wenzel-Seifert, K., Hurt, C. M., and Seifert, R. (1998a) High constitutive activity of the human formyl peptide receptor. *J. Biol. Chem.* 277:24181–24189.

Wenzel-Seifert, K., Lee, T. W., Seifert, R., and Kobilka, B. K. (1998b) Restricting mobility of $G_s\alpha$ relative to the β_2-adrenoceptor enhances adenylate cyclase activity by reducing $G_s\alpha$ GTPase activity. *Biochem. J.* 334:519–524.

Wenzel-Seifert, K., Arthur, J. M., Liu, H.-Y., and Seifert, R. (1999) Quantitative analysis of formyl peptide receptor coupling to $G_{i\alpha1}$, $G_{i\alpha2}$, $G_{i\alpha3}$. *J. Biol. Chem.* 274:33259–33266.

Wess, J. (1997) G-protein-coupled receptors:molecular mechanisms involved in receptor activation and selectivity of G-protein recognition. *FASEB J.* 11:346–354.

White, J. R., Lee, J. M., Young, P. R., Hertzberg, R. P., Jurewicz, A. J., Chaikin, M. A., Widdowson, K., Foley, J. J., Martin, L. D., Griswold, D. E., and Sarau, H. M. (1998) Identification of a potent, selective non-peptide CXCR2 antagonist that inhibits interleukin-8-induced neutrophil migration. *J. Biol. Chem.* 273:10095–10098.

Wieland, T., and Jakobs, K. H. (1989) Receptor-regulated formation of GTPγS with subsequent persistent G_s-protein activation in membranes of human platelets. *FEBS Lett.* 245:189–193.

Wieland, T., Bremerich, J., Gierschik, P., and Jakobs, K. H. (1991a) Contribution of nucleoside diphosphokinase to guanine nucleotide regulation of agonist binding to formyl peptide receptors. *Eur. J. Pharmacol.* 208:17–23.

Wieland, T., Ulibarri, I., Gierschik, P., and Jakobs, K. H. (1991b) Activation of signal-transducing guanine-nucleotide-binding regulatory proteins by guanosine 5'-[γ-thio] triphosphate. Information transfer by intermediately thiophosphorylated βγ subunits. *Eur. J. Biochem.* 196:707–716.

Wieland, T., and Jakobs, K. H. (1992) Evidence for nucleoside diphosphokinase-dependent channeling of guanosine 5'-(gamma-thio) triphosphate to guanine nucleotide-binding proteins. *Mol. Pharmacol.* 42:731–735.

Wieland, T., Gierschik, P., and Jakobs, K. H. (1992a) G protein-mediated receptor–receptor interaction:studies with chemotactic receptors in membranes of human leukemia (HL 60) cells. *Naunyn-Schmiedeberg's Arch. Pharmacol.* 346:475–481.

Wieland, T., Kreiss, J., Gierschik, P., and Jakobs, K. H. (1992b) Role of GDP in formyl-peptide-receptor-induced activation of guanine-nucleotide-binding proteins in membranes of HL 60 cells. *Eur. J. Biochem.* 205:1201–1206.

Wieland, T., Nurnberg, B., Ulibarri, I., Kaldenberg-Stasch, S., Schultz, G., and Jakobs, K. H. (1993) Guanine nucleotide-specific phosphate transfer by guanine nucleotide-binding regulatory protein β-subunits. Characterization of the phosphorylated amino acid. *J. Biol. Chem.* 268:18111–18118.

Wieland, T., and Jakobs, K.-H. (1994) Measurement of receptor-stimulated guanosine 5'-O-(γ-thio) triphosphate binding by G proteins. *Methods Enzymol.* 237:3–13.

Wieland, T., Liedel, K., Kaldenberg-Stasch, S., Meyer zu Heringdorf, D., Schmidt, M., and Jakobs, K. H. (1995) Analysis of receptor-G protein interactions in permeabilized cells. *Naunyn-Schmiedeberg's Arch. Pharmacol.* 351:329–336.

Wieland, T., Meyer zu Heringdorf, D., Schulze, R. A., Kaldenberg-Stasch, S., and Jakobs, K. H. (1996) Receptor-induced translocation of activated guanine-nucleotide-binding protein α_i subunits to the cytoskeleton in myeloid differentiated human leukemia (HL-60) cells. *Eur. J. Biochem.* 239:752–758.

Wilde, M. W., Carlson, K. E., Manning, D. R., and Zigmond, S. H. (1989) Chemoattractant-stimulated GTPase activity is decreased on membranes from polymorphonuclear leukocytes incubated in chemoattractant. *J. Biol. Chem.* 264:190–196.

Wong, A. K., Finch, A. M., Pierens, G. K., Craik, D. J., Taylor, S. M., and Fairlie, D. P. (1998) Small molecular probes for G-protein-coupled C5a receptors:conformationally constrained antagonists derived from the C terminus of the human plasma protein C5a. *J. Med. Chem.* 41:3417–3425.

Wong, Y. H., Federman, A., Pace, A. M., Zachary, I., Evans, T., Pouyssegur, J., and Bourne, H. R. (1991) Mutant α subunits of G_{i2} inhibit cyclic AMP accumulation. *Nature* 351:63–65.

Wu, D., LaRosa, G. J., and Simon, M. I. (1993) G protein-coupled signal transduction pathways for interleukin-8. *Science* 261:101–103.

Wymann, M. P., von Tscharner, V., Deranleau, D. A., and Baggiolini, M. (1987) The onset of the respiratory burst in human neutrophils. Real-time studies of H_2O_2 formation reveal a rapid agonist-induced transduction process. *J. Biol. Chem.* 262:12048–12053.

Yamamoto, Y., Kanazawa, T., Shimamura, M., Ueki, M., and Hazato, T. (1997) Inhibitory effects of spinorphin, a novel endogenous regulator, on chemotaxis, O_2^- generation, and exocytosis by *N*-formylmethionyl-leucyl-phenylalanine (FMLP)-stimulated neutrophils. *Biochem. Pharmacol.* 54:695–701.

Yokomizo, T., Izumi, T., Chang, K., Takuwa, Y., and Shimizu, T. (1997) A G-protein-coupled receptor for leukotriene B_4 that mediates chemotaxis. *Nature* 387:620–624.

10

Antimicrobial Activity of Leukocytes

BERNARD M. BABIOR, CAROLYN R. HOYAL,
ROBERT I. LEHRER, and TOMAS GANZ

The reduction of oxygen by one electron creates superoxide (O_2^-), a free radical with surprisingly little reactivity, except with itself. The reactive oxygen is reduced to water through the acceptance of three additional electrons. However, during this process the relatively inert O_2^- gives rise to a series of highly reactive oxidants. The production of these oxidants is discussed in the following.

Components and Assembly of the Oxidase

The NADPH oxidase is an oligomeric enzyme consisting of membrane-associated redox core components and cytosolic activation proteins. Some of the components have been identified through reconstitution experiments with leukocytes obtained from patients with chronic granulomatous disease (CGD). These cells are unable to form O_2^-. Four genotypes of CGD have been defined, each corresponding to the deficiency of a polypeptide component of the oxidase. The proteins that constitute the oxidase and whose deficiency gives rise to CGD include flavocytochrome b_{558}, p47^{PHOX} and p67^{PHOX}. The first component identified was the membrane-associated electron-transporting component cytochrome b_{558}, which consists of a 91 kDa glycosylated protein (the β-subunit) tightly bound to a smaller p22^{PHOX} (α-subunit; Borregaard and Tauber, 1984; Dinauer et al., 1987; Parkos et al., 1987). Cytochrome b_{558} contains three prosthetic groups; a flavin adenine dinucleotide (FAD) and two low-potential hemes of the b type. The formation of a half-reduced semiquinone of FAD supports the transfer of electrons from NADPH to FAD, and then to the heme,* which serves as the terminal electron donor for O_2. The other components of the NADPH oxidase were found in the cytosol and consist of the cytosolic proteins p47^{PHOX} (Heyworth et al., 1989) and p67^{PHOX} (Dusi et al., 1993; Jones et al., 1994). The recently discovered component p40^{PHOX} does not seem to be necessary for oxidase

---

*Some authorities believe that the hemes do not participate in electron transport by cytochrome b$_{558}$.

activity (Someya et al., 1993). An additional requirement for GTP resulted in the purification of two G-proteins involved in oxidase activation: Rac2 and Rap1A.

During the activation of the respiratory burst, p47^{PHOX} and p67^{PHOX} are phosphorylated and translocate from the cytosol to the membrane-associated cytoskeleton (Kramer et al., 1988; Rotrosen and Leto, 1990; Dusi et al., 1993; Levy et al., 1994). The C-terminal quarter of p47^{PHOX} contains a cluster of serine residues that are heavily phosphorylated during activation and are critical to NADPH oxidase activity (Rotrosen and Leto, 1990). Although four of the serine residues are located in protein kinase C consensus sequences, two others are not, implying the potential interaction with other serine-directed kinases in the activation of the p47^{PHOX}. Original studies involving the stimulation of the NADPH oxidase with anionic amphiphiles, that is, in the absence of phosphorylation, are now shown to implement C-terminal conformational changes in p47^{PHOX} similar to those observed during phosphorylation. It is proposed that the alteration reveals a cytochrome b binding site.

Whereas phosphorylation regulates the activity of p47^{PHOX}, it has been recently shown that p67^{PHOX} may contain the catalytic binding site of NADPH. There is some evidence that p67^{PHOX} regulates the transfer of electrons from NADPH to the flavin of the heme. On the other hand, p47^{PHOX} can be dispensed with if the concentration of p67^{PHOX} is high enough, suggesting that p47^{PHOX} is not indispensable for electron transport from NADPH to oxygen (Koshkin et al., 1996).

Rac2 binds guanosine triphosphate (GTP) with high affinity and cycles between active (GTP-bound) and inactive (guanosine diphosphate, or GDP-bound) forms (Abo et al., 1991). In addition, posttranslational isoprenylation is necessary for the protein to function normally (Bokoch and Prossnitz, 1992). Like p47^{PHOX} phosphorylation, the GTP/GDP bound state of Rac serves as a critical point of regulation for NADPH oxidase activity. This is evident through the action of Rac GTPase-activating proteins (GAPs), which produce a concentration-dependent inhibition of superoxide production by promoting the hydrolysis of Rac-bound GTP to GDP (Heyworth et al., 1993). Rac interacts with p67^{PHOX} and, like p67^{PHOX}, is transferred to the membrane-associated cytoskeleton when the oxidase is activated. Whether or not the transfer of Rac to the cytoskeleton depends on the transfer of p47^{PHOX} and p67^{PHOX} is controversial (El Benna et al., 1994; Heyworth et al., 1994).

Rap 1A is a membrane protein that has been demonstrated to copurify with cytochrome b_{558} and is thought to play a regulatory role in the activation of the NADPH oxidase. Rap 1A was initially identified as an anti-oncogene through the suppression of Ras function. Activation of Rap 1A in leukocytes of CGD patients has led to the conclusion that GTP cycling acts independently of oxidase activation. The ability of Rap 1A to form a complex with cytochrome b_{558} is weakened when Rap 1A is phosphorylated, suggesting a role for the phosphorylation of Rap 1A in the regulation of the oxidase (Bokoch et al., 1991).

An additional protein, p40^{PHOX}, was found to co-immunoprecipitate with p47^{PHOX} and p67^{PHOX}. Cystolic proteins p47^{PHOX}, p67^{PHOX} and p40^{PHOX} all contain src homology 3 (SH3) domains that form complexes by association with proline-rich sequences (de Mendez et al., 1994, 1996); p47^{PHOX}, p67^{PHOX} and cytochrome b_{558} all contain polyproline motifs to which SH3 domains bind. Thus, p47^{PHOX}, p67^{PHOX}, and p40^{PHOX} can form transient complexes with each other, and the polyproline motif of the α-subunit of cytochrome b_{558} may serve as a docking site for these proteins during the assembly of the NADPH oxidase. In an inactive state, the carboxyl-terminal domain of p40^{PHOX} is bound tightly to p67^{PHOX} while the SH3 domain is bound to the proline-rich region of p47^{PHOX}, possibly acting to prevent p47^{PHOX} from interacting with p67^{PHOX}. In addition, p40^{PHOX} was recently shown to be phosphorylated, suggesting a potential mode for the regulation of this inhibition (Fuchs et al., 1997). Furthermore, the binding interactions of p40^{PHOX} may regulate oxidase activity through competition among other essential oxidase components.

Oxidants

Neutrophils employ a bewildering variety of reactive oxidizing agents for the destruction of invading microorganisms. All of these arise through the action of only three enzymes: NADPH oxidase, nitric oxide synthase, and myeloperoxidase.

Oxygen-based Oxidizing Agents

Neither O_2^- nor hydrogen peroxide (H_2O_2) is particularly harmful, although O_2^- can degrade iron–sulfur clusters such as those found in the ferredoxins and the mitochondrial respiratory chain (Gardner et al., 1995), and H_2O_2 can oxidize thiols (e.g, cysteine) and thioethers (e.g, methionine) to disulfides and sulfoxides, respectively (Carr and Winterbourn, 1997). The real significance of O_2^- in the function of the neutrophil is that the O_2^- produced by the leukocyte NADPH oxidase is the precursor of all the microbicidal oxidants employed by this cell.

The first lethal oxidant recognized as a product of neutrophils is hypochlorous acid (HOCl). This is produced by *myeloperoxidase*, an enzyme that catalyzes the oxidation of chloride ion (Cl$^-$) by H_2O_2 (Thomas et al., 1982, 1995) Myeloperoxidase can also oxidize bromide (Br$^-$) and iodide (I$^-$) to the corresponding hypohalous acids, and in addition, oxidizes the pseudohalogen thiocyanate (SCN$^-$) to hypothiocyanic acid (HOSCN) but because of its abundance, Cl$^-$ is its most important substrate. The enzyme itself is a tetrameric heme protein containing two heterodimers, each composed of a 58 kDa subunit and a 14 kDa-subunit (Andrews and Krinsky, 1981). The porphyrin at its active site is protoporphyrin IX, the same as in hemoglobin and cytochrome b, but in the case of myeloperoxidase, the porphyrin is attached to the enzyme by covalent bonds involving three of the groups at the periphery of the macrocycle. As a result of these attachments, the macrocycle, planar in the free state, is forced into a dome configuration, with the central iron atom displaced toward its histidine ligand and the four pyrrole rings rotated slightly to point at the iron (Fenna et al., 1995). This anomalous conformation undoubtedly explains the very unusual green color of the enzyme, a color more characteristic of a group of partially reduced cyclic tetrapyrroles known as chlorins than of fully oxidized porphyrins, which are usually red.

For most of the oxidants to be discussed in this chapter, the mechanism of killing is known only in general terms. A very specific mechanism, however, has been described for the killing of *Escherichia coli* by HOCl (Rosen et al., 1990). The microorganism is destroyed in less than a second when it encounters a high enough concentration of HOCl (Albrich and Hurst, 1982). Killing is due to the loss of the ability of the bacterial genome to replicate itself. To replicate, the genome must be attached to a special protein complex in the plasma membrane of the cell, and HOCl destroys this complex, rendering the microorganism incapable of reproducing itself. HOCl also destroys other components of the microorganism, but the rate of killing as measured by loss of colony-forming units is virtually identical to the rate at which this essential protein complex is inactivated.

A group of agents that probably serve as a backup system for HOCl are the reactive free radicals (Halliwell, 1987). The prototype for this group is the hydroxyl radical (OH•), which is generated when a transition metal ion such as iron or copper is oxidized by H_2O_2:

$$Fe^{2+} + H_2O_2 \rightarrow Fe^{3+} + OH\bullet + OH^-.$$

The Fe^{3+} is then reduced back to Fe^{2+} by any of the abundance of reducing agents present in the cell. With ascorbate (Higson et al., 1988) as the reductant, for example,

$$Fe^{3+} + Ascorbate \rightarrow Fe^{2+} + Ascorbate \ semiquinone,$$

the net reaction is

$$H_2O_2 + RH \rightarrow OH\bullet + OH^- + R\bullet,$$

with the transition metal (in the case illustrated, iron) serving as catalyst. If the transition metal is iron and reductant should happen to be O_2^-, then the two steps are known as the Haber–Weiss reaction:

$$Fe^{2+} + H_2O_2 \rightarrow Fe^{3+} + OH\bullet + OH^-$$
$$Fe^{3+} + O_2^- \rightarrow Fe^{2+} + O_2$$

$$\overline{}$$

$$H_2O_2 + O_2^- \rightarrow OH\bullet + OH^- + O_2$$

Hydroxyl radical is an exceedingly powerful oxidant that reacts with the first molecule it encounters. Considering the vast number of different molecules inside the cell, it is easy to see how OH• can give rise to innumerable free radical species that in turn can react with other molecules, propagating a chain of free radical reactions throughout the cell:

$$OH\bullet + \equiv CH \rightarrow \equiv C\bullet + H_2O$$

$$\equiv C\bullet + \equiv C'H \rightarrow \equiv C'\bullet + \equiv CH.$$

These carbon-centered radicals can also react with oxygen to generate an alkyl peroxide radical, which can then abstract a hydrogen to form an alkyl hydroperoxide:

$$\equiv C\bullet + O_2 \rightarrow \equiv C\text{-}OO\bullet$$

$$\equiv C\text{-}OO\bullet + RH \rightarrow \equiv C\text{-}OOH + R\bullet.$$

Alkyl hydroperoxides can react with transition metals in a manner similar to the reaction of H_2O_2 with transition metals, generating alkoxy anions and OH•. From the foregoing, it is easy to see how an attack by OH• radicals can leave a cell in a shambles.

OH• can also be generated by the oxidation of O_2^- in a myeloperoxidase-dependent reaction (Kettle and Winterbourn, 1994):

$$O_2^- + HOCl \rightarrow OH\bullet + O_2 + Cl^-.$$

How much of the OH• produced by neutrophils is generated by this reaction and how much is generated by the transition metal route is not known.

Singlet oxygen ($^1O_2$) is the final oxygen-centered reactive oxidant that can be generated by phagocytes. This form of oxygen is very reactive, attacking double bonds to form peroxides that are easily broken down:

$$C = C + {}^1O_2 \rightarrow \begin{array}{c} C\text{---}C \\ | \quad | \\ O\text{---}O. \end{array}$$

Early experiments looking for $^1O_2$ production by phagocytes used singlet oxygen traps, but these experiments were difficult to interpret because these traps could also react with other oxidants to yield the same products. More recently, however, the use of cholesterol as the trapping reagent gave clear-cut evidence for the production of $^1O_2$. The product generated when cholesterol reacts with $^1O_2$ is different than the product arising from the reaction between cholesterol and OH•. Taking advantage of this difference, Karnovsky and associates (Steinbeck et al., 1992) demonstrated unequivocally that neutrophils generate $^1O_2$.

This reactive oxidant probably arises in the following reaction:

$$OCl^- + H_2O_2 \rightarrow {}^1O_2 + Cl^- + H_2O.$$

Nitrogen-Based Oxidizing Agents

Nitrogen-based reactive oxidants all arise through an interaction between an innocuous nitrogen-containing compound and one of the oxygen-containing compounds discussed in the previous section. The nitrogen-containing precursors are amines (including NH_3) and nitric oxide, and the oxygen-containing compounds that react with them are $HOCl$ and O_2^-.

The first group of reactive nitrogen-containing oxidants are the chloramines. These arise through the reaction of an amine with $HOCl$ (Thomas et al., 1982, 1983):

$$R\text{-}NH_2 + HOCl \rightarrow R\text{-}NHCl + H_2O.$$

Cells contain a huge variety of amines, so this reaction gives rise to a vast number of chloramines with widely varying properties. The more lipophilic of the chloramines, including chloramine itself ($NH_2.Cl$), are very toxic. The hydrophilic chloramines, however, are much less so, and in fact, taurine chloramine ($ClNH_2\text{-}CH_2\text{-}CH_2\text{-}SO_3^=$) is so unreactive that it is used by the neutrophil as an antidote to $HOCl$.

The other nitrogen-based reactive oxidants all arise through the action of one of the oxygen-based reactive oxidants on nitric oxide ($NO\bullet$). $NO\bullet$ for host defense is manufactured by the inducible nitric oxide synthase, a 260 kDa protein that contains heme, flavin, and tetrahydrobiopterin (Hevel et al., 1991). The inducible form also contains tightly bound calmodulin (Lee and Stull, 1998). The substrates from which $NO\bullet$ is synthesized are arginine and NADPH. In the absence of arginine, nitric oxide synthase reduces oxygen by NADPH to form O_2^- (Rodriguez-Crespo et al., 1996).

The first to be recognized of the nitrogen-based reactive oxidants was peroxynitrite ($ONOO^-$; McCall et al., 1989; Salvemini et al., 1989). Peroxynitrite is made at a diffusion-limited rate from $NO\bullet$ and O_2^-. When it is made in tissues, $ONOO^-$ leaves behind footprints in the form of 3-nitrotyrosine. The identity of the nitrating agent, however, is a puzzle. $ONOO^-$ itself is a reactive species, and it is possible that it acts directly as a nitrating agent. A second possibility is nitrocarbonate, produced in a reaction between $ONOO^-$ and CO_2 (Uppu et al., 1996):

$$ONOO^- + CO_2 \rightarrow O_2N\text{-}O\text{-}CO_2^-.$$

Yet a third possibility is nitryl chloride, made by the chlorination of nitrite by $HOCl$, the latter produced by myeloperoxidase as described previously (Eiserich et al., 1996):

$$NO_2^- + HOCl \rightarrow Cl\text{-}NO_2 + OH^-.$$

It is likely that all three nitrating agents are made and used in the complex chemical environment of the phagosome.

Oxygen-Independent Microbial Killing

The concept that the microbicidal powers of granulocytes resided in their cytoplasmic granules arose from studies performed a century ago by Metchnikoff and Ehrlich. These insights lay fallow for over 60 years, until revived by Hirsch and Spitznagel, whose descriptions of "phagocytin" (by James Hirsch) and of "lysosomal cationic proteins" (by John Spitznagel; Zeya and Spitznagel, 1963) initiated the modern era of investigating this question. During the last two decades, extractive biochemistry had delineated an array of polypeptides with microbicidal properties in the granules of neutrophils and eosinophils (Levy, 1996; Ganz and Lehrer, 1997). Electron micrographs of phagocytizing human granulocytes show that the protein-rich granule contents are not greatly diluted after their delivery to the relatively tight phagosomal space. Consequently, it is likely that very high concentrations of microbicidal and digestive granule proteins prevail in most phagosomes. Unlike granulocytes, most macrophages contain few cytoplasmic storage granules, suggesting that they may rely predominantly on oxidant production, supplemented by ongoing synthesis and translocation of microbicidal substances, to generate antimicrobial activity.

The acidification of phagocytic vacuoles was described by Metchnikoff, who noted that litmus granules turned from blue (alkaline) to pink (acid) after ingestion by granulocytes. The net pH of the vacuole is mainly determined by the balance between a vacuolar proton-pumping ATPase and the alkalinizing effect of superoxide anions generated by the activation of NADPH oxidase. In neutrophils, this balance results in early phagosome alkalinization, followed within 60 minutes by acidification to a pH of 5–6 (Cech and Lehrer, 1984). Although some microbes are inhibited by this mild acidification, many others are resistant, or may block the acidification process (Horwitz and Maxfield, 1984; Rathman et al., 1996). The connection between vacuolar acidification and the Nramp gene variants (Hackam et al., 1998) in mice is particularly intriguing since the Nramp defect is associated with a decreased ability of macrophages to inhibit intracellular pathogens such as mycobacteria.

Macrophages (and several other cell types) can also limit the intracellular multiplication of pathogens by restricting their access to nutrients essential for survival or growth. Macrophages restrict tryptophan by inducing an enzyme (indoleamine 2,3-dioxygenase) that depletes intracellular tryptophan, an amino acid essential for the survival of pathogens (Murray et al., 1989; Taylor and Feng, 1991). A similar strategy limits another essential nutrient, iron, whose transport into macrophages is diminished by macrophage activation (Byrd and Horwitz, 1989; Gebran et al., 1994).

In addition to the enzymes and transporters that modify the composition of the phagosomal environment, granulocytes also deliver to the phagosome high concentrations of preformed antimicrobial substances that directly damage their microbial targets. The best-studied granulocyte, the human neutrophil (polymorphonuclear leukocyte), contains several thousand granules that can be classified into several subtypes based on their density, com-

Table 10.1. Antimicrobial Polypeptides of Phagocytes

Polypeptide	Molecular Mass (kD)	Distribution	Probable Mechanism of Action
Myeloperoxidase (MPO) and eosinophil peroxidase (EPO)	150	MPO: neutrophils (AG), monocytes EPO: eosinophils	Generation of microbicidal hypohalites from hydrogen peroxide and halide ions
Lactoferrin	80	Neutrophils (SG)	Iron sequestration and peptide products of proteolysis
Bactericidal permeability-inducing protein (BPI)	60	Neutrophils (AG)>>eosinophils	Distruption of outer membranes of Gram-negative bacteria and ?
Serprocidins (cathepsin G, azurocidin/CAP37)	30	Neutrophils (AG)	
Calprotectin (MRP8/14, calgranulin)	11, 13	Neutrophils, macrophages (cytoplasm)	
Lysozyme	14	Neutrophils (AG,SG) monocytes, macrophages	Cleavage of glycosidic links in peptidoglycan of Gram-positive bacteria and ?
Eosinophil cationic protein (ECP)	16	Eosinophils<neutrophils	
Eosinophil-derived neurotoxin (EDN)	16	Eosinophils>neutrophils	
Major basic protein (MBP)	14	Eosinophils	
Phospholipase A2	14	Eosinophils, neutrophils	Cleavage of structural phospholipids
Secretory leukoprotease inhibitor (SLPI)	12	Macrophages	
Cathelicidin (FALL39, LL37, CAP18)	18/5*	Neutrophils (SG)	*Proteolytic products are the active agents for most cathelicidins
Defensins	4	Neutrophils (AG)	Permeabilization of microbial membranes

Note. AG = azurophil (primary) granules; SG = specific (secondary) granules.

position, time of formation, and response to various stimuli (Rice et al., 1987; Borregaard and Cowland, 1994; Egesten et al., 1994). A number of these subtypes contain substances with microbicidal properties (Table 10.1). The densest granules (dense azurophilic or dense primary granules) consist mostly of small cationic microbicidal peptides called defensins. Granules of intermediate density (classical azurophils or primary granules) contain, in addition, the larger cationic proteins myeloperoxidase, elastase, cathepsin G, azurocidin, and lysozyme. The least dense granules (secondary or specific) contain lysozyme, lactoferrin, and one or more microbicidal peptide precursors ("cathelicidins"). The generation of granule diversity is a fundamental feature of neutrophil development. Recent studies of granulogenesis favor a model of successive waves of specialized protein synthesis during the promyelocyte and myelocyte stages of the development of granulocytes in the bone marrow (Borregaard and Cowland, 1994). Granule protein synthesis begins during the promyelocyte stage, and is marked by bursts of myeloperoxidase, elastase, and cathepsin G production. These products are packaged within the classical primary (azurophil) granules. The second wave of protein synthesis occurs during the late promyelocyte stage and produces the defensins packaged in the dense primary granules. Later, during the myelocyte and metamyelocyte stages, lactoferrin and (presumably) cathelicidins are synthesized, and are packaged in the secondary (or specific) granules. Lysozyme (muramidase) is made in both promyelocytes and myelocytes, accounting for its presence in primary and secondary granule subtypes. It is presumed that the membranes of each granule subtype are decorated with specialized docking proteins that govern the movement and destination of each granule in stimulated granulocytes, by interacting with the cytoskeleton and with docking proteins on other membranes. Thus the contents of dense and intermediate primary granules can be destined predominantly for delivery to the phagosome, whereas the lighter secondary granules are largely secreted into the extracellular milieu (Leffell and Spitznagel, 1974, 1975).

Several common features of granule proteins have emerged from their biochemical characterization (Table 10.1; Nakamoto, 1996; Ganz and Lehrer, 1997; Ganz and Weiss, 1997). The granules contain a sulfated proteoglycan matrix that is negatively charged. As the major granule proteins are arginine-rich and cationic, they are probably electrostatically bound to the matrix in a dense structural array. The granule membrane fuses to the phagosome, exposing its contents to an environment that frees its cationic proteins and peptides from the matrix. Their positive charge favors interactions with the membrane phospholipids of bacteria, which tend to be more anionic than the phospholipids found in eukaryotic membranes. Myeloperoxidase, an abundant granule protein that defines light azurophil (primary) granules, is an enzyme that potentiates the toxic effects of the respiratory burst product, hydrogen peroxide. Other granule proteins have enzymatic activities that directly disrupt the integrity of bacterial cell walls and membranes. Lysozyme targets the peptidoglycan exoskeleton of bacteria, causing them to become susceptible to osmotic stress and perhaps sensitizing them to other granule substances. Both neutrophils and eosinophils contain secretory phospholipase A_2, a cationic enzyme whose preferential activity against bacterial phospholipids is believed to underlie its potent activity against gram-positive bacteria (Elsbach et al., 1990; Weinrauch et al., 1996; Ganz and Lehrer, 1997). Neutrophil elastase and proteinase 3 are proteases that can degrade proteins of microbes killed by phagocytes. Leukocyte azurocidin, an enzymatically inactive member of the serprocidin serine protease family, and cathepsin G

(Gabay and Almeida, 1993) evidently kill bacteria by a microbicidal mechanism distinct from proteolysis.

Other granule proteins act by depriving microbes of essential nutrients. Lactoferrin (Ellison, 1994) sequesters iron, making it unavailable to all but a few unusually host-adapted bacteria like *Neisseria*. Some granule proteins bind to specific structural macromolecules on microbial surfaces (e.g., lipopolysaccharide) and disrupt microbial membranes presumably by intercalating and destabilizing the interactions between essential structural elements. The bactericidal permeability-inducing protein (BPI; Elsbach and Weiss, 1993; Ganz and Weiss, 1997) of granulocytes belongs to a family of proteins that avidly bind lipids. BPI specifically interacts with lipopolysaccharide, the outer membrane constituent of Gram-negative bacteria, and disrupts the outer membrane. Two classes of small amphipathic peptide antimicrobials found in the neutrophils of many animals rely on less specific interactions with the lipid membranes. The defensins (Ganz and Lehrer, 1995) are stored in an active form and are delivered to neutrophil phagosomes at high concentrations. The cathelicidins (Ganz and Lehrer, 1995) are a highly heterogeneous group of peptides that share a common N-terminal precursor segment, cathelin. Many but not all cathelicidins require activation by small amounts of neutrophil elastase that cleaves off the cathelin moiety and liberates an active microbicidal peptide. The activation step takes place during or after secretion. The initial step in the microbicidal activity of defensins and some cathelicidins involves the formation of multimeric pores in microbial membranes. These processes have been extensively studied in artificial lipid bilayers and appear to be critically dependent on anionic phospholipids characteristic of bacterial membranes. The presence of a transmembrane electromotive force greatly facilitates the formation of pores, presumably by driving the cationic defensins into the membrane. Additional antimicrobial peptides may be generated in the phagosome by the cleavage of larger granule proteins, such as lactoferrin (Ellison, 1994) to yield the directly antimicrobial fragment lactoferricin.

The eosinophil granulocytes accumulate in tissues invaded by multicellular parasites and their microbicidal equipment is presumably specialized to destroy these pathogens (Gleich and Adolphson, 1986). Compared to the neutrophilic granulocyte, the eosinophil contains fewer but larger granules. Like neutrophilic granulocytes, the eosinophil has an NADPH oxidase that generates reactive oxygen intermediates, and its granules contain highly cationic proteins. One of the four principal proteins of eosinophil granules is eosinophil peroxidase, an enzyme similar to myeloperoxidase that amplifies the toxic effects of respiratory burst products. The other abundant granule proteins, major basic protein (MBP) and two members of the ribonuclease family (EDN, eosinophil-derived neurotoxin and ECP, eosinophil cationic protein) display in vitro activity against the parasitic worms *Trichinella spiralis* and *Schistosoma mansonii*. Evidence is increasing that eosinophils and neutrophils share several of their microbicidal proteins and functional capacities (Lehrer et al., 1989; Sur et al., 1998).

Useful insights into the role of the various microbicidal mechanisms can be gleaned from genetic diseases. With the exception of myeloperoxidase deficiency, disorders of granule composition are very rare and affect multiple granule components. In Chediak–Higashi syndrome, a disorder of granulogenesis in multiple cell types, azurophil granules of neutrophils are deficient in elastase and cathepsin G (Ganz et al., 1988). The patients suffer from frequent bacterial infections and their granulocytes manifest impaired killing ability in vitro. Another genetic condition, specific granule deficiency, can be best understood as a defect in the differentiation program of the granulocyte precursors. The components of the granules made early during the differentation process (myeloperoxidase, lysozyme, serine proteases) appear normal but defensin content is severely decreased (Ganz et al., 1988), and the secondary (specific) granule proteins (e.g., lactoferrin) are absent (Gallin et al., 1982; Johnston et al., 1992). The patients with this rare condition also suffer from recurrent bacterial infections. The complex nature of the defects in both disorders does not permit attribution of the functional defect to specific deficient neutrophil granule proteins.

The study of phagocytes in animal models has revealed a remarkable interspecies diversity of phagocytic antimicrobial arsenals. Thus, human granulocytes express a single cathelicidin gene (variously named LL-37, FALL-39 or CAP18) but bovine, sheep, and porcine granulocytes contain the products of half a dozen or more distinct genes (Zanetti et al., 1995). Defensins and BPI are abundant in the granulocytes of rabbits and humans, but mice, the experimental animals best suited for gene disruption studies, have granuloyctes that lack defensins and BPI (Eisenhauer and Lehrer, 1992). One interpretation of these findings is that the various granule proteins have overlapping and partially redundant roles in phagocytic killing, and that the evolution of the set of proteins present in each animal species may be driven by the pressures from their respective microbial pathogens. Nevertheless, transgenic experiments can be very informative when the loss or introduction of a single granule protein leads to an identifiable phenotype. Thus, the recent neutrophil elastase knockout experiments (Belaaouaj et al., 1998) have demonstrated that loss of this granule component increased the susceptibility of mice to death from *Klebsiella pneumoniae* infection, and that compared to wild-type granulocytes, the granulocytes of these mice killed *K pneumoniae* and *E coli* more slowly. It is not yet clear whether neutrophil elastase is directly microbicidal in the phagosome or whether it acts by activating other proteins or peptides (Shi and Ganz, 1998). It can be anticipated that transgenic modifications of granule composition will continue to shed light on the function of each granule component.

In addition to antimicrobial substances contained in neutrophil granules, a highly abundant neutrophil cytoplasmic protein, variously named calprotectin, MRP8/14, and L1 protein, inhibits microbial growth in vitro by a zinc-inhibitable mechanism. This protein complex is released into epithelia and epithelial fluids from neutrophils and macrophages as well as epithelial cells, and is thought to be responsible for the ability of neutrophils to inhibit the invasion of tissue by *Candida albicans* without direct contact with the yeast (Sohnle et al., 1996).

Summary

In summary, phagocytes employ a remarkably diverse arsenal of microbicidal substances that range from protons and reactive oxidants to pore-forming peptides, nutrient-binding proteins, and proteins that have recognition sites for specific bacterial macromolecules. The diverse molecular targets and overlapping antimicrobial spectra of these substances may prevent the emergence of resistance on the short time scale common to human-made antimicrobials. The complex interactions that take place within the phagosomal environment continue to be a fertile area for further investigation.

References

Abo, A., Pick, E., Hall, A., Totty, N., Teahan, C. G., and Segal, A. W. (1991) Activation of the NADPH oxidase involves the small GTP-binding protein p21rac1. *Nature* 353:668–670.

Albrich, J. M., and Hurst, J. K. (1982) Oxidative inactivation of *Escherichia coli* by hypochlorous acid. Rates and differentiation of respiratory from other reactive sites. *FEBS Lett.* 144:157–161.

Andrews, P. C., and Krinsky, N. I. (1981) The reductive cleavage of myeloperoxidase in half, producing enzymically active hemi-myeloperoxidase. *J. Biol. Chem.* 256:4211–4218.

Belaaouaj, A., McCarthy, R., Baumann, M., Gao, Z., Ley, S. N., Abraham, S. N., and Shapiro, S. D. (1998) Mice lacking neutrophil elastase reveal impaired host defense against gram negative bacterial sepsis. *Nat. Med.* 4:615–618.

Bokoch, G. M., Quilliam, L. A., Bohl, B. P., Jesaitis, A. J., and Quinn, M. T. (1991) Inhibition of Rap 1A binding to cytochrome b558 of NADPH oxidase by phosphorylation of Rap 1A. *Science* 254:1794–1796.

Bokoch, G. M., and Prossnitz, V. (1992) Isoprenoid metabolism is required for stimulation of the respiratory burst oxidase of HL-60 cells. *J. Clin. Invest.* 89:402–408.

Borregaard, N., and Tauber, A. I. (1984) Subcellular localization of the human neutrophil NADPH-oxidase:b-cytochrome and associated flavoprotein. *J. Biol. Chem.* 259:47–52.

Borregaard, N., and Cowland, J. B. (1994) Granules of the human neutrophilic polymorphonuclear leukocyte. *Blood* 89:3503–3521.

Byrd, T. F., and Horwitz, M. A. (1989) Interferon gamma-activated human monocytes downregulate transferrin receptors and inhibit the intracellular multiplication of *Legionella pneumophila* by limiting the availability of iron. *J. Clin. Invest.* 83:1457–1465.

Carr, A. C., and Winterbourn, C. C. (1997) Oxidation of neutrophil glutathione and protein thiols by myeloperoxidase-derived hypochlorous acid. *Biochem. J.* 327:275–281.

Cech, P., and Lehrer, R. I. (1984) Phagolysosomal pH of human neutrophils. *Blood* 63:88–95.

de Mendez, I., Garrett, M. C., Adams, A. G., and Leto, T. L. (1994) Role of p67-phox SH3 domains in assembly of the NADPH oxidase system. *J. Biol. Chem.* 269:16326–16332.

de Mendez, I., Adams, A. G., Sokolic, R. A., and Leto, T. L. (1996) Multiple SH3 domain interactions regulate NADPH oxidase assembly in whole cells. *EMBO J.* 15:1211–1220.

Dinauer, M. C., Orkin, S. H., Brown, R., Jesaitis, A. J., and Parkos, C. A. (1987) The glycoprotein encoded by the X-linked chronic granulomatous disease locus is a component of the neutrophil cytochrome b complex. *Nature* 327:717–720.

Dusi, S., Della Bianca, V., Grzeskowiak, M., and Rossi, F. (1993) Relationship between phosphorylation and translocation to the plasma membrane of p47phox and p67phox and activation of the NADPH oxidase in normal and Ca^{2+}-depleted human neutrophils. *Biochem. J.* 290:173–178.

Egesten, A., Breton-Gorius, J., Guichard, J., Gullberg, U., and Olsson, I. (1994) The heterogeneity of azurophil granules in neutrophil promyelocytes: immunogold localization of myeloperoxidase, cathepsin G, elastase, proteinase 3, and bactericidal/permeability increasing protein. *Blood* 70:757–765.

Eisenhauer, P. B., and Lehrer, R. I. (1992) Mouse neutrophils lack defensins. *Infect. Immun.* 60: 3446–3447.

Eiserich, J. P., Cross, C. E., Jones, A. D., Halliwell, B., and van der Vliet, A. (1996) Formation of nitrating and chlorinating species by reaction of nitrite with hypochlorous acid. A novel mechanism for nitric oxide-mediated protein modification. *J. Biol. Chem.* 271:19199–19208.

El Benna, J., Ruedi, J. M., and Babior, B. M. (1994) Cytosolic guanine nucleotide-binding protein Rac2 operates in vivo as a component of the neutrophil respiratory burst oxidase. Transfer of Rac2 and the cytosolic oxidase components p47*phox* and p67*phox* to the submembranous actin cytoskeleton during oxidase activation. *J. Biol. Chem.* 269:6729–6734.

Ellison, I.R.T. (1994) The effects of lactoferrin on gram-negative bacteria. *Adv. Exp. Med. Biol.* 357:71–90.

Elsbach, P., Weiss, J., Wright, G., Forst, S., van den Bergh, C. J., and Verheij, H. M. (1990) Regulation and role of phospholipases in host–bacteria interaction. *Prog. Clin. Biol. Res.* 349:1–9.

Elsbach, P., and Weiss, J. (1993) Bactericidal/permeability increasing protein and host defense against gram-negative bacteria and endotoxin. *Curr. Opin. Immunol.* 5:103–107.

Fenna, R., Zeng, J., and Davey, C. (1995) Structure of the green heme in myeloperoxidase. *Arch. Biochem. Biophys.* 316:653–656.

Fuchs, A., Bouïn, A.-P., Rabilloud, T., and Vignais, P. V. (1997) The 40-kDa component of the phagocyte NADPH oxidase (p40*phox*) is phosphorylated during activation in differentiated HL60 cells. *Eur. J. Biochem.* 249 :531–539.

Gabay, J. E., and Almeida, R. P. (1993) Antibiotic peptides and serine protease homologs in human polymorphonuclear leukocytes: defensins and azurocidin. *Curr. Opin. Immunol.* 5:97–102.

Gallin, J. I., Fletcher, M. P., Seligmann, B. E., Hoffstein, S., Cehrs, K., and Mounessa, N. (1982) Human neutrophil-specific granule deficiency: A model to assess the role of neutrophil-specific granules in the evolution of the inflammatory response. *Blood* 59:1317–1329.

Ganz, T., Metcalf, J. A., Gallin, J. I., Boxer, L. A., and Lehrer, R. I. (1988) Microbicidal/cytotoxic proteins of neutrophils are deficient in two disorders: Chediak–Higashi syndrome and "specific" granule deficiency. *J. Clin. Invest.* 82:552–556.

Ganz, T., and Lehrer, R. I. (1995) Defensins. *Pharmacol. Ther.* 66:191–205.

Ganz, T., and Lehrer, R. I. (1997) Antimicrobial peptides of leukocytes. *Curr. Opin. Hematol.* 4: 53–58.

Ganz, T., and Weiss, J. (1997) Antimicrobial peptides of phagocytes and epithelia. *Semin. Hematol.* 34:343–354.

Gardner, P. R., Rainer, I., Epstein, L. B., and White, C. W. (1995) Superoxide radical and iron modulate aconitase activity in mammalian cells. *J. Biol. Chem.* 270:13399–13405.

Gebran, S. J., Newton, C., Yamamoto, Y., Widen, R., Klein, T. W., and Friedman, H. (1994) Macrophage permissiveness for *Legionella pneumophila* growth modulated by iron. *Infect. Immun.* 62:564–568.

Gleich, G. J., and Adolphson, C. R. (1986) The eosinophilic leukocyte: structure and function. *Adv. Immunol.* 39:177–253.

Hackam, D. J., Rotstein, O. D., Zhang, W., Gruenheid, S., Gros, P., and Grinstein, S. (1998) Host resistance to intracellular infection: mutation of natural resistance-associated macrophage protein 1 (Nramp1) impairs phagosomal acidification. *J. Exp. Med.* 188:351–364.

Halliwell, B. (1987) Oxidants and human disease: some new concepts. *FASEB J.* 1:358–364.

Hevel, J. M., White, K. A., and Marletta, M. A. (1991) Purification of the inducible murine macrophage nitric oxide synthase. *J. Biol. Chem.* 266:22789–22791.

Heyworth, P. G., Shrimpton, C. F., and Segal, A. W. (1989) Localization of the 47 kDa phosphoprotein involved in the respiratory-burst NADPH oxidase of phagocytic cells. *Biochem. J.* 260: 243–248.

Heyworth, P. G., Knaus, U. G., Settleman, J., Curnutte, J. T., and Bokoch, G. M. (1993) Regulation of NADPH oxidase activity by Rac GTPase activating protein(s). *Mol. Biol. Cell* 4:1217–1223.

Heyworth, P. G., Bohl, B. P., Bokoch, G. M., and Curnutte, J. T. (1994) Rac translocates independently of the neutrophil NADPH oxidase components p47*phox* and p67*phox*. Evidence for its interaction with flavocytochrome b_{558}. *J. Biol. Chem.* 269:30749–30752.

Higson, F. K., Kohen, R., and Chevion, M. (1988) Iron enhancement of ascorbate toxicity. *Free Radic. Res. Commun.* 5:107–115.

Horwitz, M. A., and Maxfield, F. R. (1984) *Legionella pneumophila* inhibits acidification of its phagosome in human monocytes. *J. Cell Biol.* 99:1936–1943.

Johnston, J. J., Boxer, L. A., and Berliner, N. (1992) Correlation of messenger RNA levels with protein defects in specific granule deficiency. *Blood* 80:2088–2091.

Jones, S. A., Wood, J. D., Coffey, M. J., and Jones, O.T.G. (1994) The functional expression of p47-*phox* and p67-*phox* may contribute to the generation of superoxide by an NADPH oxidase-like system in human fibroblasts. *FEBS Lett.* 355:178–182.

Kettle, A. J., and Winterbourn, C. C. (1994) Superoxide-dependent hydroxylation by myeloperoxidase. *J. Biol. Chem.* 269:17146–17151.

Koshkin, V., Lotan, O., and Pick, E. (1996) The cytosolic component p47*phox* is not a *sine qua non* participant in the activation of NADPH oxidase but is required for optimal superoxide production. *J. Biol. Chem.* 271:30326–30329.

Kramer, I.J.M., Verhoeven, A. J., van der Bend, R. L., Weening, R. S., and Roos, D. (1988) Purified protein kinase C phosphorylates a 47 kDa protein in control neutrophil cytoplasts but not in neutrophil cytoplasts from patients with the autosomal form of chronic granulomatous disease. *J. Biol. Chem.* 263:2352–2357.

Lee, S. J., and Stull, J. T. (1998) Calmodulin-dependent regulation of inducible and neuronal nitric-oxide synthase. *J. Biol. Chem.* 273:27430–26437.

Leffell, M. S., and Spitznagel, J. K. (1974) Intracellular and extracellular degranulation of human polymorphonuclear azurophl and specific granules induced by immune complexes. *Infect. Immun.* 10:1241–1249.

Leffell, M. S., and Spitznagel, J. K. (1975) Fate of human lactoferrin and myeloperoxidase in-phagocytizing human neutrophils: effects of immunoglobulin G subclasses and immune complexes coated on latex beads. *Infect. Immun.* 12:813–820.

Lehrer, R. I., Szklarek, D., Barton, A., Ganz, T., Hamann, K. J., and Gleich, G. J. (1989) Antibacterial properties of eosinophil major basic protein and eosinophil cationic protein. *J. Immunol.* 142:4428–4434.

Levy, O. (1996) Antibiotic proteins of polymorphonuclear leukocytes. *Eur. J. Haematol.* 56:263–277.

Levy, R., Dana, R., Leto, T. L., and Malech, H. L. (1994) The requirement of p47 phosphorylation for activation of NADPH oxidase by opsonized zymosan in human neutrophils. *Biochim. Biophys. Acta Mol. Cell Res.* 1220:253–260.

McCall, T. B., Boughton-Smith, N. K., Palmer, R. M., Whittle, B. J., and Moncada, S. (1989) Synthesis of nitric oxide from L-arginine by neutrophils. Release and interaction with superoxide anion. *Biochem. J.* 261:293–296.

Murray, H. W., Szuro-Sudol, A., Wellner, D., Oca, M. J., Granger, A. M., Libby, D. M., Rothermel, C. D., and Rubin, B. Y. (1989) Role of tryptophan degradation in respiratory burst-independent antimicrobial activity of gamma interferon-stimulated human macrophages. *Infect. Immun.* 57:845–849.

Nakamoto, R. K. (1996) Mechanisms of active transport in the $F_0.F_1$ ATP synthase. *J. Membr. Biol.* 151:101–111.

Parkos, C. A., Allen, R. A., Cochrane, C. G., and Jesaitis, A. J. (1987) Purified cytochrome b from human granulocyte plasma membrane is comprised of two polypeptides with relative molecular weights of 91,000 and 22,000. *J. Clin. Invest.* 80:732–742.

Rathman, M., Sjaastad, M. D., and Falkow, S. (1996) Acidification of phagosomes containing *Salmonella typhimurium* in murine macrophages. *Infect. Immun.* 64:2765–2773.

Rice, W. G., Ganz, T., Kinkade J. M. Jr., Selsted, M. E., Lehrer, R. I., and Parmley, R. T. (1987) Defensin-rich dense granules of human neutrophils. *Blood* 70:757–765.

Rodriguez-Crespo, I., Gerber, N. C., and Ortiz de Montellano, P. R. (1996) Endothelial nitric-oxide synthase. Expression in *Escherichia coli*, spectroscopic characterization, and role of te-trahydrobiopterin in dimer formation. *J. Biol. Chem.* 271:11462–11467.

Rosen, H., Orman, J., Rakita, R. M., Michel, B. R., and VanDevanter, D. R. (1990) Loss of DNA-membrane interactions and cessation of DNA synthesis in myeloperoxidase-treated *Escherichia coli. Proc. Natl. Acad. Sci.* 87:10048–10052.

Rotrosen, D., and Leto, T. L. (1990) Phosphorylation of neutrophil 47-kDa cytosolic oxidase factor. Translocation to membrane is associated with distinct phosphorylation events. *J. Biol. Chem.* 265:19910–19915.

Salvemini, D., Nucci, G., Gryglewski, R. J., and Vane, J. R. (1989) Human neutrophils and mono-nuclear cells inhibit platelet aggregation by releasing a nitric oxide-like factor. *Proc. Natl. Acad. Sci.* 86:6328–6332.

Shi, J., and Ganz, T. (1998) The role of protegrins and other elastase-activated polypeptides in the bactericidal properties of porcine inflammatory fluids. *Infect. Immun.* 66:3611–3617.

Sohnle, P. G., Hahn, B. L., and Santhanagopalan, V. (1996) Inhibition of *Candida albicans* growth by calprotectin in the absence of direct contact with the organisms. *J. Infect. Dis.* 174:1369–1372.

Someya, A., I. Nagaoka, and T. Yamashita (1993). Purification of the 260 kDa cytosolic complex involved in the superoxide production of guinea pig neutrophils. *FEBS Lett.* 330:215–218.

Steinbeck, M. J., Khan, A. U., Karnovsky, M. J., and Hegg, G. G. (1992) Intracellular singlet oxy-gen generation by phagocytosing neutrophils in response to particles coated with a chemical trap. *J. Biol. Chem.* 267:13425–13433.

Sur, S., Glitz, D. G., Kita, H., Kujawa, S. M., Peterson, E. A., Weiler, D. A., Kephart, G. M., Wagner, J. M., George, T. J., Gleich, G. J., and Leiferman, K. M. (1998) Localization of eosinophil-drived neurotoxin and eosinophil cationic protein in neutrophilic leukocytes. *J. Leukoc. Biol.* 63:715–722.

Taylor, M. W., and Feng, G.-S. (1991) Relationship between interferon-gamma, indoleamine 2,3-dioxygenase, and tryptophan catabolism. *FASEB J.* 5:2516–2522.

Thomas, E. L., Jefferson, M. M., and Grisham, M. (1982) Myeloperoxidase-catalyzed incorpora-tion of amino acids into proteins: Role of hypochlorous acid and chloramines. *Biochemistry* 21:6299–6308.

Thomas, E. L., Grisham, M. B., and Jefferson, M. M. (1983) Myeloperoxidase-dependent effect of amines on functions of isolated neutrophils. *J. Clin. Invest.* 72:441–454.

Thomas, E. L., Bozeman, P. M., Jefferson, M. M., and King, C. C. (1995) Oxidation of bromide by the human leukocyte enzymes myeloperoxidase and eosinophil peroxidase. Formation of bromamines. *J. Biol. Chem.* 270:2906–2913.

Uppu, R. M., Squadrito, G. L., and Pryor, W. A. (1996) Acceleration of peroxynitrite oxidations by carbon dioxide. *Arch. Biochem. Biophys.* 327:335–343.

Weinrauch, Y., Elsbach, P., Madsen, L. M., Foreman, A., and Weiss, J. (1996) The potent anti-*Staphylococcus aureus* activity of a sterile rabbit inflammatory fluid is due to a 14-kD phospho-lipase A2. *J. Clin. Invest.* 97:250–257.

Zanetti, M. R., Gennaro, R., and Romeo, D. (1995) Cathelicidins: a novel protein family with a common proregion and a variable C-terminal antimicrobial domain. *FEBS Lett.* 374:1–5.

Zeya, H. I., and Spitznagel, J. K. (1963) Antibacterial and enzymic basic proteins from leukocyte lysosomes: separation and identification. *Science* 142:1085–1087.

11

In Vitro Flow Models of Leukocyte Adhesion

MICHAEL B. LAWRENCE

The expression and regulation of adhesive interactions between the leukocyte and the endothelium are critical for directing leukocytes to sites of inflammatory challenge. In vitro flow experiments that replicate circulatory hydrodynamics in simplified form have shed considerable light on the functional relationship between different types of adhesion mechanisms used by leukocytes to interact with endothelium. In conjunction with in vivo studies, a model of the basic regulatory architecture of an acute inflammatory response has emerged in which leukocyte interactions with endothelium under flow conditions consist of an initial rolling interaction followed by β_2/β_1 integrin mediated arrest (Springer, 1994). This chapter describes methods of studying leukocyte adhesion under flow conditions and illustrates the key differences among measurement techniques that incorporate shear into the assessment of leukocyte adhesive interactions.

Adhesion Assays to Characterize Leukocyte–Endothelial Cell Interactions

Cell surface receptors that signal and those that mediate adhesion must be able to interact with ligands on the apposing cell membrane. However, adhesion receptors, unlike cell surface signaling receptors, must be able to form bonds that withstand mechanical stresses. Therefore, to quantify cell–cell adhesion and the consequences of adhesive interactions, it is necessary to apply force to separate cells from each other. Several types of shearing systems have been developed to introduce forces into adhesion assays in a controlled fashion: the capillary tube, the parallel plate chamber, the cone and plate viscometer, and the radial flow chamber. Shear flow assays introduce two related parameters into adhesion assays: the element of force acting on the molecular cross-bridges and the reduction in cell-substrate or cell–cell contact times by fluid motion. The magnitude of the applied force and how rapidly it is applied may have significant consequences for the interpretation of adhesion experiments. The most common types of adhesion assays are listed in Table 11.1 along with a brief comment on the type of force applied and a representative citation.

Table 11.1. Cell–Cell and Cell-Substrate Adhesion Assays

Assay	Contacting Method	Reference
Stamper–Woodruff	Leukocyte suspension layered onto rotating tissue specimen (nonstatic), shear force	Stamper and Woodruff, 1976
Plate-binding	Cells allowed to settle in wells of an ELISA plate (static), normal and shear forces	Dustin and Springer, 1989
Smith–Hollers chamber	Cells injected into sealed chamber, allowed to settle, then chamber inverted (1G), normal force	Smith et al., 1988, 1991
Centrifugation assay	Cells in sealed ELISA plates are centrifuged, force depends on the rotation speeds, normal force	McClay et al., 1981; Ward et al., 1995; Piper et al., 1998
Cone & plate viscometer	Suspension of cells exposed to uniform shear, shear and normal force on aggregated cells	Taylor et al., 1996
Couette viscometer	Suspension of cells exposed to uniform shear	Xia and Frojmovic, 1994
Capillary tube	Suspension of cells exposed to varying shear forces; exposure of anchored cells to defined shear force; some designs employ a recirculating loop	Bell et al., 1989; Bargatze et al., 1994
Radial flow chamber	Leukocytes interacting with adhesive substrates experience fluid shear force based on position from center of disk, shearing force	Kuo and Lauffenburger, 1993
Parallel plate flow chamber	Leukocytes are perfused over adhesive substrates or endothelial cells at defined shear stress, shearing force	Sung et al., 1985; Palecek et al., 1997

Note. ELISA, enzyme-linked immunosorbent assay.

Static and Centrifugation Assays

Static assays dominate the literature on leukocyte–endothelial cell interactions for good reasons: the assays are simple, require relatively inexpensive microtitre plates or petri dishes, and allow many variables to be studied because a number of assays can be conducted in parallel. In most cases, a suspension of leukocytes is pipetted into the well or dish and allowed to settle by gravity. Alternatively, the plate may be centrifuged to bring the leukocytes down more quickly (Luscinskas et al., 1989). Leukocyte adhesion is frequently quantified by microscopic visualization or by measuring bound fluorescence or radioactivity. One point that is frequently overlooked is how few "static" adhesion assays are truly static. Whenever a plate or microtitre well is washed to remove unbound leukocytes, a broad spectrum of fluid shear forces with spatial- and time-varying components is imparted onto the adherent leukocytes.

To surmount the variable washing conditions inherent in most static adhesion assays, the Smith–Hollers chamber (Smith and Hollers, 1980; Smith et al., 1988) and the centrifugation chamber (McClay et al., 1981; Lotz et al., 1989) have been developed to impart a uniform normal force to detach the leukocyte from its substrate. The force acting on the leukocyte is the force of gravity or of the centrifugation field times the difference between the cell's weight and that of the media it displaces. However, selectin or integrin tether lifetimes and leukocyte rolling cannot be directly characterized in either system due to the lack of a shear flow component, although some dynamical measures are still possible on populations of bound leukocytes. (Piper et al., 1998).

Stamper–Woodruff Assay

In the Stamper–Woodruff assay, a small dish is placed on an orbital or rotating plate. Typically, a thin frozen section of peripheral lymph node is immobilized on the bottom of the dish and a suspension of lymphocytes is layered over the tissue. (Stamper and Woodruff, 1976). After allowing time for an interaction to take place, fixative is added to link lymphocytes to the substrate. One of the strengths of the Stamper–Woodruff assay is the ability to contact leukocytes with tissue samples. The assay can also be adapted to study leukocyte interactions with extralymphoid thin-sectioned tissue, allowing even pathological samples to be studied (Grober et al., 1993; Symon et al., 1996). The Stamper–Woodruff adhesion assay introduces fluid shear as a parameter in adhesion, although the flow is not well defined. As the plate or dish rotates, the centrifugal forces acting on the fluid create significant secondary flows that roll some leukocytes to the center of the disk and a significant number to the very outside edge of the dish because of the development of convection cells. After some minutes, the majority of leukocytes are no longer in contact with the surface of interest, hence assay times could potentially be shortened considerably. The intent of the assay design was to use the fluid rotation to facilitate interactions of leukocytes with the lymph node tissue section.

Cone and Plate (Viscometer) Assays

The cone and plate viscometer generates a constant shear gradient (Fig. 11.1). As the cone or plate rotates, the two surfaces move at a constant relative velocity that generates a linear shear field. Because the velocity gradient (change of velocity with position) is constant, the fluid shear stress is uniform throughout the fluid volume and on any surfaces. The shear rate, (γ), that characterizes the fluid flow is defined as the change in velocity (distance/time) divided by the change in position perpendicular to the flow (distance) as shown in Equation 1:

$$\gamma = \frac{\Delta \; velocity}{\Delta \; position} = \frac{dv}{dx}. \tag{1}$$

A

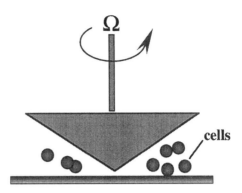

B

Shear Rate = $(v_2\text{-}v_1)/h$

Leukocyte or platelet
aggregates

Tumbling neutrophil

Rolling neutrophil

Fig. 11.1. Schematic of the cone and plate viscometer used in cell aggregation and adhesion assays: A. Rotation of either the cone or the plate generates a velocity gradient that creates a shear field; cells such as platelets or neutrophils encounter each other with the same relative velocity; all cells in the volume are uniformly accessible (view is through the top of the cone and plate viscometer). B. The fluid velocity gradient is constant and uniform; the velocity gradient causes the cells in suspension to rotate.

Consequently, units of shear rate are reciprocal seconds (s^{-1}). In the cone and plate geometry (Ley et al., 1989), the shear rate is described by

$$\gamma = \frac{2\pi f}{\alpha}. \tag{2}$$

In Equation 2, f is the rotation frequency in units of radians per second and α is the angle in radians between the cone and plate. The shear stress is the product of the shear rate (s^{-1}) times the viscosity, μ (dyn $-$ s/cm^2), such that $\tau = \gamma \cdot \mu$. In centimeter-gram-second (cgs) units the shear stress is therefore dyn/cm^2. The shear stress in the cone and plate viscometer is:

$$\tau = \frac{2\mu\pi f}{\alpha} = \gamma \cdot \mu. \tag{3}$$

Although the cone and plate viscometer assay requires more specialized equipment and consequently is not used as frequently as perfusion shear assays, it has several significant strengths. Leukocytes or platelets tumbling in the flow field will encounter each other moving at the same relative velocity; hence the time for bond formation is strictly a function of shear rate (Fig 11.1). The encounter rates of objects in the uniform shear field can be modeled by hydrodynamic equations to extract a collision frequency, which then can be used to define adhesion efficiencies (Tees et al., 1993; Taylor et al., 1996). Additionally, adhesion mechanisms may be analyzed at different shear stresses (Kroll et al., 1996). One consideration in the design of experiments using the cone and plate assay is the existence of secondary flows due to the centrifugal force acting on the rotating fluid. In the Stamper–Woodruff assay, the induced secondary flows are critical for moving cells across the rotating adhesive surface. Cone and plate viscometers will generate secondary flows at a significant level at rotational rates necessary to generate shear stresses greater than 10dyn/cm^2. A number of investigators have used the cone and plate to study platelet aggregation (Chow et al., 1992; Xia and Frojmovic, 1994), leukocyte–platelet aggregation (Konstantopoulos et al., 1998), neutrophil aggregation (Taylor et al., 1996), and leukocyte–endothelial interactions (Ley et al., 1989).

Shear Flow Assays

In the radial flow, parallel plate, and capillary tube assays, the level of flow of the rinsing media determines the forces acting on a leukocyte and is typically controlled by a syringe pump. The flow is laminar under most experimental conditions (Reynolds number on the order of 1 or less) in order to simulate the nonturbulent flows in the microcirculation. The Reynolds number (Re) is defined as $Dv\rho/\mu$, where D is the chamber gap, v is the mean velocity of the fluid, ρ is the density, and μ is the viscosity. In essence, the Re number is a dimensionless group that indicates the relative importance of fluid momentum versus the damping effect of fluid viscosity. The viscous drag of the plasma on the leukocyte under in vitro flow assay conditions or in vivo is so great that there is no "coasting" upon cessation of flow. Stenosed vessels and heart valves are the principle locations of high Re flows in vivo where turbulence might exist due to the high inertial forces created by the high blood flow velocities.

Specification of the wall shear stress makes it possible to compare data from two shear perfusion assays having a different geometry and flow rates because the wall shear stress is the major determining factor in whether a leukocyte or other cell type will adhere. Several significant differences exist in experimental approach between the shear perfusion assays and the previously described cone and plate assay. For one, shear flow assays typically have a continuous exchange of media during the experiment (unless a recirculating flow path is used) so reactants secreted by cells do not accumulate. In contrast, the cone and plate system has a fixed volume of media and cells that continuously mix, so that the system is closed and any factors released by the sheared cells accumulate. Another advantage of the perfusion assays is that leukocytes can be tracked visually, thereby allowing dynamics of cell–surface interactions to be quantified. In the perfusion assays, it is important to note that the shear stress is not uniform in the flow channel as in the cone and plate assay, but is at a maximum at the wall. The flow profile is parabolic, so the shear stress decreases linearly with distance from the wall. In the center of flow, the shear rate is zero and therefore the shear stress is zero as well.

The Radial Flow Assay

From the dimensions of the radial flow chamber, the wall shear stress is calculated assuming that the suspending media is a Newtonian fluid and then performing a momentum balance. The radial flow assay has not been used as extensively as the parallel plate or capillary tube flow assays, in part because of the more complex chamber design required (Fig. 11.2), but nevertheless has several useful characteristics. In the radial flow assay, unlike the cone and plate assay, leukocytes and/or particles can be directly visualized, so their dynamic behavior is accessible. Additionally, because the wall shear stress varies with the radius, a spectrum of wall shear stresses can be sampled by a leukocyte as it flows through the gap between the two plates rather than having to perform a separate experiment for each flow condition (Kuo and Lauffenburger, 1993). The wall or surface shear stress is a function of the flow rate, the gap between the surfaces, and the distance from the center of the radial flow chamber. The wall shear stress is therefore defined as

$$\tau = 3Q\mu/\pi r h^2. \tag{4}$$

This geometry is particularly valuable in the study of particle or cell detachment as a function of force, because, upon the initiation of flow, a population of cells will experience a range of forces depending on initial position.

Parallel Plate Flow Chamber

As with the radial flow chamber, the formula for the wall shear stress is derived assuming the suspending media is a Newtonian fluid and performing a momentum balance on the flowing fluid (Fig. 11.3). The components of the equation for wall shear stress in a parallel plate flow chamber are viscosity (μ, g cm^{-1} sec^{-1} Poise), flow rate (Q, cm^3/sec), chamber width (b, cm), and channel half height (a, cm). The geometry is defined so that $x = 0$ is the center of the channel and at the wall, $x = a$ (see Fig. 11.3A, B). The shear

A

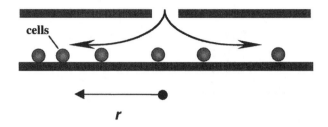

B

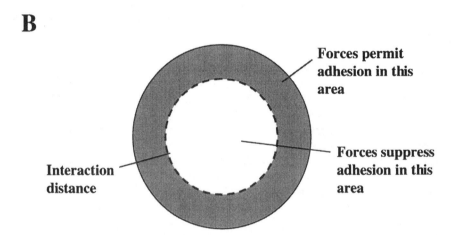

Fig. 11.2. Schematic of the radial flow assay: A. Fluid flow enters the center of the two disks and spreads from the center to the outer edges of the parallel disks; because the flow diverges, the shear rate and wall shear stress fall with increased distance from the center of the chamber. B. View from the top of the radial flow chamber; at a certain distance from the fluid inlet port, shear forces are low enough to allow interactions of cells with the substrate as depicted by the circle marked "interaction distance."

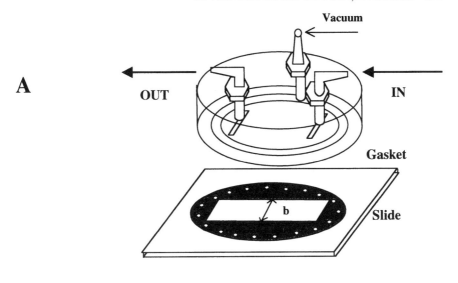

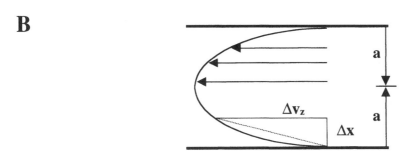

Fig. 11.3. Schematic of a parallel plate flow chamber and velocity profile: A. A gasket separating two flat plates forms the channel (width b); the narrow gap allows the flow field to be approximated by the equations for flow between two infinite parallel plates. B. The fluid velocity profile is parabolic with a maximum at the center of flow while the shear stress is at a maximum at the wall; the channel gap half-height (a) is indicated by the two arrows.

stress (Eq. 5) is given by the following relationship in which the velocity gradient is multiplied by the viscosity of the suspending media:

$$\tau_{xz} = \mu \frac{dv_z}{dx} = \mu \cdot \gamma = \frac{3\mu Q x}{2ba^3}.$$ (5)

Therefore, at the wall of the parallel plate flow chamber, where shear rate (Eq. 6) is defined as γ_{wall}, the wall shear stress is also specified (Eq. 7):

$$\gamma_{wall} = \frac{3Q}{2ba^2}, \tag{6}$$

$$\tau_{wall} = \frac{3\mu Q}{2ba^2}. \tag{7}$$

The formula for fluid velocity in the parallel plate chamber is presented to emphasize the dependence of velocities of free-flowing leukocytes, platelets, and red blood cells on their positions relative to the wall. Equation 8 describes the parabolic velocity profile in a parallel plate flow chamber as a function of distance from the wall and volumetric flow rate:

$$v_z = \frac{3Q}{4ab}\left[1 - \left(\frac{x}{a}\right)^2\right]. \tag{8}$$

Note that at the wall, where $x = a$, v_z equals 0 to satisfy the "no-slip" boundary condition, that is, the layer of fluid molecules next to the wall is stationary. The parabolic velocity profile generated in a parallel plate flow chamber can be approximated close to the wall as a linear function of the wall shear rate. For example, if the wall shear rate is 100 s^{-1}, a small fluid element that is 1 micron from the wall will be moving at approximately 100 μm/s. Similarly, a fluid element 4 microns from the wall, approximating the position of the center of a leukocyte very near the vessel wall, would move at a velocity of 400 μm/s.

Capillary Tube Flow Assay

The equation for a capillary tube has slightly different coefficients but shares the same functional dependence on position as the parallel plate flow chamber (Fig. 11.3). The formulas for the velocity profile (Eq. 9) and the wall shear stress (Eq. 10) for flow in a tube with radius (R) are:

$$v_z = \frac{2Q}{\pi R^2}\left[1 - \left(\frac{r}{R}\right)^2\right], \text{ and} \tag{9}$$

$$\tau(r)_{rz} = \mu \cdot \frac{dv_z}{dr} = \frac{4\mu Qr}{\pi R^2}. \tag{10}$$

Therefore, at the wall of the capillary tube, the shear stress is:

$$\tau_{wall} = \frac{4\mu Q}{\pi R^3}. \tag{11}$$

The pressure gradient, $(-dP/dx)$ is related to the velocity of fluid flow in a tube geometry by the Hagen–Poiseulle equation:

$$-\frac{dp}{dx} = \frac{32\mu v_{av}}{D^2}. \tag{12}$$

The differential $(-dP/dx)$ under most experimental conditions is simply the change in pressure over a fixed length such that $(P_2 - P_1)/(x_2 - x_1)$.

Critical Velocity Indicates Leukocyte–Substrate Interactions

Near the wall, spherical objects are tumbling end over end because of the differences in fluid velocity (Fig. 11.1), with the fluid nearer the wall moving more slowly than the fluid in the center of flow. Consequently, a tumbling leukocyte will rotate as if rolling on a selectin, but the tumbling is much faster. In the case of L-selectin mediated adhesive events, pauses are so brief that leukocyte interactions in shear flow appear to be rapid skips, resulting in an overall reduction in velocity relative to a free-flowing leukocyte (Jung et al., 1996). The distance of the cell from the wall and its diameter are the critical parameters that establish the velocity of a sphere near a wall in a shear flow (Goldman et al., 1967a, 1967b). An estimate of critical velocity (*Vcrit*) can be made by direct measurement of tumbling leukocytes and checked by calculation using the appropriate formulas. Some groups use the equivalent term of a leukocyte's hydrodynamic velocity to indicate the velocity of nonadherent leukocytes in shear flow. If the velocity of a spherical particle is lower than the *Vcrit* (knowing its size and average distance from the wall), then it may be assumed that there is an adhesive interaction. A small particle such as a platelet has a lower *Vcrit* than a leukocyte because it is much smaller and occupies slower moving fluid streamlines closer to the wall. For a spherical object the size of a neutrophil 100 nanometers from the wall, the *Vcrit* is 70% of the velocity of a fluid element one neutrophil radius from the wall. Therefore, at a shear rate of 100 s^{-1}, the *Vcrit* for a neutrophil (4 μm radius) would be approximately 280 μm/s, whereas for a platelet (1.0 μm radius) the *Vcrit* would be approximately 70 μm/s. The shear force (*F*) and torque (*T*) acting on a spherical particle (cell) next to a surface are described by equations 13 and 14: (see Fig. 11.4):

$$F = C_s 6\pi\mu R^2(\gamma) \tag{13}$$

$$T = C_t 4\pi\mu R^3(\gamma) \tag{14}$$

where γ is the shear rate in s^{-1}, μ is the viscosity, R is the radius of the leukocyte, and C_s and C_t are integration constants that depend on the difference between the cell's radius and the distance from the center of the cell to the wall. When the cell is more than a diameter away from the wall, the integration constants C_s (eq. 13) and C_t (eq. 14) both are equal to 1. The closer the cell is to the wall, the greater the flow disturbance created by the sphere and the larger C_s becomes, reaching a value of 1.7 when the cell is within 1 nanometer of the wall. C_t for the cell 1 nanometer from the wall is approximately 0.94. Values for the integration constants C_s and C_t have been tabulated as a function of the ratio of sphere radius to the distance between the wall and the centroid of the sphere (Goldman et al., 1967a, 1967b; Alon et al., 1997).

Experimental Design Considerations of Perfusion/Shear Assays

Two general types of experiments are typically performed using parallel plate flow chambers. The detachment or shear resistance assay can be used to

A

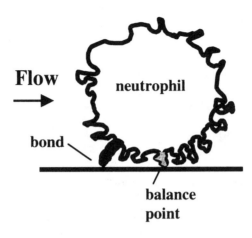

B

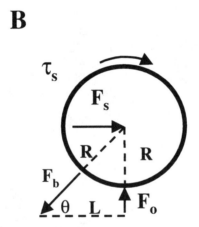

Fig. 11.4. Free body diagram of neutrophil in static equilibrium: A. Schematic of a neutrophil interacting with a substrate through one attachment point as indicated by the heavy black microvillus while the balancing point is at the center and is colored gray because no bond has formed yet. B. A force balance on a sphere the same size as the neutrophil that allows estimation of the force acting on a single bond holding the neutrophil stationary. The sum of the forces in the x-direction (the shear flow directions) gives $F_s = F_t \cos \theta$, and the sum of the forces in the y-direction gives $F_o = F_b \sin \theta$. The sum of the moments about the point of contact at F_b gives $\tau_s + F_s R = (F_s \sin \theta) L$. For a leukocyte 8.5 microns in diameter, $F_s = 60$ pN per dyn/cm² wall shear stress and $F_b = 124$ pN per dyn/cm² wall shear stress (Alon et al., 1997; Goldman et al., 1967b). The estimate of the force on the bond or bond cluster is very dependent on the lever arm estimate, L.

evaluate leukocyte–endothelial cell or leukocyte–matrix–receptor interactions (with any number or combination of receptor–ligand pairs). In this format, either proteins or cells such as endothelial, epithelial, or an anchorage-dependent cell expressing transfected receptors are immobilized or cultured on one wall of the chamber. Leukocytes are introduced into the flow chamber flow and allowed to settle onto the lower wall of the flow chamber under quiescent conditions (Chan et al., 1991; Carr et al., 1996; Puri et al., 1997). The sedimentation velocity for leukocytes is approximately 1μm/s, but can be estimated from Stoke's law: $v_t = 2R^2 (\rho_p - \rho_s)/9\mu$, where ρ_p is the density of the cell, ρ_s is the density of the suspending media, μ is the viscosity of the suspending media, R is the radius of the spherical particle or cell, and v_t is the cell's sedimentation velocity. Since most flow chambers are transparent to allow microscopic visualization, the number of input cells can be directly counted and their fates determined. Among the critical variables that must be controlled are the magnitude of the flow and its duration. The force acting on the adherent leukocyte can be roughly estimated by multiplying the wall shear stress by the surface area of the cell. Calculation of the magnitude of the stresses acting on an adherent cell depends in part on the geometry of the cell. However, in the case of comparative studies of a specific cell type, adherent cells experience nearly the same level of detachment force.

The second experimental approach to probe the role of forces in leukocyte adhesion with a flow chamber is to use continuous flow to create contact time constraints on leukocyte adhesion, similar to that imparted by blood flow (Lawrence et al., 1997). Higher flow rates exert higher levels of stress on the initial bonds formed, and concurrently, limits the contact time because the fluid velocity is greater. If a bond creates a strong enough cross-bridge to hold a cell under physiologic levels of shear, the time for the association of the ligand–receptor pair may be too brief for the second binding event to take place. The time available for bond formation is approximately one-tenth the reciprocal of the shear rate (0.1/G; Capo et al., 1982; Taylor et al., 1996). Modeling studies have proposed relationships between shear stress, receptor kinetics, and leukocyte topography that predict whether a leukocyte will be successful at forming an adhesion or not (Hammer and Apte, 1992; Tozeren and Ley, 1992; Damiano et al., 1996; Chang and Hammer, 1999).

Data from flow chamber assays are typically presented as number of leukocytes bound per unit area of visualized substrate. In continuous flow assays, the rate of accumulation as a function of time and area can be determined, creating an adhesion parameter of cells/area/time (Puri et al., 1995). When cell accumulation is linear with time this can be a useful parameter, but attachment of cells may create nonlinear effects due to coverage of the surface's binding sites and cell adhesion to previously adhered leukocytes (Bargatze et al., 1994; Walcheck et al., 1996). Additionally, if flow rates are low enough, sedimentation will have an effect on the number of cells near the wall (Munn et al., 1994).

Among the selectins, there are at least order-of-magnitude differences in bond lifetimes and rolling velocities, and apparently significant differences between their capture rates (Puri et al., 1997; Alon et al., 1998; Smith et al., 1999). The number of rapidly skipping leukocytes interacting through L-selectin will plateau quickly with an in vitro flow assay, and the time the leukocyte is within the microscope's field of view may be less than 5 seconds. In contrast, P-selectin and E-selectin rolling is much slower, residence times are longer, and the time required to equilibrate on the observation surface is much longer (Lawrence and Springer, 1993; Lawrence et al., 1995). It is hypothesized that differences in leukocyte rolling velocity and skipping parameters may reflect intrinsic bond lifetimes (Bell, 1978; Kaplanski et al., 1993).

Adhesion Receptor Bond Lifetimes in Shear Flow

A number of methods have been applied to measure the effect of forces on biologic adhesive bonds, including micromanipulation (Evans et al., 1995), shear flow chambers and centrifugation assays (Kaplanski et al., 1993; Piper et al., 1998), optical trapping (Schmidt et al., 1993), atomic force microscopy (Fritz et al., 1998), surface force apparatus (Leckband et al., 1994), and more recently, dynamic force probes (Merkel et al., 1999). In contrast to micromechanical approaches, direct measures of molecular equilibrium and kinetics by methods such as surface plasmon resonance cannot readily include the effect of forces on bond lifetimes (van der Merwe and Barclay, 1996; Mehta et al., 1998). The insight that adhesive bond dissociation constants can be estimated from singular leukocyte adhesive interactions has been used to quantify the effect of force on bond lifetimes (Kaplanski et al., 1993; Alon et al., 1995) and determine molecular mechanical properties based on the Bell and Hookean spring models of force-driven molecular dissociation (Bell, 1978; Dembo et al., 1988; Kuo et al., 1997, see Table 11.2).

In an approach pioneered by Bongrand and co-workers (Kaplanski et al., 1993), it was hypothesized that pauses in the motion of leukocytes flowing over substrates expressing low densities of adhesion receptors would represent single bonds. The duration of pauses could then be measured by counting the number of video frames in which a leukocyte remained stationary, and after enough interactions were collected, the distribution of pause times could then be analyzed by the appropriate model. If the pauses represent single-bond events, or at least single-bond cluster-mediated pauses, then the rate of bond dissociation can be described by $k_{off}C = -(dC/dt)$, which can be integrated, giving the equation $ln(C) = -k_{off}t + C_0$, with C_0 equal to the initial number of bonds (the y-intercept). The dissociation constant, k_{off} can then be determined from the natural log of the number of interactions versus the bond lifetime. A linear regression suggests whether the distribution of pause times supports the single-bond hypothesis.

As a bond experiences stress, energy barriers to bond dissociation are lowered and the probability of dissociation becomes greater (Bell, 1978; Dembo et al., 1988). In order to describe the change in a bond's dissociation prob-

Table 11.2. Estimates of Selectin Bond Lifetimes Based on High-Speed Video Analysis

Substrate	Frame Rate (fps)	Bell Model Stressed (100pN) k_{off} (s^{-1})	Bell Model Unstressed k_{off}^0 (s^{-1})	Bell Model Bond Separation Length (σ) (Å)	Hookean Spring Model Unstressed k_{off}^0 (s^{-1})	Hookean Spring Model Spring Constant/Fractional Slippage κ/f_κ (N/m)
P-selectin	48	6.3	2.4 ± 0.47	0.39 ± 0.08	3.70 ± 0.51	2.50 ± 0.61
E-selectin	48	5.0	2.6 ± 0.45	0.18 ± 0.03	3.35 ± 0.47	9.12 ± 1.9
L-selectin	240	36	2.8 ± 0.72	1.11 ± 0.12	8.20 ± 0.17	0.90 ± 0.1
PNAd	240	16	3.8 ± 0.97	0.59 ± 0.10	7.42 ± 1.27	1.80 ± 0.37

Neutrophil interactions were tracked by computer software using a digital camera at the indicated frame rates (frames per second; fps) and observed at 20X magnification. Measures of reactive bond compliance (bond separation distance; σ) as defined in the Bell model (Bell, 1978) (see text) and $f\kappa/\kappa$ (fractional slippage divided by the bond spring constant) in the Hookean spring model (Dembo et al., 1988; Ward et al., 1995) were derived by a nonlinear least squares fit of the dependence of k_{off} on the force/bond over the range of 37 pN to 125 pN. The Hookean model assumes that the bond behaves like a spring and that a fraction of the energy applied to the bond as it is stressed goes into breaking the bond, hence a higher f_κ/κ indicates the bond is less likely to break as force is applied, (i.e., stiffer). The chi-square value for a Levenberg–Marquardt fit of the Bell model for P-selectin was 1.43; for E-selectin, 0.32; for PNAd, 9.93; and for L-selectin (interacting with the neutrophil L-selectin ligand), 4.9. χ^2 derived for the Hookean model for E-selectin was 0.2; for P-selectin, 2.11; for PNAd, 8.65; and for the L-selectin substrate, 0.69. For the calculation of the force on the bond, the lever arm was assumed to be 3 µm, with the neutrophil radius set at 4.25 µm, resulting in an estimate of F_b as 125 pN per 1 dyn/cm^2 wall shear stress (Smith et al., 1999).

ability with force, the bond lifetime may be linked to the force on the bond (F_b) through an exponential relationship proposed by Bell:

$$k_{off} = k_{off}^o \exp\left(\frac{\sigma F_b}{k_B T}\right). \tag{15}$$

The work done on the bond is scaled by the thermal energy, which is the product of the Boltzmann constant and the temperature $(k_B T)$ (Bell, 1978). Under stress, the height of the potential well barrier to dissociation decreases approximately by the energy term represented by σF_b, where σ is defined as the bond separation distance in Angstroms (Å), or the distance between the strained bond interfaces; a larger σ correlates with a higher bond compliance (the bond's susceptibility to force-driven dissociation). Dissociation constants (k_{off}) determined at several different forces are analyzed by various regression methods to extract the bond interaction distance, σ, and the zero shear dissociation constant, $k^0 off$. A free body diagram of neutrophil in static equilibrium is shown to illustrate how the estimate of the force on the bond or bond cluster is derived (Fig. 11.4). The force on the bond is very dependent on the lever arm estimate, L. Recent work using a high-speed digital camera to quantitate pause times of flowing neutrophils indicates that even among the selectins, there are large differences in their respective mechanical properties (see Table 11.2; Smith et al., 1999). L-selectin is much more susceptible to force-driven dissociation than P-selectin or E-selectin, but appears to compensate by higher cellular tethering rates (Alon et al., 1998; Smith et al., 1999). Interestingly, all three selectins appear to have similar zero shear stress dissociation constants, but their large differences in stressed dissociation constants illustrate the physiologic significance of selectin bond mechanical properties. Analysis of selectin bond mechanics and the mechanical properties of microvilli will be critical for understanding both the carbohydrate regulation of selectin recognition and the detection of the effects of receptor valence, clustering, and cytoskeletal anchorage on leukocyte adhesion.

Conclusions

Shear flow assays give the investigator an opportunity to study the dynamic behavior of leukocyte–endothelial cell interactions. In addition to the further understanding of selectin-mediated adhesive interactions, flow systems allow the transition for rolling to β_2/β_1-mediated firm adhesion to be quantified, with clear indications of integrin bond engagement. The study of the role of immobilized and soluble chemokine triggering of leukocyte arrest is also likely to generate valuable insights into the dynamics of inside-out signaling of integrins and the requirements for cytoskeletal rearrangements to stabilize leukocyte firm adhesion.

Support of the National Institutes of Health, Heart, Lung, and Blood Division and the American Heart Association is gratefully acknowledged.

References

Alon, R., Hammer, D. A., and Springer, T. A. (1995) Lifetime of the P-selectin–carbohydrate bond and its response to tensile force in hydrodynamic flow. *Nature (Lond.)* 374:539–542.

Alon, R., Chen, S., Puri, K. D., Finger, E. B., and Springer, T. A. (1997) The kinetics of L-selectin tethers and the mechanics of selectin-mediated rolling. *J. Cell. Biol.* 138:1169–1180.

Alon, R., Chen, S., Fuhlbrigge, R. C., Puri, K. D., and Springer, T. A. (1998) The kinetics and shear threshold of transient and rolling interactions of L-selectin with its ligand on leukocytes. *Proc. Natl. Acad. Sci. USA* 95:11631–11636.

Bargatze, R. F., Kurk, S., Butcher, E. C., and Jutila, M. A. (1994) Neutrophils roll on adherent neutrophils bound to cytokine-induced endothelial cells via L-selectin on the rolling cells. *J. Exp. Med.* 180:1785–1792.

Bell, G. I. (1978) Models for the specific adhesion of cells to cells. *Science* 200:618–627.

Bell, D. N., Spain, S., and Goldsmith, H. L. (1989) Adenosine disphosphate-induced aggregation of human platelets in flow through tubes. I. Measurement of concentration and size of single platelets and aggregates. *Biophys. J.* 56:817–828.

Capo, C., Garrouste, F., Benoliel, A.-M., Bongrand, P., Ryter, A., and Bell, G. I. (1982) Concanavalin-A-mediated thymocyte agglutination: A model for a quantitative study of cell adhesion. *J. Cell. Sci.* 56:21–48.

Carr, M. W., Alon, R., and Springer, T. A. (1996) The C-C chemokine MCP-1 differentially modulates the avidity of b1 and b2 integrins on T lymphocytes. *Immun.* 4:179–187.

Chan, P.-Y., Lawrence, M. B., Dustin, M. L., Ferguson, L. M., Golan, D. E., and Springer, T. A. (1991) Influence of receptor lateral mobility on adhesion strengthening between membranes containing LFA-3 and CD2. *J. Cell. Biol.* 115:245–255.

Chang, K. C., and Hammer, D. A. (1999) The forward rate of binding of surface-tethered reactants: effect of relative motion between two surfaces. *Biophys. J.* 76:1280–1292.

Chow, T. W., Hellukrolms, J. D., Moake, J. L., and Kroll, M. H. (1992) Shear stress-induced von Willebrand factor binding to platelet glycoprotein Ib initiates calcium influx associated with aggregation. *Blood* 80:113–120.

Damiano, E. R., Westheider, J., Tozeren, A., and Ley, K. (1996) Velocity, deformation, and adhesion energy density of leukocytes rolling within venules. *Circ. Res.* 79, 1122–1130.

Dembo, M., Torney, D. C., Saxman, K., and Hammer, D. A. (1988) The reaction limited kinetics of membrane-to-surface adhesion and detachment. *Proc. R. Lond. B. Sci.* 234:55–83.

Dustin, M. L., and Springer, T. A. (1989) T-cell receptor cross-linking transiently stimulates adhesiveness through LFA-1. *Nature (Lond.)* 341:41–46.

Evans, E. A., Ritchie, K., and Merkel, R. (1995) Sensitive force technique to probe molecular adhesion and structural linkages at biological interfaces. *Biophys. J.* 68:2580–2587.

Fritz, J., Katopoidis, A. G., Kolbinger, F., and Anselmetti, D. (1998) Force-mediated kinetics of single P-selectin/ligand complexes observed by atomic force microscopy. *Proc. Natl. Acad. Sci. USA* 95:12283–12288.

Goldman, A. J., Cox, R. G., and Brenner, H. (1967a) Slow viscous motion of a sphere parallel to a plane wall-I. Motion through a quiescent fluid. *Chem. Eng. Sci.* 22:637–651.

Goldman, A. J., Cox, R. G., and Brenner, H. (1967b) Slow viscous motion of a sphere parallel to a plane wall-II. Couette flow. *Chem. Eng. Sci.* 22:653–660.

Grober, J. S., Bowen, B. L., Ebling, H., Athey, B., Thompson, C. B., Fox, D. A., and Stoolman, L. M. (1993) Monocyte-endothelial adhesion in chronic rheumatoid arthritis: in situ detection of selectin and integrin-dependent interactions. *J. Clin. Invest.* 91:2609–2619.

Hammer, D. A., and Apte, S. M. (1992) Simulation of cell rolling and adhesion on surfaces in shear flow: General results and analysis of selectin-mediated neutrophil adhesion. *Biophys. J.* 63:35–57.

Jung, U., Bullard, D. C., Tedder, T. F., and Ley, K. (1996) Velocity differences between L-selectin and P-selectin dependent neutrophil rolling in venules of the mouse cremaster muscle in vivo. *Am. J. Physiol.* 271:H2740–H2747.

Kaplanski, G., Farnarier, C., Tissot, O., Pierres, A., Benoliel, A.-M., Alessi, M. C., Kaplanski, S., and Bongrand, P. (1993) Granulocyte–endothelium initial adhesion. Analysis of transient binding events mediated by E-selectin in a laminar shear flow. *Biophys. J.* 64:1922–1933.

Konstantopoulos, K., Neelamegham, S., Burns, A. R., Hentzen, E., Kansas, G. S., Snapp, K. R., Berg, E. L., Hellums, J. D., Smith, C. W., McIntire, L. V., and Simon, S. I. (1998) Venous levels of shear support neutrophil-platelet adhesion and neutrophil aggregation in blood via P-selectin and β2-integrin. *Cir.* 98:873–882.

Kroll, M. H., Hellums, J. D., McIntire, L. V., Schafer, A. I., and Moake, J. L. (1996) Platelets and shear stress. *Blood* 88:1525–1541.

Kuo, S. C., and Lauffenburger, D. A. (1993) Relationship between receptor/ligand binding affinity and adhesion strength. *Biophys. J.* 65:2191–2200.

Kuo, S. C., Hammer, D. A., and Lauffenburger, D. A. (1997) Simulation of detachment of specifically bound particles from surfaces by shear flow. *Biophys. J.* 73:517–531.

Lawrence, M. B., and Springer, T. A. (1993) Neutrophils roll on E-selection. *J. Immunol.* 151:6338–6346.

Lawrence, M. B., Berg, E. L., Butcher, E. C., and Springer, T. A. (1995) Rolling of lymphocytes and neutrophils on peripheral node addressin and subsequent arrest on ICAM-1 in shear flow. *Eur. J. Immunol.* 25:1025–1031.

Lawrence, M. B., Kansas, G. S., Kunkel, E. J., and Ley, K. (1997) Threshold levels of fluid shear promote leukocyte adhesion through selectins (CD62L, P, E). *J. Cell Biol.* 136:717–727.

Leckband, D. E., Schmitt, F.-J., Israelachvili, J. N., and Knoll, W. (1994) Direct force measurements of specific and nonspecific protein interactions. *Biochem.* 33:4611–4624.

Ley, K., Lundgren, E., Berger, E. M., and Arfors, K.-E. (1989) Shear-dependent inhibition of granulocyte adhesion to cultured endothelium by dextran sulfate. *Blood* 73:1324–1330.

Lotz, M. M., Burdsal, C. A., Erickson, H. P., and McClay, D. R. (1989) Cell adhesion to fibronectin and tenascin: Quantitative measurements of initial binding and subsequent strengthening response. *J. Cell Biol.* 109:1795–1805.

Luscinskas, F. W., Brock, A. F., Arnaout, M. A., and Gimbrone, M. A. Jr. (1989) Endothelial–leukocyte adhesion molecule-1–dependent and leukocyte (CD11/CD18)-dependent mechanisms contribute to polymorphonuclear leukocyte adhesion to cytokine-activated human vascular endothelium. *J. Immunol.* 142:2257–2263.

McClay, D. R., Wessel, G. M., and Marchase, R. B. (1981) Intercellular recognition: Quantitation of initial binding events. *Proc. Natl. Acad. Sci. USA* 78:4975–4979.

Mehta, P., Cummings, R. D., and McEver, R. P. (1998) Affinity and kinetic analysis of P-selectin binding to P-selectin glycoprotein ligand-1. *J. Biol. Chem.* 273:32506–32513.

Merkel, R., Nassoy, P., Leung, A., Ritchie, K., and Evans, E. A. (1999) Energy landscapes of receptor–ligand bonds explored with dynamic force spectroscopy. *Nature (Lond.)* 397:50–53.

Munn, L. L., Melder, R. J., and Jain, R. K. (1994) Analysis of cell flux in the parallel plate flow chamber:Implications for cell capture studies. *Biophys. J.* 67:889–895.

Palecek, S. P., Loftus, J. C., Ginsberg, M. H., Lauffenburger, D. A., and Horwitz, A. F. (1997) Integrin–ligand binding properties govern cell migration speed through cell-substratum adhesiveness. *Nature (Lond.)* 385:537–540.

Piper, J. W., Swerlick, R. A., and Zhu, C. (1998) Determining force dependence of two-dimensional receptor–ligand binding affinity by centrifugation. *Biophys. J.* 74:492–513.

Puri, K. D., Finger, E. B., Gaudernack, G., and Springer, T. A. (1995) Sialomucin CD34 is the major L-selectin ligand in human tonsil high endothelial venules. *J. Cell. Biol.* 131:261–270.

Puri, K. D., Finger, E. B., and Springer, T. A. (1997) The faster kinetics of L-selectin than of E-selectin and P-selectin rolling at comparable binding strength. *J. Immunol.* 158:405–413.

Schmidt, C. E., Horwitz, A. F., Lauffenburger, D. A., and Sheetz, M. P. (1993) Integrin–cytoskeletal interactions in migrating fibroblasts are dynamic, asymmetric, and regulated. *J. Cell. Biol.* 123:977–991.

Smith, C. W., and Hollers, J. C. (1980) Motility and adhesiveness in human neutrophils:Redistribution of chemotactic factor induced adhesion sites. *J. Clin. Invest.* 65:804–812.

Smith, C. W., Rothlein, R., Hughes, B. J., Mariscalco, M. M., Schmalstieg, F. C., and Anderson, D. C. (1988) Recognition of an endothelial determinant for CD18-dependent neutrophil adherence and transendothelial migration. *J. Clin. Invest.* 82:1746–1756.

Smith, C. W., Kishimoto, T. K., Abbassi, O., Hughes, B. J., Rothlein, R., McIntire, L. V., Butcher, E. C., and Anderson, D. C. (1991) Chemotactic factors regulate lectin adhesion molecule 1

(LECAM-1)-dependent neutrophil adhesion to cytokine-stimulated endothelial cells in vitro. *J. Clin. Invest.* 87:609–618.

Smith, M. J., Berg, E. L., and Lawrence, M. B. (1999) Direct comparison of selectin bond lifetimes using high temporal resolution. *Biophys. J.* 77:3371–3383.

Springer, T. A. (1994) Traffic signals for lymphocyte recirculation and leukocyte emigration: The multistep paradigm. *Cell* 76:301–314.

Stamper, H. B. Jr., and Woodruff, J. J. (1976) Lymphocyte homing into lymph nodes:in vitro demonstration of the selective affinity of recirculating lymphocytes for high-endothelial venules. *J. Exp. Med.* 144:828–833.

Sung, L. A., Kabat, E. A., and Chien, S. (1985) Interaction energies in lectin-mediated erythrocyte aggregation. *J. Cell. Biol.* 101:652–659.

Symon, F. A., Lawrence, M. B., Williamson, M. L., Walsh, G. M., Watson, S. R., and Wardlaw, A. J. (1996) Functional and structural characterization of the eosinophil P-selectin ligand. *J. Immunol.* 157:1711–1719.

Taylor, A. D., Neelamegham, S., Hellums, J. D., Smith, C. W., and Simon, S. I. (1996) Molecular dynamics of the transition from L-selectin to β2 integrin dependent neutrophil adhesion under defined hydrodynamic shear. *Biophys. J.* 71:3488–3500.

Tees, D.F.J., Coenen, O., and Goldsmith, H. L. (1993) Interaction forces between red cells agglutinated by antibody. IV. Time and force dependence of break-up. *Biophys. J.* 65:1318–1334.

Tozeren, A., and Ley, K. (1992) How do selectins mediate leukocyte rolling in venules? *Biophys. J.* 63:700–709.

van der Merwe, P. A., and Barclay, A. N. (1996) Analysis of cell-adhesion molecule interactions using surface plasmon resonance. *Curr. Opinion Immunol.* 8:257–261.

Walcheck, B., Moore, K. L., McEver, R. P., and Kishimoto, T. K. (1996) Neutrophil–neutrophil interactions under hydrodynamic shear stress involve L-selectin and PSGL-1:a mechanism that amplifies initial leukocyte accumulation on P-selectin in vitro. *J. Clin. Invest.* 98:1081–1087.

Ward, M. D., Dembo, M., and Hammer, D. A. (1995) Kinetics of cell detachment:Effect of ligand density. *Ann. Biomed. Eng.* 23:322–331.

Xia, Z., and Frojmovic, M. M. (1994). Aggregation efficiency of activated normal or fixed platelets in a simple shear field:Effect of shear and fibrinogen occupancy. *Biophys. J.* 66:2190–2201.

12

Selectins and Their Ligands in Inflammation

GEOFFREY S. KANSAS

Research over the last 10 years has greatly enhanced our understanding of the molecular basis for the regulation of leukocyte traffic in inflammation and other settings. This chapter deals with one family of adhesion molecules termed *selectins*, which play a crucial role in leukocyte recruitment during inflammation. Other chapters focus on other parts of the adhesion cascade that lead to leukocyte recruitment.

Expression of Selectins

There are three known selectins, each with a highly specific pattern of cellular expression. Although the individual selectins have each had several names through their scientific history, they are known today by single letters designating the cell type on which they are expressed or were first identified. Thus, L-selectin (CD62L) is expressed exclusively on cells of the hematopoietic system (i.e., leukocytes), including neutrophils and other granulocytes, monocytes, and T, B, and NK lymphocytes (Gallatin et al., 1983; Kansas et al., 1985b). However, erythrocytes and platelets do not express L-selectin. E-selectin expression is limited to endothelial cells, and P-selectin is expressed on both activated platelets and activated endothelium. As detailed in the following, L-selectin is constitutively expressed on most leukocytes, whereas expression of both E- and P-selectin on endothelium and expression of P-selectin on platelets are inducible.

L-selectin is expressed on essentially all blood-borne granulocytes and monocytes, consistent with its expression on hematopoietic precursors (Griffin et al., 1990). L-selectin is also expressed on all naive, immunocompetent T and B lymphocytes (Kansas et al., 1985a, 1985b). However, on all types of leukocytes, L-selectin is shed from the cell surface by a proteolytic mechanism that is activated by diverse cellular stimuli (Jung et al., 1988; Kishimoto et al., 1989). The function of this shedding mechanism is unknown. On T and B lymphocytes, this loss of L-selectin is reflected in a stable population of L-selectin-negative cells, both in the blood and in secondary lymphoid organs. Within lymphoid organs, L-selectin-negative cells are found almost exclusively within the germinal centers, sites of T-cell-dependent B-cell activation, proliferation, and differentiation into memory B cells and plasma cells. However, under conditions that have still not been adequately defined, but are likely related to the precise microenvironment in which lymphocyte activation occurs (Picker et al., 1993), a subset of activated T and B cells either retains or reexpresses L-selectin following activation. Thus, an absence or low level of L-selectin expression is indicative of a memory lymphocyte, but not all memory lymphocytes fail to express L-selectin.

E-selectin expression is induced on most cultured endothelium as well as most postcapillary endothelium in vivo by a number of stimuli, with the best known being inflammatory mediators such as TNF, IL-1, or bacterial lipo-plysaccharide (LPS:(Bevilacqua et al., 1989). Induction of E-selectin by these cytokines occurs exclusively at the transcriptional level, and requires proteasome-dependent activation of NF-κB for maximal expression (Collins et al., 1995; Read et al., 1995). E-selectin mRNA is first detectable approximately 2 hours after initial exposure to cytokine. In cultured endothelium, expression peaks in 4–8 hours, and subsequently declines slowly, reaching baseline levels by 24 hours, even in the continued presence of the cytokine. In vivo, however, E-selectin can be chronically expressed at sites of continued inflammation, especially in the skin (Picker et al., 1991a). This difference in the duration of expression may be related to differences in mRNA structure, with alternative 3' untranslated regions responsible for these differences in the pattern of expression (Chu et al., 1994).

The nature and pattern of P-selectin expression in both endothelium and platelets are quite distinct. Unlike L-selectin, which is expressed constitutively at the cell surface, or E-selectin, which is transcriptionally induced, P-selectin is expressed in resting endothelium and resting platelets, and is stored in the secondary granules of these cells, the α-granules of platelets and the Weibel–Palade bodies of endothelium (Bonfanti et al., 1989; McEver et al., 1989). Exposure of either of these two cell types to a variety of agonists induces very rapid (i.e., seconds to minutes) fusion of the P-selectin–containing granules with the outer membrane of the cell, thereby exposing P-selectin at the cell surface. In the case of endothelial cells, histamine released from tissue mast cells in response to inflammatory insult is one of the physiologic inducers of rapid P-selectin expression (Kubes and Kanwar, 1994). For platelets, many of the known platelet activators, including thrombin and collagen, will induce rapid P-selectin expression at the cell surface.

In addition to this rapid expression at the cell surface of preformed P-selectin, P-selectin is also transcriptionally induced, similar to E-selectin. In the mouse, P-selectin is strongly induced over a period of hours by inflammatory cytokines (Gotsch et al., 1994; Weller et al., 1992). Similarly, P-selectin can be chronically expressed at sites of long-standing inflammation, such as rheumatoid synovium (Grober et al., 1993). The transcriptional and posttranscriptional mechanisms that govern P-selectin expression are poorly understood.

Structure of Selectins

The selectins are type I integral membrane proteins composed of a unique arrangement of distinct tandem protein domains (Fig. 12.1). At the amino-terminal is a C-type (Ca^{2+}–requiring) lectin domain of 119 residues. Following the lectin domain is a single epidermal growth factor (EGF)-like domain of 36 residues, followed by a series of 62 residue short-concensus-repeat (SCR) domains, the number of which varies depending on the selectin and the species. L-selectin from all species examined has 2 SCR domains, whereas E- and P-selectin have 4–9. Domain swapping experiments have demonstrated that SCR domains from different selectins can functionally substitute for each other, and that the number of SCR domains is not crucial for selectin function (Kansas et al., 1991, 1994). Selectin SCR domains differ from those found in other proteins, such as complement regulatory proteins, in having one extra conserved disulfide bond, but are otherwise structurally similar. Between the SCR domains and the membrane-spanning domain is a short stretch of residues in which the L-selectin cleavage site is located, followed by the transmembrane domain and a relatively short cytoplasmic tail. The lectin, EGF, and SCR domains are quite homologous to the corresponding domains in different selectins and species, although the lectin and EGF domains are more homologous for the same selectin between species than for different selectins within a single species (Kansas, 1996). Additionally, both the transmembrane and cytoplasmic domains are quite homologous for the same selectin between species, but not at all between different selectins, suggesting selectin-specific functions of these regions.

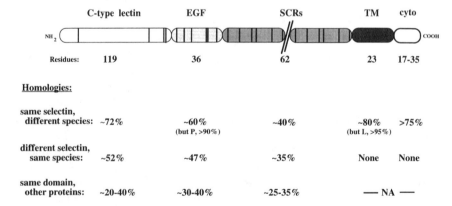

Figure 12.1. *Structure of selectins.* Individual domains are indicated by ovals, with vertical black lines indicating conserved cysteines participating in disulfide bonds. The double slash between the two SCR domains indicates the variable number of such domains in selectins. The number of amino acid residues in each domain is given below the domain, and the amino acid identity ("homologies") for each domain is indicated.

The structure of the genes that encode selectins is concordant with this domain structure, with each of the individual domains in the extracellular portion of the molecule encoded by a separate exon (Johnston et al., 1990; Ord et al., 1990; Collins et al., 1991). Interestingly, although there is no sequence homology between the cytoplasmic domains of the different selectins, each is encoded by two distinct exons. The genes for the selectins are arranged in tandem in syntenic positions on chromosome 1 of both mouse and human, strongly suggesting that they arose by gene duplication (Watson et al., 1990).

An extensive series of studies has shown that each domain plays some role in cell adhesion by selectins. The precise role of the EGF and SCR domains is not clear, but as mentioned above domain-swapping studies have demonstrated that ligand specificity is not imparted by these domains. However, deletion of either the EGF or SCR domains abolishes adhesion, indicating some essential function. In contrast, it is quite clear that the lectin domain is solely responsible for ligand specificity and recognition (Bowen et al., 1990; Kansas et al., 1994). Hence, selectin ligands are carbohydrate in nature, and are therefore among the very few cell adhesion molecules that recognize carbohydrates. The crystal structure of the lectin and EGF domains of E-selectin (Graves et al., 1994) suggests little interaction of the lectin and EGF domains, consistent with recognition of carbohydrate ligand solely by the lectin domain. However, modeling studies based on small carbohydrate model ligands is inconsistent with the known requirements for selectin-mediated recognition of physiologic ligands (discussed later). Precisely how selectin lectin domains interact physically with their carbohydrate ligands remains incompletely understood.

Studies involving mutational analysis of selectins, their ligands, and related proteins are carried out in stably transfected cell lines that have been engineered to express the normal or mutated protein of interest at levels at, or slightly above, the level found in normal leukocytes. As described in more detail elsewhere in this book, these stably transfected cell lines can then be analyzed under defined shear flow in parallel plate flow chambers, in vivo by means of intravital microscopy, by flow cytometry using recombinant soluble selectins as antibody-like reagents, or in more specialized assays, such as the Stamper–Woodruff frozen section assay for L-selectin–mediated adhesion to high endothelial venules (HEV). This gain-of-function somatic cell genetics approach has been instrumental in defining the molecular basis for adhesion by selectins, and is an essential complement to loss-of-function experiments such as genetically deficient mice.

The Nature of Cell Adhesion by Selectins

As described in Chapter 16, selectins mediate the initial steps of a cascade of leukocyte interaction with endothelium. Adhesion by selectins takes the form of initial attachment and rolling along the luminal surface of the endothelium, at velocities considerably below that of flowing blood elements

(Ley and Tedder, 1995). As such, the very nature of cell adhesion mediated by selectins differs fundamentally from that mediated by most other classes of adhesion molecules (e.g., integrins). In particular, rolling by selectins necessarily involves a "rapid-on, rapid-off" mode of interaction in which bonds between the leukocyte and the endothelium must form rapidly at the leading edge of the cell in order for rolling to initiate, and must break at the trailing edge of the cell in order for the cell to release and continue rolling (Tozeren and Ley, 1992). Selectins are highly specialized to perform this function, and are clearly far more efficient at initial "capture" and rolling than other molecules, such as very late antigen-4 (VLA-4) or CD44 which can also support rolling under certain circumstances (Berlin et al., 1995; DeGrendele et al., 1996). Rolling adhesion is obviously quite different from the firm adhesion mediated by integrins. The precise molecular and biophysical basis for the ability of selectins to mediate rolling is under intense investigation, but this form of adhesion appears to involve rapid cellular on and off rates, and a relative insensitivity of these parameters to increasing shear. In addition, unlike most, if not all, other cell adhesion molecules, selectins actually require shear force for their function (Finger et al., 1996; Lawrence et al., 1997). Although a discussion of the extremely complex biophysical basis for selectin-mediated rolling is beyond the scope of this chapter, these considerations have important practical implications for how one studies selectins, and for the identification of physiologic selectin ligands.

Functions of Selectins in Leukocyte Traffic

Numerous studies by many investigators have clearly established an essential role for selectins in the recruitment of virtually all types of leukocytes from the blood to essentially all target sites. Broadly speaking, these pathways can be separated into two main categories:those that are constitutively active and are required for maintenance of a specific immune function; and those that are inducible and are involved in recruitment to a specific site of inflammation or tissue injury. The best studied of the former is that of the crucial role of L-selectin in lymphocyte recirculation, the constant movement of T and B cells from the blood into lymphoid tissues and/or sites of chronic inflammation, from there through the efferent lymph, and finally back through the thoracic duct into the blood-stream. Entry of T and B lymphocytes from the blood into lymph nodes occurs exclusively through specialized postcapillary venules (high endothelial venules, or (HEV), and L-selectin is absolutely required for binding to HEV and subsequent entry into lymph nodes. Thus, monoclonal antibodies (mAb) to L-selectin completely block homing of intravenously injected lymphocytes to lymph nodes. Lymph nodes from L-selectin–deficient mice are extremely hypocellular because of the absence of the normal lymphocyte population of these organs (Gallatin et al., 1983; Arbones et al., 1994; Bradley et al., 1994). In addition, L-selectin–deficient mice, although generally healthy, have impaired immune responses as a direct result of this impaired lymphocyte recirculation (Catalina et al.,

1996). These studies collectively demonstrate the critical role of L-selectin in lymphocyte recirculation and effective immunity.

In contrast, P- and E-selectin, as inducible endothelial adhesion molecules, are critical for leukocyte, particularly neutrophil, recruitment, to sites of inflammation, especially acute inflammation. The two endothelial selectins have overlapping but not identical functions, mostly because of their overlapping but not identical patterns of expression. As a result of its very rapid mode of expression, P-selectin will be expressed at the surface of endothelium at sites of inflammation or tissue injury within minutes of the original insult. P-selectin therefore serves as a rapid response to inflammatory stimuli. If the stimulus is sustained and magnified, as would be the case for a site of bacterial inflammation for example, both P- and E-selectin will be transcriptionally induced, and their expression will be maintained for hours, resulting (along with other changes in the endothelium) in a rapid and huge influx of leukocytes, initially nearly all neutrophils, but with monocytes and some T cells at later time points. Expression of both E- and P-selectin can also be constitutively maintained in certain sites of chronic inflammation, including the skin and rheumatoid synovium (Grober et al., 1993; Chu et al., 1994).

These points are exemplified by the phenotypes of mice deficient in E-selectin, P-selectin, or both (Mayadas et al., 1993; Labow et al., 1994; Bullard et al., 1996; Frenette et al., 1996). Mice deficient in either endothelial selectin alone are generally healthy, show either no or only mild leukocytosis, and have either no (E-selectin) or mild (P-selectin) impairments in neutrophil recruitment to peritoneal inflammation. The overlapping function is exemplified by the nearly complete inhibition of neutrophil recruitment in E-selectin mice administered anti–P-selectin mAb. In contrast to the mild phenotypes of mice deficient in a single selectin, knockout (KO) mice deficient in both endothelial selectins (E/P KO) develop a chronic bacterial dermatitis, have extremely high circulating leukocyte counts, exhibit alterations in hematopoiesis, have a greatly expanded and activated B-cell compartment, and show a nearly absent recruitment of neutrophils to peritoneal and other sites of inflammation (Bullard et al., 1996; Frenette et al., 1996). The phenotype of these E/P KO mice is therefore far more severe than that of any of the single-selectin KO mice, and illustrates the crucial role for the endothelial selectins in leukocyte recruitment to sites of inflammation.

Although the endothelial selectins predominate in an inflammatory setting, a contribution by L-selectin is also detectable. L-selectin mediates rolling on endothelium at sites of inflammation, which is easily detectable in the absence of P-selectin (Ley et al., 1995). L-selectin–deficient mice show a mild impairment of neutrophil recruitment in the inflamed peritoneum that persists for longer times than the corresponding defect in P-selectin–deficient mice (Arbones et al., 1994). However, L-selectin is also important for neutrophil aggregation (Simon et al., 1992, 1993), which is an important feature of certain inflammatory disorders. The ability of L-selectin to mediate interactions between leukocytes may also be important for leukocyte recruitment to sites of inflammation, especially in smaller vessels or in settings where the endothelium is "paved" with adherent leukocytes. Inhibition of these "secondary" interactions may underlie the defects exhibited by L-selectin–deficient mice in certain inflammatory models.

Recently, it has been shown that the endothelial selectins also participate in a novel homing pathway, that of hematopoietic stem cells (HSC) to bone marrow (Frenette et al., 1998). Like other tissues, the bone marrow sinusoids are lined with a continuous endothelial cell layer that must be traversed to enter the extravascular regions of the marrow in which hematopoiesis occurs. Similar to lymphocyte homing, this pathway appears to be constitutively active, permitting transplanted or otherwise blood-borne HSC to efficiently enter the bone marrow. In both mice and humans, E-selectin is constitutively expressed on the bone marrow endothelium (Schweitzer et al., 1996), whereas P-selectin is not detectable, suggesting that E-selectin may be more important in this pathway. Interestingly, vascular cell adhesion molecule-1 (VCAM-1), another endothelial adhesion molecule that is inducible on endothelial cells in all other tissues examined (see Chapter 14), is also constitutively expressed on bone marrow endothelium, and is involved in homing of HSC (Papayannopoulou et al., 1995; Schweitzer et al., 1996; Frenette et al., 1998). The role of E-selectin and VCAM-1 in HSC homing to bone marrow therefore offers a parallel to that of L-selectin in lymphocyte homing to lymph nodes.

P-selectin expressed on activated platelets is an important mediator of leukocyte–platelet adhesion. Although platelet aggregation and adhesion to subendothelial matrix does not require P-selectin, recruitment of monocytes into a developing thrombus, which is important for thrombin deposition, involves P-selectin expressed on activated platelets within the clot (Palabrica et al., 1992). P-selectin–deficient mice do not exhibit a significant bleeding disorder, although alterations in certain hemostatic parameters are detectable (Johnson et al., 1995). Hence, P-selectin may play an important role in the interface between the inflammatory and hemostatic systems.

Finally, it is worth mentioning the functional cooperativity between different selectins and between different classes of adhesion receptors. Apart from naive T and B lymphocytes, most leukocytes, particularly neutrophils, monocytes, and other myeloid cells, express L-selectin as well as functional ligands for both E- and P-selectin. Hence, engagement of all three selectins is likely in a site of intense inflammation. Under these circumstances, leukocytes typically roll with a velocity characteristic of E-selectin, which mediates the slowest rolling at site densities that prevail in vivo (Kunkel et al., 1995; Kunkel and Ley, 1996). Blocking mAb directed against L- or P-selectin reduces the number of cells interacting with the endothelium, demonstrating the involvement of these other two selectins as well. Detailed analysis of leukocyte rolling under these circumstances reveals that L-selectin is most efficient at initial attachment, and mediates the fastest characteristic rolling velocities, P-selectin is intermediate for these parameters, and E-selectin is the least efficient at initial attachment but mediates the slowest rolling and occasional arrest. Thus, interacting cells can sequentially (or perhaps simultaneously) utilize all three selectins in the process of decelerating from the high velocities typical of noninteracting cells. The activity of selectins therefore, spans a large velocity range (>400 μm/sec to nearly 1–2 μm/sec). This ensures that circulating leukocytes can be efficiently captured from the circulation and readily exposed to activating stimuli on the surface of the endothelium, thereby guaranteeing an opportunity for the leukocytes to undergo integrin-mediated arrest and transmigration into the tissue.

In summary, the different selectins have overlapping but distinct functions in the recruitment of all types of leukocytes from the blood into the tissues. In addition, each selectin has a unique role in specific leukocyte adhesion events:L-selectin in lymphocyte recirculation, E-selectin in HSC homing to bone marrow, and P-selectin in leukocyte–platelet adhesion. These molecules are thus responsible for an array of cell adhesion events occuring under the shear force present within the vasculature.

Ligands for Selectins

In discussing the ligands for selectins, it is important to understand that the term *ligand* can mean the entire molecule with which the selectin interacts, or can refer to only that part of the entire molecule with which the selectin directly makes physical contact. In this regard, consistent with the presence of the lectin domain, all known selectin ligands are carbohydrates. However, for at least some selectin ligands, the relevant carbohydrates must be displayed on the appropriate protein backbone. Thus, at least some physiologic selectin ligands are glycoproteins. In addition, it is important to emphasize that the putative "identification" of selectin ligands is heavily dependent on the assay systems used. Thus, given the nature of cell adhesion by selectins and the role that shear force plays in selectin-mediated adhesion, studies of "ligands" in essentially static assays are often misleading.

This point is especially relevant when considering the relationship between carbohydrate ligands of selectins and anticarbohydrate monoclonal antibodies (mAb). In early studies of selectin ligands, it was found that mAb to the tetrasaccharide sialyl Lewis X (sLex) inhibited adhesion by all three selectins (Phillips et al., 1990; Walz et al., 1990; Polley et al., 1991; Foxall et al., 1992). Subsequent work, however, showed that the actual physiologic recognition structures seen by selectins were both more complex, and restricted to only one or a few glycoproteins among the many that carried sLex. Thus, although the sLex moiety itself is a simple prototype of structures recognized by selectins, and is consistent with the requirements for both fucose and sialic acid, mAbs to sLex do not block adhesion when the assays are carried out under shear (Knibbs et al., 1998; Sanders et al., 1999). Thus, sLex per se is not necessarily the physiologic ligand for any of the selectins. However, the presence of sLex, as detected by appropriate mAb such as HECA-452 and CSLEX1, signifies the expression of certain enzymes required for expression of such ligands, and is therefore a good marker of cells capable of binding to selectins, in particular, E-selectin, (Picker et al., 1991a; Knibbs et al., 1996; Wagers et al., 1997). As discussed in the following, it remains unclear precisely which carbohydrate moieties directly interact with the lectin domains of selectins, and how they do so at the molecular level.

Prior to the identification of specific glycoprotein ligands for selectins or the enzymes (glycosyltransferases) responsible for the biosynthesis of selectin ligands, it was shown that neuraminidase treatment of ligand-bearing cells abrogated or substantially reduced adhesion to selectins. Although first shown for L-selectin (Rosen et al., 1985), this observation was subsequently extended to E- and P-selectin as well (Zhou et al., 1991; Varki, 1997). Thus, all selectins require sialic acid for cell adhesion, probably in an $\alpha2,3$ linkage. The sialyltransferases that carry out this modification have not yet been definitively identified, but four enzymes capable of adding sialic acid in an $\alpha2,3$ linkage have been cloned (Tsuji, 1996). Which of these is responsible for biosynthesis of selectin ligands, whether one or more such enzyme participates in construction of such ligands, and whether these are the same for each selectin, is currently unknown.

In contrast, $\alpha1,3$ fucosyltransferases controlling selectin ligand biosynthesis have been definitively identified. Two such enzymes are expressed in leukocytes, designated FucT-IV and FucT-VII. Myeloid cells, including neutrophils, monocytes, and their precursors, constitutively express high levels of both enzymes, whereas only FucT-VII is expressed at significant levels in T lymphocytes, and only following activation in the presence of appropriate cytokines (Smith et al., 1996; Knibbs et al., 1998; Wagers et al., 1998). At least in the mouse, activated B cells also express FucT-VII, but the stimuli that induce FucT-VII in activated B cells have not been identified. Naive T and B cells do not express detectable FucT-VII. In humans but not in mice, three other $\alpha1,3$ fucosyltransferases have been identified, but these enzymes are expressed in epithelial and other tissues, not in hematopoietic cells.

Transfections of essentially any cell type with cDNA encoding FucT-VII confers the ability to bind E-selectin, and is required for binding to P-selectin (Knibbs et al., 1996; Snapp et al., 1996; Wagers et al., 1997). T cells that are activated by engagement of their T-cell receptor (TCR) in the presence of either IL-12 or TGF-β1 express high levels of FucT-VII and bind to both E- and P-selectin (Wagers et al., 1998). Most convincingly, mice with targeted disruption of the FucT-VII gene exhibit a nearly complete loss of leukocyte ligands for all three selectins as well as impaired homing to lymph nodes, consequent to loss of L-selectin ligands in HEV (Maly et al., 1996). Consistent with the role of selectins in leukocyte recruitment described above, mice deficient in FucT-VII have sharply impaired accumulation of leukocytes in sites of inflammation. The degree of impairment exhibited by FucT-VII mice is considerably higher than is exhibited by mice deficient in any single selectin, and is comparable to that seen in mice deficient in all those selectins. Taken together, these data firmly establish a critical role for FucT-VII in biosynthesis of ligands for all three selectins.

The importance of FucT-VII, in addition to what was just outlined, also lies in the fact that among glycosyltransferases known to be involved in selectin ligand biosynthesis, only FucT-VII exhibits any form of regulation in T lymphocytes. As mentioned before, naive T cells do not express detectable FucT-VII mRNA, and activation of T cells in the presence of either IL-12 or transforming growth factor (TGF-β) strongly activates FucT-VII transcription.

In addition, FucT-VII mRNA levels, and therefore enzyme expression levels, can be sharply down-regulated by IL-4, providing a means for restricting the homing ability of activated T cells, especially Th2 cells (Austrup et al., 1997; Wagers et al., 1998). In contrast, sialyltransferases and other enzymes that are also involved in selectin ligand biosynthesis are constitutively expressed in all leukocytes and do not appear to undergo significant regulation of expression, although C2GnT-(see next paragraph) expression increases with T-cell activation. Similarly, expression of P-selectin glycoprotein ligand-1 (PSGL-1), which functions as P-and L-selectin ligand also does not change significantly during T-cell activation. Expression of FucT-VII is therefore a crucial control point in the regulation of T-cell migration.

A second enzyme required for biosynthesis of selectin ligands is the O-linked carbohydrate-branching enzyme, core 2 β1,6 glucosaminyltransferase (C2GnT); Bierhuizen et al., 1992; Kumar et al., 1996; Li et al., 1996). Mice deficient for C2GnT exhibit impaired or absent rolling of neutrophils in vitro on all three selectins, although the degree of impairment varies among selectins (Ellies et al., 1998). In addition, these mice have sharply impaired recruitment of neutrophils to the inflamed peritoneum, comparable to that seen in mice deficient in FucT-VII, and clearly significantly greater than that observed with single-selectin deficient mice. In part, this may be due to the fact that PSGL-1, which serves as a leukocyte ligand for both P-and L-selectin (see the following), requires the action of C2GnT. Thus, a deficiency in this enzyme directly abolishes ligands for both P-selectin, which is important in an acute inflammatory response, and L-selectin, which mediates leukocyte–leukocyte interactions in the same setting.

The main leukocyte ligand for P-selectin has been clearly established to be a homodimeric sialomucin designated PSGL-1 (Sako et al., 1993; Moore et al., 1995). MAb directed against certain epitopes of PSGL-1 abolish binding of all classes of leukocytes to P-selectin (Moore et al., 1995; Snapp et al., 1998b), and transfection of cell lines (which also express FucT-VII and C2GnT) with PSGL-1 cDNA confers the ability to bind P-selectin. PSGL-1 has a tyrosine sulfate motif at the amino-terminus, and mutational analysis has shown that at least one of the three tyrosines in the motif must be sulfated for recognition (Pouyani and Seed, 1995; Sako et al., 1995). In addition, a threonine residue just downstream from the tyrosine sulfate motif is also required (Liu et al., 1998), presumably for attachment of the sialylated, fucosylated, and branched oligosaccharides, which are also involved in recognition of P-selectin. Dimerization of PSGL-1 through the single cysteine in the ectodomain is also required for recognition (Snapp et al., 1998a). PSGL-1 also serves as a ligand for L-selectin (Walchek et al., 1996), with the same requirements for posttranslational modifications and glycosyltransferases as for P-selectin binding. MAb directed against PSGL-1 which block binding to P-selectin also block binding to L-selectin. Thus, both P- and L-selectin see the same or closely overlapping site at the amino-terminus of PSGL-1, which consists of at least one tyrosine sulfate juxtaposed with both sialic acid and fucose in a three-dimensional configuration dependent on both the action of C2GnT and the dimerization of PSGL-1.

PSGL-1 has also been reported to function as a ligand for E-selectin, on the basis of the ability of recombinant soluble E-selectin to affinity capture PSGL-1 (Sako et al., 1993 Lenter et al., 1994), and the high density of epitopes recognized by human endothelial cell antigen-452 (HECA-452) mAb on PSGL-1 (Fuhlbrigge et al., 1997). However, mAb against PSGL-1 do not affect direct interaction of neutrophils with E-selectin (Snapp et al., 1998b), and proteases that destroy PSGL-1 do not affect binding to E-selectin (Larsen et al., 1992). In addition, PSGL-1 knockout mice closely resemble P-selectin knockout mice, with no obvious defect in rolling on E-selectin (Yang et al., 1999). Whether PSGL-1 functions as a physiologic ligand for E-selectin remains to be determined.

Ligands for L-selectin can be functionally detected on leukocytes, on HEV, and on endothelium at sites of inflammation. On leukocytes, PSGL-1 is the principal ligand, although other ligands may also exist (Ramos et al., 1998). L-selectin ligands on non-HEV endothelium have not been defined at the molecular level. On HEV, however, a number of molecular species have been identified by affinity capture and subsequently shown to support leukocyte rolling when isolated and immobilized on plastic. One of these, GlyCAM-1, is a soluble mucin-like molecule that is apparently secreted from HEV and may play a role in activation of the integrin LFA-1 on naive lymphocytes (Lasky et al., 1992; Hwang et al., 1996). A second L-selectin ligand is an HEV-specific glycoform of CD34, a mucin-like molecule universally expressed on endothelium and on HSC (Puri et al., 1995). A third molecule, sgp200, has not been identified at the molecular level. The fourth molecule identified as a possible HEV ligand is podocalyxin, previously found on kidney podocytes (Sassetti et al., 1998). Which of these glycoproteins actually function as L-selectin ligands in vivo has yet to be definitively determined.

As indicated above, FucT-VII expression in HEV is required for L-selectin ligand activity and homing in vivo (Maly et al., 1996), suggesting that FucT-VII may modify each of the previously listed glycoproteins. In contrast, although branched O-linked structures, which would require C2GnT activity, are also thought to be required for biosynthesis of L-selectin ligands, mice deficient in C2GnT exhibit little impairment in homing of lymphocytes to lymph nodes in vivo (Ellies et al., 1998). Whether this is due to expression in HEV of other enzymes with similar activity or to a diminished requirement for the core 2 structure is unclear. L-selectin ligand activity on HEV also requires sulfation, but unlike PSGL-1, this sulfation is a modification of oligosaccharides. In addition, sialylation of HEV ligands is essential for L-selectin activity. A candidate-capping structure that can account for all of these requirements is the 6-sulfo-sLex structure, which occurs in HEV. MAb against this structure block binding of lymphocytes in an ex vivo HEV binding assay (Hemmerich and Rosen, 1994; Mitsuoka et al., 1997, 1998). Thus, expression of 6-sulfo-sLex on any or all of the glycoproteins mentioned above may constitute the physiologic ligands for L-selectin on HEV.

A number of cell surface molecules have been proposed to serve as E-selectin ligands, including PSGL-1 (discussed above), L-selectin (Picker et al., 1991b), and ESL-1 (Steegmaier et al., 1995), a variant of a fibroblast growth factor (Burruss et al., 1992). However, mAb to these molecules either do not block direct interaction of cells with E-selectin (PSGL-1 and L-selectin), or have not been produced or characterized (E-selectin ligand-1 or ESL-1). Transfection of cells with cDNA encoding any of these three molecules does not confer or enhance binding to E-selectin. However, each of these molecules can be affinity captured by recombinant E-selectin, suggesting that they may serve as ligands under some circumstances. Interestingly, binding of cells to E-selectin is resistant to a spectrum of proteases, suggesting that some physiologic E-selectin ligands are glycolipids (Alon et al., 1995). In addition, E-selectin ligands do not appear to require sulfate, in sharp contrast to both L- and P-selectin. The precise identity of functional, physiologic ligands for E-selectin remains unclear.

Given this information, it is worth considering exactly how the various carbohydrate moieties implicated in selectin ligand structure might interact with the lectin domain of selectins. The crystal structure of the E-selectin lectin plus EGF domains has been solved (Graves et al., 1994), and mutagenesis of specific residues defines a face of the molecule at the "top" of the lectin domain, on the opposite face from the EGF-like domain, which can accomodate the binding of sLex and is consistent with the calcium requirement and with epitopes defined by mAb blocking studies. A few of these residues are positively charged amino acids that are completely conserved among all three selectins and across species, and are likely to interact directly with carbohydrate ligand atoms. However, certain mutations block binding of soluble E-selectin to immobilized sLex without affecting cell adhesion to E-selectin (Erbe et al., 1992). In addition, other studies have identified residues predicted to lie on the opposite face of P-selectin that are also apparently involved in ligand binding. Furthermore, although no crystal structure is available for L- and P-selectin, it seems reasonable to assume that the structure will be quite similar, as the E-selectin lectin domain structure is quite similar to that of the mannose-binding protein (MBP), which is obviously much less closely related to E-selectin than are the other two selectins. Yet both L- and P-selectin also recognize sulfate (unlike E-selectin), and there is no obvious way to accomodate a sulfate moiety in the cleft of the lectin domain putatively responsible for binding sLex. Hence, the precise way in which the lectin domain of selectins interacts with their physiologic carbohydrate ligands remains unclear, and is an important topic for future investigation.

Cell Biology of Selectins and Their Ligands

Certain cell biologic aspects of selectins are of interest in understanding how selectins function. One of these is the subcellular localization of these "rolling receptors." On normal leukocytes and many cell lines, L-selectin is localized predominantly to the tips of microvilli, which are thought to be the first portion of a cell to contact the endothelium (Hasslen et al., 1995; von Andrian et al., 1995). At least on neutrophils, PSGL-1 is also localized to the microvilli. Similarly, VLA-4, an integrin that can mediate attachment and rolling of T cells under some circumstances (Berlin et al., 1995), is localized to microvilli on lymphocytes and transfected cell lines (Abitorabi et al., 1997). These observations have given rise to the intuitively very appealing hypothesis that this localization is in some way essential to the ability of selectins or other rolling receptors to facilitate capture and rolling of freely flowing leukocytes. However, CD44, which on activated T cells can also mediate attachment and rolling on its ligand hyaluronate (DeGrendele et al, 1996), is localized in an essentially opposite manner to the planar cell body (von Andrian et al., 1995). Therefore, localization to microvilli cannot be essential for attachment and rolling. L-selectin mutants confined to the cell body impair attachment but not rolling which replace the transmembrane plus cytoplasmic domains with those of CD44, redirect the localization of the chimeric molecules from microvilli to the cell body and impair attachment but not rolling (von Andrian et al., 1995), consistent with this localization being important for the function of L-selectin. Localization of VLA-4 to microvilli of transfected K562 cells depends on the ectodomain (Abitorabi et al., 1997). No similar studies have been reported for PSGL-1, but PSGL-1 does not localize to microvilli of certain transfected cell lines that do localize L-selectin to microvilli. Thus, distinct mechanisms control the sorting of these different molecules to microvilli, and the individual molecules may rely, to different extents, on this localization.

Adhesion by selectins and their ligands may be regulated by association with the actin cytoskeleton. Treatment of cells with high doses of cytochalasins, which disrupt the actin cytoskeleton, blocks cell adhesion (Kansas et al., 1993). L-selectin interacts constitutively with the cytoskeletal linker protein α-actinin, and mutations within the L-selectin cytoplasmic domain that block this interaction also block cell adhesion (Pavalko et al., 1995). However, L-selectin is not constitutively associated with the actin cytoskeleton in lymphocytes; rather, this attachment is rapidly induced upon initial engagement of ligand (Evans et al., 1999). The mechanisms leading to this rapid attachment to the actin cytoskeleton are unknown. However, neutrophils from mice deficient in the small GTPase rac2 have normal L-selectin expression, but greatly impaired attachment and rolling in vitro (Roberts et al., 1999). In contrast, these mice exhibit normal attachment and rolling on P-selectin, indicating that PSGL-1 activity is unimpaired. Given the role of the rho subfamily of GTPases in controlling cytoskeletal remodeling and actin dynamics (Hall, 1998), it is tempting to speculate that rac2 regulates the attachment of L-selectin to the cytoskeleton and/or other essential aspects of interactions between L-selectin and the actin cytoskeleton.

The E-selectin cytoplasmic domain is not required for cell adhesion per se, but adhesion of neutrophils to endothelium through E-selectin induces association of E-selectin with several cytoskeletal and signaling molecules (Yoshida et al., 1996). This adhesion-induced association of E-selectin with cytoskeletal molecules may be important for downstream events, including firm adhesion and transmigration. Interaction of P-selectin with the cytoskeleton has not been reported, and the effects of actin-disrupting agents (e.g., cytochalasins) on adhesion to P-selectin is unknown.

Signaling by Selectins and Their Ligands

Mounting evidence suggests that selectins and their (glycoprotein) ligands have signaling functions as well as cell-adhesion functions. On neutrophils, engagement of L-selectin by mAb or artificial ligands (e.g., sulfatide) can initiate tyrosine phosphorylation, mitogen-activated protein (MAP) kinase activation, up-regulation of cytokine mRNA levels, and activation of calcium ion influx and the oxidative burst (Laudanna et al., 1994; Waddell et al., 1994, 1995). In addition, engagement of L-selectin can induce integrin activation on both neutrophils and T lymphocytes, as does binding of neutrophils to E-selectin (Lo et al., 1991; Simon et al., 1995; Hwang et al., 1996). The time scale of these effects, however, is in minutes, making it less likely that these signaling events are relevant for interaction with endothelium within the vasculature.

Engagement of PSGL-1 by P-selectin on platelets also has important signaling consequences. This interaction initiates phagocytosis and induces the expression of tissue factor on monocytes, and can also potentiate cytokine synthesis and release (Elstad et al., 1995; Weyrich et al., 1995, 1996). These events appear to be related to activation of NF-κB. Binding to PSGL-1 can also activate leukocyte integrins, similar to L-selectin. Taken together, these observations suggest that engagement of rolling receptors on leukocytes can contribute to the control of leukocyte traffic apart from their direct function in rolling.

Conclusions

Selectins are key adhesion molecules in the control of leukocyte traffic and in the maintenance of effective immunity. Initiation of recognition of endothelium by selectins is crucial to effective leukocyte recruitment in most settings of inflammation, and in normal lymphocyte traffic and probably in hematopoietic stem cell traffic. Blockade of selectin-mediated cell adhesion may prove to be beneficial in treatment of inflammatory, autoimmune, and metastatic disease.

References

Abitorabi, M. A., Pachynski, R. K., Ferrando, R. E., Tidswell, M., and Erle, D. J. (1997) Presentation of integrins on leukocyte microvilli: A role for the extracellular domain in determining membrane localization. *J. Cell. Biol.* 139:563–571.

Alon, R., Feizi, T., Yuen, C. T., Fuhlbrigge, R. C., and Springer, T. A. (1995) Glycolipid ligands for selectins support leukocyte tethering and rolling under physiologic flow conditions. *J. Immunol.* 154:5356–5366.

Arbones, M. L., Ord, D. C., Ley, K., Ratech, H., G., Maynard-Curry, C., Otten, G., Capon, D. J., and Tedder, T. F. (1994) Lymphocyte homing and leukocyte rolling and migration are impaired in L-selectin (CD62L) deficient mice. *Immun.* 1:247–260.

Austrup, F., Vestweber, D., Borges, E., Lohning, M., Brauer, R., Herz, U., Renz, H., Hallmann, R., Scheffold, A., Radbruch, A., and Hamann, A. (1997) P-and E-selectin mediate recruitment of T helper 1 but not T helper 2 cells into inflamed tissues. *Nature* 385:81–83.

Berlin, C., Bargatze, R. F., Campbell, J. J., von Andrian, U. H., Szabo, M. C., Hasslen, S. R., Nelson, R. D., Berg, E. L., Erlandsen, S. L., and Butcher, E. C. (1995) α4 Integrins mediate lymphocyte attachment and rolling under physiologic flow. *Cell* 80:413–422.

Bevilacqua, M. P., Stengelin, S., Gimbrone, Jr., M. A., and Seed, B. (1989) Endothelial leukocyte adhesion molecule 1: an inducible receptor for neutrophils related to complement regulatory proteins and lectins. *Science* 243:1160–1164.

Bierhuizen, M. F., and Fukuda, M. (1992) Expression cloning of a cDNA encoding UDP-GlcNAc: Gal beta 1-3-GalNAc-R (GlcNAc to GalNAc) beta 1-6GlcNAc transferase by gene transfer into CHO cells expressing polyoma large tumor antigen. *Proc. Natl. Acad. Sci. USA* 89:9326–330.

Bonfanti, R., Furie, B. C., Furie, B., and Wagner, D. D. (1989) PADGEM is a component of Weibel–Palade bodies in endothelial cells. *Blood* 73:1109–1112.

Bowen, B. R., Fennie, C., and Lasky, L. A. (1990) The MEL-14 antibody binds to the lectin domain of the murine peripheral lymph node homing receptor. *J. Cell. Biol.* 110:147–153.

Bradley, L. M., Watson, S. R., and Swain, S. L. (1994) Entry of naive CD4 T cells into peripheral lymph nodes requires L-selectin. *J. Exp. Med.* 180:2401–2406.

Bullard, D. C., Kunkel, E. J., Kubo, H., Hicks, M. J., Lorenzo, I., Doyle, C. A., Doerschuk, C. M., Ley, K., and Beaudet, A. L. (1996) Infectious susceptibility and severe deficiency of leukocyte rolling and recruitment in E-selectin and P-selectin double mutant mice. *J. Exp. Med.* 183: 2329–2337.

Burruss, L. W., Zuber, M. E., Lueddecke, B. A., and Olwin, B. B. (1992) Identification of a cysteine-rich receptor for fibroblast growth factors. *Mol. Cell. Biol.* 12:5600–5609.

Catalina, M. D., Carroll, M. C., Arizpe, H., Takashima, A., Estess, P., and Siegelman, M. H. (1996) The route of antigen entry determines the requirement for L-selectin during immune responses. *J. Exp. Med.* 184:2341–2351.

Chu, W., Presky, D. H., Swerlick, R. A., and Burns, D. K. (1994) Alternatively processed human E-selectin transcripts linked to chronic expression of E-selectin in vivo. *J. Immunol.* 153:4179–4189.

Collins, T., Williams, A., Johnston, G. I., Kim, J., Eddy, R., Shows, T., Gimbrone, M. A., and Bevilacqua, M. P. (1991) Structure and chromosomal location of the gene for endothelial–leukocyte adhesion molecule-1. *J. Biol. Chem.* 266:2466–2478.

Collins, T., Read, M. A., Neish, A. S., Whitley, M. Z., Thanos, D., and Maniatis, T. (1995) Transcriptional regulation of endothelial cell adhesion molecules: NF-kappa B and cytokine-inducible enhancers. *FASEB J.* 9:899–909.

DeGrendele, H. C., Estess, P., Picker, L. J., and Siegelman, M. H. (1996) CD44 and its ligand hyaluronate mediate rolling under physiologic flow: a novel lymphocyte–endothelial cell primary adhesion pathway. *J. Exp. Med.* 183:1119–1130.

Ellies, L. G., Tsuboi, S., Petryniak, B., Lowe, J. B., Fukuda, M., and Marth, J. D. (1998) Core 2 oligosaccharide biosynthesis distinguishes between selectin ligands essential for leukocyte homing and inflammation. *Immun.* 9:881–890.

Elstad, M. R., La Pine, T. R., Cowley, F. S., McEver, R. P., McIntyre, T. M., Prescott, S. M., and Zimmerman, G. A. (1995) P-selectin regulates platelet-activating factor synthesis and phagocytosis by monocytes. *J. Immunol.* 155:2109–2122.

Erbe, D. V., Wolitzky, B. A., Presta, L. G., Norton, C. R., Ramos, R. J., Burns, D. K., Rumberger, J. M., Rao, B.N.N., Foxall, C., Brandley, B. K., and Lasky, L. A. (1992) Identification of an E-selectin region critical for carbohydrate recognition and cell adhesion. *J. Cell. Biol.* 119:215–227.

Evans, S. S., Bowman, L., Schleider, D. M., Kansas, G. S., and Black, J. D. (1999) Dynamic association of L-selectin with the lymphocyte cortical cytoskeleton. *J. Immunol.* 162:3615–3624.

Finger, E. B., Puri, K. D., Alon, R., Lawrence, M. B., von Andrian, U. H., and Springer, T. A.

(1996) Adhesion through L-selectin requires a threshold hydrodynamic shear. *Nature* 379: 266–269.

Foxall, C., Watson, S. R., Dowbenko, D., Fennie, C., Lasky, L. A., Kiso, M., Hasegawa, A., Asa, D., and Brandley, B. K. (1992) The three members of the selectin receptor family recognize a common carbohydrate epitope, the sialyl lewis^x oligosaccharide. *J. Cell. Biol* 117:895–902.

Frenette, P. S., Mayads, T. N., Rayburn, H., Hynes, R. O., and Wagner, D. D. (1996) Susceptibility to infection and altered hematopoiesis in mice deficient in both P- and E-selectins. *Cell* 84: 563–574.

Frenette, P. S., Subbarao, S., Mazo, I. B., von Andrian, U. H., and Wagner, D. D. (1998) Endothelial selectins and vascular adhesion molecule-1 promote hematopoietic progenitor homing to bone marrow. *Proc. Natl. Acad. Sci. USA* 195:14423–14428.

Fuhlbrigge, R. C., Kieffer, J. D., Amerding, A., and Kupper, T. S. (1997) Cutaneous lymphocyte antigen is a specialized form of PSGL-1 expressed on skin-homing T cells. *Nature* 389:978–981.

Gallatin, W. M., Weissman, I. L., and Butcher, E. C. (1983) A cell-surface molecule involved in organ-specific homing of lymphocytes. *Nature* 304:30–34.

Gotsch, U., Jager, U., Dominis, M., and Vestweber, D. (1994) Expression of P-selectin on endothelial cells is upregulated by LPS and TNF-alpha in vivo. *Cell Adhesion & Commun.* 2:7–14.

Graves, B. J., Crowther, R. L., Chadran, C., Rumberger, J. M., Li, S., Huang, K.-S., Presky, D. M., Familetti, P. C., Wolitzky, B. A., and Burns, D. (1994) Insight into the E-selectin/ligand interaction from the crystal structure and mutagenesis of the lec/EGF domains. *Nature* 367: 532–538.

Griffin, J. D., Spertini, O., Ernst, T. J., Belvin, M. P., Levine, H. B., Kanakura, Y., and Tedder, T. F. (1990) GM-CSF and other cytokines regulate surface expression of the leukocyte adhesion molecule-1 on human neutrophils, monocytes, and their precursors. *J. Immunol.* 145: 576–584.

Grober, J. S., Bowen, B. L., Ebling, H., Athey, B., Thompson, C. B., Fox, D. A., and Stoolman, L. M. (1993) Monocyte–endothelial adhesion in chronic rheumatoid arthritis. In situ detection of selectin and integrin-dependent interactions. *J. Clin. Invest.* 91:2609–2619.

Hall, A. (1998) Rho GPases and the actin cytoskeleton. *Science* 279:509–514.

Hasslen, S. R., von Andrian, U. H., Butcher, E. C., Nelson, R. D., and Erlandsen, S. L. (1995) Spatial distribution of L-selectin (CD62L) on human lymphocytes and transfected murine L1-2 cells. *Histochem. J.* 27:547–554.

Hemmerich, S., and Rosen, S. D. (1994) 6'-sulfated sialyl Lewis^x is a major capping group of GlyCAM-1. *Biochem.* 33:4830–4835.

Hwang, S. T., Singer, M. S., Giblin, P. A., Yednock, T. A., Bacon, K. B., Simon, S. I., and Rosen, S. D. (1996) GlyCAM-1, a physiologic ligand for L-selectin, activates beta 2 integrins on naive peripheral lymphocytes. *J. Exp. Med.* 184:1343–1348.

Johnson, R. C., Mayadas, T. N., Frenette, P. S., Mebius, R. E., Subramaniam, M. Lacasce, A. Hynes, R. O., and Wagner, D. D. (1995) Blood cell dynamics in P-selectin deficient mice. *Blood* 86:1106–1114.

Johnston, G. I., Bliss, G. A., Newman, P. J., and McEver, R. P. (1990) Genomic structure of GMP-140, a member of the selectin family of adhesion receptors for leukocytes. *J. Biol. Chem.* 34: 21381–21385.

Jung, T. M., Gallatin, W. M., Weissman, I. L., and Dailey, M. O. (1988) Down-regulation of homing receptors after T-cell activation. *J. Immunol.* 141:4110–4117.

Kansas, G. S., Wood, G. S., and Engleman, E. G. (1985a) Maturational and functional diversity of human B lymphocytes delineated with anti–Leu-8. *J. Immunol.* 134:3003–3006.

Kansas, G. S., Wood, G. S., Fishwild, D. M., and Engleman, E. G. (1985b) Functional characterization of human T-lymphocyte subsets distinguished by monoclonal anti–Leu-8. *J. Immunol.* 134:2995–3002.

Kansas, G. S., Spertini, O., Stoolman, L. M., and Tedder, T. F. (1991) Molecular mapping of functional domains of the leukocyte receptor for endothelium, LAM-1. *J. Cell Biol.* 114:351–358.

Kansas, G. S., Ley, K. Munro, J. M., and Tedder, T. F. (1993) Regulation of leukocyte rolling and adhesion to HEV through the cytoplasmic domain of L-selectin. *J. Exp. Med.* 177:833–838.

Kansas, G. S., Saunders, K. B., Ley, K., Zakrzewicz, A., Gibson, R. M., Furie, B. C., Furie, B., and Tedder, T. F. (1994) A role for the epidermal growth factor-like domain of P-selectin in ligand recognition and cell adhesion. *J. Cell. Biol.* 124:609–618.

Kansas, G. S. (1996) Selectins and their ligands: current concepts and controversies. *Blood* 88: 3259–3286.

Kishimoto, T. K., Julita, M. A., Berg, E. L., and Butcher, E. C. (1989) Neutrophil Mac-1 and MEL-14 adhesion proteins inversely regulated by chemotactic factors. *Science* 245:1238–1241.

Knibbs, R. N., Craig, R. A., Maly, P., Smith, P. L., Wolber, F. M., Faulkner, N. E., Lowe, J. B., and Stoolman, L. M. (1998) α1,3-Fucosyltransferase VII dependent synthesis of P- and E-selectin ligands on cultured T lymphoblasts. *J. Immunol.* 161:6305–6315.

Knibbs, R. N., Craig, R. A., Natsuka, S., Chang, A., Cameron, M., Lowe, J. B., and Stoolman L. M. (1996) The fucosyltransferase FucT-VII regulates E-selectin ligand synthesis in human T cells. *J. Cell. Biol.* 133:911–920.

Kubes, P., and Kanwar S. (1994). Histamine induces leukocyte rolling in postcapillary venules. A P-selectin-mediated event. *J. Immunol.* 152:3570–3577.

Kumar, R., Camphausen, R. T., Sullivan, F. X., and Cumming, D. A. (1996) Core 2 β-1,6-N-Acetylglucosaminyltransferase enzyme activity is critical for P-selectin glycoprotein ligand-1 binding to P-selectin. *Blood* 88:3872–3879.

Kunkel, E. J., Jung, U. Bullard, D. C. Norman, K. E. Wolitzky, B. A. Vestweber, D. Beaudet, A. L. and Ley K. (1995) Absence of trauma-induced leukocyte rolling in mice deficient in both P-selectin and intercellular adhesion molecule-1 (ICAM-1). *J. Exp. Med.* 183:57–65.

Kunkel, E. J., and Ley K. (1996) Distinct phenotype of E-selectin-deficient mice. E-selectin is required for slow leukocyte rolling in vivo. *Circ. Res.* 79:1196–1204.

Labow, M. A., Norton, C. R., Rumberger, J. M., Lombard-Gilloly, K. M., Shuster, D. J., Hubbard, J., Bertko, R., Knaack, P. A., Terry, R. W., Harbison, M. L. et al. (1994) Characterization of E-selectin–deficient mice demonstration of overlapping function of the endothelial selectins. *Immun.* 1:709–720.

Larsen, G. R., Sako, D., Ahern, T. J., Shaffer, M., Erban, J., Sajer, S. A., Gibson, R. M., Wagner, D. D., Furie, B. C., and Furie, B. (1992) P-selectin and E-selectin. Distinct but overlapping leukocyte ligand specificities. *J. Biol. Chem.* 267:11104–11110.

Lasky, L. A., Singer, M. S., Dowbenko, D. Imai, Y., Henzel, W. J., Grimley, C. Fennie, C. Gillett, N. Watson, S. R., and Rosen, S. D. (1992) An endothelial ligand for L-selectin is a novel mucin-like molecule. *Cell* 69:927–938.

Laudanna, C., Constantin, G., Baron, P., Scarpini, E., Scarlato, G., Cabrini, G. Dechecchi, C. Rossi, F. Cassatella, M. A., and Berton G. (1994) Sulfatides trigger increase of cytosolic free calcium and enhanced expression of tumor necrosis factor-alpha and interleukin-8 mRNA in human neutrophils. Evidence for a role of L-selectin as a signaling molecule. *J. Biol chem.* 269:4021–4026.

Lawrence, M. B., Kansas, G. S., Kunkel, E. J., and Ley, K. (1997) Threshold levels of fluid shear promote leukocyte adhesion through selectins (CD62L, P,E). *J. Cell Biol.* 136:717–727.

Lenter, M., Levinovitz, A., Isenmann, S., Vestwebber D. (1994) Monospecific and common glycoprotein ligands for E- and P-selectin on myeloid cells. *J. Cell. Biol.* 125:471–481.

Ley, K., Bullard, D., Arbones, M. L., Bosse, R., Vestweber, D., Tedder, T. F., and Beaudett, A. L. (1995) Sequential contribution of L- and P-selectin to leukocyte rolling in vivo. *J. Exp. Med* 181:669–675.

Ley, K., and Tedder, T. F. (1995) Leukocyte interactions with vascular endothelium. New insights into selectin-mediated attachment and rolling. *J. Immunol.* 155:525–528.

Li, F., Wilkins, P. P., Crawley, S., Weinstein, J., Cummings, R. D., and McEver. R. P. (1996) Post-translational modifications of recombinant P-selectin glycoprotein ligand-1 required for binding to P- and E-selectin. *J. Biol. Chem.* 271:3255–3264.

Liu, W., Ramachandran, V., Kang, J., Kishimoto, T. K., Cummings, R. D., and McEver, R. P. (1998) Identification of N-terminal residues on P-selectin glycoprotein ligand-1 required for binding to P-selectin. *J. Biol. Chem.* 273:7078–7087.

Lo, S. K., Lee, S., Ramos, R. A., Lobb, R., Rosa, M., Chi-Rosso, G., and Wright, S. D. (1991)

Endothelial–leukocyte adhesion molecule 1 stimulates the adhesive activity of leukocyte integrin CR3 (CD11b/CD18, Mac-1, $\alpha_m\beta_2$) on human neutrophils. *J. Exp. Med.* 173:1493–1500.

Maly, P., Thall, A. D., Petryniak, B., Rogers, C. E., Smith, P. L., Marks, R. M., Kelly, R. J., Gersten, K. M., Cheng, G., Saunders, T. L. et al. (1996) The $\alpha(1,3)$ fucosyltransferase FucT-VII controls leukocyte trafficking through an essential role in L-, E-, and P-selectin ligand biosynthesis. *Cell* 86:643–653.

Mayadas, T. N., Johnson, R. C., Rayburn, H., Hynes, R. O., and Wagner, D. D. (1993) Leukocyte rolling and extravasation are severely compromised in P-selectin–deficient mice. *Cell* 74:541–554.

McEver, R. P., Beckstead, J. H., Moore, K. L., Marshal-Carlson, L., Bainton, D. F. (1989) GMP-140, a platelet alpha granule membrane protein, is also synthesized by vascular endothelial cells and is localized in Weibel–Palade bodies. *J. Clin. Invest.* 84:92–99.

Mitsuoka, C., Kawakami-Kimura, N., Kasugai-Sawada, M., Hiraiwa, N., Toda, K., Ishida, H., Kiso, M., Hasegawa, A., and Kannagi, R., (1997) Sulfated sialyl Lewis X, the putative L-selectin ligand, detected on endothelial cells of high endothelial venules by a distinct set of anti-sialyl Lewis X antibodies. *Biochem. Biophys. Res. Comm.* 230:546–551.

Mitsuoka, C., Sawada-Kasugai, M., Ando-Furui, K., Izawa, M., Nakanishi, H., Nakamura, S., Ishida, H., Kiso, M., and Kannagi, R. (1998) Identification of a major carbohydrate capping group of the L-selectin ligand on high endothelial venules in human lymph nodes as 6-sulfo-sialyl X. *J. Biol. Chem* 273:11225–11233.

Moore, K. L., Patel, K. D., Breuhl, R. E., Fugang, L., Johnson, D. L., Lichenstein, H. S., Cummings, R. D., Bainton, D. F., and McEver, R. P., (1995) P-selectin glycoprotein ligand-1 mediates rolling of human neutrophils on P-selectin. *J. Cell. Biol.* 128:661–671.

Ord, D. C., Ernst, T. J., Zhou, L. J., Rambaldi, A., Spertini, O., Griffin, J. D., and Tedder, T. F. (1990) Structure of the gene encoding the human leukocyte adhesion molecule-1 (TQ1, Leu-8) of lymphocytes and neutrophils. *J. Biol. Chem.* 265:7760–7767.

Palabrica, T., Lobb, R., Furie, B. C. Aronovitz, M. Benjamin, C. M. Hsu, Y.-M. Sajer, S. A. and Furie, B. (1992) Leukocyte accumulation promoting fibrin deposition is mediated in vivo by P-selectin on adherent platelets. *Nature* 359:848–851.

Papayannopoulou, T., Craddock, C. Nakamoto, B. Priestley, G. V. and Wolf, N. S. (1995) The VLA4/VCAM-1 adhesion pathway defines contrasting mechanisms of lodgement of transplanted murine hemopoietic progenitors between bone marrow and spleen. *Proc. Natl. Acad. Sci. USA* 92:9647–9651.

Pavalko, F. M., Walker, D. M. Graham, L. Doerschuk, C. M. and Kansas, G. S. (1995) The cytoplasmic domain of L-selectin interacts with cytoskeletal proteins via α-actinin: receptor positioning in microvilli does not require interaction with α-actinin. *J. Cell. Biol.* 129:1155–1164.

Phillips, M. L., Nudelman, E. Gaeta, F.C.A. Perez, M. Singhal, A. K. Hakomori, S.-I. and Paulson, J. C. (1990) ELAM-1 mediates cell adhesion by recognition of a carbohydrate ligand, sialyl-Le^x. *Science* 250:1130–1132.

Picker, L. J., Kishimoto, T. K. Smith, C. W. Warnock, R. A. and Butcher, E. C. (1991a) ELAM-1 is an adhesion molecule for skin-homing T cells. *Nature* 349:796–799.

Picker, L. J., Treer, J. R. Ferguson-Darnell, B. Collins, P. A. Buck, D. and Terstappen, L. W. (1991b) Control of lymphocyte recirculation in man. I. Differential regulation of the peripheral lymph node homing receptor L-selection on T cells during the virgin to memory cell transition. *J. Immunol.* 150:1105–1121.

Picker, L. J., Warnock, R. A. Burns, A. R. Doerschuk, C. M., Berg, and Butcher, E. C. (1993) The neutrophil selectin LECAM-1 presents carbohydrate ligands to the vascular selectins ELAM-1 and GMP-140. *Cell* 66:921–933.

Polley, M. J., Phillips, M. L. Wayner, E. Nudelman, E. Singhal, A. K. Hakomori, S.-I. and Paulson, J. C. (1991) CD62 and endothelial cell–leukocyte adhesion molecule-1 (ELAM-1) recognize the same carbohydrate ligand, sialyl-Lewis X. *Proc. Natl. Acad. Sci. USA* 88:6224–6228.

Pouyani, T., and Seed, B. (1995) PSGL-1 recognition of P-selectin is controlled by a tyrosine sulfation consensus at the PSGL-1 amino terminus. *Cell* 83:333–343.

Puri, K. D., Finger, E. B. Gaudernack, G. and Springer, T. A. (1995) Sialomucin CD34 is the major L-selectin ligand in human tonsil high endothelial venules. *J. Cell. Biol* 131:261–270.

Ramos, C. L., Smith, M. J. Snapp, K. R. Kansas, G. S. Stickney, G. W. Ley, K. and Lawrence, M. B.

(1998) Functional characterization of L-selectin ligands on human neutrophils and leukemia cell lines: evidence for mucinlike ligand activity distinct from P-selectin glycoprotein ligand-1 *Blood* 91:1067–1075.

Read, M. A., Neish, A. S. Luscinskas, F. W. Palombella, V. J. Maniatis, T. and Collins, T. (1995) The proteosome pathways is required for cytokine-induced endothelial–leukocyte adhesion molecule expression. *Immun.* 2:493–506.

Roberts, A. W. Kim, C. Zhen, L. Lowe, J. B. Kapur, R. Petryniak, B. Spaetti, A. Pollock, J. D. Borneo, J. B. Bradford, G. B. Atkinson, S. J. et al. (1999) Deficiency of hematopoietic cell specific Rho family GTPase rac2 is characterized by abnormalities in neutrophil function and host defense. *Immun.* 10:183–196.

Rosen, S. D., Singer, M. S. Yehnock, Y. A. and Stoolman, L. M. (1985) Involvement of sialic acid on endothelial cells in organ-specific lymphocyte recirculation. *Science* 228:1005–1007.

Sako, D., Chang, X.-J. Barone, K. M. Vachino, G. White, H. M. Shaw, G. Veldman, G. M. Bean, K. B. Ahern, T. J. Furie, B. et al. (1993) Expression cloning of a functional glycoprotein ligand for P-selectin. *Cell* 75:1179–1186.

Sako, D., Comess, K. M. Barone, K. M. Camphausen, R. T. Cumming, D. A. and Shaw, G. D. (1995) A sulfated peptide segment at the amino terminus of PSGL-1 is critical for P-selectin binding. *Cell* 83:323–331.

Sassetti, C., Tangemann, K. Singer, M. S. Kershaw, D. B. and Rosen S. D. (1998) Identification of podocalyxin-like protein as a high endothelial venule ligand for L-selectin: parallels to CD34. *J. Exp Med.* 187:1965–1975.

Schweitzer, K. M., Drager, A. M. van der Valk, P. Thijsen, S.F.T. Zevenbergen, A. Theijsmeijer, A. P. van der Schoot, C. E. and Langenhuijsen, M.M.A.A. (1996) Constitutive expression of E-selectin and vascular cell adhesion molecule-1 on endothelial cells of hematopoietic tissues. *Am. J. Path.* 148:165–175.

Simon, S. I. Burns, A. R. Taylor, A. D. Gopalan, P. K. Lynam, E. B. Sklar, L. A. and Smith, C. W. (1995) L-selectin (CD62L) cross-linking signals neutrophil adhesive functions via the Mac-1 (CD11b/Cd18) beta 2-integrin. *J. Immunol.* 155:1502–1514.

Simon, S. I. Chambers J. D. Butcher E. C., and Sklar L. A. (1992) Neutrophil aggregation is β_2-integrin– and L-selectin–dependent in blood and isolated cells. *J. Immunol.* 149:2765–2771.

Simon, S. I. Rochon, Y. P. Lynam, E. B. Smith, C. W. Anderson, D. C. and Sklar, L. A. (1993) β_2 Integrin and L-selectin are obligatory receptors in neutrophil aggregation. *Blood* 82:1097–1103.

Smith, P. L., Gersten, K. M. Petryniak, B. Kelly, R. J. Rogers, C. Natsuka, N. Alford III, Scheideger, P. Natsuka, S. and Lowe J. B. (1996) Expression of the $\alpha 1,3$ fucosyltransferase Fuc-TVII in lymphoid aggregate high endothelial venules correlates with expression of L-selectin ligands. *J. Biol. Chem.* 271:8250–8255.

Snapp, K. R., Craig, R. Herron, M. Nelson, R. D. Stoolman, L. M. and Kansas, G. S. (1998a) Dimerization of P-selectin glycoprotein ligand-1 (PSGL-1) required for optimal recognition of P-selectin. *J. Cell. Biol.* 142:263–270.

Snapp, K. R., Ding, H. Atkins, K. Warnke, R. Luscinskas, F. W. and Kansas, G. S. (1998b) A novel P-selectin glycoprotein ligand-1 (PSGL-1) monoclonal antibody recognizes an epitope within the tyrosine sulfate motif of human PSGL-1 amd blocks recognition of both P-and L-selectin. *Blood* 91:154–164.

Snapp, K. R., Wagers A. J. Craig R., Stoolman L. M., and Kansas G. S. (1996) P-selectin glycoprotein ligand-1 (PSGL-1) is essential for adhesion to P-selectin but not E-selectin in stably transfected hematopoietic cell lines *Blood* 89:896–901.

Steegmaier, M., Levinovitz A., Isenmann I., Borges E., Lenter M., Kocher H. P. Kleuser B. and Vestweber D. (1995). The E-selectin ligand ESL-1 is a variant of a receptor for fibroblast growth factor. *Nature* 373:615–620.

Tozeren, A., and Ley, K. (1992) How do selectins mediate leukocyte rolling in venules? *Biophys. J.* 63:700–709.

Tsuji, S. (1996) Molecular cloning and functional analysis of sialyltransferases. *J. Biochem.* 120:1–13.

Varki, A. (1997) Selectin ligands: will the real ones please stand up? *J. Clin. Invest.* 99:1–5.

von Andrian, U. H., Hasslen, S. R., Nelson, R. D. Erlandsen, S. L., and Butcher. E. C. (1995) A central role for microvillous receptor presentation in leukocyte adhesion under flow. *Cell* 82: 989–999.

Waddell, T. K., Fialkow, L. Chan, C. K. Kishimoto, T. K. and Downey, G. P. (1994) Potentiation of the oxidative burst of human neutrophils. A signaling role for L-selectin. *J. Biol. Chem.* 269:18485–18491.

Waddell, T. K., Fialkow, L. Chan, C. K. Kishimoto, T. K. and Downey, G. P., (1995) Signaling functions of L-selectin. Enhancement of tyrosine phosphorylation and activation of MAP kinase. *J. Biol. Chem.* 270:15403–15411.

Wagers, A. J., Stoolman, L. M. Kannagi, R. Craig, R. and Kansas, G. S. (1997) Expression of leukocyte fucosyltransferases regulates binding to E-selectin. Relationship to previously implicated carbohydrate epitopes. *J. Immunol.* 159:1917–1929.

Wagers, A. J., Waters, C. M. Stoolman, L. M. and Kansas G. S. (1998) IL-12 and IL-4 control T-cell adhesion to endothelial selectins through opposite effects on Fuc T-VII gene expression. *J. Exp. Med.* 188:2225–2231.

Walchek, B., Moore, K. L. McEver, R. P. and Kishimoto, T. K. (1996) Neutrophil–neutrophil interactions under hydrodynamic shear stress involve L-selectin and PSGL-1. *J. Clin. Invest.* 98:1081–1087.

Walz, G., Aruffo, A. Kolanus, W. Bevilacqua, M. and Seed, B. (1990) Recognition by ELAM-1 of the Sialyl-Le^x determinant on myeloid and tumor cells. *Science.* 250:1132–1134.

Watson, M. L., Kingsmore, S. F. Johnston, G. I. Siegelman, M. H. Le Beau M. M. Lemons, R. S. Bora, N. S. Howard, T. A. Weissman, I. L. McEver, R. P. and Seldin, M. F. (1990) Genomic organization of the selectin family of leukocyte adhesion molecules on human and mouse chromosome 1. *J. Exp. Med.* 172:263–272.

Weller, A., Isenmann, S. and Vestweber, D. (1992) Cloning of the mouse endothelial selectins: expression of both E- and P-selectin is inducible by TNF-α *J. Biol. Chem.* 267:15176–15183.

Weyrich, A. S. Elstad, M. R. McEver, R. P. McIntyre, T. M. Moore, K. L. Moorissey, J. M. (1995) Prescott, S. M. and Zimmerman, G. A. (1996) Activated platelets signal chemokine synthesis by human monocytes. *J. Clin. Invest.* 97:1525–1534.

Weyrich, A. S., McIntyre, T. M. McEver, R. P. Prescott, S. M. and Zimmerman, G. A. (1995) Monocyte tethering by P-selectin regulates monocyte chemotactic protein-1 and tumor necrosis factor-α secretion. Signal integration and NF-KB translocation. *J. Clin. Invest.* 95:2297–2303.

Yang, J., Hirata, T. Croce, K. Merrill-Sokoloff, G. Tchernychev, B. Williams, E. Flaumenhaft, R. Furie, B. C. and Furie, B. (1999) Targeted gene disruption demonstrates that PSGL-1 is required for P-selectin–mediated but not E-selectin–mediated neutrophil rolling and migration. *J. Exp. Med.* 190:1769–1782.

Yoshida, M., Westlin, W. F. Wang, N. Ingber, D. E. Rosenzweig, A. Resnick, N. and Gimbrone, M. A. (1996) Leukocyte adhesion to vascular endothelium induces E-selectin linkage to the actin cytoskeleton. *J. Cell. Biol.* 133:445–455.

Zhou, Q., Moore, K.L. Smith, D. F. Varki, A. McEver, R. P. and Cummings, R. D. (1991) The selectin GMP-140 binds to sialylated, fucosylated lactosaminoglycans on both myeloid and nonmyeloid cells. *J. Cell. Biol.* 115:557–564.

13

β$_2$ Integrins and Their Ligands in Inflammation

MICHAEL L. DUSTIN

The physiology of inflammatory reactions depends on the entry of leukocytes into tissues. Members of the leukocyte integrin family of adhesion molecules play an important role in this process. Integrins mediate firm adhesion and locomotion by interacting with ligands on cells and in tissues with a dependence on divalent cations (Springer, 1994). The term *integrin* reflects the hypothesis that these receptors form an integral membrane linkage between the cytoskeleton and the extracellular matrix (Tamkun et al., 1986). This is an important concept for leukocyte location because the linkage of extracellular matrix to cytoplasmic force generation is a central process in cell movement within tissues. Thus, cellular physiology plays an important role in the regulation of leukocyte integrins. The physiological importance of leukocyte integrins is illustrated by leukocyte adhesion deficiency-type 1 (LAD-1) (Springer et al., 1984; Anderson et al., 1995). In this disease the four members of the leukocyte integrin subfamily are decreased or absent on all leukocytes. The resulting defects in leukocyte entry into tissue sites leave patients highly susceptible to bacterial infections of the skin and mucous membranes. This chapter will relate the expression pattern, structure, and function of this adhesion receptor family to the process of inflammation and tissue repair.

Integrins are a large family of cell surface adhesion molecules that participate in all aspects of development from fertilization onward. Leukocyte integrins are a subset of the integrin family exclusively expressed on cells of the hematopoietic lineage. Integrins are noncovalent heterodimers of type 1 transmembrane glycoproteins. The integrin subfamilies are organized around particular subunits that are shared among multiple functional complexes. Figure 13.1 illustrates the current organization of integrins into the β$_1$, β$_2$, and α$_V$ subfamilies. All the leukocyte integrins share a common small subunit (β$_2$). There are at least four larger (α) subunits that can combine with the β$_2$ subunit to form unique receptors. The α and β subunits are expressed from different genes and thus can be independently expressed on different cell types. Table 13.1 identifies the subunits for the four character-

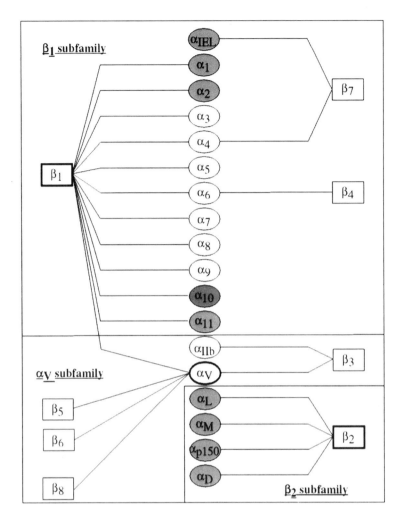

Fig. 13.1. The integrin family: The lines represent observed $\alpha\beta$ complexes. Initially the subfamilies were defined by β_1, β_2, and β_3, but the large number of complexes involving α_V have led to incorporation of the β_3 complexes in an α_V subfamily. Both the α and β subunits define ligand specificity. Shaded and subunits have "I" domains.

ized leukocyte integrins along with other useful statistics. Note that the β_2 subunit antibody epitopes define the CD18 cluster in the Leukocyte Differentiation Workshop nomenclature. The α-subunit epitopes are defined as CD11a, b, c, and d. The leukocyte integrins mediate adhesion by interacting with ligands in the extracellular matrix or the cell surface. The integrins' interaction with ligands is dependent on divalent cations and is regulated by leukocyte activation.

Table 13.1. Leukocyte Integrins, Their Ligands, and Distribution

Integrin	Integrin Distribution	Ligands	Ligand Distribution	Assays
$\alpha_L\beta_2$ CD11a/CD18, LFA-1 (180 kd/95 kd)	all leukocytes	ICAM-1 (95 kd) ICAM-2 (50 kd) ICAM-3 (120 kd) other ICAMs	endo*, epi*, leuk* endo resting leuk RBC, neuro	Leuk, aggregation coated plate $\alpha_L\beta_2$ coated plate IFN act. epi layer
$\alpha_M\beta_2$, CD11b/CD18, Mac-1 (170 kd/95 kd)	neutrophils, monocytes, macrophages eosinophils	C3bi Factor X Fibrinogen ICAM-1 (d3)	act. complement plasma leakage plasma leakage endo*, epi*, leuk*	C3bi coated RBC C3bi coated plate $\alpha_M\beta_2$ coated plate endo layer
$\alpha_x\beta_2$, CD11c/CD18, p150,95 (150 kd/95 kd)	resident macrophages, dendritic cells, some CD8 T cells	C3bi	act. complement	C3bi coated RBC C3bi coated plate
$\alpha_D\beta_2$, CD11d/CD18 (167 kd, 95 kd)	some tissue macro- phages foam cells, some CD8 T cells, IL-5 act eosinophil	ICAM-3 VCAM-1	resting leuk. endo*	ICAM-3 Fc flow, act. endo layer (VCAM-1)

Note. endo, endothelial cells; epi, epithelial cells; leuk, leukocytes;* (asterisk), activated cells; act., activated.
$\alpha_L\beta_2$ Interacts with ICAM immunoglobulin domain 1, $\alpha_M\beta_2$ interacts with ICAM-1 through domain 3 (d3). $\alpha_L\beta_2$ Interaction with ICAMs is the dominant adhesion mechanism for phorbol ester stimulated B lymphoblastoid cell aggregation. *Coated plate* is static adhesion assay of leukocyte adhesion to purified molecule coated plate; *flow* is flow cytometry. IFN-interfeon.

Leukocyte Activation

The following discussion of integrin activity will make frequent reference to resting and activated leukocytes. It is important to define this concept clearly. A resting leukocyte could be defined as a cell suspended in blood, or a cell that is carefully isolated from tissues. Resting leukocytes are nonmotile and display a round morphology with many small surface projections or micro-villi. The cortical cytoskeleton of these cells actively maintains this shape as the cells are propelled through the blood or are jostled in the hematopoietic or lymphoid tissues. Activation of a leukocyte is a broad concept that covers both transient and reversible processes in the developmental sequence of long-lived lymphocytes and macrophages, or can be the beginning of an irreversible process for cells like neutrophils and some dendritic cells. For these latter cells, the process of activation initiates a program of directed migration, differentiation, and death in 1 to 2 days. Activation results in a dramatic change in the cortical cytoskeleton that can begin with a transient increase in tension, but is rapidly followed by an increase in surface activity, irregular membrane projections, and acquisition of a more irregular or po-larized overall cell shape. Stimuli for this process in lymphocytes include a variety of diverse chemoattractants, chemokines, cytokines, antigens for B and T cells, and surfaces coated with complement products or immunoglobulins. The activity of integrins is closely linked to the cytoskeletal changes of leukocyte activation.

Expression of Leukocyte Integrins and Their Ligands

LFA-1 (α_L β_2; CD11a/CD18)

Lymphocyte function-associated antigen (LFA-1) is the most broadly expressed leukocyte integrin. It is expressed on early hemotopoietic progenitor cells and on all mature leukocytes. LFA-1 has only been found to interact with cell surface ligands known as intercellular adhesion molecules (ICAMs). ICAMs are type I transmembrane glyocoproteins and belong to the immunoglobulin superfamily. While LFA-1 is expressed on the surface of resting leukocytes, it is essentially inactive. The activation process results in a reversible increase in LFA-1 activity (Dustin and Springer, 1989). ICAM-1 is expressed on resting endothelium and is induced on many cell types of inflammatory cytokines (see Table 13.1 and Fig. 13.2). It is notable that ICAM-1 expression in epidermal keratinocytes of a transgenic mouse did not induce inflammation (Williams and Kupper, 1994). Thus, ICAM-1 expression does not induce inflammation, hence other factors are required. In vitro, ICAM-1 expression on epithelial cells is induced by interferon. ICAM-2 and ICAM-3 are mainly expressed on endothelial cells and leukocytes, respectively. As for activity, ICAM-1 is a more active LFA-1 ligand than ICAM-2 or ICAM-3 (de Fougerolles and Springer, 1991).

Mac-1 ($\alpha_M\beta_2$; CD11b/CD18)

(Mac)-1 is restricted to mature neutrophils, monocytes, and macrophages. Mac-1 interacts with a wider variety of ligands compared to LFA-1. Mac-1 is the receptor for the C3bi fragment of the third component of complement (Wright et al., 1983). This complement fragment forms covalent bonds to surfaces when triggered through immunoglobulin (classical complement pathway) or microbial surfaces (alternative complement pathway). Particles coated with C3bi are referred to as opsonized and are readily phagocytosed by neutrophils and macrophages. Mac-1 also interacts with a site in ICAM-1 distinct from the LFA-1 binding site and with provisional matrix proteins such as clotting factor X and fibrinogen (Diamond et al., 1991 and chapter 19). Mac-1 also participates in a number of adhesion reactions where the nature of the ligand is not known, such as adhesion of neutrophils and macrophages to plastic surfaces. Ligands for this type of adhesion may be secreted attachment factors from the leukocyte, although this is not clear. In addition to displaying regulated ligand binding on the cell surface, Mac-1 is stored in endosome-like vesicles in neutrophils that are translocated to the surface following certain types of activation allowing increased Mac-1 expression following activation of neutrophils and monocytes (Borregaard et al., 1987).

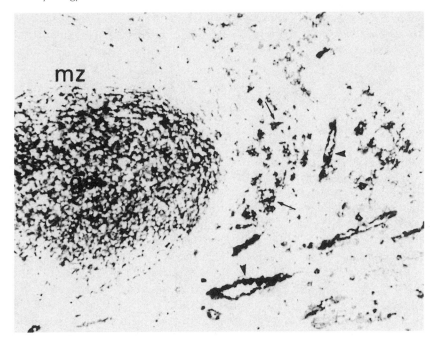

Fig. 13.2. ICAM-1 expression in inflammation: Immunoperoxidase staining of ICAM-1 expression in inflamed tonsil (Dustin et al., 1986). ICAM-1 expression is strong on cells in the mantle zone (mz) and germinal center (gc) of the follicle. ICAM-1 expression is also strong on endothelial cells (arrowhead) and dentritic cells in the T-cell areas (arrows). Although not shown here, ICAM-1 expression is also dramatically increased on epithelial cells in the skin, gut, and lungs in response to inflammation (Vejlsgaard et al., 1989; Parkos et al., 1996; Taguchi et al., 1998).

Mac-1, like LFA-1, is less active on resting cells than activated cells. Increases in Mac-1 expression further augment the activation-dependent increase in activity, but are not necessary to observe increased Mac-1 dependent adhesion. It has also been suggested that newly up-regulated Mac-1 is not competent to participate in adhesion unless the cell undergoes further stimulation, for example, by an incremental increase in chemoattractant concentration (Hughes et al., 1992). Finally, a scavanger receptor-like function of Mac-1 is suggested by the finding that Mac-1 can interact with a variety of denatured proteins (Davis, 1992).

P150,95 ($\alpha_x\beta_2$; CD11c/Cd18)

P150,95 is expressed on tissue macrophages, dendritic cells and some chronically activated lymphocytes. Like Mac-1, p150,95 is a receptor for the C3bi complement product. Beyond this, p150,95 biology is poorly understood because the cells that express it are not readily accessible. P150,95 is strongly expressed on hairy cell leukemia (Miller et al., 1987). It is possible that expression of p150,95 contributes to the localization of this malignancy to the spleen. Like Mac-1, p150,95 also interacts with a variety of denatured proteins (Davis, 1992).

$\alpha_D\beta_2$ (CD11d/Cd18)

The most recently defined member of the leukocyte integrin family is expressed on tissue macrophages and eosinophils and binds to ICAM-3 and vascular cell adhesion molecule-1 VCAM-1 (Van der Vieren et al., 1995; Grayson et al., 1998). $\alpha_D\beta_2$ interacts with ICAM-3 more avidly than does LFA-1; $\alpha_D\beta_2$ on eosinophils interacts with the inducible endothelial adhesion molecules VCAM-1. Thus, $\alpha_D\beta_2$ may contribute to recruitment of eosinophils to inflamed airways.

Other Leukocyte Integrins

Whereas β_2 integrins are only expressed on leukocytes, not all integrins on leukocytes are of the β_2 family (Hemler, 1990). Although Mac-1 and LFA-1 are the major integrins on neutrophils, neutrophils also express a small amount of $\alpha_V\beta_3$, a receptor for provisional matrix components like vitronectin, fibronectin, and fibrinogen. Neutrophils also express $\alpha_4\beta_1$ following activation, which may play an important role, with $\alpha_V\beta_3$, in neutrophil migration through tissues (Reinhardt et al., 1997). Provisional matrix components are defined as those molecules present only in special circumstances such as wounding or inflammation. In contrast, monocytes, eosinophils, and lymphocytes express several β_1 integrins including $\alpha_4\beta_1$ that interact with fibronectin and VCAM-1, an inflammation-induced endothelial cell ligand. Activated lymphocytes can express increased levels of other β_1 integrins including collagen or laminin receptors $\alpha_1\beta_1$, $\alpha_2\beta_1$, $\alpha_3\beta_1$, $\alpha_6\beta_1$ and the provisional matrix receptor, $\alpha_V\beta_3$. Understanding the array of integrins expressed by different leukocyte subtypes is important in understanding the pathology of leukocyte integrin deficiencies.

Structure of Leukocyte Integrins

α-Subunit

The α-subunits are large, approximately 1060 amino acids. The most prominent features of the α-subunits are a series of seven repeats interrupted by an inserted domain (I domain). The inserted domain has been independently expressed in a variety of expression systems. The LFA-1 and Mac-1 inserted domains retain the ability to interact with ligands. This interaction is generally weaker than that of the intact integrin. The LFA-1 and Mac-1 inserted domains are structurally homologous to enzymes and G-protein α-subunits that assume a dinucleotide fold as characterized by X-ray crystallography (Lee et al., 1995; Qu and Leahy, 1995). The integrin inserted domains contain a unique type of divalent cation binding site referred to as a *metal ion dependent adhesion site* (MIDAS), which may participate directly in ligand binding. The structure of the seven repeats has not been solved, but a highly credible model has been proposed (Springer, 1997). It has been determined by modeling that the repeats may form into a seven-bladed β-propeller structure similar to the heterotrimeric G-protein β-subunit. The β-propeller structure is predicted to have four divalent cation binding sites. Unlike the inserted domain, the seven repeats do not fold or maintain their native structure in the absence of the β-subunit. Based on the model, the inserted domain appears to sit on top of the β-propeller (Fig. 13.3). This organization is remarkably similar to the noncovalent interaction of the α- and β-subunits of heterotrimeric G-proteins. The sequence between the β-propeller and the transmembrane domain may constitute a stalk that is visible in electron micrographs of purified integrins (Carrell et al., 1985). The C-terminal half of the transmembrane domain and the membrane proximal segment of the cytoplasmic domain are highly conserved and appear to play an important

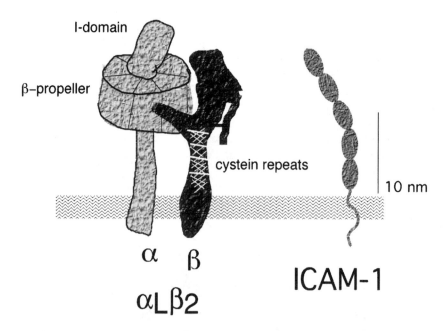

I-domain

β–propeller

cystein repeats

10 nm

α   β

αLβ2

ICAM-1

Fig. 13.3. Schematic structure of β_2 integrin and ICAM-1: A model for the relative position of the α-subunit inserted (I) domain and β-propeller domain in an intact integrin. The interaction of the β-subunit with the β-propeller is based on the interaction of the heterotrimeric G-protein γ- and β-subunits. Integrin and ICAM-1 size (scale bar) is based on electron microscopy. The only positively identified ligand-binding sites are in the I domain, the only component of the integrin that can fold independently. Mutagenic data also suggest a ligand-binding site in the β-subunit.

role in conformational changes that regulate affinity. The membrane distal segments of the short cytoplasmic domain are not conserved and may link different integrins to the cytoskeleton.

β-Subunit

Most of the β-subunits have approximately 769 amino acids. The pattern of cystein residues in the ectodomain is highly conserved. The cytoplasmic domains are also well conserved with differences corresponding to differential regulation. The folding of integrin β-subunits is not well understood. The amino-terminus of the β-subunit contains a highly conserved region that is implicated in ligand binding and is associated with the α-subunit. The highly conserved region does not assume its native structure in the absence of the α-subunit. Regions of the β-subunit may interact with the α-subunit β-propeller in a manner similar to interaction of heterotrimeric G-protein γ and β-subunits (Figure 13.3, Springer, 1997). This region also contains a series of functionally important amino acids with similarity to the MIDAS motif of the inserted domain; however, there is no compelling evidence that the highly conserved region is I-domain-like in other aspects (Goodman and Bajt, 1996). Many mutations in leukocyte-adhesion deficiency (LAD) patients cluster in the highly conserved regions and disrupt association of α- and β-subunits (Anderson et al., 1995). The dissociated subunits are not transported to the surface and are eventually degraded in the endoplasmic reticulum. Between the highly conserved region and the transmembrane domain there are four cysteine-rich repeats that may form part of a rigid stalk structure. The carboxy-terminal end of the transmembrane domain and the entire cytoplasmic domain are well conserved. This suggests that the β-subunit may mediate a conserved interaction of integrins with the cytoskeleton.

Function of Leukocyte Integrins

Adhesion molecules function in a manner that is integrated with cellular physiology and therefore has been refractory to biochemical analysis. Although enormous progress has been made in understanding structure–function relationships in integrins and their ligands, we are only beginning to appreciate the cellular mechanisms that regulate integrin function. Changes in integrin expression can be important in adjusting thresholds for adhesion, but this effect is superimposed on dominant mechanisms that act without altering receptor expression levels. An important concept that can be distilled from examining integrin regulation across the entire family of molecules is that the relatively rigid structural framework of integrins allows for a surprising adaptability to different physiological situations and demands. Thus, lessons learned from one integrin must be tested in other integrins to determine if or how they apply. Some key characteristics that allow this flexibility are described in the following, and a current working model that integrates these characteristics is presented.

Affinity Change

Inside-Out Signaling

Affinity change models are based on the platelet paradigm for integrin regulation. The integrin $\alpha_{IIb}\beta_3$ is a major platelet surface protein that binds fibrinogen on activated platelets, but not on resting platelets. The affinity of $\alpha_{IIb}\beta_3$ for fibrinogen is increased by at least 100-fold on activation (Ginsberg et al., 1993). The range of the affinity change is well matched to the physiological concentrations of fibrinogen to allow a switchlike response. This process of affinity change in response to signals within the cell has been referred to as inside-out signaling. Interaction of thrombin with its receptor on the platelet surface triggers signals in the cytoplasm that lead to assembly of an integrin-activating complex that induces a conformational change in $\alpha_{IIb}\beta_3$ to increase affinity. Because the biologically important ligands for β_2 integrins are typically presented on surfaces or in a three-dimensional matrix, rather than in solution-like fibrinogen, the physiological demands on β_2 integrins are different, and thus, they appear to emphasize a different type of regulation than the platelet integrin. The β_2 integrins that have been most closely studied are LFA-1 and Mac-1. LFA-1 and Mac-1 have a low affinity for soluble ICAM-1 and C3bi respectively, whether or not the cell is activated (Cai and Wright, 1995; Stewart et al., 1996; Ganpule et al., 1997). Thus, unlike platelet $\alpha_{IIb}\beta_3$, β_2 integrins do not display simple affinity regulation in response to activation, but nonetheless, their activity on the cell surface is rapidly increased.

Ligand-Induced Conformational Change

A distinct mode of affinity regulation is induced by ligand itself. Interestingly, this mode of regulation was also discovered during study of $\alpha_{IIb}\beta_3$ (Ginsberg et al., 1993). It was found that incubating the purified integrin with a ligand mimetic peptide actually increased the affinity of $\alpha_{IIb}\beta_3$ for fibrinogen. Subsequently, this general phenomenon was also demonstrated for LFA-1 interaction with ICAM-1 (Cabanas and Hogg, 1993). The mechanism of the ligand-induced conformational change is not known, but it appears to produce both a change in affinity and a change in the conformation of the transmembrane or cytoplasmic domain that can lead to cytoskeletal association (Felsenfeld et al., 1996). Thus, the ligand-induced change both increases affinity for ligand and produces an outside-in signal based on ligand binding. Whereas ligand-induced conformational change results in a high affinity conformation of the integrin, the net affinity observed when incubating cells with soluble ICAM-1 is low because the ligand must first interact with a low affinity form of the integrin to have a possibility to induce the high affinity conformation. The efficiency with which the high affinity form is generated is also low. When LFA-1 is saturated with soluble ICAM-1, only 20% of LFA-1 molecules are shifted to the high affinity conformation (Dustin, 1998).

Affinity and Divalent Cations

Integrin interactions are divalent cation-dependent. The physiological divalent cation milieu is approximately 1 mM each of $MgCl_2$ and $CaCl_2$. When the Ca^{2+} concentration is decreased below 1 μM with a calcium chelator in the presence of 1 mM $MgCl_2$ the affinity of many LFA-1 molecules to ICAM-1 is dramatically increased (Stewart et al., 1996; Ganpule et al., 1997). Similarly, 200 μM Mn^{2+} can induce a high affinity form of many integrins. Although these experiments have offered some structural insights into how cation binding sites in integrins relate to various integrin conformations, they have not provided insight into physiological regulation because these conditions are not likely to be encountered in vivo.

The Importance of Affinity in Cell Adhesion Systems

What is the significance of affinity in the contact area between two cells? It is possible to determine or estimate the solution affinity of integrins for their ligands in both the low and high affinity conformations. For example, the low affinity form of LFA-1 binds ICAM-1 with a Kd nearly equal to 100 μM, whereas the high affinity form has a Kd nearly equal to 100 nM, a 1000-fold difference (Knorr and Dustin, 1997; Dustin, 1998; Labadia et al., 1998). This is the most dramatic difference for any integrin; a more typical difference is on the order of 10- to 100-fold between low and high affinity forms. The Kd for a bimolecular interaction is the product of the concentrations of the free receptor and ligand divided by the concentration of the complex. A lower Kd corresponds to a higher affinity. Two-dimensional interaction can be predicted from the solution Kd if the lateral mobility of receptor and ligands and confinement length, defined as the height of the space in which the adhesion molecules encounter each other, is known (Bell et al., 1984). Direct measurements of receptor–ligand interactions in contact areas has revealed that low affinity interactions with solution Kd of 1–10 μM can align interacting membranes to within a confinement length of 5 nm, resulting in a highly efficient interaction in the contact area (Dustin et al., 1997). This effect begins to degrade for interactions with lower affinity (Kd > 50 μM). Therefore, the low affinity interaction of LFA-1 would not be able to create an effective adhesion domain on its own, whereas the high affinity form would be very effective at aligning apposed membranes and creating adhesive domains.

Cytoskeletal Control: Dual Role of the Actin Cytoskeleton

Lateral Mobility

Receptor-ligand interactions can be broken into two steps: The reactants must encounter one another in the first step, and then react in the second step. Interactions in solution are reaction limited, meaning that diffusion results in many encounters, it is the reaction following encounter that is rate limiting. In contrast, interactions in cell–cell interfaces may be diffusion limited, meaning that the encounter of receptor and ligand is rate limiting. Thus, regulation of lateral mobility of adhesion molecules may have a large effect on interactions. It has been shown that LFA-1 is largely immobile on the surface of resting lymphocytes, but that activation results in increased LFA-1 mobility that correlates with increased adhesion (Kucik et al., 1996). These studies led to the hypothesis that the low activity of LFA-1 was actively maintained in the resting cell by linking LFA-1 to the cytoskeleton of the resting lymphocyte. The actin-disrupting drug cytochalasin D was used to test this hypothesis. Low concentrations of cytochalasin D increased LFA-1 mobility and increased adhesion as predicted by the hypothesis. However, when the cytochalasin D concentration was further increased, the adhesion-activating effect was lost. These results suggest a dual role for the actin cytoskeleton (Kucik et al., 1996; Lub et al., 1997; Yauch et al., 1997). Actin filaments are involved in many structures within the cell. Actin filaments participate in active suppression of LFA-1 activity, but different populations of actin filaments are also required for strong adhesion. Actin usually does not interact directly with membrane proteins, rather the actin filaments are linked to adhesion molecules by linker molecules. The linker molecules responsible for the suppression of LFA-1 diffusion in resting cells are not known.

Stabilization of Adhesion

As demonstrated previously, the actin cytoskeleton plays an important positive role in integrin-mediated adhesion. The paradigm for stabilization of adhesion by the actin cytoskeleton is actin-mediated clustering of the engaged integrins (van Kooyk et al., 1994). Clustering increases the peak force needed to disrupt adhesion molecule interactions and thus increases the effective strength. The archetype for this process is the focal adhesion of fibroblasts. These structures contain multiple proteins that link actin bundles to integrin cytoplasmic domains including α-actinin, vinculin, and talin (Burridge and Chrzanowska-Wodnicka, 1996). Focal adhesions are enriched in kinases and phosphatases, suggesting an important role of signaling pathways in adhesion formation. There is evidence that LFA-1 clusters at the cell surface are important for regulation of adhesion. Although lymphocytes do not form focal adhesions, the focal adhesion component talin is localized to sites of LFA-1 engagement in T-cell contacts. Talin may act as a linker between LFA-1 and actin following ligand engagement.

Integrating Affinity Regulation and Cytoskeletal Controls

We can integrate all the elements of LFA-1 regulation described previously in a working model (Dustin, 1998). Unlike the platelet-integrin regulation where avid binding of ligand is accomplished in one inside-out signaling step, this model requires multiple steps with bidirectional communication across the plasma membrane (Fig. 13.4). The resting state is characterized by laterally immobile, low affinity LFA-1.

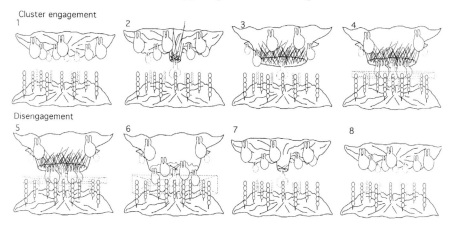

Fig. 13.4. Multistep model for leukocyte integrin engagement and disengagement (LFA-1 molecules are indicated in two forms—low affinity as two-legged lollipop and high affinity as two-legged lollipop with deep notch): (1) laterally mobile integrins and ligands in apposed membrane patches; (2) engagement and ligand-induced conformational change (conformational change takes place in 20% of encounters); (3) cytoskeletal response to ligand-induced conformational change induces local molding of the membrane/cytoskeleton to the substrate; (4) low affinity integrins are recruited into cluster due to membrane alignment (box); (the aligned domains act by increasing the effective concentration of ICAM-1 and LFA-1 proximal to the initial high affinity interaction); (5) stable cluster to be disengaged; (6) cytoskeletal change relaxes alignment of apposed membranes (larger box) and low affinity integrin–ligand interactions are lost; (7) the isolated high affinity interaction is broken within bond lifetime (~30 seconds); and (8) detachment is complete.

1. Activation results in increased lateral mobility of low affinity LFA-1 leading to more encounters with ligand.
2. Twenty percent of the resulting low affinity interactions can be converted to high affinity interactions. One important property of the high affinity interaction is that it is much longer-lived than the low affinity interaction (30 seconds vs. less than 1 second); this allows time for a cellular response to LFA-1 engagement.
3. The high affinity conformation is recognized by unknown cytoplasmic proteins to produce a direct linkage to the cytoskeleton or local signals that organize the cytoskeleton.
4. Local actin remodeling at the site of initial LFA-1 engagement promotes cell spreading onto the ligand-bearing surface to promote precise membrane alignment.

Thus, this pioneer high affinity interaction acts as a nucleus for cytoskeletal remodeling, and the resulting membrane alignment allows recruitment of many low affinity LFA-1/ICAM-1 interactions to the site of initial LFA-1 engagement. If more than four low affinity interactions are recruited, the cluster becomes self-perpetuating in that new high affinity interactions will be generated (with 20% efficiency) to replace the first high affinity interaction once its finite lifetime is over. This structure is dependent on a constant cytoskeletal contribution to membrane alignment to keep the low affinity interactions in the cluster, such that the clusters can be rapidly dissolved in response to changes in cytoskeletal organization.

The global organization of the actin cytoskeleton then regulates the outcome of integrin engagement. In migrating cells, the actin cytoskeleton is transported rearward, and when linked to stationary substrate attachments, propels the cell forward. In this case the engaged integrins accumulate toward the rear of the trailing edge of the moving cell's contact with the substrate. A distinct organization of the actin cytoskeleton is observed during antigen-receptor stimulated cell–cell interaction, in which the actin movement is toward a central point in the stationary junction, and engaged integrins accumulate near the center of the contact. This is the organization of the "immunological synapse" observed in antigen-specific T-cell interactions with antigen-presenting cells (Monks et al., 1998; Wülfing and Davis, 1998; Grakoui et al., 1999). This model for leukocyte integrin regulation is testable, but only by experimentation in the context of intact cells where the cellular physiology behind this process is retained.

Outside-In Signaling

It is widely believed that integrins play an important role in control of cell differentiation, proliferation, and death through processes on outside-in signaling. A number of potential signaling modes and specific biochemical pathways have been identified. The most generalized signaling mode is addressed by the tensegrity models (Ingber, 1997). The biochemical effectors of mechanotransduction in the tensegrity model are not known, but may include the cytoskeletal regulation of low molecular weight G-proteins (Nobes and Hall, 1995). It has also been demonstrated that integrins regulate the duration of signals generated by growth factor receptors (Miyamoto et al., 1996). There is a current notion that an integrin-based scaffolding for T-cell interactions with antigen-presenting cells (the immunological synapse) may play an important role in sustaining T-cell receptor signals (Grakoui et al., 1999). Integrins have also been implicated in control of cell survival, possibly by a signaling pathway involving oxygen free radicals (Coxon et al., 1996).

Physiology of Leukocyte Integrins and Their Ligands

Leukocyte integrins contribute to leukocyte localization and thus host defense. On the other hand, pathological situations develop when leukocytes mediate tissue damage, and in these situations the blockade of leukocyte integrins becomes therapeutic.

The Role of Leukocyte Integrins in Host Defense

Leukocyte Adhesion Deficiency Type-1 (LAD-1)

Leukocyte adhesion deficiency is the result of genetic lesions in the β_2-subunit that lead to failure to express the β_2-subunit protein or in a mutated form of β_2 that cannot associate with the α-subunits (Anderson et al., 1995). Thus, all four leukocyte integrins are absent or reduced on all cells in LAD-1. Individuals who are heterozygous for defective β_2 genes are normal, but individuals homozygous for defective β_2 genes suffer from recurrent and life-threatening bacterial infections of the mucous membranes and skin. There is a marked absence of pus formation that reflects the near total absence of neutrophil recruitment to wound sites despite the presence of bacteria, but there are high levels of circulating neutrophils. Other chapters in this book describe the multistep paradigm for leukocyte interactions with endothelial cells involving selectin-mediated rolling adhesion, recognition of an activating stimulus while rolling, and integrin-mediated arrest. Rolling adhesion is normal in LAD-1 patients, but the integrin-dependent arrest is completely abrogated. Thus, neutrophils are completely dependent on β_2 integrins for entry into skin and some mucous membrane sites. In contrast, entry of leukocytes into the peritoneal cavity is relatively normal in the mouse model for LAD-1.

Lymphocytes and monocytes express a β_1 integrin, $\alpha_4\beta_1$, that interacts with the endothelial cell ligand VCAM-1. This interaction appears to compensate partly for loss of β_2 intgrins in these cells. The cellular immune response to viruses and responses to active immunizations are within the normal range in LAD-1 patients. However, if untreated, the disease is usually fatal in childhood, so the long-term effects of decreased β_2 integrin in humans are not known. The only effective treatment at this time is bone marrow transplantation (Le Deist et al., 1989; Fischer et al., 1991). Interestingly, human leukocyte antigen (HLA)-mismatched transplants are more successful in LAD-1 patients than in individuals with a normal immune system, thus some reduction in alloreactivity may exist due to absence of LFA-1 on lymphocytes or β_2 integrins on host antigen-presenting cells.

Role of LFA-1 in Tumor Immunity

A potential role of LFA-1 in the response to immunogenic tumors was revealed in studies with LFA-1 knockout mice (Schmits et al., 1996). Lymphocytes from LFA-1–deficient mice show striking deficits in responses to mitogens and model antigens. There is also a striking reduction in adhesion between T cells and antigen-presenting cells. These results are consistent with early in vitro studies on human and mouse lymphocytes that demonstrated a major role for LFA-1 in stable adhesion between T cells and antigen-presenting cells. LFA-1 mutant mice were bred with T-cell receptor transgenic mice, a model that allows the sensitivity to antigens to be dissected in great detail. It was found that mice lacking LFA-1 were 10-fold less sensitive to antigen in vivo and in vitro (Bachmann et al., 1997). Thus, LFA-1 appears to promote the ability of T cells to respond to small amounts of antigen, but is not essential for in vivo antiviral responses where antigens are abundant in infected cells. A striking phenotype of the LFA-1 mutant mice was the inability to clear immunogenic tumors. Thus, LFA-1 may play an important role in tumor immunity. It is possible that the tumor antigen in the model examined was of lower abundance than the viral antigen, or that the tumor immune response places greater demands on lymphocyte adhesion.

The Role of Leukocyte Integrins in Inflammatory Tissue Damage

Reperfusion Injury

Ischemia (lack of blood flow to the tissue) and reperfusion result in endothelial cell activation and massive neutrophil recruitment. Whereas leukocytes are essential for healing, this initial recruitment can lead to exacerbation of the immediate damage and to expansion of the damaged areas and destruction of the microcirculation, leading to necrosis (Hernandez et al., 1987). Striking examples of this are seen in animal models where an area is made ischemic and then allowed to undergo reperfusion in the absence or presence of function-blocking antiβ_2 antibodies (Vedder et al., 1990). In the absence of the antibodies, the affected tissue becomes necrotic and nonfunctional. The presence of the antibodies at the time of reperfusion can result in complete protection and recovery of the tissues. The essential role of leukocytes in the tissue repair process argues that the single-dose administration of the anti-β_2 antibody does not completely inhibit leukocyte entry over an extended period, but blunts the acute, massive leukocyte adhesion to the reperfused vasculature. Thus, judicious inhibition of leukocyte recruitment can clearly improve long-term tissue healing following certain types of injury.

Endotoxin Shock

Endotoxin shock is an animal model for some forms of acute sepsis. In this model, the injection of endotoxin results in a systemic activation of leukocytes. Pathology is mostly focused in the liver, which can lose function with fatal consequences. Neutrophils that enter the liver form clusters that may have a role in focal damage. Mice that are genetically deficient in ICAM-1 are resistant to endotoxin shock (Xu et al., 1994). Whereas the same number of neutrophils are observed in the liver, the cells do not form clusters and the hepatotoxicity is not as severe. Thus, β_2 integrins and their ligands may have roles in both leukocyte recruitment and cell–cell interactions within tissues that have an impact on pathology.

Motheaten Mice: A Case of Leukocyte Integrin Hyperactivity?

Motheaten and the motheaten viable mice have mutations in the tyrosine phosphatase SHP-1 (Shultz et al., 1993). This mutation causes an inflammatory disease characterized by chronic leukocyte infiltration of the skin and lungs. A hypothesis for the motheaten pathology has been proposed based on defects in adhesion (Roach et al., 1998). In leukocytes the src family kinases lyn and hck form a complex that maintains activity of phosphatidyl inositol 3-kinase. The products of the latter enzyme are required for integrin activity, possibly due to their role in recruiting molecules with pleckstrin homology domains. The activity of this protein-kinase/lipid-kinase complex is counteracted by SHP-1. Thus, mutations in SHP-1 block an important regulatory circuit that sets the basal activity level for integrins. Hyperactive integrins may then act in several ways to perpetuate inflammation. First, integrin engagement may keep leukocytes from exiting tissues. Second, integrin engagement may amplify cytokine signals, making leukocytes more sensitive to pro-inflammatory cytokines. Third, more active integrins may induce leukocyte aggregation that may also amplify local pro-inflammatory circuits. This hypothesis proposes an important role for integrin regulation in the control of physiological inflammatory processes. Importantly, the motheaten mouse pathology is alleviated by early administration of inhibitory anti-α_M (CD11b) antibodies (Koo et al., 1993). These antibodies may act to keep the leukocytes out of the tissues, and also may act to suppress pro-inflammatory interactions within the tissues. The motheaten mouse is an important model for chronic inflammation.

Methods Used to Study Leukocyte Integrins

Adhesion Assays

Cell adhesion assays are as diverse as the adhesion molecules and biological situations that the assays are designed to study. Table 13.1 includes information on assays that have been to used to measure the activity of leukocyte integrins. There are two general types of experiments, those that examine interactions of leukocytes with cells of biological interest, for example, endothelial cells, or with a complex extracellular matrix of biological origin. These experiments typically involve many adhesion mechanisms operating in parallel and are usually designed to describe what mechanisms are used, or to test a hypothesis about the use of a particular mechanism. These experiments frequently derive specificity from use of adhesion-blocking monoclonal antibodies or from genetic manipulations. The other major class of adhesion experiments are those that isolate a particular interaction. There are some cell–cell adhesion models dominated by one adhesion mechanism, but more frequently, this type of isolation is accomplished by attaching a single purified or recombinant ligand to a solid phase and testing cell adhesion to the substrate. Specificity in these systems must also be established on a case-by-case basis using blocking monoclonal antibodies or genetically altered cells because multiple cell surface receptors may interact with the same purified or recombinant ligands. Once specificity is established, these assays are excellent for studying regulation of a single adhesion mechanism. As a note, the latter type of assay can be difficult to establish for neutrophils and monocytes as these cells can attach to plastic that has been coated with seemingly irrelevant proteins. Thus, studies with neutrophils and monocytes will often examine adhesion to treated surfaces that are β_2-integrin–dependent, but for which the ligands are unknown. This is a decided disadvantage for quantitative study of cell adhesion. Recently, it has also been possible to examine adhesion in vivo as described in detail in Chapter 16.

Molecular Interaction Assays

Adhesion assays necessarily measure avidity, and typically are not used to measure affinity. Even when two-dimensional affinity values are obtained from adhesion experiments, it is always useful to have a solution affinity value for comparison.

Interactions of Purified Molecules

The most important methods in current use are surface plasmon resonance (SPR) and differential scanning calorimetry (DSC). These methods supply important information about real-time kinetics, equilibrium affinity, and enthalpy. Together, these methods allow a complete analysis of the interaction of soluble purified molecules. There are two technical hurdles. First, it must be possible to purify the molecules in a native state. Second, many adhesion molecule interactions have such low affinities that they are marginal even for these sensitive methods. The first issue is particularly significant for integrins that are large complex molecules that are readily denatured. For example, purified $\alpha_L\beta_2$ is locked in the high affinity state, and efforts to isolate the low affinity form have only been partially successful. Purified $\alpha_M\beta_2$, in contrast, can be isolated in low and high affinity forms. This is an empirical issue and is most related to the reagents available for purification of a particular integrin. SPR and DSC methods provide limited capacity for screening many conditions because each measurement is time consuming. Enzyme-linked or radioligand-binding assays have been developed for high affinity forms of LFA-1. These assays lack the quantitative rigor of SPR and DSC, but, in principle, are more amenable to high throughput screening.

Interactions with Intact Cells

Whereas experiments that measure interaction of soluble ligands with intact cells are less accurate than those with purified molecules and usually do not allow examination of real-time interactions, they are often important because the integrin can be left in its natural environment. Usually, soluble adhesion molecule interactions are of too low affinity to result in stable binding. Dimeric forms of ICAM-1 bind to cells expressing high affinity $\alpha_L\beta_2$ that is generated through nonphysiological cation manipulations as detected by flow cytometry. However, no interaction of ICAM-1 dimers with cells is detected in flow cytometry assays under physiological activating conditions. Lower affinity interactions with faster off-rates can be directly measured by performing radioligand-binding assays with separation of bound and free ligand by centrifugation through an oil cushion. This method readily allows measurements of interactions in the 1–10 µM Kd range, but has not been successful with low affinity $\alpha_L\beta_2$ with a Kd nearly equal to 100 µM. An even more sensitive approach is to examine the competition between the low affinity ligand and a higher affinity labeled Fab that binds stably. The Fab (fragment, antigen-binding) is added at a concentration equivalent to its Kd (typically about 10 nM), while the unlabeled competitor is added at a range of concentrations up to two times its own Kd. The point at which the unlabeled competitor decreases the binding of the labeled Fab fragment by 50% (IC_{50}) is then determined and can be used to calculate the Kd of the competitor by using the equation: Kd (competitor) = $IC_{50} \div [1 + ($concentration of the Fab$) \div$ Kd (Fab)] (Cheng and Prusoff, 1973). This approach allows an estimate of the Kd for low affinity $\alpha_L\beta_2$ and the isolated inserted domain (Lollo et al., 1993; Knorr and Dustin, 1997). However, it is dependent on the assumption of direct competitive inhibition between the Fab and biological ligand that has not been proven for any anti-integrin antibodies. It is just as likely that blocking anti-integrin antibodies work by allosteric mechanisms (induced conformational changes). In a system where direct competition can be proven, this approach should be accurate.

Summary

Leukocyte integrins play an important role in the recruitment of leukocytes to tissues. Ligands for leukocyte integrins are present or up-regulated at sites of tissue injury or inflammation. The cellular mechanisms by which leukocyte intgrins are regulated are poorly understood, but are likely to be closely linked to cytoskeletal regulation. The strongest evidence for the physiological role of leukocyte integrins is the immunodeficiency disease LAD-1. In LAD-1 the acute response of neutrophil infiltration is profoundly defective. However, leukocyte integrins may also play important roles in adaptive immunity including the antitumor response. Excessive integrin activation (leukocyte activation) plays a role in tissue injury in acute and chronic inflammation.

I thank C. Spencer for assisting with research for this chapter. I would also like to thank B. Tillman and R. L. White for critically reading the chapter.

References

Anderson, D. C., Kishimoto, T. K., and Smith, C. W. (1995) Leukocyte adhesion deficiency and other disorders of leukocyte adherence and motility. In: *The Metabolic and Molecular Basis of Inherited Disease.* C. R. Scriver, A. L. Beaudet, W. S. Sly, and D. Valle, eds. New York: McGraw-Hill, pp. 3955–3994.

Bachmann, M. F., McKall-Faienza, K., Schmits, R., Bouchard, D., Beach, J., Speiser, D. E., Mak, T. W., and Ohashi, P. S. (1997) Distinct roles for LFA-1 and CD28 during activation of naive T cells: adhesion versus costimulation. *Immunity* 7:549–557.

Bell, G. I., Dembo, M., and Bongrand, P. (1984) Cell adhesion: Competition between nonspecific repulsion and specific binding. *Biophys J.* 45:1051–1064.

Borregaard, N., Miller, L. J., and Springer, T. A. (1987) Chemoattractant-regulated fusion of a novel, mobilizable intracellular compartment with the plasma membrane in human neutrophils. *Science* 237:1204–1206.

Burridge, K., and Chrzanowska-Wodnicka, M. (1996) Focal adhesions, contractility, and signaling. *Annu. Rev. Cell. Dev. Biol.* 12:463–518.

Cabanas, C., and Hogg, N. (1993) Ligand intercellular adhesion molecule I has a necessary role in activation of integrin lymphocyte function associated molecule 1. *Proc. Natl. Acad. Sci. USA* 90:5838–5842.

Cai, T. Q., and Wright, S. D. (1995) Energetic of leukocyte integrin activation. *J. Biol. Chem.* 270: 14358–14365.

Carrell, N. A., Fitzgerald, L. A., Steiner, B., Erickson, H. P., and Phillips, D. R. (1985) Structure of human platelet membrane glycoproteins IIb and IIIa as determined by electron microscopy. *J. Biol. Chem.* 260:1743–1749.

Cheng, Y. C., and Prusoff, W. H. (1973) Relationship between the inhibition constant (Ki) and the concentration of inhibitor which causes 50 per cent inhibition (I50) of an enzymatic reaction. *Biochem. Pharmaco.* 22:3099–3108.

Coxon, A., Rieu, P., Barkalow, F. J., Askari, S., Sharpe, A. H., von Andrian, U. H., Arnaout, M. A., and Mayadas, T. N. (1996) A novel role for the beta 2 integrin CDIIb/CD18 in neutrophil apoptosis: a homeostatic mechanism in inflammation. *Immunity* 5:653–666.

Davis, G. E. (1992) The Mac-1 and p150,95 beta 2 integrins bind denatured proteins to mediate leukocyte cell-substrate adhesion. *Exp. Cell. Res.* 200:242–252.

de Fougerolles, A. R., and Springer, T. A. (1991) ICAM-3, a third adhesion counter-receptor for LFA-1 on resting lymphocytes. *J. Exp. Med.* 175:185–195.

Diamond, M. S., Staunton, D. E., Marlin, S. D., and Springer, T. A. (1991) Binding of the integrin Mac-1 (CD11b/CD18) to the third immunoglobulin-like domain of ICAM-1 (CD54) and its regulation by glycosylation. *Cell* 65:961–971.

Dustin, M. L., Rothlein, R., Bhan, A. K., Dinarello, C. A., and Springer, T. A. (1986) Induction by IL-1 and interferon, tissue distribution, biochemistry, and function of a natural adherence molecule (ICAM-1). *J. Immuno.* 137:245–254.

Dustin, M. L., and Springer, T. A. (1989) T-cell receptor cross-linking transiently stimulates adhesiveness through LFA-1. *Nature* 341:619–624.

Dustin, M. L., Golan, D. E., Zhu, D. M., Miller, J. M., Meier, W., Davies, E. A., and van der Merwe, P. A. (1997) Low affinity interaction of human or rat T-cell adhesion molecule CD2 with its ligand aligns adhering membranes to achieve high physiological affinity. *J. Biol. Chem.* 272: 30889–30898.

Dustin, M. L. (1998) Making a little affinity go a long way: a topological view of LFA-1 regulation. *Cell. Adhes. Commun.* 6:255–262.

Dustin, M. L. and Shaw, A. S. (1999). Costimulation: building an immunological synapse. *Science* 283:649–650.

Felsenfeld, D. P., Choquet, D., and Sheetz, M. P. (1996) Lingand binding regulates the directed movement of betal integrins on fibroblasts. *Nature* 383:438–440.

Fischer, A., Friedrich, W., Fasth, A., Le Deist, F., Girault, D., Veber, F., Vossen, J., Lopez, M., Griscelli, C., and Hirn, M. (1991) Reduction of graft failure by a monoclonal antibody (anti–LFA-1 CD11a) after HLA nonindentical bone marrow transplantation in children with immunodeficiencies, osteopetrosis, and Fanconi's anemia (a European Group for Immunodeficiency/European Group for Bone Marrow Translation Report). *Blood* 77:249–256.

Ganpule, G., Knorr, R., Miller, J. M., Carron, C. P., and Dustin, M. L. (1997) Low affinity of cell surface LFA-1 generates selectivity for cell–cell interactions. *J. Immunol.* 159:2685–2692.

Ginsberg, M. H., Xiaoping, D., O'Toole, T. E., Loftus, J. C., and Plow, E. F. (1993) Platelet integrins. *Thrombo. Haemost.* 70:87–93.

Goodman, T. G., and Bajt, M. L. (1996) Identifying the putative metal ion-dependent adhesion site in the β_2 (CD18) subunit required for $\alpha_L\beta_2$ and $\alpha_M\beta_2$ ligand interactions. *J. Biol. Chem.* 271:23729–23736.

Grakoui, A., Bromley, S. K., Sumen, C., Davis, M. M., Shaw, A. S., Allen, P. M., and Dustin, M. L. (1999) The immunological synapse: A molecular machine controlling T-cell activation. *Science* 285:221–227.

Grayson, M. H., Van der Vieren, M., Sterbinsky, S. A., Michael Gallatin, W., Hoffman, P. A., Staunton, D. E., and Bochner, B. S. (1998) Alpha d beta 2 integrin is expressed on human eosinophils and functions as an alternative ligand for vascular cell adhesion molecule 1 (VCAM-1). *J. Exp. Med.* 188:2187–2191.

Hemler, M. E. (1990) VLA proteins in the integrin family: Structures, functions, and their role on leukocytes. *Ann. Rev. Immunol.* 8:365–400.

Hernandez, L. A., Grishma, M. B., Twohig, B., Arfors, K. E., Harlan, J. M., and Granger, D. N. (1987) Role of neutrophils in ischemia-reperfusion-induced microvascular injury. *Am. J. Physiol.* 253:H669–H703.

Hughes, B. J., Hollers, J. C., Crockett-Torabi, E., and Smith, C. W. (1992) Recruitment of CD11b/CD18 to the neutrophil surface and adherence-dependent cell locomotion. *J. Clin. Invest.* 90: 1687–1696.

Ingber, D. E. (1997) Tensegrity: the architectural basis of cellular mechanotransduction. *Ann. Rev. Physiol.* 59:575–599.

Knorr, R., and Dustin, M. L. (1997) The LFA-1 I domain is a transient binding module for ICAM-1 and ICAM-3 in hydrodynamic flow. *J. Exp. Med.* 186:719–730.

Koo, G. C., Rosen, H., Sirotina, A., Ma, X. D., and Shultz, L. D. (1993) Anti-CD11b antibody prevents immunopathologic changes in viable moth-eaten bone marrow chimeric mice. *J. Immunol.* 151:6733–6741.

Kucik, D. F., Dustin, M. L., Miller, J. M., and Brown, E. J. (1996) Adhesion activating phorbol ester increases the mobility of leukocyte integrin LFA-1 in cultured lymphocytes. *J. Clin. Invest.* 97:2139–2144.

Labadia, M. E., Jeanfavre, D. D., Caviness, G. O., and Morelock, M. M. (1998) Molecular regulation of the interaction between leukocyte function-associated antigen-1 and soluble ICAM-1 by divalent metal cations. *J. Immunol.* 161:836–842.

Le Deist, F., Blanche, S., Keable, H., Gaud, C., Pham, H., Descamp-Latscha, B., Wahn, V., Griscelli, C., and Fischer, A. (1989) Successful HLA non-identical bone marrow transplantation in three patients with the leukocyte adhesion deficiency. *Blood* 74:512–516.

Lee, J. O., Rieu, P., Arnaout, M. A., and Liddington, R. (1995) Crystal structure of the A domain from the alpha subunit of integrin CR3 (CD11b/CD18). *Cell* 80:631–638.

Lollo, B. A., Chan, K.W.H., Hanson, E. M., Moy, V. T., and Brian, A. A. (1993) Direct evidence for two affinity states for lymphocyte function-associated antigen-1 on activated T cells. *J. Biol. Chem.* 268:21693–21700.

Lub, M., van Kooyk, Y., van Vliet, S. J., and Figdor, C. G. (1997) Dual role of the action cytoskeleton in regulating cell adhesion mediated by the integrin lymphocyte function associated antigen-1. *Mol. Biol. Cell* 8:341–351.

Miller, L. J., Weibe, M., and Springer, T. A. (1987) Purification and alpha subunit N-terminal sequences of human Mac-1 and p150,95 leukocyte adhesion proteins. *J. Immunol.* 138:2381–2383.

Miyamoto, S., Teramoto, H., Silvio, G., and Yamada, K. M. (1996) Integrins can collaborate with growth factors for phosphoryltion of receptor tyrosine kinases and MAP kinase activation: roles of integrin aggregation and occupancy of receptors. *J. Cell Biol.* 135:1633–1642.

Monks, C. R., Freiberg, B. A., Kupfer, H., Sciaky, N., and Kupfer, A. (1998) Three-dimensional segregation of supramolecular activation clusters in T cells. *Nature* 395:82–86.

Nobes, C. D., and Hall, A. (1995) Rho, Rac, and Cdc42 GTPases regulate the assembly of multimolecular focal complexes associated with actin stress fibers, lamellipodia, and filipodia. *Cell* 81:53–62.

Parkos, C. A., Colgan, S. P., Diamond, M. S., Nusrat, A., Liang, T. W., Springer, T. A., and Madara, J. L. (1996) Expression and polarization of intercellular adhesion molecule-1 on human intestinal epithelia: consequences for CD11b/CD 18-mediated interactions with neutrophils. *Mol. Med.* 2:489–505.

Qu, A., and Leahy, D. J. (1995) Crystal structure of the I-domain from the CD11a/CD 18 (LFA-1,alphaLbeta2) integrin. *Proc. Natl. Acad. Sci. USA* 92:10277–10281.

Reinhardt, P. H., Elliott, J. F., and Kubes, P. (1997) Neutrophils can adhere via alpha4beta1-integrin under flow conditions. *Blood* 89:3837–3846.

Roach, T. I., Slater, S. E., White, L. S., Zhang, X., Majerus, P. W., Brown, E. J., and Thomas, M. L. (1998) The protein tyrosine phosphatase SHP-1 regulates integrin-mediated adhesion of macrophages. *Curr. Biol.* 8:1035–1038.

Schmits, R., Kündig, T. M., Baker, D. M., Shumaker, G., Simard, J.J.L., van der Heiden, A., Bachmann, M. F., Ohashi, P. S., Mak, T. W., and Hickstein, D. D. (1996) LFA-1-deficient mice show normal CTL responses to virus but fail to reject immunogenic tumor. *J. Exp. Med.* 183:1415–1426.

Shultz, L. D., Schweitzer, P. A., Rajan, T. V., Taolin, Y., Ihle, J. N., Matthews, R. J., Thomas, M. L., and Beier, D. R. (1993) Mutations at the murine motheaten locus are within the hematopoietic cell protein-tyrosine phosphatase (Hcph) gene. *Cell* 73:1445–1454.

Springer, T. A., Thompson, W. S., Miller, L. J., Schmalstieg, F. C., and Anderson, D. C. (1984) Inherited deficiency of the Mac-1, LFA-1, pl50,95 glycoprotein family and its molecular basis. *J. Exp. Med.* 160:1901–1918.

Springer, T. A. (1994) Traffic signals for lymphocyte recirculation and leukocyte emigration: the multistep paradigm. *Cell* 76:301–314.

Springer, T. A. (1997) Folding of the N-terminal, ligand-binding region of integrin alpha-subunits into a beta-propeller domain. *Proc. Natl. Acad. Sci. USA* 94:65–72.

Stewart, M. P., Cabanas, C., and Hogg, N. (1996) T-cell adhesion to intercellular adhesion molecule-1 (ICAM-1) is controlled by cell spreading and the activation of integrin LFA-1. *J. Immuno.* 156:1810–1817.

Taguchi, M., Sampath, D., Koga, T., Castro, M., Look, D. C., Nakajima, S., and Holtzman, M. J. (1998) Patterns for RANTES secretion and intercellular adhesion molecule 1 expression mediate transepithelial T-cell traffic based on analyses in vitro and in vivo. *J. Exp. Med.* 187:1927–40.

Tamkun, J. W., DeSimone, D. W., Fonda, D., Patel, R. S., Buck, C., Horwitz, A. F., and Hynes, R. O. (1986) Structure of integrin, a glycoprotein involved in the transmembrane linkage between fibronectin and actin. *Cell* 46:271–282.

Van der Vieren, M., Le Trong, H., Wood, C. L., Moore, P. F., St. John, T., Staunton, D. E., and Gallatin, W. M. (1995) A novel leukointegrin, alpha d beta 2, binds preferentially to ICAM-3. *Immunity* 3:683–690.

van Kooyk, Y., Weder, P., Heije, K., and Figdor, C. G. (1994) Extracellular calcium modulates leukocyte function-associated antigen-1 cell surface distribution on T lymphocytes and consequently affects cell adhesion. *J. Cell. Biol.* 124:1061–1070.

Vedder, N. B., Winn, R. K., Rice, C. L., Chi, E. Y., Arfors, K. E., and Harlan, J. M. (1990) Inhibition of leukocyte adherence by anti-CD 18 monoclonal antibody attenuates reperfusion injury in the rabbit ear. *Proc. Nat. Acad. Sci. USA* 87:2643–2646.

Vejlsgaard, G. L., Ralfkiaer, E., Avnstorp, C., Czajkowski, M., Marlin, S. D., and Rothlein, R. (1989) Kinetics and characterization of intercellular adhesion molecule-1 (ICAM-1) expression on keratinocytes in various inflammatory skin lesions and nalignant cutaneous lymphomas. *J. Am. Acad. Dermatol.* 20:782–790.

Williams, I. R., and Kupper, T. S. (1994) Epidermal expression of intercellular adhesion molecule 1 is not a primary inducer of cutaneous inflammation in transgenic mice. *Proc. Natl. Acad. Sci. USA* 91:9710–9714.

Wright, S. D., Rao, P. E., Van Voorhis, W. C., Craigmyle, L. S., Iida, K., Talle, M. A., Westberg, E. F., Goldstein, G., and Silverstein, S. C. (1983) Identification of the C3bi receptor of human monocytes and macrophages with monoclonal antibodies. *Proc. Nat. Acad. Sci. USA* 80:5699–5703.

Wülfing, C., and Davis, M. M. (1998) A receptor/cytoskeletal movement triggered by costimulation during T-cell activation. *Science* 282:2266–2269.

Xu, H., Gonzalo, J. A., St. Pierre, Y., Williams, I. R., Kupper, T. S., Cotran, R. S., Springer, T. A., and Gutierrez-Ramos, J. C. (1994) Leukocytosis and resistance to septic shock in intercellular adhesion molecule–deficient mice. *J. Exp. Med.* 180:95–109.

Yauch, R. L., Felsenfeld, D. P., Kraeft, S. K., Chen, L. B., Sheetz, M. P., and Hemler, M. E. (1997) Mutational evidence for control of cell adhesion through integrin diffusion/clustering, independent of ligand binding. *J. Exp. Med.* 186:1347–1355.

14

VCAM-1 and Its Ligands

SHARON J. HYDUK and MYRON I. CYBULSKY

VCAM-1 Identification, Structure, Genomic Organization and Alternative Splicing

The discovery of vascular cell adhesion molecule-1 (VCAM-1) depended largely on the development of an efficient and reproducible technique for culturing human umbilical vein endothelial cells and on the demonstration that treatment with inflammatory cytokines, interleukin-1 (IL-1), and tumor necrosis factor (TNF) α activates endothelium (Pober & Cotran, 1990). Activated endothelium becomes hyperadhesive for leukocytes through a process dependent on protein synthesis. VCAM-1 was identified in activated endothelium through the use of monoclonal antibodies (Rice & Bevilacqua, 1989, Carlos et al., 1990) and expression cloning (Osborn et al., 1989). The former studies involved immunizing mice with activated endothelium and screening for monoclonal antibodies that recognized cytokine-inducible epitopes. The monoclonal antibodies were then used to identify a unique protein by immunoprecipitation and leukocyte adhesion function with adhesion-blocking assays. Expression cloning was done with a subtracted cytokine-activated human umbilical vein endothelial cell library packaged in a eukaryotic expression vector that was expressed in transiently transfected COS cells. Complementary DNA (cDNA) was extracted for reamplification and rescreening from cells exhibiting increased leukocyte adhesion (Osborn et al., 1989).

VCAM-1 is a type I transmembrane glycoprotein and member of the immunoglobulin (Ig) gene superfamily. Expression cloning identified a form with 6 extracellular C2 or H-type Ig domains (Osborn, 1989); however, cDNAs were subsequently isolated from cytokine-activated endothelium that contained an additional Ig domain, designated domain 4 (the remaining domains were designated 5–7; (Cybulsky et al., 1991a; Hession et al., 1991; Polte et al., 1991; (Fig. 14.1). Both 6 and 7Ig VCAM-1 transcripts were detected in IL-1-stimulated human umbilical vein endothelial cells by polymerase chain reaction, but the 7 domain form was much more abundant and was the only form detected on the activated endothelial cell surface by immunoprecipitation (Cybulsky et al., 1991a). Cloning of the human *VCAM1* gene determined that 6 and 7Ig domain forms arise by alternative RNA splicing (Cybulsky et al., 1991b).

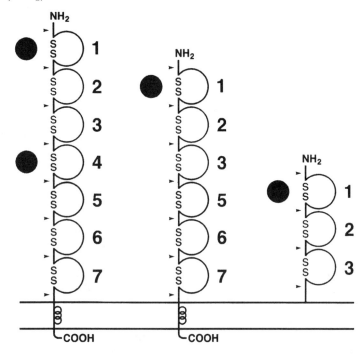

Fig. 14.1. Schematic illustration of different forms of VCAM-1 generated by alternative RNA splicing. Binding sites of α_4 integrins to Ig domains 1 and 4 are indicated by solid circles. Loops represent disulfide-linked Ig domains (numbered) and arrowheads point to exon splice junctions. The three-domain form of VCAM-1 (far right) does not have a transmembrane region and is attached to the membrane by a glycerophosphatidylinositol linkage.

Genomic clones encoding the human and murine *VCAM1* genes revealed that each of the extracellular Ig domains is contained in a separate exon. All splice junctions occur after the first nucleotide of a codon (type I; Cybulsky et al., 1991b, 1993), therefore any exon can be spliced in or out without disturbing the reading frame of the messenger RNA (mRNA). The structure of the gene and homology of Ig domains 1–3 and 4–6 (55%–75% amino acid identity, highest between domains 1 and 4) is consistent with the proposal that exon duplication played a role in the formation of the gene. This explains why the 7Ig domain form has two ligand-binding sites, in Ig domains 1 and 4 (Osborn et al., 1994; Vonderheide et al., 1994; Fig. 14.1). VCAM-1 binds to $\alpha_4\beta_1$ (VLA-4, CD49d/CD29) and weakly to $\alpha_4\beta_7$ integrins (LPAM-1; see the following). ICAM-1, which has a very similar structure, also has two ligand-binding domains and binds $\alpha_L\beta_2$ integrins (LFA-1, CD11a/CD18) via Ig domain 1 and $\alpha_M\beta_2$ (Mac-1, CD11b/CD18) via Ig domain 3 (see Springer, 1994).

The murine *VCAM1* gene contains an additional exon that is unique to rodents and is located between Ig domains 3 and 4 (Cybulsky et al., 1993; Moy et al., 1993; Terry et al., 1993). This exon contains a stop codon and polyadenylation signal, but does not encode a transmembrane domain, therefore, alternatively spliced forms of VCAM-1 with this exon consist of 3Ig domains (domains 1–3) that are attached to the cell membrane by a glycerophosphatidylinositol linkage (Fig. 14.1). Rabbit VCAM-1 has 7 or 8Ig domains. The additional Ig domain is located in position 8 and is homologous to domains 3, 6, and 7.

VCAM-1 Expression In Vitro and In Vivo

VCAM-1 expression is low or absent on unactivated cultured human umbilical vein endothelium. IL-1, TNF, or bacterial lipopolysaccharide (LPS) rapidly induce endothelial cell surface expression to maximum at 10 to 24 hours, then it gradually declines (Rice & Bevilacqua, 1989; Carlos et al., 1990). These stimuli activate the NF-κB signal transduction pathway (See Ghosh et al., 1998) in endothelium, which is essential for induced VCAM-1 expression. The human and murine *VCAM1* promoters contain two adjacent consensus elements for binding of NF-κB transcription factor family members (Cybulsky et al., 1991b, 1993). The functional significance of these cis-elements was revealed through in vitro studies (reviewed in Collins et al., 1995). Transient transfection experiments with segments of human *VCAM1* 5' flanking sequence coupled to a reporter defined a −258 bp region capable of directing full cytokine-induced expression in endothelial cells. Mutational analysis and further deletion experiments revealed that the integrity of both NF-κB cis-elements (−73 and −58 bp) was necessary but not sufficient for full cytokine-mediated transcription activation (Iademarco et al., 1992; Neish et al., 1992). In TNF-activated endothelial cells, the *VCAM1* promoter NF-κB cis-elements bound primarily p50/p65 heterodimers, and NF-κB interacted with other transcription factors, including interferon regulatory factor-1 and Sp1 in transactivating VCAM-1 expression (Neish, 1995a, 1995b).

In addition to IL-1 and TNF, many other stimuli can induce endothelial cell expression of VCAM-1. These include binding of ligands to receptor for advanced glycation end products (RAGE; Schmidt et al., 1996; Cines et al., 1998), binding of CD154, the 39 kD CD40 ligand on activated T cells, to endothelial CD40 (Hollenbaugh et al., 1995; Karmann et al., 1995; Yellin et al., 1995), and exposure of endothelium to lysophosphatidylcholine, a component of oxidized low-density lipoprotein (Kume et al., 1992). The latter up-regulates VCAM-1 expression in cultured arterial, but not venous, endothelium. IL-4 induces low levels of VCAM-1 without inducing expression of ICAM-1 or E-selectin, and in combination with TNF enhances VCAM-1 and partly suppresses ICAM-1 and E-selectin expression (Masinovsky, 1990; Thornhill and Haskard, 1990). The combination of TNF and IL-4 induces a synergistic increase and prolongation of VCAM-1 expression on the cell surface. This results from a combination of transcriptional activation by TNF and stabilization of transcripts by IL-4 (Iademarco, 1995).

IL-1 and TNF-inducible expression of VCAM-1 in endothelium can be inhibited by a variety of compounds that affect NF-κB signal transduction. These include various antioxidants (Marui et al., 1993; Weber et al., 1994) which inhibit the activity of IκB kinases (Spiecker et al., 1997), gallates (Murase et al., 1999), proteasome inhibitors (Read et al., 1995), which prevent degradation of IκBα (an inhibitory component of NF-κB), and nitric oxide (De Caterina et al., 1995; Khan et al., 1996), which augments IκBα expression (Spiecker et al., 1997). The mechanism by which docosahexaenoate, an omega-3 fatty acid, reduces cytokine-induced endothelial cell expression of VCAM-1 and other adhesion molecules is not known (De Caterina et al., 1994).

In addition to inducible expression on vascular endothelium, VCAM-1 can be expressed constitutively on a variety of cell types. In normal tissues, endothelial cell VCAM-1 expression is generally absent, although occasional blood vessels show positive immunohistochemical staining. VCAM-1 is constitutively expressed on some epithelial and monocyte-derived cells, including dendritic cells in lymphoid tissues and skin and Kupffer cells in liver (Rice et al., 1991). Cultured bone marrow stromal cells and skeletal muscle cells during myogenesis also express VCAM-1 (Miyake et al., 1991a; Rosen et al., 1992; Simmons et al., 1992). Constitutive expression of VCAM-1 may not be dependent on NF-κB activation. Absence of VCAM1 NF-κB cis-elements did not affect constitutive VCAM-1 expression in mouse myoblasts (Iademarco, 1993).

VCAM-1 expression is induced in many acute and chronic inflammatory conditions and other pathological processes. In patients with these conditions, a soluble form of VCAM-1, which most likely arises by proteolytic cleavage of the transmembrane form expressed on the cell surface, is often elevated in the plasma. The conditions associated with VCAM-1 expression are too numerous to review comprehensively and only examples will be listed. VCAM-1 is induced on vascular endothelium in acute appendicitis, acute diverticulitis, sarcoidosis, cat scratch lymphadenitis, a variety of dermatoses, rheumatoid and osteoarthritis, allograft rejection, various vasculitides, in tumors, and during atherosclerotic lesion formation. VCAM-1 expression can also be induced in a variety of other vascular cells, including intimal smooth muscle and macrophages (during atherogenesis) and nonvascular cells, including mesothelial, synovial, and renal tubular epithelial cells.

Structure of α₄ Integrins

The mature α_4 subunit (CD49d) is a 999 amino acid, type I transmembrane glycoprotein with a molecular mass of 150 kDa (Takada et al., 1989). The N-terminal extracellular domain is formed from 944 amino acids, and 32 amino acids make up the short cytoplasmic tail. Variable cleavage of the α_4 subunit produces two fragments of 70 and 80 kDa that remain noncovalently associated and retain full biological function (Berdnarczyk et al., 1992; Teixido et al., 1992). Features shared with other α-subunits include seven homologous repeats in the extracellular domain and three divalent cation-binding sites. The cytoplasmic domain also contains the membrane-proximal GFFKR sequence, which is highly conserved within the integrin α-subunits. In contrast to the α-subunits of several other integrins, including all members of the β_2 family, the α_4-subunit does not contain the inserted (I) domain, which is believed to be a recognition site involved in ligand binding (see chapter 13; Fig. 14.2).

The α_4 *integrin* is a single-copy gene on the long arm of human chromosome 2 (2q31–q32), a region that may contain a cluster of integrin genes including α_V (Zhang et al., 1991; Fernadex-Ruiz et al., 1992, 1993). DNA regulatory elements including an AP-1 site, MyoD regulatory sequence and PU-box, which may function as an enhancer, are present in the 5' flanking region and first exon of the gene (Rosen et al., 1991). The sequence of the

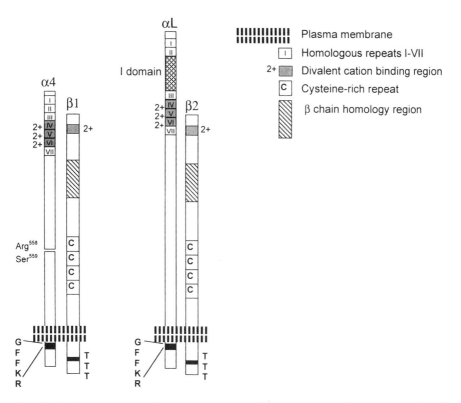

Fig. 14.2. A comparison of the basic structural elements of $\alpha_4\beta_1$ integrin and $\alpha_L\beta_2$ integrin. The similarities and differences in the structures of $\alpha_4\beta_1$ and $\alpha_L\beta_2$ integrin are highlighted. The major differences include the absence of an inserted domain in the α_4 subunit and cleavage of the α_4 subunit to produce two noncovalently associated fragments of 70 and 80 kDa (diagram is not to scale).

murine α_4 integrin is 84% homologous to the human gene (Neuhaus et al., 1991; De Meirsman et al., 1996).

The α_4-subunit associates with either the β_1 (CD29)- or β_7-subunits (Hemler et al., 1987; Holzmann and Weisman, 1989), which are type I transmembrane glycoproteins of 116 kDa and 100 kDa, respectively. Their extracellular domains contain four cysteine-rich repeats located in a segment of 180 amino acids adjacent to the transmembrane domain that is common to all β chains and a highly conserved 100–200 amino acid sequence (Argraves et al., 1987). Their relatively short cytoplasmic tails (47 and 52 amino acids, respectively) interact with cytoskeletal proteins such as talin and α actinin (Horwitz et al., 1986; Otey et al., 1990) and contain three highly conserved threonine residues essential for receptor function (Fig. 14.2).

Expression of α_4 Integrins

The $\alpha_4\beta_1$ and $\alpha_4\beta_7$ integrins are expressed on many leukocytes. Human T cells, B cells, and mast cells express both $\alpha_4\beta_1$ and $\alpha_4\beta_7$, and eosinophils, natural killer cells, monocytes, and hematopoietic progenitor cells express $\alpha_4\beta_1$. During development in the bone marrow, neutrophils express high levels of α_4 integrins, although as they mature and are released from the bone marrow, they have very low expression of α_4 (Taooka et al., 1999). In addition, human neutrophils can be induced to express α_4 following transendothelial migration or treatment with dihydrocytochalasin B (Reinhardt, 1997a, 1997b). Rodent neutrophils express moderate to low levels of α_4 integrins that mediate adhesion to VCAM-1 and MAdCAM-1 in in vitro assays (Issekutz et al., 1996b; Davenpeck et al., 1998).

Expression of $\alpha_4\beta_1$ and $\alpha_4\beta_7$ is differentially regulated during thymocyte maturation and following the activation of mature T cells. Double negative (CD4−CD8−) thymocytes express higher levels of $\alpha_4\beta_1$ than double positive (CD4+CD8+) or single positive cells (Sawada et al., 1992). Naive CD4+ and CD8+ T cells express moderate levels of both α_4 integrins (Picker et al., 1990; Erle et al., 1994). Upon T-cell activation by their specific antigens, the expression of α_4 integrins is increased, with preferential up-regulation of $\alpha_4\beta_7$ on gut-associated lymphocytes (Schweighoffer et al., 1993). Increased expression of many integrins (including α_4) is observed following long-term activation of lymphocytes in vitro and on chronically activated lymphocytes in vivo, such as those localized to the joint synovium in patients with rheumatoid arthritis (Laffon et al., 1991).

The expression of $\alpha_4\beta_7$ is restricted to cells of hematopoietic origin, but $\alpha_4\beta_1$ is also expressed on nonhematopoietic cells including smooth muscle cells, neural crest cells (Kil et al., 1998), and cells of the chorioallantois (Gurtner et al., 1995). The embryonic lethality of VCAM-1 and α_4 integrin knockout mice underscores the importance of interactions between these molecules during development (Gurtner et al., 1995; Yang et al., 1995).

The α_4 Integrin Ligands

The primary ligands for $\alpha_4\beta_1$ integrin are VCAM-1 (Elices et al., 1990) and fibronectin. Unlike other fibronectin-binding integrins ($\alpha_5\beta_1$, $\alpha_v\beta_1$, $\alpha_v\beta_3$, $\alpha_{IIb}\beta_3$), $\alpha_4\beta_1$ does not bind to the RGD sequences within fibronectin. The $\alpha_4\beta_1$ binding sites in fibronectin are within the CS-1 and CS-5 regions generated by alternative splicing and the heparin-binding (Hepll) domain (Guan and Hynes, 1990; Mould and Humphries, 1991; Mould et al., 1991). The primary ligand for $\alpha_4\beta_7$ integrin is MAdCAM-1, a ligand expressed on Peyer's patch high endothelial venules (HEV; Berlin et al., 1993). The $\alpha_4\beta_7$ integrin also binds weakly to VCAM-1 and the CS-1 fragment of fibronectin. The α_4 integrin recognition sites within its ligands are well characterized. The α_4 integrin binds to different, yet homologous sequences in each ligand: EILDV in CS-1, REDV in CS-5, IDAPS in Hepll, IDSP in VCAM-1, and LDTSL in MAdCAM-1 (Eble, 1997). The ligand-binding site within α_4 integrin is less well characterized than that of other leukocyte integrins because α_4 integrins do not contain an inserted domain. By mapping the epitopes recognized by function-blocking monoclonal antibodies, residues 108–268 of the α_4-subunit and Asp 130 of the β_1-subunit have been identified as essential regions for VCAM-1 and CS-1 binding (Kamata et al., 1995). Osteopontin, casein, and propolypeptide of von Willebrand factor have been identified as alternative ligands for $\alpha_4\beta_1$ integrin (Davis et al., 1997; Isobe et al., 1997; Bayless et al., 1998).

Signaling via α_4 Integrin

Inside-Out Signaling (Avidity/Affinity Regulation)

Integrins on circulating leukocytes generally cannot bind ligands, yet during the process of emigration from blood into tissues, they become "activated" and rapidly acquire ligand-binding capacity. During leukocyte migration in tissues, integrin activity may fluctuate. Intracellular signals that up-regulate integrin–ligand binding are termed *inside-out signals.* Engagement of a wide array of cell surface receptors including the T-cell receptor complex (TCR) and costimulatory proteins (Chan et al., 1991), G-protein–coupled chemokine receptors (Burke-Gaffney and Hellewell, 1996; Kitayama et al., 1998), or cytokine and growth factor receptors (Kitazawa et al., 1997; Sung et al., 1997; Yuan et al., 1997) leads to alterations in integrin–ligand binding activity.

Ligand-binding activity can be regulated by changes in integrin affinity or avidity or both. Alterations in affinity are the result of conformational changes that allow persistent binding of soluble ligand. Epitopes unique to high affinity β_1 integrins can be detected with monoclonal antibodies. The divalent cation Mn^{2+} is extensively used as an exogenous mechanism for increasing the affinity of α_4 integrins for their soluble ligands (Bazzoni and

Hemler, 1998). Avidity changes, which include integrin clustering, association with the cell cytoskeleton and activation-dependent cell spreading, up-regulate integrin–ligand binding without affecting affinity. Although affinity and avidity are distinct processes, it is likely that both are involved in leukocyte integrin regulation in vivo.

For many of the aforementioned physiological regulators of α_4 integrin activity, it has not been determined whether affinity or avidity changes are involved in increasing ligand-binding capacity. Cross linking the TCR complex induces cell flattening, association of integrins with cytoskeletal proteins, and adhesion to immobilized VCAM-1 without altering the affinity for VCAM-Ig fusion protein, yet stimulates binding of soluble fibronectin (Faull et al., 1994; Jakubowski et al., 1995). The regulation of $\alpha_4\beta_1$ integrin activity on human eosinophils by the chemokines RANTES, MCP-3, or the complement peptide C5a is mediated through cytoskeletal alterations and does not involve changes in α_4 integrin affinity (Weber et al., 1996). Ligation of L-selectin on T cells generates intracellular signals that regulate $\alpha_4\beta_1$ integrin affinity for soluble fibronectin (Giblin et al., 1997). Thus, in a physiological setting, affinity and avidity changes likely contribute to an increase in the activity of the $\alpha_4\beta_1$ integrin.

Molecules and Signal Transduction Cascades Involved in Inside-Out Signalling

Reciprocal co-immunoprecipitations have established associations of several integrins including $\alpha_4\beta_1$ with a family of transmembrane proteins (transmembrane 4 superfamily (TM4SF) that includes CD53, CD63, CD81, and CD82. CD81 and CD82 colocalize with $\alpha_4\beta_1$ integrin in cell surface clusters. Furthermore, in α_4 adhesion-deficient mutants, α_4 integrins no longer associate with CD81, implicating TM4SF members as adhesion modulators (Mannion et al., 1996). CD98, an early T-cell activation marker, is a transmembrane protein that associates with α_4 integrin. A genetic complementation approach was used to identify CD98 as a regulator of β_1 integrin function (Fenczik et al., 1997).

The molecular mechanisms leading to alterations in α_4 integrin avidity or affinity are not well defined. Several potential signal transduction pathways have been identified. A role for P13 kinase has been described in activation of many of the integrins by various stimulators. CD28 cross linking stimulates $\alpha_4\beta_1$ integrin-mediated adhesion to fibronectin in a P13 kinase-dependent manner as illustrated using specific P13 kinase inhibitors (Zell et al., 1996). The rho family of GTPases is important for chemokine-induced increases in $\alpha_4\beta_1$ adhesion to VCAM-1 as illustrated using inhibitor studies (Laudanna et al., 1996). Activation of $\alpha_4\beta_1$ integrin by IL-3 stimulation requires the GTP-binding proteins H-ras; dominant negative constructs of H-ras inhibit IL-3–induced adhesion and transfection with constitutively active constructs is sufficient to stimulate adhesion to fibronectin (Shibayama et al., 1999). Similarly, constitutively active R-ras converts cells that grow in suspension to an adherent phenotype (Zhang et al., 1996). Phorbol ester treatment of T cells triggers β_1 integrin-mediated adhesion and cell spreading, implicating an important role for protein kinase C (PKC) in integrin activation. The effects of phorbol esters are mediated by avidity changes (integrin clustering, Faull et al., 1994) and affinity changes as demonstrated by binding of activation reporter antibodies (Yednock et al., 1995) and soluble VCAM-1 (S. Hyduk, unpublished observations 1999). CD3-activated adhesion of T cells to VCAM-1 is blocked by PKC inhibitors, illustrating a physiological role for PKC in integrin regulation (MacKenzie et al., 1999). The molecular mechanisms that regulate integrin affinity are currently a topic of intensive study.

Relevance of Affinity and/or Avidity Changes to α_4 Integrin Function

The ability of some activators to alter integrin affinity and others to alter avidity may have important implications for leukocyte trafficking. Low affinity interactions mediate the tethering and rolling of T cells on VCAM-1, but are unable to mediate firm adhesion. High affinity α_4 integrin is required for adhesion strengthening. Locking α_4 integrin in a high affinity state with Mn^{2+} inhibits tethering and rolling interactions, and leads to immediate arrest (Chen et al., 1999).

Outside-In Signaling

In addition to their adhesive functions, integrins also participate in multiple cellular signaling events and transmit signals to the cell from the surrounding environment. These outside-in signals allow the extracellular matrix to regulate cellular proliferation and differentiation, induce gene transcription, and provide survival signals. The integrin cytoplasmic tails themselves have no intrinsic enzymatic activity; however, integrins associate with and activate a number of nonreceptor tyrosine kinases (for a recent review, see Schlaepfer and Hunter, 1998). In addition, ligation of α_4 integrins induces Ca^{2+} transients (Ricard et al., 1997; Weismann et al., 1997), modulates intracellular pH levels (Rich et al., 1998), activates PKC, JNK, and MAP kinases (McGilvray et al., 1997; Mainiero et al., 1998), activates phospholipase C (PLC), and induces redistribution and activation of P13 kinase. Many integrin-dependent signaling pathways require the assembly of multimolecular signaling complexes that link the actin cytoskeleton and signaling proteins to integrins. These large aggregations provide a high local concentration of cytoskeletal elements and signaling proteins to coordinate integrin-mediated signals. One of the earliest steps in α_4 integrin-mediated signal transduction is tyrosine phosphorylation of cellular proteins including focal adhesion kinase (p125 FAK; Lin et al., 1995; Maguire et al., 1995; Nojima et al., 1995). FAK interacts with Src, Grb2, and P13 kinase in an adhesion-dependent manner and may serve as a docking protein involved in the assembly of these multimolecular signaling complexes. FAK may play a critical role in α_4 integrin-mediated activation of signal transduction cascades including P13 kinase and MAP kinase (Chen and Guan, 1994; Schlaepfer and Hunter, 1998).

Integrin-mediated signals play an important role in the development of an inflammatory response by participating in lymphocyte activation and the production of inflammatory mediators. In addition to the costimulatory role demonstrated for $\alpha_L\beta_2$ integrin, $\alpha_4\beta_1$ integrin costimulates CD3-dependent proliferation of mature T cells (Nojima et al., 1990; Shimizu et al., 1990), mature thymocytes, and immature double-negative thymocytes (Halvorson et al., 1998) through interactions with fibronectin and VCAM-1 (Burkly et al., 1991). In addition, in B cells, T cells, NK cells, and monocytes, $\alpha_4\beta_1$ integrin-initiated signals induce the expression of a number of inflammatory mediator genes including matrix metalloproteinases and cytokines (Damle and Aruffe, 1991; Yurochko et al., 1992; Lin et al., 1995; Dackiw et al., 1996; McCarthy et al., 1997; Mainiero et al., 1998).

Other VCAM-1 Ligands

In addition to α_4 integrins, several other integrins have been identified as alternative ligands of VCAM-1 including $\alpha_9\beta_1$ and $\alpha_D\beta_2$ (Grayson et al., 1998; Taooka et al., 1999). The α_9-subunit is 41% homologous to the α_4-subunit and pairs with the β_1 chain to form a single integrin. The $\alpha_9\beta_1$ integrin also binds to the third fibronectin type III repeat of the extracellular matrix protein tenascin-C. CHO cells transfected with $\alpha_9\beta_1$ adhere to immobilized recombinant VCAM-1 and TNF-α–stimulated endothelium. Flow cytometric analysis revealed expression of $\alpha_9\beta_1$ integrin on human peripheral blood neutrophils, and to a lesser degree on monocytes. In addition, $\alpha_9\beta_1$ integrin mediates neutrophil transmigration across recombinant VCAM-1–coated filters or TNF-α–activated endothelial monolayers (Taooka et al., 1999).

The $\alpha_D\beta_2$ integrin, a member of the leukocyte integrin family (see Chapter 13) is expressed by human eosinophils and supports the adhesion of eosinophils to endothelial VCAM-1 in static adhesion assays (Grayson et al., 1998). In addition, expression of $\alpha_D\beta_2$ in an α_4 integrin-null Jurkat cell line confers the ability to adhere to VCAM-1 under flow conditions (Van der Vieren et al., 1999). The $\alpha_D\beta_2$ integrin interacts with a region of VCAM-1 that overlaps with the binding site for α_4 integrin. The ligand-binding site in $\alpha_D\beta_2$ is believed to be within the inserted domain (Van der Vieren et al., 1999), which is not present in α_4 integrins.

Potential Physiological and Developmental Roles of VCAM-1 and α_4 Integrins

As was implied previously, VCAM-1 expressed on activated vascular endothelium may participate in the emigration of α_4 integrin-bearing leukocytes during infections and inflammatory conditions. In normal animals, the temporal and spatial patterns of VCAM-1 and α_4 integrin expression suggest that these adhesion molecules may participate in a variety of physiological and developmental processes. Knockout mice have clearly defined a critical developmental role for these molecules during fusion of the allantois to the chorion, which results in the formation of the umbilical cord and placenta. VCAM-1 is expressed on the tip of the allantois and $\alpha_4\beta_1$ integrin on the inner surface of the chorionic plate (Gurtner et al., 1995; Kwee et al., 1995; Yang et al., 1995). Virtually all VCAM-1 knockout (VCAM-1$^{-/-}$) mouse embryos died in utero due to this placentation defect (Gurtner et al., 1995; Kwee et al., 1995). Less than 3% of VCAM-1$^{-/-}$ embryos survived development, presumably by circumventing the placentation defects; as adults these VCAM-1$^{-/-}$ mice were healthy, fertile, and had organs with normal histological features (Gurtner et al., 1995). Mice deficient in α_4 integrins displayed a morphologically similar chorioallantoic fusion defect (Yang et al., 1995).

VCAM-1 and α_4 integrins participate in hematopoiesis and lymphocyte homing. Immunolocalization studies demonstrated VCAM-1 expression in bone marrow stroma reticular and sinusoidal endothelial cells (Miyake et al., 1991a; Simmons et al., 1992; Jacobsen et al., 1996). In vitro antibody blocking studies suggest that VCAM-1 and α_4 integrins mediate adherence of lymphoid precursors and CD34$^+$ hematopoietic progenitor cells to stromal cells (Miyake et al., 1991a; Simmons et al., 1992) and support proliferation of lymphoid cells in long-term bone marrow cultures (Miyake et al., 1991b). In vitro injection of antibodies stimulates release of progenitor cells into the circulation in mice and primates (Papayannopoulou and Nakamoto, 1993; Funk et al., 1994; Craddock et al., 1997). Mice with markedly reduced VCAM-1 expression (see the following) did not have hematopoietic insufficiencies in myeloid or lymphoid compartments (Friedrich et al., 1996), but had a higher level of hematopoietic progenitor cells (Papayannopoulou et al., 1998). In Dexter-type long-term bone marrow cultures, VCAM-1–deficient stromal cells supported normal myeloid differentiation and proliferation (Friedrich et al., 1996). Studies with α_4 integrin chimeric mice revealed that T-cell development was dependent on α_4 integrins after birth, but not in the fetus (Arroyo et al., 1996). These investigators also demonstrated that both B-cell and T-cell precursors, but not monocytes or natural killer cells, require α_4 integrins for normal development in the bone marrow. In peripheral tissues, α_4 integrins participate in T-cell homing to Peyer's patches (Arroyo et al., 1996; Berlin-Rufenach et al., 1999).

Other roles of VCAM-1 and α_4 integrins in development and physiology are still not well defined, and some are even controversial. Embryos deficient in α_4 integrin or VCAM-1 exhibited dissolution of the forming epicardium and coronary vessels leading to pericardial edema and hemorrhage. This defect temporally followed the chorioallantoic fusion defect, and thus, may be a secondary event, at least in VCAM-1–deficient mice, because occasional VCAM-1$^{-/-}$ mice that survived development and VCAM-1 domain 4 deficient mice with hypomorphic VCAM-1 expression ($< 8\%$ of wild-type) had normal pericardium and coronary arteries (Gurtner et al., 1995, Cybulsky unpublished observations, 2000).

The role of VCAM-1 and α_4 integrins in myogenesis is controversial. Myogenesis is a biphasic process, in which primary myoblasts fuse to form primary myotubes, then secondary myoblasts align along the primary myotubes and form secondary myotubes that comprise most of the skeletal muscle in adult mammals. In vivo immunolocalization demonstrated expression of α_4 integrins on primary and secondary myotubes and VCAM-1 on secondary myoblasts. Antibodies to either molecule inhibited myotube formation in culture (Rosen et al., 1992). However, subsequent studies using α_4 integrin null cells derived from chimeric mice, demonstrated normal myogenesis (Yang et al., 1996).

VCAM-1 on antigen-presenting cells and α_4 integrins on lymphocytes may participate in immune processes. For example, α_4 ligation may provide a costimulatory pathway in T-lymphocyte activation (Burkly et al., 1991; Damle and Aruffo, 1991; van Seventer et al., 1991). In lymphoid germinal centers, VCAM-1 expressed on dendritic cells may mediate B-lymphocyte adhesion (Freedman et al., 1990).

VCAM-1 and α_4 Integrin-Mediated Leukocyte–Endothelial Interactions During Emigration

The process of leukocyte emigration from blood into tissues has been subdivided by many investigators into tethering, rolling, arrest, stable or firm adhesion, and transendothelial migration (Springer, 1994; Butcher and Picker, 1996). VCAM-1 and α_4 integrins have been shown to participate to various degrees in all steps of leukocyte emigration. In contrast, ICAM-1 and β_2 integrins promote firm adhesion and transmigration of all leukocyte types, but do not mediate tethering or rolling (Springer, 1994) except at very low shear.

Tethering and rolling are initial adhesive interactions of leukocytes with endothelium. Tethering is the first adhesive interaction, which slows the velocity of a leukocyte as it makes contact with the endothelial monolayer. Both tethering and rolling are mediated by binding of E-, P- or L-selectin to their respective ligands (reviewed in Springer, 1994). VCAM-1 and α_4 integrins can promote tethering and rolling of lymphocytes at low shear stress (Alon et al., 1995b; Berlin et al., 1995; Luscinskas et al., 1995). It is essential that bonds that mediate tethering and rolling have rapid binding and release rates (high k_{on} and k_{off}) (Alon et al., 1995; 1997). Rolling leukocytes are in close proximity to endothelium and are exposed to chemokines presented on the endothelial cell surface (Middleton et al., 1997; Tanaka et al., 1993). Chemokine binding to receptors on leukocytes initiates signals that up-regulate β_1 and β_2 integrin–ligand binding capability and allow them to interact with VCAM-1 and ICAM-1 (Campbell et al., 1996; Lloyd et al., 1996; Campbell et al., 1998) to induce firm adhesion.

Arrest, firm adhesion, and transendothelial migration (diapedesis) are mediated by leukocyte integrins that bind to members of the Ig gene superfamily, including VCAM-1 and ICAM-1. Although these steps are mediated by the same adhesion molecules, it is likely that the molecules are utilized in different ways. The arrest of a spherical leukocyte that is rolling is a sudden and persistent event that likely is mediated by relatively few molecular bonds that persist. Recent studies demonstrated that high affinity α_4 integrins mediate arrest of rolling leukocytes (Labor et al., 1997; Chen et al., 1999); however, in the context of inflammation, it is not known if, when, or how α_4 integrin affinity is up-regulated. Campbell and colleagues demonstrated that chemoattractants and chemokines rapidly and transiently increased the arrest of leukocytes rolling on immobilized VCAM-1 or ICAM-1 (Campbell et al., 1996, 1998), but it is not known if this was mediated by increased integrin affinity.

Stabilization of adhesion and transendothelial migration are kinetically slower steps associated with leukocyte shape changes and migration. Integrin avidity changes, which are associated with cytoskeletal reorganization, are likely important in mediating these steps. Recently, Chan et al., (1999) demonstrated that binding of α_4 integrins to VCAM-1 induces a signal transduction pathway in leukocytes that up-regulates β_2 integrin avidity and increases the strength of adhesion to ICAM-1. The role of VCAM-1 and α_4 integrins in leukocyte transendothelial migration has been confirmed by several laboratories using in vitro models (Chuluyan et al., 1995; Meerschaert & Furie, 1995).

Function-blocking monoclonal antibodies were used in a variety of inflammatory, allergic, and immune in vivo models to evaluate the roles of α_4 integrins in monocyte and lymphocyte emigration and compare them to β_2 integrins (Issekutz, 1995; Issekutz et al., 1996a; Li, 1998; Issekutz, 1999). Blockade of α_4 and β_2 integrins resulted in reduced monocyte and lymphocyte recruitment and/or tissue injury. The relative contributions of each integrin depended on the inflammatory stimulus and tissue.

We produced VCAM-1 domain 4-deficient (D4D) mice, which partially circumvented the embryonic lethality of VCAM-1 knockout mice (Cybulsky unpublished data, 2000). VCAM-1$^{D4D/D4D}$ mice express a 6Ig domain form of VCAM-1 and lack Ig domain 4, which contains an α_4 integrin-binding site (Figure 14.1). Thus, the 6Ig domain form has only one ligand-binding site, unlike two found in wild-type mice. Also, the expression levels of D4D VCAM-1 are markedly reduced or hypomorphic (3%–8% of wild-type). VCAM-1$^{D4D/D4D}$ and ICAM-1$^{-/-}$ mice were used to demonstrate VCAM-1–dependent and independent recruitment of mononuclear leukocytes. Lymphocyte recruitment in an ovalbumin immunization model was significantly reduced in VCAM-1$^{D4D/D4D}$, but not ICAM-1$^{-/-}$ mice. In contrast, macrophage accumulation in thioglycollate-induced peritonitis was normal in VCAM-1$^{D4D/D4D}$ and ICAM-1$^{-/-}$, but was reduced in mice with combined VCAM-1$^{D4D/D4D}$ + ICAM-1$^{-/-}$ (Cybulsky, unpublished data, 2000).

Summary

The temporal and spatial patterns of VCAM-1 and α_4 integrin expression suggest that these adhesion molecules participate in a variety of physiological and developmental processes. They play a critical role during fusion of the allantois to the chorion, and may play roles in myogenesis and pericardial development. In the context of inflammation, VCAM-1 and α_4 integrins have been shown to participate to various degrees in all steps of leukocyte emigration, provide a costimulatory pathway for T-lymphocyte activation, and participate in hematopoiesis and lymphocyte homing. VCAM-1 expression is induced in many acute and chronic inflammatory conditions and other pathological processes. Expression of α_4 integrins is increased following T-cell activation by their specific antigens. In addition, α_4 integrins become activated and rapidly acquire ligand-binding capacity following the generation of inside-out signals by a wide variety of stimuli including engagement of T-cell receptor and costimulatory proteins and chemokine, cytokine, and growth factor receptors. Integrin-mediated signals may play an important role in the development of an inflammatory response by participating in lymphocyte activation and the production of inflammatory mediators.

References

Alon, R., Kassner, P. D., Carr, M. W., Finger, E. B., Hemler, M. E., and Springer, T. A. (1995b) The integrin VLA-4 supports tethering and rolling in flow on VCAM-1. *J. Cell Biol.* 128:1243–1253.

Alon, R., Hammer, D. A., and Springer, T. A. (1995a) Lifetime of the P-selectin–carbohydrate bond and its response to tensile force in hydrodynamic flow. *Nature* 374:539–542.

Alon, R., Chen, S., Puri, K. D., Finger, E. B., and Springer, T. A. (1997). The kinetics of L-selectin tethers and the mechanics of selectin-mediated rolling. *J. Cell Biol.* 138:1169–1180.

Argraves, W. S., Suzuki, S., and Arai. H. (1987) Amino acid sequence of the human fibronectin receptor. *J. Cell Biol.* 105:1183–1190.

Arroyo, A. G., Yang, J. T., Rayburn, H., and Hynes, R. O. (1996) Differential requirements for integrins during fetal and adult hematopoiesis. *Cell* 85:997–1008.

Bayless, K. J., Meininger, G. A., Scholtz, J. M., and Davis, G. E. (1998) Osteopontin is a ligand for the $\alpha_4\beta_1$ integrin. *J. Cell Sci.* 111:1165–1174.

Bazzoni, G., and Hemler. M. E. (1998) Are changes in integrin affinity and conformation over-emphasized? *Trends Biol. Sci.* 23:30–34.

Berdnarczyk, J. L., Szabo, M. C., and McIntyre, B. W. (1992) Post-translational processing of the leukocyte integrin $\alpha_4\beta_1$. *J. Biol. Chem* 267:25274–25281.

Berlin, C., Berg, E. L., Briskin, M. J., Andrew, D. P., Kilshaw, P. J., Holzmann, B., Weissman, I. L., Hamann, A., and Butcher, E. C. (1993) $\alpha_4\beta_7$ integrin mediates lymphocyte binding to the mucosal vascular addressin MAdCAM-1. *Cell* 74:185–195.

Berlin, C., Bargatze, R. F., Campbell, J. J., von Andrian, U. H., Szabo, M. C., Hasslen, S. R., Nelson, R. D., Berg, E. L., Erlandsen, S. L., and Butcher, E. C. (1995) α_4 integrins mediate lymphocyte attachment and rolling under physiologic flow. *Cell* 80:413–422.

Berlin-Rufenach, C., Otto, F., Mathies, M., Westermann, J., Owen, M. J., Hamann, A., and Hogg, N. (1999) Lymphocyte migration in lymphocyte function-associated antigen (LFA)-1–deficient mice. *J. Exp. Med.* 189:1467–1478.

Burke-Gaffney, A., and Hellewell, P. G. (1996) Eotaxin stimulates eosinophil adhesion to human lung microvascular endothelial cells. *Biochem. Biophys. Res. Commun.* 227:35–40.

Burkly, L. C., Jakubowski, A., Newman, B. M., Rosa, M. D., Chi-Rosso, G., and Lobb, R. R. (1991)

Signaling by vascular cell adhesion molecule-1 (VCAM-1) through VLA-4 promotes CD3-dependent T-cell proliferation. *Eur. J. Immunol.* 21:2871–2875.

Butcher, E. C., and Picker, L. J. (1996) Lymphocyte homing and homeostasis. *Science* 272:60–66.

Campbell, J. J., Qin, S., Bacon, K. B., Mackay, C. R., and Butcher, E. C. (1996) Biology of chemokine and classical chemoattractant receptors: differential requirements for adhesion-triggering versus chemotactic responses in lymphoid cells. *J. Cell Biol.* 134:255–266.

Campbell, J. J., Hedrick, J., Zlotnik, A., Siani, M. A., Thompson, D. A., and Butcher, E. C. (1998) Chemokines and the arrest of lymphocytes rolling under flow conditions. *Science* 279:381–384.

Carlos, T. M., Schwartz, B. R., Kovach, N. L., Yee, E., Rosa, M., Osborn, L., Chi-Rosso, G., Newman, B., Lobb, R., and Harlan, J. M. (1990) Vascular cell adhesion molecule-1 mediates lymphocyte adherence to cytokine-activated cultured human endothelial cells. *Blood* 76:965–970. [Published erratum appears in *Blood* (1990) 76(11):2420]

Chan, B.M.C., Wong, J.G.P., Rao, A., and Hemler, M. E. (1991) T cell receptor-dependent, antigen-specific stimulation of a murine T-cell clone induced a transient, VLA-4 protein-mediated binding to extracellular matrix. *J. Immunol.* 147:398–404.

Chan, J. R., Hyduk, S. J., and Cybulsky, M. I. (1999) $\alpha_4\beta_1$ integrin/VCAM-1 interaction activates $\alpha_L\beta_2$ integrin-mediated adhesion to ICAM-1 in human T cells. *J. Immunol.* 164:746–753.

Chen, H.-C., and Guan, J.-L. (1994). Association of focal adhesion kinase with its potential substrate phosphatidylinositol 3-kinase. *Proc. Nat. Acad. Sci. USA* 91:10148–10152.

Chen, C., Mobley, J. L., Dwir, O., Shimron, F., Grabovsky, V., Lobb, R. R., Shimizu, Y., and Alon, R. (1999) High affinity very late antigen-4 subsets expressed on T cells are mandatory for spontaneous adhesion strengthening but not for rolling on VCAM-1 in shear flow. *J. Immunol.* 162:1084–1095.

Chuluyan, H. E., Schall, T. J., Yoshimura, T., and Issekutz, A. C. (1995) IL-1 activation of endothelium supports VLA-4 (CD49d/CD29)-mediated monocyte transendothelial migration to C5a, MIP-1 alpha, RANTES, and PAF but inhibits migration to MCP-1: a regulatory role for endothelium-derived MCP-1. *J. Leuko. Biol.* 58:71–97.

Cines, D. B., Pollak, E. S., Buck, C. A., Loscalzo, J., Zimmerman, G. A., McEver, R. P., Pober, J. S., Wick, B. A., Konkle, B. A., Schwartz, B. S., et al. (1998) Endothelial cells in physiology and in the pathophysiology of vascular disorders. *Blood* 91:3527–3561.

Collins, T., Read, M. A., Neish, A. S., Whitley, M. Z., Thanos, D., and Maniatis, T. (1995) Transcriptional regulation of endothelial cell adhesion molecules: NF-kappa B and cytokine-inducible enhancers. *FASEB J.* 9:899–909.

Craddock, C. F., Nakamoto, B., Andrews, R. G., Priestley, G. V., and Papayannopoulou, T. (1997) Antibodies to VLA-4 integrin mobilize long-term repopulating cells and augment cytokine-induced mobilization in primates and mice. *Blood* 90:4779–4788.

Cybulsky, M. I., Fries, J. W., Williams, A. J., Sultan, P., Davis, V. M., Gimbrone, M. A., Jr., and Collins, T. (1991a) Alternative splicing of human VCAM-1 in activated vascular endothelium. *Am. J. Pathol.* 138:815–820.

Cybulsky, M. I., Fries, J. W., Williams, A. J., Sultan, P., Eddy, R., Byers, M., Shows, T., Gimbrone, M. A., Jr., and Collins, T. (1991b) Gene structure, chromosomal location, and basis for alternative mRNA splicing of the human VCAM1 gene. *Proc. Nat. Acad. Sci. USA* 88:7859–7863.

Cybulsky, M. I., Allan-Motamed, M., and Collins, T. (1993) Structure of the murine VCAM1 gene. *Genomics* 18:387–391.

Dackiw, A. P., Nathens, A. B., Marshall, J. C., and Rotstein, O. D. (1996) Integrin engagement induces monocyte procoagulant activity and tumor necrosis factor production via induction of tyrosine phosphorylation. *J. Surg. Res.* 64:210–215.

Damle, N. K., and Aruffo, A. (1991) Vascular cell adhesion molecule-1 induces T-cell antigen receptor-dependent activation of CD4+ T lymphocytes. *Proc. Natl. Acad. Sci. USA* 88:6403–6407.

Davenpeck, K. L., Sterbinsky, S. A., and Bochner, B. S. (1998) Rat neutrophils express α_4 and β_1 integrins and bind to vascular cell adhesion molecule-1 (VCAM-1) and mucosal addressin cell adhesion molecule-1 (MAdCAM-1). *Blood* 91:2341–2346.

Davis, G. E., Thomas, J. S., and Madden, S. (1997). The $\alpha_4\beta_1$ integrin can mediate leukocyte adhesion to casein and denatured protein substrates. *J. Leukoc. Biol.* 62:18–328.

De Caterina, R., Cybulsky, M. I., Clinton, S. K., Gimbrone, M. A., Jr., and Libby, P. (1994) The omega-3 fatty acid docosahexaenoate reduces cytokine-induced expression of proatherogenic and proinflammatory proteins in human endothelial cells. *Arteriosci. Thromb.* 14:1829–1836.

De Caterina, R., Libby, P., Peng, H. B., Thannickal, V. J., Rajavashisth, T. B., Gimbrone, M. A., Jr., Shin, W. S., and Liao, J. K. (1995) Nitric oxide decreases cytokine-induced endothelial activation. Nitric oxide selectively reduces endothelial expression of adhesion molecules and proinflammatory cytokines. *J. Clin. Inves.* 96:60–68.

De Meirsman, C., Jaspers, M., Schollen, E., and Cassiman, J.-J. (1996) The genomic structure of the murine α_4 integrin gene. *DNA Cell Biol.* 15:595–603.

Eble, J. A. (1997) The ligand recognition motifs of α_4 integrins and leukocyte integrins. In: *Integrin–Ligand Interaction.* J. A. Eble and K. Kuhn, eds. Austin: R. G. Landes, pp. 123–131.

Elices, M. J., Osborn, L., Takada, Y., Crouse, C., Luhowskyj, S., Hemler, M. E., and Lobb, R. R. (1990) VCAM-1 on activated endothelium interacts with the leukocyte integrin VLA-4 at a site distinct from the VLA-4/fibronectin binding site. *Cell* 60:577–584.

Erle, D. J., Briskin, M. J., Butcher, E. C., Garcia Pardo, A. Lazarovits, A., and Tidswell, M. (1994) Expression and function of the MAdCAM-1 receptor, integrin $\alpha_4\beta_7$ on human leukocytes. *J. Immunol.* 153:717–729.

Faull, R. J., Kovach, N. L., Harlan, J. M., and Ginsberg, M. H. (1994) Stimulation of integrin-mediated adhesion of T lymphocytes and monocytes: two mechanisms with divergent biological consequences. *J. Exp. Med.* 179:1307–1316.

Fenczik, C. A., Sethi, T., Ramos, J. W., Hughes, P. E, and Ginsberg, M. H. (1997) Complementation of dominant suppression implicates CD98 in integrin activation. *Nature* 390:81–85.

Fernadez-Ruiz, E., Pardo-Manuel de Villena, F., and Rubio, M. A. (1992) Mapping of the human VLA-α_4 gene to chromosome 2q31-q32. *Eur. J. Immunol.* 22:587–590.

Fernadez-Ruiz, E., Pardo-Manuel de Villena, F., and Rodriguez de Cordoba, S. (1993) Regional localization of the human vitronectin receptor α subunit gene (VNRA) to chromosome 2q31-q32. *Cytogene Cell Genetics* 62:26–28.

Freedman, A. S., Munro, J. M., Rice, G. E., Bevilacqua, M. P., Morimato, C., McIntyre, B. W., Rhynhart, K., Pober, J. S., and Nadler, L. M. (1990) Adhesion of human B cells to germinal centers in vitro involves VLA-4 and INCAM-110. *Science* 249:1030–1033.

Friedrich, C., Cybulsky, M. I., and Gutierrez-Ramos, J. C. (1996) Vascular cell adhesion molecule-1 expression by hematopoiesis-supporting stromal cells is not essential for lymphoid or myeloid differentiation in vivo or in vitro. *Eur. J. Immunol.* 26:2773–2780.

Funk, P. E., Kincade, P. W., and Witte, P. L. (1994) Native associations of early hematopoietic stem cells and stromal cells isolated in bone marrow cell aggregates. *Blood* 83:361–369.

Ghosh, S., May, M. J., and Kopp, E. B. (1998) NF-kappa B and Rel proteins:evolutionarily conserved mediators of immune responses. *Ann. Rev. Immunol.* 16:225–260.

Giblin, P. A., Hwang, S. T., Katsumoto, T. R., and Rosen, S. D. (1997) Ligation of L-selectin on T lymphocytes activates β_1 integrins and promotes adhesion to fibronectin. *J. Immunol.* 159: 3498–3507.

Grayson, M. H., Van der Vieren, M., Sterbinsky, A., Gallatin, W. M., Hoffman, P. A., Staunton, D. E., and Bochner, B. S. (1998) $\alpha_D\beta_2$ Integrin is expressed on human eosinophils and functions as an alternative ligand for vascular cell adhesion molecule-1 (VCAM-1). *J. Exp. Med.* 188:2187–2191.

Guan, J. L., and Hynes, R. O. (1990) Lymphoid cells recognize an alternatively spliced segment of fibronectin via the integrin receptor $\alpha_4\beta_1$. *Cell* 60:53–61.

Gurtner, G. C., Davis, V., Li, H., McCoy, M. J., Sharpe, A., and Cybulsky, M. I. (1995) Targeted disruption of the murine VCAM-1 gene:essential role of VCAM-1 in chorioallantoic fusion and placentation. *Genes & Dev.* 9:1–14.

Halvorson, M. J., Magner, W., and Coligan, J. E. (1998) α_4 and α_5 integrins costimulate the CD3-dependent proliferation of fetal thymocytes. *Cell. Immunol.* 189:1–9.

Hemler, M. E., Huang, C., Takada, Y., Schwarz, L., Strominger, J. L., and Clabby, M. L. (1987) Characterization of the cell surface heterodimer VLA-4 and related peptides. *J. Biol. Chem.* 262:11478–11485.

Hession, C., Tizard, R., Vassallo, C., Schiffer, S. B., Goff, D., Moy, P., Chi-Rosso, G., Luhowskyj,

S., Lobb, R., and Osborn, L. (1991) Cloning of an alternate form of vascular cell adhesion molecule-1 (VCAM-1). *J. Biol. Chem.* 266:6682–6685.

Hollenbaugh, D., Mischel-Petty, N., Edwards, C. P., Simon, J. C., Denfeld, R. W., Kiener, P. A., and Aruffo, A. (1995) Expression of functional CD40 by vascular endothelial cells. *J. Exp. Med.* 182:33–40.

Holzmann, B., and Weisman, I. L. (1989) Peyer's patch-specific lymphocyte homing receptors consist of a VLA-4–like α chain associated with either of two integrin β chains, one of which is novel. *EMBO J.* 8:1735–1741.

Horwitz, A., Duggan, K., and Buck, C. (1986) Interaction of plasma membrane fibronectin receptor with talin; a transmembrane linkage. *Nature* 320:531–533.

Iademarco, M. F., McQuillan, J. J., Rosen, G. D., and Dean, D. C. (1992) Characterization of the promoter for vascular cell adhesion molecule-1 (VCAM-1). *J. Biol. Chem.* 267:16323–16329.

Iademarco, M. F., McQuillan, J. J., and Dean, D. C. (1993) Vascular cell adhesion molecule 1: contrasting transcriptional control mechanisms in muscle and endothelium. *Proc. Nat. Acad. Sci. USA* 90:3943–3947.

Iademarco, M. F., Barks, J. L., and Dean, D. C. (1995) Regulation of vascular cell adhesion molecule-1 expression by IL-4 and TNF-alpha in cultured endothelial cells. *J. Clin. Invest.* 95: 264–271.

Isobe, T., Hisaoka, T., Shimizu, A., Okuno, M., Aimoto, S., Takada, Y., Saito, Y., and Takagi, J. (1997) Propolypeptide of von Willebrand factor is a novel ligand for very late antigen-4 integrin. *J. Biol. Chem.* 272:8447–8453.

Issekutz, T. B. (1995) Leukocyte adhesion and the anti-inflammatory effects of leukocyte integrin blockade. *Agents Actions Suppl.* 46:85–96.

Issekutz, A. C., Ayer, L., Miyasaka, M., and Issekutz, T. B. (1996a) Treatment of established adjuvant arthritis in rats with monoclonal antibody to CD18 and very late activation antigen-4 integrins suppresses neutrophil and T-lymphocyte migration to the joints and improves clinical disease. *Immunol.* 88:569–576.

Issekutz, T. B., Miyasaka, M., and Issekutz, A. C. (1996b) Rat blood neutrophils express very late antigen 4 and it mediates migration to arthritic joint and dermal inflammation. *J. Exp. Med.* 183:2175–2184.

Issekutz, T. B. (1999) Integrins regulating the interaction of lymphocytes with vascular endothelium. *Transplant. Proc.* 31:1600–1601.

Jacobsen, K., Kravitz, J., Kincade, P. W., and Osmond, D. G. (1996) Adhesion receptors on bone marrow stromal cells:in vivo expression of vascular cell adhesion molecule-1 by reticular cells and sinusoidal endothelium in normal and gamma-irradiated mice. *Blood* 87:73–82.

Jakubowski, A., Rosa, M. D., Bixler, S., Lobb, R., and Burkly, L. C. (1995) Vascular cell adhesion molecule (VCAM)-lg fusion protein defines distinct affinity states of the very late antigen-4 (VLA-4) receptor. *Cell Adhesion Commun.* 3:131–142.

Kamata, T., Puzon, W., and Takada, Y. (1995) Identification of putative ligand-binding sites of the integrin $\alpha_4\beta_1$ (VLA-4, CD49d/CD29). *Biochem. J.* 305:945–951.

Karmann, K., Hughes, C. C., Schechner, J., Fanslow, W. C., and Pober, J. S. (1995) CD40 on human endothelial cells:inducibility by cytokines and functional regulation of adhesion molecule expression. *Proc. Natl. Acad. Sci. USA* 92:4342–4346.

Khan, B. V., Harrison, D. G., Olbrych, M. T., Alexander, R. W., and Medford, R. M. (1996) Nitric oxide regulates vascular cell adhesion molecule 1 gene expression and redox-sensitive transcriptional events in human vascular endothelial cells. *Proc. Natl. Acad. Sci. USA* 93:9114–9119.

Kil, S. H., Krull, C. E., Cann, G., Clegg, D., and Bronner-Fraser, M. (1998) The α4 subunit of integrin is important for neural crest cell migration. *Dev. Biol.* 202:29–42.

Kitayama, J., Mackay, C. R., Ponath, P. D., and Springer, T. A. (1998) The C-C chemokine receptor CCR3 participates in stimulation of eosinophil arrest on inflammatory endothelium in shear flow. *J. Clin. Invest.* 101:2017–2024.

Kitazawa, H., Muegge, K., Badolato, R., Wang, J.-M., Foler, W. E., Ferris, D. K., Lee, C.-K., Candeias, S., Smith, M. R., Oppenheim, J. J., and Durum, S. K. (1997) IL-7 activates α4β1 integrin in murine thymocytes. *J. Immunol.* 159:2259–2264.

Kume, N., Cybulsky, M. I., and Gimbrone, M. A., Jr. (1992) Lysophosphatidylcholine, a component of atherogenic lipoproteins, induces mononuclear leukocyte adhesion molecules in cultured human and rabbit arterial endothelial cells. *J. Clin. Inves.* 90:1138–1144.

Kwee, L., Baldwin, H. S., Shen, H. M., Stewart, C. L., Buck, C., Buck, C. A., and Labow, M. A. (1995) Defective development of the embryonic and extraembryonic circulatory systems in vascular cell adhesion molecule (VCAM-1) deficient mice. *Dev.* 121:489–503.

Laffon, A., Garcia-Vicuna, R., and Humbrial, A. (1991) Up-regulated expression and function of VLA-4 fibronectin receptor on human activated T cells in rheumatoid arthritis. *J. Clin. Invest.* 88:546–552.

Lalor, P. F., Clements, J. M., Pigott, R., Humphries, M. J., Spragg, J. H., and Nash, G. B. (1997) Association between receptor density, cellular activation, and transformation of adhesive behavior of flowing lymphocytes binding to VCAM-1. *Eur. J. Immunol.* 27:1422–1426.

Laudanna, C., Campbell, J. J., and Butcher, E. C. (1996) Role of Rho in chemoattractant-activated leukocyte adhesion through integrins. *Science* 271:981–983.

Li, X. C., Miyasaka, M., and Issekutz, T. B. (1998) Blood monocyte migration to acute lung inflammation involves both CD11/CD18 and very late activation antigen-4–dependent and independent pathways. *J. Immunol.* 161:6258–6264.

Lin, T. H., Rosales, C., Mondal, K., Bolen, J. B., Haskill, S., and Juliano, R. L. (1995) Integrin-mediated tyrosine phosphorylation and cytokine message induction in monocytic cells. A possible signaling role for the Syk tyrosine kinase. *J. Biol. Chem.* 270:16189–16197.

Lloyd, A. R., Oppenheim, J. J., Kelvin, D. J., and Taub, D. D. (1996) Chemokines regulate T-cell adherence to recombinant adhesion molecules and extracellular matrix proteins. *J. Immunol.* 156:932–938.

Luscinskas, F. W., Ding, H., and Lichtman, A. H. (1995) P-selectin and vascular cell adhesion molecule 1 mediate rolling and arrest, respectively, of CD4+ T lymphocytes on tumor necrosis factor alpha-activated vascular endothelium under flow. *J. Exp. Med.* 181:1179–1186.

MacKenzie, W. M., Hoskin, D. W., and Blay, J. (1999) The adhesion of anti-CD3–activated mouse T cells to syngeneic colon adenocarcinoma cells is differentially regulated by protein tyrosine kinase-, protein kinase C-, and cAMP-dependent pathways in the effector cell. *Biochem. Biophys. Res. Commun.* 255:460–465.

Maguire, J. E., Danahey, K. M., Burkly, L. C., and van Seventer, G. A. (1995) T cell receptor- and β_1 integrin-mediated signals synergize to induce tyrosine phosphorylation of focal adhesion kinase (pp125FAK) in human T cells. *J. Exp. Med.* 182:2079–2090.

Mainiero, F., Gismondi, A., Soriani, A., Cipitelli, M., Palmiero, G., Jacobelli, J., Piccoli, M., Frati, L., and Santoni, A. (1998) Integrin-mediated Ras-extracellular regulated kinase (ERK) signaling regulates interferon γ production in human natural killer cells. *J. Exp. Med.* 188:1267–1275.

Mannion, B. A., Berditchevski, F., Kraeft, S. K., Chen, L. B., and Hemler, M. E. (1996) Transmembrane-4 superfamily proteins CD81 (TAPA-1), CD82, CD63, and CD53 specifically associated with integrin $\alpha_4\beta_1$ (CD49d/CD29). *J. Immunol.* 157:2039–2047.

Marui, N., Offermann, M. K., Swerlick, R., Kunsch, C., Rosen, C. A., Ahmad, M., Alexander, R. W., and Medford, R. M. (1993) Vascular cell adhesion molecule-1 (VCAM-1) gene transcription and expression are regulated through an antioxidant-sensitive mechanism in human vascular endothelial cells. *J. Clin. Invest.* 92:1866–1874.

Masinovsky, B., Urdal, D., and Gallatin, W. M. (1990) IL-4 acts synergistically with IL-1β to promote lymphocyte adhesion to microvascular endothelium by induction of vascular cell adhesion molecule-1. *J. Immunol.* 145:2886–2895.

McCarthy, J. B., Vachhani, B. V., Wahl, S. M., Finbloom, D. S., and Feldman, G. M. (1997). Human monocyte binding to fibronectin enhances IFN-gamma-induced early signaling events. *J. Immunol.* 159:2424–2430.

McGilvray, I. D., Lu, Z., Bitar, R., Dackiw, A.P.B., Davreux, C. J., and Rotstein, O. D. (1997). VLA-4 integrin cross-linking on human monocytic THP-1 cells induces tissue factor expression by a mechanism involving mitogen-activated protein kinase. *J. Biol. Chem.* 272:10287–10294.

Meerschaert, J., and Furie, M. B. (1995). The adhesion molecules used by monocytes for migration across endothelium include CD11a/CD18, CD11b/CD18, and VLA-4 on monocytes and ICAM-1, VCAM-1, and other ligands on endothelium. *J. Immunol.* 154:4099–5112.

Middleton, J., Neil, S., Wintle, J., Clark-Lewis, I., Moore, H., Lam, C., Auer, M., Hub, E., and

Rot, A. (1997). Transcytosis and surface presentation of IL-8 by venular endothelial cells. *Cell* 91:385–395.

Miyake, K., Medina, K., Ishihara, K., Kimoto, M., Auerbach, R., and Kincade, P. W. (1991a) A VCAM-like adhesion molecule on murine bone marrow stromal cells mediates binding of lymphocyte precursors in culture. *J. Cell Biol.* 114:557–565.

Miyake, K., Weissman, I. L., Greenberger, J. S., and Kincade, P. W. (1991b) Evidence for a role of the integrin VLA-4 in lympho-hemopoiesis. *J. Exp. Med.* 173:599–607.

Mould, A. P., and Humphries, M. J. (1991) Identification of a novel recognition sequence for the integrin α4β1 in the COOH-terminal heparin-binding domain of fibronectin. *EMBO J.* 10:4089–4095.

Mould, A. P., Komoriya, A., Yamada, K. M., and Humphries, M. J. (1991) The CS5 peptide is a second site in the IIICS region of fibronectin recognized by the integrin $\alpha_4\beta_1$. Inhibition of $\alpha_4\beta_1$ function by RGD peptide homologues. *J. Biol. Chem.* 266:3579–3585.

Moy, P., Lobb, R., Tizard, R., Olson, D., and Hession, C. (1993) Cloning of an inflammation-specific phosphatidyl inositol-linked form of murine vascular cell adhesion molecule-1. *J. Biol. Chem.* 268:8835–8841.

Murase, T., Kume, N., Hase, T., Shibuya, Y., Nishizawa, Y., Tokimitsu, I., and Kita, T. (1999) Gallates inhibit cytokine-induced nuclear translocation of NF-kappaB and expression of leukocyte adhesion molecules in vascular endothelial cells. *Arterioscl. Thromb. Vasc. Biol.* 19:1412–1420.

Neish, A. S., Williams, A. J., Palmer, H. J., Whitley, M. Z., and Collins, T. (1992) Functional analysis of the human vascular cell adhesion molecule 1 promoter. *J. Exp. Med.* 176:1583–1593.

Neish, A. S., Khachigian, L. M., Park, A., Baichwal, V. R., and Collins, T. (1995a) Sp1 is a component of the cytokine-inducible enhancer in the promoter of vascular cell adhesion molecule-1. *J. Biol. Chem.* 270:28903–28909.

Neish, A. S., Read, M. A., Thanos, D., Pine, R., Maniatis, T., and Collins, T. (1995b) Endothelial interferon regulatory factor 1 cooperates with NF-kappa B as a transcriptional activator of vascular cell adhesion molecule 1. *Mol. Cell. Biol.* 15:2558–2569.

Neuhaus, H., Hu, M.C.T., Hemler, M. E., Takada, Y., Holzmann, B., and Weissman, I. L. (1991) Cloning and expression of cDNAs for the α subunit of the murine lymphocyte-Peyer's patch adhesion molecule. *J. Cell Biol.* 4:1149–1158.

Nojima, Y., Humphries, M. J., Mould, A. P., Komoriya, A., Yamada, K. M., Schlossman, S. F., and Morimoto, C. (1990) VLA-4 mediates CD3-dependent CD4+ T-cell activation via the CS1 alternatively spliced domain of fibronectin. *J. Exp. Med.* 172:1185–1192.

Nojima, Y., Tachibana, K., Sato, T., Schlossman, S. F., and Morimoto, C. (1995) Focal adhesion kinase (pp125FAK) is tyrosine phosphorylated after engagement of $\alpha_4\beta_1$ and $\alpha_5\beta_1$ integrins on human T-lymphoblastic cells. *Cell. Immunol.* 161:8–13.

Osborn, L., Hession, C., Tizard, R., Vassallo, C., Luhowskyj, S., Chi-Rosso, G., and Lobb, R. (1989) Direct expression cloning of vascular cell adhesion molecule 1, a cytokine-induced endothelial protein that binds to lymphocytes. *Cell* 59:1203–1211.

Osborn, L., Vassallo, C., Browning, B. G., Tizard, R., Haskard, D. O., Benjamin, C. D., Dougas, I., and Kirchhausen, T. (1994) Arrangement of domains, and amino acid residues required for binding of vascular cell adhesion molecule-1 to its counter-receptor VLA-4 ($\alpha_4\beta_1$). *J. Cell Biol.* 124:601–608.

Otey, C. A., Pavalko, F. M., and Burridge, K. (1990) An interaction between α-actinin and the β1 integrin subunit in vitro. *J. Cell Biol.* 111:721–729.

Papayannopoulou, T., and Nakamoto, B. (1993) Peripheralization of hemopoietic progenitors in primates treated with anti-VLA4 integrin. *Proc. Natl. Acad. Sci. USA* 90:9374–9378.

Papayannopoulou, Th., Priestley, G., Scott, L., Cybulsky, M. I. and Nakamoto, B. (1998) Role of VCAM-1 in mobilization and in homing of hematopoietic progenitor cells (HPC): distinct features. *Blood* 92 (suppl. 1):152a.

Picker, L. J., Terstappen, L. W., Rott, L. S., Streeter, P. R., Stein, H., and Butcher, E. C. (1990) Differential expression of homing-associated adhesion molecules by T-cell subsets in man. *J. Immunol.* 145:3247–3255.

Pober, J. S., and Cotran, R. S. (1990) Cytokines and endothelial cell biology. *Physiol. Rev.* 70:427–451.

Polte, T., Newman, W., Raghunathan, G., and Gopal, T. V. (1991) Structural and functional studies of full-length vascular cell adhesion molecule-1: internal duplication and homology to several adhesion proteins. *DNA & Cell Biol.* 10:349–357.

Read, M. A., Neish, A. S., Luscinskas, F. W., Palombella, V. J., Maniatis, T., and Collins, T. (1995) The proteasome pathway is required for cytokine-induced endothelial–leukocyte adhesion molecule expression. *Immun.* 2:493–506.

Reinhardt, P. H., Elliott, J. F., and Kubes, P. (1997a) Neutrophils can adhere via $\alpha 4\beta 1$-integrin under flow conditions. *Blood* 89:3837–3846.

Reinhardt, P. H., Ward, C. A., Giles, W. R., and Kubes, P. (1997b) Emigrated rat neutrophils adhere to cardiac myocytes via $\alpha 4$ integrin. *Circ. Res.* 81:196–201.

Ricard, I., Payet, M. D., and Dupuis, G. (1997) Clustering the adhesion molecules VLA-4 (CD49d/CD29) in Jurkat cells or VCAM-1 (CD106) in endothelial cells activates the phosphoinositide pathway and triggers Ca^{2+} mobilization. *Eur. J. Immunol.* 27:1530–1538.

Rice, G. E., and Bevilacqua, M. P. (1989) An inducible endothelial cell surface glycoprotein mediates melanoma adhesion. *Science* 246:1303–1306.

Rice, G. E., Munro, J. M., Corless, C., and Bevilacqua, M. P. (1991) Vascular and nonvascular expression of INCAM-110. A target for mononuclear leukocyte adhesion in normal and inflamed human tissues. *Am. J. Pathol.* 138:385–393.

Rich, I. N., Brackmann, I., Worthington-White, D., and Dewey, M. J. (1998) Activation of the sodium/hydrogen exchanger via the fibronectin–integrin pathway results in hematopoietic stimulation. *J. Cell. Physiol.* 177:109–122.

Rosen, G. D., Birkenmeier, T. M., and Dean, D. C. (1991) Characterization of the $\alpha 4$ integrin gene promoter. *Proc. Natl. Acad. Sci. USA* 68:4094–4098.

Rosen, G. D., Sanes, J. R., LaChance, R., Cunningham, J. M., Roman, J., and Dean, D. C. (1992) Roles for the integrin VLA-4 and its counter receptor VCAM-1 in myogenesis. *Cell* 69:1107–1119.

Sawada, M., Nagamine, J., Takeda, K., Utsumi, K., Kosugi, A., Tatsumi, Y., Hamaoka, T., Miyake, K., Nakajima, K., Watanabe, T., et al. (1992) Expression of VLA-4 on thymocytes: maturation stage-associated transition and its correlation with their capacity to adhere to thymic stromal cells. *J. Immunol.* 149:3517–3524.

Schlaepfer, D. D., and Hunter, T. (1998) Integrin signalling and tyrosine phophorlyation: just the FAKs? *Trends Cell Biol.* 8:151–157.

Schmidt, A. M., Hori, O., Cao, R., Yan, S. D., Brett, J., Wautier, J. L., Ogawa, S., Kuwabara, K., Matsumoto, M., and Stern, D. (1996) RAGE: a novel cellular receptor for advanced glycation end products. *Diabetes* 45:S77–80.

Schweighoffer, T., Tanaka, Y., Tidswell, M., Erle, D. J., Horgan, K. J., Ginther Luce, G. E., Lazarovits, A. I., Buck, D., and Shaw, S. (1993) Selective expression of integrin $\alpha_4\beta_7$ on a subset of human CD4+ memory T cells with hallmark of gut-tropism. *J. Immunol.* 151:717–729.

Shibayama, H., Anzai, N., Braun, S. E., Fukuda, S., Mantel, C., and Broxmeyer, H. E. (1999) H-Ras is involved in the inside-out signaling pathway of interleukin-3-induced integrin activation. *Blood* 93:1540–1548.

Shimizu, Y., van Seventer, G. A., Horgan, K. J., and Shaw, S. (1990) Costimulation of proliferative responses of resting CD4+ T cells by the interaction of VLA-4 and VLA-5 with fibronectin or VLA-6 with laminin. *J. Immunol.* 145:59–67.

Simmons, P. J., Masinovsky, B., Longenecker, B. M., Berenson, R., Torok-Storb, and Gallatin, W. M. (1992) Vascular cell adhesion molecule-1 expressed by bone marrow stromal cells mediates the binding of hematopoietic progenitor cells. *Blood* 80:388–395.

Spiecker, M., Peng, H. B., and Liao, J. K. (1997) Inhibition of endothelial vascular cell adhesion molecule-1 expression by nitric oxide involves the induction and nuclear translocation of IkappaBalpha. *J. Biol. Chem.* 272:30969–30974.

Springer, T. A. (1994) Traffic signals for lymphocyte recirculation and leukocyte emigration: the multistep paradigm. *Cell* 76:301–314.

Sung, K.-L. P., Yang, L., Elices, M., Jin, G., Sriramarao, P., and Broide, D. H. (1997) Granulocyte–

macrophage colony-stimulating factor regulates the functional adhesive state of very late antigen-4 expressed by eosinophils. *J. Immunol.* 158:919–927.

Takada, Y., Elices, M. J., Crouse, C., and Hemler, M. E. (1989) The primary structure of the α4 subunit of VLA-4: homology to other integrins and a possible cell–cell adhesion function. *EMBO J* 8:1361–1368.

Tanaka, Y., Adams, D. H., Hubscher, S., Hirano, H., Siebenlist, U., and Shaw, S. (1993) T-cell adhesion induced by proteoglycan-immobilized cytokine MIP-1β. *Nature* 361:79–82.

Taooka, Y., Chen, J., Yednock, T., and Sheppard, D. (1999) The integrin α9β1 mediates adhesion to activated endothelial cells and transendothelial neutrophil migration through interaction with vascular cell adhesion molecule-1. *J. Cell Biol.* 145:413–420.

Teixido, J., Parker, C. M., and Kassner, P. D. (1992) Functional and structural analysis of VLA-4 integrin α4 subunit cleavage. *J. Biol. Chem.* 267:1786–1791.

Terry, R. W., Kwee, L., Levine, J. F., and Labow, M. A. (1993) Cytokine induction of an alternatively spliced murine vascular cell adhesion molecule (VCAM) mRNA encoding a glycosylphosphatidylinositol-anchored VCAM protein. *Proc. Natl. Acad. Sci. USA* 90:5919–5923.

Thornhill, M. H., and Haskard, D. O. (1990) IL-4 regulates endothelial cell activation by IL-1, tumor necrosis factor, or IFN-gamma. *J. Immunol.* 145:865–872.

Van der Vieren, M., Crowe, D. T., Hoekstra, D., Vazeux, R., Hoffman, P. A., Grayson, M. H., Bochner B. S., Gallatin, W. M., and Staunton, D. E. (1999) The leukocyte integrin α_Dβ_2 binds VCAM-1: evidence for a binding interface between I domain and VCAM-1. *J. Immunol.* 163:1984–1990.

van Seventer, G. A., Newman, W., Shimizu, Y., Nutman, T. B., Tanaka, Y., Horgan, K. J., Gopal, T. V., Ennis, E., O'Sullivan, D., Grey, H., et al. (1991) Analysis of T-cell stimulation by superantigen plus major histocompatibility complex class II molecules or by CD3 monoclonal antibody: costimulation by purified adhesion ligands VCAM-1, ICAM-1, but not ELAM-1. *J. Exp. Med.* 174:901–913.

Vonderheide, R. H., Tedder, T. F., Springer, T. A., and Staunton, D. E. (1994) Residues within a conserved amino acid motif of domains 1 and 4 of VCAM-1 are required for binding to VLA-4. *J. Cell Biol.* 125:215–222.

Weber, C., Erl, W., Pietsch, A., Strobel, M., Ziegler-Heitbrock, H. W., and Weber, P. C. (1994) Antioxidants inhibit monocyte adhesion by suppressing nuclear factor-kappa B mobilization and induction of vascular cell adhesion molecule-1 in endothelial cells stimulated to generate radicals. *Arterioscl. Thromb.* 14:1665–1673.

Weber, C., Kitayama, J., and Springer, T. A. (1996) Differential regulation of β1 and β2 integrin avidity by chemoattractants in eosinophils. *Proc. Natl. Acad. Sci. USA* 93:10939–10944.

Weismann, M., Guse, A. H., Sorokin, L., Broker, B., Frieser, M., Hallmann, R., and Mayr, G. W. (1997) Integrin-mediated intracellular Ca^{2+} signaling in Jurkat T lymphocytes. *J. Immunol.* 158:1618–1627.

Yang, J. T., Rayburn, H., and Hynes, R. O. (1995) Cell adhesion events mediated by α4 integrins are essential in placental and cardiac development. *Dev.* 121:549–560.

Yang, J. T., Rando, T. A., Mohler, W. A., Rayburn, H., Blau, H. M., and Hynes, R. O. (1996) Genetic analysis of α_4 integrin functions in the development of mouse skeletal muscle. *J. Cell Biol.* 135:829–835.

Yednock, T. A., Cannon, C., Vandevert, C., Goldbach, E. G., Shaw, G., Ellis, D. K., Liaw, C., Fritz, L. C., and Tanner, L. I. (1995) α_4β_1 Integrin-dependent cell adhesion is regulated by a low affinity receptor pool that is conformationally responsive to ligand. *J. Biol. Chem.* 270:28740–28750.

Yellin, M. J., Brett, J., Baum, D., Matsushima, A., Szabolcs, M., Stern, D., and Chess, L. (1995) Functional interactions of T cells with endothelial cells: the role of CD40L-CD40–mediated signals. *J. Exp. Med.* 182:1857–1864.

Yuan, Q., Austen, K. F., Friend, D. S., Heidtman, M., and Boyce, J. A. (1997) Human peripheral blood eosinophils express a functional c-kit receptor for stem cell factor that stimulates very late antigen 4 (VLA-4)-mediated cell adhesion to fibronectin and vascular cell adhesion molecule 1 (VCAM-1). *J. Exp. Med.* 186:313–323.

Yurochko, A. D., Liu, D. Y., Eierman, D., and Haskill, S. (1992) Integrins as a primary signal transduction molecule regulating monocyte immediate-early gene induction *Proc. Natl. Acad. Sci. USA* 89:9034–9038.

Zell, T., Hunt, S. W., III, Mobley, J. L., Finkelstein, L. D., and Shimizu, Y. (1996) CD28-mediated up-regulation of β_1-integrin adhesion involves phosphatidylinositol 3-kinase. *J. Immunol.* 156: 883–886.

Zhang, Z., Vekemans, S., and Aly, M. S. (1991) The gene for the $\alpha 4$ subunit of the VLA-4 integrin maps to chromosome 2q31-q32. *Blood* 78:2396–2399.

Zhang, Z., Vuori, K., Wang, H.-G., Reed, J. C., and Ruoslahti, E. (1996) Integrin activation by R-ras. *Cell* 85:61–69.

15

Soluble Leukocyte–Endothelial Adhesion Molecules

CHRISTOPHER D. BUCKLEY, DAVID H. ADAMS,
and DAVID L. SIMMONS

The leukocyte–endothelial interface is a dynamic place. There are dramatic, often whole-scale changes in the expression of cell surface molecules during the lifetime of these cells. This is particularly the case as their activation state changes, resulting in both the loss and acquisition of different cell surface receptors (Brown, 1997)

During the cellular response to developmental and pathogenic cues, cell surface proteins, receptors, ligands, and enzymes as well as the extracellular matrix are altered by pericellular proteolysis (Werb, 1997; Shapiro, 1998). Moreover, during leukocyte transendothelial migration, there is tight regulation of leukocyte adhesion and activation, resulting in the induction and loss of a number of cell surface adhesion receptors (Carlos and Harlan, 1994; Imhof and Dunon, 1995; Springer, 1995). How this refurbishment of the cell surface is regulated has remained unclear until recently, but it has now emerged that integral membrane proteinases, known as *secretases* or *sheddases*, are involved in the cleavage and shedding of the ectodomains of these proteins from the cell surface (Hooper et al., 1997).

This shedding process is an ancient and conserved pathway, present from worms to humans, that plays a fundamental role in development, immunity, and disease pathology (Black and White, 1998; Werb and Yang, 1998). The demonstration that adhesion molecule expression is tightly regulated by proteolytic shedding, has caused a reappraisal of the function of soluble leukocyte–endothelial cell adhesion molecules in normal physiological responses, as well as during disease pathology. It now seems likely that the production of such soluble ectodomains does not just represent waste products: cleavage and shedding of membrane proteins not only alters the adhesive properties of cells, but also resets the signaling pathways in these cells and their neighbors (Werb, 1997).

What are Soluble Leukocyte–endothelial Cell Adhesion Molecules?

The ability to clone leukocyte and endothelial cell surface molecules has led to the isolation and cataloging of a large number of cell surface proteins that play important roles in interleukocyte and leukocyte–endothelial cell adhesion (Butcher and Picker, 1996; Brown, 1997; Buckley and Simmons, 1997). Fortunately, these proteins fall into a small number of discrete families with well-defined structural and functional features (Horwitz and Hunter, 1996).

Soon after these cell adhesion molecules were cloned, it became apparent that soluble isoforms could be detected both in vitro and in the circulation (Gearing and Newman, 1993). In most cases these soluble isoforms appear to be proteolytically processed extracellular domains; however, in some cases, for example, platelet–endothelial cell adhesion molecule-1 (PECAM-1; CD31), soluble isoforms consisting of the ectodomain linked directly to the cytoplasmic domain have been discovered (Goldberger et al., 1995). The distinction between primary adhesion receptors and primary signaling receptors is not always possible because some proteins are capable of mediating adhesion and activating signaling pathways. A particularly striking example is the cell surface-tethered chemokine fractalkine, which, in addition to its role as a soluble chemokine, can also mediate direct, integrin-independent leukocyte capture and firm adhesion (Bazan et al., 1997; Fong et al., 1998).

For the purposes of this chapter, we have restricted the discussion to well-defined adhesion receptors known to play a role in leukocyte–endothelial interactions (Table 15.1). Most of these fall into the selectin–selectin receptor and immuglobin super families (IgSF) but members of the syndecan, glipican, and other proteoglycan and sialoglycoprotein receptors such as CD44 and CD43 also exist in soluble forms (Bazil and Strominger, 1993; Crocker and Feizi, Suguri et al., 1996; Subramanian et al., Kato et al., 1998; Ostberg et al., 1998). In addition, adhesion receptors, which are also ectoenzymes (VAP-1, CD73; Airas et al., 1997 Kurkijarvi et al., 1998), have been found in soluble forms, as have members of the disintegrin and metalloprotease (ADAM) family (Wolfsberg et al., 1995).

Although endothelial cells are capable of laying down an extensive extracellular matrix, which is actively degraded and remolded during inflammation and repair, for the purposes of this chapter we will concentrate only on soluble cell–cell adhesion molecules known to be involved in leukocyte–endothelial interactions. Soluble extracellular matrix molecules can also modulate leukocyte and endothelial cell function, but we will not consider them further here. There are a number of excellent reviews that detail the role of soluble extracellular matrix molecules in regulating leukocyte and endothelial cell function (Basbaum and Werb, 1996; Gumbiner, 1996; Chapman, 1997; Werb, 1997; Boudreau and Bissell, 1998)

Table 15.1. Soluble Leukocyte–Endothelial Cell Adhesion Molecules

Receptor	Source	Function
L-selectin	leukocytes	rolling
P-selectin	endothelium	rolling
E-selectin	endothelium	rolling
PSGL-1/CLA	leukocytes	selectin ligand
GlyCAM-1	endothelium HEVs	selectin ligand
CD34	endothelium	
MadCAM	gut mucosal endothelium	rolling triggering
PECAM-1 (CD31)	leuko–endo	adhesion migration
ICAM-1	leuko–endo	adhesion
ICAM-2	leuko–endo	adhesion
ICAM-3	leukocytes	immune responses
VCAM-1	endothelium	rolling adhesion
L1	leukocytes	? adhesion
Syndecan (1–4)	leukocytes	adhesion ? signaling
CD44	leuko–endo	rolling adhesion
CD43	leukocyte	de-adhesion
VAP-1	leuko–endo	adhesion
CD73		ecto-enzyme

What is the Role of Soluble Cell Adhesion Molecules?

Many integral plasma membrane proteins are released from the lipid bilayer by proteolysis (Hooper et al., 1997). Although the physiological significance of this ectodomain shedding has remained unclear until recently, there are at least four ways in which shedding might modulate biological function. First, it may be a mechanism for the rapid down-regulation of proteins from the cell surface. Second, it may provide a soluble functional form of the protein that has properties identical with, or subtly different from, those of the membrane form. Third, it provides a potential mechanism by which cells can detach from other cells or the extracellular matrix. Finally, shed ligands may serve to regulate the biological activity of their receptors by acting as agonists or antagonists (Fig. 15.1).

Significant progress has been made toward characterizing the proteases responsible for releasing/shedding these proteins. The same family of proteases responsible for cleaving growth factor, cytokine, and other cell surface ligands and receptors is also responsible for the shedding of adhesion recep-

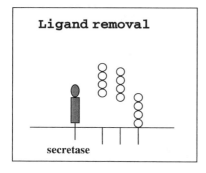

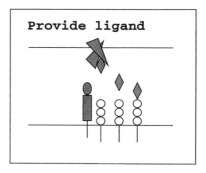

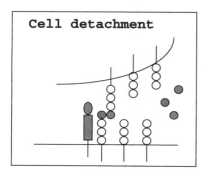

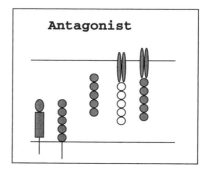

Fig. 15.1. Possible roles for soluble cell adhesion molecules (sCAMs): Proteolytic cleavage of cell adhesion molecules' ectodomains by secretases can potentially reomove ligands, provide ligands, antagonize ligand binding, or result in cell detachment.

tors, despite the fact that cleavage sites are often nonconserved (Hooper et al., 1997). Assessing the physiological significance of these soluble adhesion molecules (sCAMS) in vivo is difficult for two main reasons. First, the levels of sCAMs in blood may not be as meaningful as their concentrations within microenvironments. Second, it remains unclear whether sCAMs exist primarily as monomeric or multimeric species.

Whereas initial studies using immunoblotting and enzyme-linked immunosorbent assays (ELISAs) suggested that many sCAMs existed in monomeric forms, it has now become clear that it is more likely that the biologically relevant forms of sCAMs are dimeric. For example intercellular adhesion molecule-1 (ICAM-1) has been shown to exist in both its native membrane-bound and shed forms as a noncovalent dimer. Furthermore, only dimeric and not monomeric forms of ICAM-1 are able to bind LFA-1 with measurable affinity (Kd 8nM; Miller et al., 1995; Reilly et al., 1995). Studies using surface plasmon resonance, with other sCAMs, have shown that oligomerization or clustering of sCAMs is important in suppressing the net dissociation of sCAMs from their receptors. (Van der Merwe et al., 1993).

Soluble CAMs as Decoy and Signaling Receptors

There are two possible ways in which circulating adhesion molecules may have physiological effects on cell signaling: one is by competing for cell–cell interactions by acting as a decoy receptor; the other is by triggering a response in a ligand-bearing cell. Given the wide range of functions regulated by leukocyte–endothelial cell adhesion molecules such as leukocyte homing, migration, and costimulation, it is not surprising that examples exist of sCAMs acting as decoys as well as signaling receptors. Most sCAMS are produced by proteolytic cleavage at sites very close to the cell membrane. However, in some cases cleavage at or near the ligand-binding site has been shown to abolish binding, as in the case of the P-selectin ligand PSGL-1 (De Luca et al., 1995).

The sCAMs produced by proteolysis are often functional, retaining the ability to bind both ligand–receptor and antibodies. Soluble-ICAM-1, sVCAM-1, and sE- and sP-selectin are able to support cell adhesion (Rothlein et al., 1991; Dunlop et al., 1992; Newman et al., 1993; Wellicome et al., 1993), and sL-selectin inhibits lymphocyte binding to endothelium (Schleiffenbaum et al., 1992). In addition, sICAM-1 has been shown to block the in vitro proliferation of T cells from patients with insulin-dependent diabetes mellitus in response to an islet cell autoantigen. The ability to retain ligand binding after shedding may be particularly important for those molecules, such as ICAM-1, that are used as portals of entry for pathogens such as *P falciparum* and rhinovirus. The shedding of cell surface ICAM-1 may have a dual role, not only reducing the cell surface receptor through which the pathogen gains entry, but also providing a soluble receptor to bind and neutralize circulating pathogens (Greve et al., 1989; Staunton et al., 1992; Martin et al., 1993; Simmons, 1995).

Role of sCAMs in the Regulation of Cell Migration and Angiogenesis— Cross-Talk Between Adhesion Receptors

Cell adhesion mechanisms play an important role during cell migration (Gumbiner, 1996) and angiogenesis (Hanahan and Folkman 1996; Stromblad and Cheresh, 1996). Whether sCAMs are involved in these processes in vivo remains unclear. However, studies using soluble recombinant E-selectin and VCAM-1 have demonstrated that these sCAMs can act as potent angiogenic factors (Koch et al., 1995). In addition, a soluble form of PECAM-1 (CD31) has been shown to inhibit leukocyte transendothelial migration in vitro (Liao et al., 1997). Although not strictly relevant to leukocyte–endothelial interactions, the best examples of how sCAMs regulate cell migration and guidance have come from studies of axon and neurite outgrowths, which are dramatically affected by sCAMs such as neural cell adhesion molecule (NCAM-1) and N-cadherin (Fields and Itoh, 1996; Tessier-Lavigne and Goodman, 1996).

In addition to their possible role in modulating cell motility, a new and as yet largely unexplored role of sCAMs relates to the ability of many cell-adhesion receptors to converse with each other via cis-interactions within the plane of the same cell membrane (Buckley and Simmons, 1997). In the case of integrins, it is now clear that as well as interacting with molecules on neighboring cells, integrins can form associations with a wide variety of other receptors expressed on the same cell, forming large multireceptor complexes. For example $\alpha_v\beta_3$ can associate with growth factor receptors, the matrix metalloproteinase MMP-2, as well as the glycoslyphosphatidylinositol (GPI)-linked recptor, uPAR (Porter and Hogg, 1998). Some integrins such as $\alpha_4\beta_1$ have been shown to associate with members of the transmembrane-4 superfamily (TM4SF) via residues on the extracellular divalent cation-binding region of the integrin (Hemler, 1998). This opens the possibility that sIg-CAMs binding to their integrin receptors might be able to regulate these cis-interactions and thereby modulate cell function.

In some cases, proteolysis of extracellular matrix (ECM) and shedding of ectodomains may release cryptic epitopes with different biological activities. For example, once cleaved, ECM fragments may bind to different integrins and mediate distinct functions compared to native, mature matrix. Proteolytic cleavage of laminin-5 by MMP-2 exposes a promigratory site on laminin-5 that triggers integrin-mediated cell motility (Gianelli et al., 1997). In addition, shedding the ectodoamin of syndecan-1 converts it from a fibroblast growth factor co-receptor into a potent inhibitor of FGF-2 (Kato et al., 1998). Both these examples show that in addition to providing growth factor ligands that regulate cell proliferation and survival, cell surface shedding can also down-regulate ligands and therefore modulate cell behavior in a manner remarkably similar to the TNF/NGF death receptor superfamily (Orlinick and Chao, 1998).

Soluble Cell Adhesion Molecules with Enzymatic Activity

An intriguing complication of the role of sCAMs has come from the recent observations that two endothelial CAMs, VAP-1 and CD73, both have specific enzyme activity that is preserved in the soluble form and can modulate their adhesive function. Vascular adhesion protein-1 (VAP-1) is a 170 kD homodimeric transmembrane glycoprotein that is largely confined to high endothelial venules (HEV) of lymph nodes and hepatic endothelium where it mediates tissue-selective lymphocyte adhesion in a sialic acid-dependent manner. It is induced at other sites including the gut, skin, and joints during inflammation. Soluble VAP-1 can be detected in serum as a dimer with the same molecular weight as the transmembrane form, and like the transmembrane form, sVAP-1 is also heavily sialidated. Soluble VAP-1 is probably derived from the transmembrane form by proteolytic cleaving close to the cell membrane (Salmi and Jalkanen, 1997).

The recent finding that VAP-1 is a semicarbazide-sensitive monoamine oxidase (SSAO) was unexpected. Recent unpublished studies suggest that sVAP-1 accounts for most if not all of the MAO activity in serum. The physiological role of sVAP-1 may be to regulate leukocyte–endothelial interactions, and it probably does this in a complex manner rather than by simple competition with the membrane-bound form. Evidence that the relationship is complex comes from studies in which sVAP-1 was added to VAP-1–dependent adhesion assays. Rather than inhibiting adhesion, the soluble molecule appeared to increase adhesion further, presumably by activating other adhesion molecules. How this mechanism operates and whether it is related to the enzymatic activity of sVAP-1 remain to be determined.

Another adhesion molecule with intrinsic enzymatic activity is CD73, which is a 5'-nucleotidase that catalyses the dephosphorylation of purine and pyrimidine ribo- and deoxyribonucleoside monophosphates to their corresponding nucleosides. This function of CD73 may be important for the conversion of adenosine monophosphate (AMP) to adenosine, which is then available as a substrate or ligand for cell surface adenosine receptors. CD73 is expressed on both lymphocytes and endothelium, and mediates binding between B cells and follicular dendritic cells as well as between lymphocytes and endothelium. It is rapidly shed from the cell surface of lymphocytes after monoclonal antibody (mAb) engagement, but not from endothelial cells where it appears to be internalized. The relevance of the enzymatic activity to adhesion is unclear at present. Neither the ability of CD73 to act as a costimulatory molecule, nor its adhesive function are affected by inhibiting the 5' nucleotidase activity (Salmi and Jalkanen, 1997).

How Are sCAMs Produced and How Is Production Regulated?

The major enzymes that degrade extracellular matrix and cell surface proteins are the matrix metalloproteinases (MMPs), the adamolysin-related proteinases (ADAMs), and tissue serine proteinases such as tissue plasminogen activator (tPA), urokinase (uPA), and plasmin. It is thought that sCAMs are released from the cell surface either by secretion of specific isoforms or proteolytic cleavage near the membrane (Fig. 15.2). For example, alternative splicing of messenger RNA (mRNA) generates a soluble secreted form of P-selectin in plasma lacking the transmembrane domain (Dunlop et al., 1992). However, for L-selectin, a membrane-proximal cleavage site with a well-defined amino acid motif close to the plasma membrane results in rapid shedding from activated leukocytes (Schleiffenbaum et al., 1992; Kahn et al., 1994). The soluble forms of ICAM-1, ICAM-3, VCAM-1, and E-selectin all have sizes consistent with the absence of transmembrane and cytoplasmic domains. Because there is no current evidence of alternatively spliced mRNA for any of these molecules in humans, proteolytic cleavage seems more likely (Rothlein et al., 1991; Newman et al., 1993; Wellicome et al., 1993; del Pozo et al., 1994; Pino-Otin et al., 1995). A glycolipid-anchored splicing variant of mouse VCAM-1 has been identified that is shed by a mechanism independent of the one involved in the release of the transmembrane form (Hahne et al., 1994).

Despite nonconserved cleavage sites, most sCAMS appear to be released

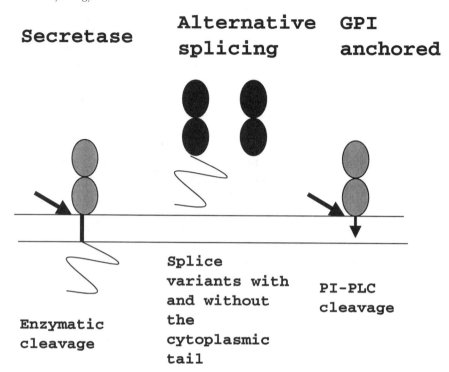

Secretase

Alternative splicing

GPI anchored

Enzymatic cleavage

Splice variants with and without the cytoplasmic tail

PI-PLC cleavage

Fig. 15.2. Principle pathways by which soluble cell adhesion molecules (sCAMs) are generated.

in a similar manner so that the bulk of the protein is released, often in a functional form (Hooper et al., 1997). In the majority of cases it is likely that cleavage occurs at a single, unique site defined both by the specificity of the secretase and the topology of the protein substrate with steric access to a stalk region close to the membrane surface being an important determining factor (Fig. 15.3).

One of the best-understood examples of sCAM shedding is L-selectin shedding. The biophysical properties of L-selectin–receptor bond formation allows it to capture leukocytes from flowing blood and roll on endothelium prior to activation (Alon et al., 1995). Recent studies have shown that this rolling phase is crucial to allow leukocytes to integrate chemoattractant signals from the endothelial surface prior to firm adhesion (Jung et al., 1998). It has been suggested that the rapid loss of L-selectin allows leukocytes to de-adhere from the luminal surface and start migrating under the endothelium (Kishimoto et al., 1989; Kahn et al., 1998).

The stimuli that induce shedding of L-selectin are varied, but, in general, relate to cell activation. For example, chemotactic factors such as IL-8 and fMLP, TNF-α, PMA, and reagents that cross-link L-selectin all stimulate L-selectin release with slightly differing time courses. The site of cleavage

Release

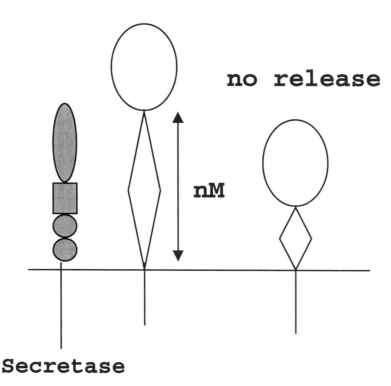

no release

nM

Secretase

Fig. 15.3. Selectivity of secretase action appears to be determined partly by the length of the membrane-proximal stalk region such that susceptiblity to cleavage depends on steric access of the secretase.

within L-selectin has been mapped to Lys 321–Ser 322, 11 amino acid residues distal to the membrane region (Kahn et al., 1994). Replacing the cleavage site in L-selectin with the corresponding sequence from E-selectin, which is not secreted, prevents L-selectin release; however, point mutations at the cleavage site did not significantly affect release (Migaki et al., 1995). Further studies have also shown that the length of the membrane-proximal region was critical because truncation of this region completely abolished cleavage (Chen et al., 1995). Together, these results suggest that the L-selectin secretase requires a minimum stalk length and may have a relaxed sequence specificity.

The secretase responsible for L-selectin shedding has been biochemically characterized using a number of protease inhibitors. Serine, metallo, and thiol protease inhibitors do not affect shedding. However, a hydroxaminic acid inhibitor blocks both the release of L-selectin and reduces neutrophil rolling velocity under conditions of hydrodynamic flow (Kahn et al., 1994;

Feehan et al., 1996; Walcheck et al., 1996). Further biochemical characterization suggests that L-selectin shedding is mediated by an enzyme with functional similarities to MMPs, but distinct from known MMPs.

Recent genetic studies have shown that one of the enzymes responsible for L-selectin shedding is the TNF-α convertase (TACE), a member of the ADAM family (ADAM 17; Peschon et al., 1998). In fact, this same MMP-disintegrin (TACE) is also responsible for the proteolytic cleavage of TGF-α. Despite the divergence in the structure, distribution, membrane topology, and cleaveage site sequence of TNF-α, TGF-α, and L-selectin, genetic studies in mice lacking TACE have pointed to an expanded role for ADAMs in ectodomain shedding in vivo (Black and White, 1998; Werb and Yang, 1998) The processing of L-selectin and probably many other sCAMs requires both the membrane-anchored enzyme (ADAM 17) and its substrate to be present in cis on the same cell (Preece et al., 1996). This presents a number of potential problems, particularly with regard to how the activity of the shedding enzyme (ADAM 17) is regulated in terms of specificity, location, and timing (Werb and Yang, 1998). So far, it appears that cytoskeletal interactions are required for the activation of ADAM 17 and coclustering of active ADAM with its substrate (Fig. 15.4). Although the activation of L-selectin shedding is both rapid and complete, for most processing there appears to be a basal level of ectodomain shedding. This finding and the phenotype of the TACE-null mice suggests that shedding of ectodomains may be necessary to provide paracrine growth and survival factors, for example, TGF-α, as well as to remove ligands such as L-selectin from leukocytes (Fig. 15.1).

The natural physiological activators of ADAMs remain to be elucidated. Upon treatment with PMA, ADAMs are brought together, leading to autocatalytic activation that can have different consequences depending on whether the cell is adherent or not. Adherent cells may be induced to detach from processed ligands, whereas the same mechanism can promote cell attachment as demonstrated by the ability of the disintegrin domains of ADAM 15 to bind to integrins $\alpha_v\beta_3$ and $\alpha_5\beta_1$ (Nath et al., 1999). The different responses of adherent and nonadherent cells to PMA may reflect differential effects on ADAM activation in adherent and nonadherent cells.

As well as being affected by the state of activation or adherence of the cell, shedding of CAMs can differ among different cell types. This is best illustrated by CD73, the cell surface expression of which is regulated differently on lymphocytes and endothelium. On lymphocytes, CD73 is shed from the cell surface of metabolically active cells after ligand binding, whereas endothelial CD73 is not shed but can be internalized into cytoplasmic pools, where it can be reexpressed on the cell surface. Triggering of lymphocyte CD73 leads to changes in tyrosine phosphorylation of several intracellular proteins, whereas there are no demonstrable effects on signal transduction following engagement of endothelial CD73. These distinct responses are unlikely to be due to structural differences because the protein appears to be identical at the protein, mRNA, and cDNA levels in both cell types (Airas et al., 1997).

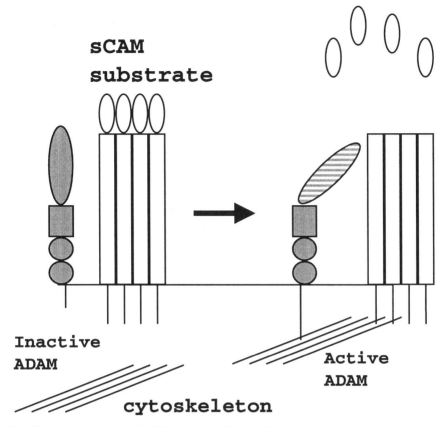

Fig. 15.4. Activation of (ADAMs; secretases) depends on cytoskeletal attachments and clustering of substrate within the same cell surface membrane (cis-interactions).

Applications of Soluble Cell Adhesion Molecules
Diagnostics—Clinical Markers of Disease Activity/Damage

There has been great interest in the measurement of sCAMs as indicators of disease activity in a wide variety of inflammatory and infectious diseases. Measurement of circulating sCAMS is increasing as ELISA kits become available, and in many cases, elevated levels of these sCAMs have been found to be associated with both disease activity and damage. In some cases, for example, the endothelial marker VCAM in renal graft rejection and ICAM-1 for coronary artery disease, show elevated levels prior to other clinical markers of activity or damage (Gearing and Newman, 1993; Wenzel et al., 1996).

The concept that measuring sCAMs may allow one to detect patients at risk before they develop clinical signs of disease is clearly exciting and has enormous potential implications for screening and early intervention in atherosclerosis. However, as with so many of the early studies reporting the use of sCAMs as disease markers, confirmation of specificity and sensitivity in larger studies is required before they can be considered for routine use. Several such large-scale studies are currently underway in patients at risk for atherosclerosis.

Only one sCAM has been shown to display a marked degree of disease specificity and that is VAP-1. A recent study has demonstrated that elevated serum levels of soluble VAP-1 are found almost exclusively in inflammatory liver disease (Kurkijarvi et al., 1998). Levels were not elevated in other inflammatory conditions including inflammatory bowel disease and rheumatoid arthritis. These findings are consistent with the distribution of VAP-1 in vivo, which under normal conditions is largely confined to the liver endothelial bed. Larger studies are required to determine whether this apparent tissue specificity is correct and whether levels of sVAP-1 have any prognostic use in liver disease.

Assessing the diagnostic or physiological significance of sCAMs in vivo is difficult because the average level in blood may not be as meaningful as the levels at the site of inflammation or in the rejecting organ. To illustrate this, a previous study has shown that levels of sICAM in serum were elevated in liver allograft rejection but lacked specificity, whereas elevated levels in bile (which comes directly from the rejecting liver) were highly specific (Adams et al., 1993). Similar findings have been reported in urinary sICAM-1 in renal transplantation. It remains unclear whether ELISA kits can distinguish between biologically active or inactive material, and whether these ELISAs distinguish between circulating free sCAMs and those bound to their counterligands (Gearing and Newman, 1993). In addition, as with other serum proteins, the levels in the blood reflect a balance among synthesis, release, and clearance.

Therapeutics—Treating Disease with Immunoadhesins

Fusion proteins that combine the constant region of an immunoglobulin (Fc region) with the ligand-binding region of an adhesion molecule or cytokine involved in immune reactions have been termed *immunoadhesins* (Ashkenazi and Chamow, 1997). Such constructs have proved to be immensely powerful in vitro tools for identifying unknown ligand receptors and for elucidating the molecular interactions regulating cell–cell interactions. However, these Fc-fusion proteins are likely to have different functional effects in vivo compared to soluble adhesion proteins, especially since they are multimeric, have a higher avidity, and may be cleared via different pathways compared to naturally occurring soluble proteins.

Recent studies have show that immunoadhesins are also powerful therapeutic agents capable of modulating autoimmune and inflammatory diseases because they have both exquisite target specificity and pharmacokinetic stability. For example, immunoadhesins based on the TNF receptor (TNFR) have been successfully used in both acute and chronic inflammatory models such as rheumatoid arthritis and experimental models of asthma (Lukacs et al., 1995; Gater et al., 1996) uveitis (Dick et al., 1996), and experimental allergic encephalomyelitis (EAE; Korner et al., 1995). Recently, long-term inhibition of chronic murine EAE has also been achieved with a CTLA-4Fc immunoadhesin (Cross et al., 1995). More dramatically, the combination of a CTLA-4 immunoadhesin and anti-CD40 antibody has been shown to lead to long-term acceptance of skin or cardiac allografts in mice (Larsen et al., 1996).

Both sVCAM-1 and sPECAM-1 exhibit biological activities in vivo: in the case of sVCAM-1, delaying the onset of diabetes in non obese diabetic (NOD) mice in an adoptive transfer model (Jakubowski et al., 1995); and in the case of PECAM-1, inhibiting leukocyte transmigration (Liao et al., 1997). In addition to their effects in inflammatory models, it is likely that other immunoadhesins based on cell adhesion molecules will be useful in other disease processes, for example, the entry of infectious agents such as viruses (sICAM-1), bacteria (sCD66), and parasites (sICAM-1) into cells (Staunton et al., 1992; Martin et al., 1993; Meyer et al., 1995). Immunoadhesins are also likely to play an emerging role in the treatment of cancer, both through the effects on metastatic spread and angiogenesis (Simmons, 1995; Hanahan and Folkman, 1996).

Structure–function Studies—Investigating Immune Function with Immunoadhesins

One obvious application of sCAMs is their use in structural studies. To date, site-directed mutagenesis studies in combination with crystal structures for ICAM-1, ICAM-2, VCAM, MadCAM, and E-selectin have revealed important short, linear motifs essential for their interaction with receptors (de-Fougerolles and Springer, 1995; Jones, 1996). Definition of these specificity residues is a key area for research to allow for the development of discriminatory peptide therapeutics targeted at either IgSF members or selectins (Buckley and Simmons, 1997).

Immunoadhesins are potent and specific blocking agents, and an increasing number of in vitro studies are taking advantage of their neutralizing activity to elucidate the role of sCAMs in complex biological systems. The best examples come from the TNFR/NGFR family, where an unexpected role for NGF in peripheral hypersensitivity to pain was demonstrated by blocking NGF action with an immunoadhesin based on its receptor trkA, a member of the trk family of tyrosine kinases (McMahon et al., 1995; Chamow and Ashkenazi, 1996).

Soluble CAMs have also proven to be very useful tools in delineating functional effects in autoimmune and inflammatory processes. The major limitation, which partly explains why immunoadhesins based on cytokines and their receptors have proven to be more useful so far, is that the affinity and association rates of monomeric adhesion ligands for their receptors are weak. We also remain relatively ignorant about the stoichiometry of the ligand–receptor interaction (Buckley et al., 1998). The use of multimeric sCAMs, perhaps as small membrane vesicles, may turn out to be one way around this obstacle, rather like the way that HLA-tetramers have revolutionized the study of T-cell receptor specificities (Ogg and McMichael, 1998).

Key Methods of Investigation and Measurement

The majority of studies on sCAMs have used ELISAs with biological fluid, such as serum or the conditioned media from cells grown in culture. Although these studies have been very informative, the use of specific inhibitors that block sCAM shedding and production has permitted the biochemical characterization of the enzymes involved in their production. Combined with the molecular characterization of the growing members of the MMP and ADAMolysins, it has now become clear that membrane protein secretases/sheddases/proteinases are vitally important in the regulation of ECM cell surface ecology (Werb, 1997). Genetic approaches (overexpression and deletion)in mice have confirmed the functional importance of these shedding mechanisms in many biological processes ranging from the regulation of cell development and death to neoplastic transformation, immunity, and signal transduction.

Proteolytic cleavage has turned out to be a useful strategy for regulating many biological processes as diverse as the coagulation cascade, complement activation, and the triggering of apoptosis through caspase activation. Many of the biochemical and molecular tools that have been successfully used to examine these pathways are likely to help elucidate the principles by which the wardrobe of leukocyte–endothelial cell surface adhesion molecules are changed and discarded.

References

Adams, D. H., Mainolfi, E., Elias, E., Neuberger, J. M., and Rothlein, R. (1993) Detection of circulating intercellular adhesion molecule-1 after liver transplantation: evidence of local release within the liver during graft rejection. *Transplantation* 55:83–87.

Airas, L., Salmi, M., Puurunen, T., Smith, D. J., and Jalkanen, S. (1997) Differential regulation and function of CD73, a GPI-linked 70Kda adheison molecule on lymphocytes and endothelium. *J. Cell. Biol.* 136:421–431.

Alon, R., Hammer, D. A., and Springer, T. A. (1995) Lifetime of the P-selectin-carbohydrate bond and its response to tensile force in hydrodynamic flow. *Nature* 374:539–542.

Ashkenazi, A., and Chamow, S. M. (1997) Immunoadhesins as research tools and therapeutic agents. *Curr. Opion. Rheumatol.* 9:195–200.

Basbaum, C. B., and Werb, Z. (1996) Focalized proteolysis: spatial and temporal regulation of extracellular matrix degradation at the cell surface. *Curr. Opin. Cell. Biol.* 8:731–738.

Bazan, J. F., Bacon, K. B., Hardiman, G., Wang, W., Soo, K., Rossi, D., Greaves, D. R., Zlotnik, A., and Schall, T. J. (1997) A new class of membrane-bound chmeokine with a CX_3C motif. *Nature* 385:640–644.

Bazil, V., and Strominger, J. L. (1993) CD43, the major sialoglycoprotein of human leukocytes, is proteolytically cleaved from the surface of stimulated lymphocytes and granulocytes. *Proc. Natl. Acad. Sci. USA* 90:3792–3796.

Black, A. B., and White, J. M. (1998) ADAMs: focus on the protease domain. *Curr. Opion. Cell. Biol.* 10:654–659.

Boudreau, N., and Bissell, M. J. (1998) Extracellular matrix signaling: integration of form and function in normal and malignant cells. *Curr. Opin. Cell Biol.* 10:640–646.

Brown, E. J. (1997) Adhesive interactions in the immune system. *Trends Cell Biol.* 7:289–295.

Buckley, C. D., Rainger, G. E., Bradfield, P. F., Nash, G. B., and Simmons, D. L. (1998) Cell adhesion: more than just glue (Review). *Mol. Membr. Biol.* 15:167–176.

Buckley, C. D., and Simmons, D. L. (1997) Cell adhesion: a new target for therapy. *Mol. Med. Today* 3:449–456.

Butcher, E. C., and Picker, L. J. (1996) Lymphocyte homing and homeostasis. *Science* 272:60–66.

Carlos, T. M., and Harlan, J. M. (1994) Leukocyte–endothelial adhesion molecules. *Blood* 84: 2068–2101.

Chamow, S. M., and Ashkenazi, A. (1996) Immunoadhesions: principles and applications. *Trends Biotechnol.* 14:52–60.

Chen, W., Knapp, W., Majdic, O., Stockinger, H., Bohmig, G., and Zlabinger, G. J. (1995) Co-ligation of CD31 and FcγRII induces cytokine production in human monocytes. *J. Immunol.* 152:3991–3997.

Chapman, H. A. (1997) Plasminogen activators, integrins, and the coordinated regulation of cell adhesion and migration. *Curr. Opin. Cell Biol.* 9:714–724.

Crocker, P. R., and Feizi, T. (1996) Carbohydrate recognition systems: functional triads in cell–cell interactions. *Curr. Opion. Struct. Biol.* 6:679–691.

Cross, A., Girard, T., Giacoletto, K., Evans, R., Keeling, R., Lin, R., Trotter, J., and Karr, R. (1995) Long-term inhibition of murine experimental autoimmune encephalomyelitis using CTLA-4-Fc supports a key role for CD28 costimulation. *J. Clin. Invest.* 95:2783–2789.

De Fougerolles, A., and Springer, T. A. (1995) Ideas crystallized in immunoglobulin superfamily–integrin interactions. *Chem. Biol.* 2:639–643.

De Luca, M., Dunlop, L. C., Andrews, R. K., Flannery, J. V., Jr., Ettling, R., Cumming, D. A., Veldman, G. M. and Berndt, M. C. (1995) A novel cobra venom metalloproteinase, mocar-hagin, cleaves a 10-amino acid peptide from the mature N terminus of P-selectin glycoprotein ligand receptor, PSGL-1 and abolishes P-selectin binding. *J. Biol. Chem.* 10:270:26734–26737.

del Pozo, M. A., Pulido, R., Munoz, C., (1994) Regulation of ICAM-3 (CD50) membrane expression on human neutrophils through a proteolytic shedding mechanism. *Eur. J. Immunol.* 24:2586–2594.

Dick, A., McMenamin, P. G., Korner, H., Scallon, B., Ghrayeb, J., Forrester, J., and Sedgwick, J. (1996) Inhibition of tumor necrosis factor activity minimizes target organ damage in experimental autoimmune uveoretinitis despite quantitatively normal activated T-cell traffic to the retina. *Eur. J. Immunol.* 26:1018–1025.

Dunlop, L. C., Skinner, M. P., and Bendall, L. J., et al. (1992) Characterization of GMP-140 (P-selectin) as a circulating plasma protein. *J. Exp. Med.* 175:1147–1150.

Feehan, C., Darlak, K., Kahn, J., Spatola, B.A.F., and Kishimoto, T. K. (1996) Shedding of the lymphocyte L-selectin adhesion molecule is inhibited by a hydroxamic acid-based protease inhibitor. Identification with an L-selectin-alkaline phosphatase reporter. *J. Biol. Chem.* 271: 7019–7024.

Fields, D., and Itoh, K. (1996) Neural cell adhesion molecules in activity-dependent development and synaptic plasticity. *Trends Neurosci.* 19:473–480.

Fong, A. M., Robinson, L. A., Steeber, D. A., Tedder, F. T., Yoshie, O., Toshio, I., and Patel, D. D. (1998) Fractaline and CX₃CR1 mediate a novel mechanism of leukocyte capture, firm adhesion and activation under physiologic flow. *J. Exp. Med.* 188:1413–1419.

Gater, P., Wasserman, M., Paciorek, P., and Renzetti, L. (1996) Inhibition of Sephadex-induced lung injury in the rat by Ro 45-2081, a tumour necrosis factor receptor fusion protein. *Am. J. Respir. Cell Mol. Biol.* 14:454–460.

Gearing, A.J.H., and Newman, W. (1993) Circulating adhesion molecules in disease. *Immunol. Today.* 14:506–512.

Giannelli, G., Falk-Marzillier, J., Schiraldi, O., Stetler-Stevenson, W. G., and Quaranta, V. (1997) Induction of cell migration by matrix metalloprotease-2 cleavage of laminin-5. *Science* 277: 225–228.

Goldberger, A., Middleton, K. A., Oliver, J. A., Paddock, C., Yan, H-C., DeLisser, H. M., Albelda, S. M., and Newman, P. J. (1994) Biosynthesis and processing of the cell adhesion molecule PECAM-1 includes production of a soluble form. *J. Biol. Chem.* 25:17183–17191.

Greve, J. M., Davis, G., Meyer, A. M., Forte, C. P., Yost, S. C., Marlor, C. W., Kamarck, M. E., and McClelland, A. (1989) The major human rhinovirus receptor is ICAM-1. *Cell* 56: 839–847.

Gumbiner, B. M. (1996) Cell adhesion: The molecular basis of tissue architecture and morphogenesis. *Cell* 84:345–357.

Hahne, M., Lenter, M., Jager, U., and Vestweber, D. (1994) A novel soluble form of mouse VCAM-1 is generated from a glycolipid-anchored splicing variant. *Eur. J. Immunol.* 24:421–428.

Hanahan, D., and Folkman, J. (1996) Patterns and emerging mechanisms of the angiogenic switch during tumorigenesis. *Cell* 86:353–364.

Hemler, M. E. (1998) Integrin associated proteins. *Curr. Opin. Cell Biol.* 10:578–585.

Hooper, N. M., Karran, E. H., and Turner, A. J. (1997) Membrane protein secretases. *Biochem. J.* 321:265–279.

Horwitz, A. F., and Hunter, T. (1996) Cell adhesion: integrating circuitry. *Cell Biol.* 6:460–461.

Imhof, B. A., and Dunon, D. (1995) Leukocyte migration and adhesion. *Adv. Immunol.* 58:345–415.

Jakubowski, A., Rosa, M. D., Bixler, S., Lobb, R., and Burkly, L. C. (1995) Vascular cell adhesion molecule-Ig fusion protein seletively targets activated α4-integrin receptors in vivo: inhibition of autoimmune diabetes in an adoptive transfer model in nonobese diabetic mice. *J. Immunol.* 155:938–946.

Jones Y. E. (1996) Three-dimensional structure of cell adhesion molecules. *Curr. Opin. Cell Biol.* 8:602–608.

Jung, U., Norman, K. E., Scharffetter-Kochanek, K., Beaudet, A. L., and Ley, K. (1998) Transit time of leukocytes rolling through venules controls cytokine-induced inflammatory cell recruitment in vivo. *J. Clin. Invest.* 102:1526–1533.

Kahn, J., Ingraham, R. H., Shirley, F., Migaki, G. I., and Kishimoto, T. K. (1994) Membrane proximal cleavage of L-selectin: identification of the cleavage site and a 6-kD transmembrane peptide fragment of L-selectin. *J. Cell Biol.* 125:461–470.

Kahn, J., Walcheck, B., Migaki, G. I., Jutila, M. A., and Kishimoto, T. K. (1998) Calmodulin regulates L-selectin adhesion molecule expression and function through a protease-dependent mechanism. *Cell* 92:809–818.

Kato, M., Wang, H., Kainulainen, V., Fitzgerald, M. L., Ledbetter, S., Ornitz, D. M., and Bernfield, M. (1998) Physiological degradation converts the soluble syndecan-1 ectodomain from an inhibitor to a potent activator of FGF-2. *Nat. Med.* 4:691–697.

Kishimoto, T. K., Jutila, M. A., Berg, E. L., and Butcher, E. C. (1989) Neutrophil Mac-1 and MEL-14 adhesion proteins inversely regulated by chemotactic factors. *Science* 245:1238–1241.

Koch, A. E., Halloran, M. M., Haskell, C. J., Shah, M. R., and Polverini, P. J. (1995) Angiogenesis mediated by soluble forms of E-selectin and vascular cell adhesion molecule-1. *Nature* 376: 517–519.

Korner, H., Goodsall, A., Lemckert, F., Scallon, B., Ghrayeb, J., Ford, A., and Sedgwick, J. (1995) Unimpaired autoreactive T-cell traffic within the central nervous system during tumor necrosis factor receptor-mediated inhibition of experimental autoimmune encephalomyelitis. *Proc. Natl. Acad. Sci.* 92:11066–11070.

Kurkijarvi, R., Adams, D. H., Leino, R., Mottonen, T., Jalkanen, S., and Salmi, M. (1998) Circulating form of human vascular adhesion protein-1 (VAP-1): increased serum levels in inflammatory liver diseases. *J. Immunol.* 161:1549–1557.

Larsen, C., Elwood, E., Alexander, D., Richie, S., Hendrix, R., Tucker-Burden, C., Cho, H., Aruffo, A., Hollenbaugh, D., and Lindsey, P. et al. (1996) Long-term acceptance of skin and cardiac allografts after blocking CD40 and CD28 pathways. *Nature*, 381:434–438.

Liao, F., Jahanara, A., Greene, T., and Muller, W. A. (1997) Soluble domain 1 of platelet–endothelial cell adhesion molecule (PECAM) is sufficient to block transendothelial migration in vitro and in vivo. *J. Exp. Med.* 185:1349–1357.

Lukacs, N., Strieter, R., Chensue, S., Widmer, M., and Kunkel, S. (1995) TNF-alpha mediates recruitment of neutrophils and eosinophils during airway inflammation. *J. Immunol.* 154: 5411–5417.

Martin, S., Casasnovas, J. M., Staunton, D. E., and Springer, T. A. (1993) Efficient neutralization and disruption of rhinovirus by chimeric ICAM-1/immunoglobulin molecules. *J. Virol.* 67: 3561–3568.

McMahon, S., Bennett, D., Priestley, J., and Shelton, D. (1995) The biological effects of endogenous nerve growth factor on adult sensory neurons revealed by a TrkA-IgG fusion molecule. *Nat. Med.* 1:774–780.

Meyer, D. M., Dustin, M. L., and Carron, C. P. (1995) Characterization of intercellular adhesion molecule-1 ectodomain (sICAM-1) as an inhibitor of lymphocyte function-associated molecule-1 interaction with ICAM-1. *J. Immunol.* 155:3578–3594.

Migaki, G. I., Kahn, J., and Kishimoto, T. K. (1995) Mutational analysis of the membrane-proximal cleavage site of L-selectin: relaxed sequence specificity surrounding the cleavage site. *J. Exp. Med.* 182:549–557.

Miller, J., Knorr, R., Ferrone, M., Houdei, R., Carron, C. P., and Dustin, M. L. (1995) Intercellular adhesion molecule-1 dimerization and its consequences for adhesion mediated by lymphocyte function associated-1. *J. Exp. Med.* 182:1231–1241.

Nath, D., Slocombe, P. M., Stephens, P. E., Warn, A., Hutchinson, G. R., Yamada, K. M., Docherty, A. J., and Murphy, G. (1999) Interaction of metargidin (ADAM-15) with $\alpha_v\beta_3$ and $\alpha_5\beta_1$ integrins on different haemopoietic cells. *J. Cell. Sci.* 112:579–587.

Newman, W., Beall, L. D., Carson, C. W., Hunder, G. G., Graben, N., Randhawa, Z. I., Gopal, T. V., Wiener-Kronish, J., and Matthay, M. A. (1993) Soluble E-selectin is found in supernatants of activated endothelial cells and is elevated in the serum of patients with septic shock. *J. Immunol.* 150:644–654.

Ogg G. S., and McMichael, A. J. (1998) HLA-peptide tetrameric complexes. *Curr. Opin. Immunol.* 10:393–396.

Orlinick, J. R., and Chao, M. V. (1998) TNF-related ligands and their receptors. *Cell Signal* 10: 543–551.

Ostberg, J. R., Barth, R. K., and Frelinger, J. G. (1998) The Roman god Janus: a paradigm for the function of CD43. *Immunol. Today* 19:12:456–450.

Peschon, J. J., Slack, J. L., Reddy, P., Stocking, K. L., Sunnarborg, S. W., Lee, D. C., Russell, W. E., Castner, B. J., Johnson, R. S., Fitzner, J. N., et al. (1998) An essential role for ectodomain shedding in mammalian development. *Science* 282:1281–1284.

Pino-Otin, M. R., Vinas, O., and de la Fuente, M. A., et al. (1995) Existence of a soluble form of CD50 (intercellular adhesion molecule-3) produced upon human lymphocyte activation. Present in normal human serum and levels are increased in the serum of systemic lupus erythematosus patients. *J. Immunol.* 154:33015–3023.

Porter, J. C., and Hogg, N. (1998) Integrins take partners: cross-talk between integrins and other membrane receptors. *Cell Biol.* 8:390–396.

Preece, G., Murphy, G., and Ager, A. (1996) Metalloproteinase-mediated regulation of L-selectin levels on leucocytes. *J. Biol. Chem.* 271:11 634–11640.

Reilly, P. L., Woska, J. R., Jr., Jeanfavre, D. D., McNally, E., Rothlein, R., and Bormann, B. J. (1995) The native structure of intercellular adhesion molecule-1 (ICAM-1) is a dimer. *J. Immunol.* 155:529–532.

Rothlein, R., Mainolfi, E. A., Czajkowski, M., and Marlin, S. D. (1991) A form of circulating ICAM-1 in human serum. *J. Immunol.* 147:3788–3793.

Salmi, M., and Jalkanen, S. (1997) How do lymphocytes know where to go: current concepts and enigmas of lymphocyte homing. *Adv. Immunol.* 64:139–218.

Schleiffenbaum, B. O., Spertini, O., and Tedder, T. F. (1992) Soluble L-selectin is present in human plasma at high levels and retains funtional activity. *J. Cell Biol.* 119:229–238.

Shapiro, S. D. (1998) Matrix metalloproteinase degradation of extracellular matric: biological consequences. *Curr. Opin. Cell Biol.* 10:602–608.

Simmons, D. L. (1995) The role of ICAM expression in immunity and disease. *Cancer Surveys, Cell Adhesion and Cancer* 24:141–155.

Springer, T. A. (1995) Traffic signals on endothelium for lymphocyte recirculation and leukocyte emigration. *Annu. Rev. Physiol.* 57:827–872.

Staunton D. E., Ockenhouse, C. F., and Springer, T. A. (1992) Soluble intercellular adhesion molecule-1–immunoglobulin G1 immunoadhesion mediates phagocytosis of malaria-infected erythrocytes. *J. Exp. Med.* 176:1471–1476.

Stromblad, S., and Cheresh, D. A. (1996) Cell adhesion and angiogenesis. *Trends Cell Biol.* 6:462–468.

Subramanian, S. V., Fitzgerald, M. L., Bernfield, M., et al. (1997) Regulated shedding of syndecan-1 and α_4 ectodomains by thrombin and growth factor receptor activation. *J. Biol. Chem.* 272:14712–14720.

Suguri, T., Kikuta, A., Iwagaki, H., Yoshino, T., Tanaka, N., Orita, K. (1996) Increased plasma GlyCAM-1, a mouse L-selectin ligand, in response to an inflammatory stimulus. *J. Leukoc. Biol.* 60:593–598.

Tessier-Lavigne, M., and Goodman, C. S. (1996) The molecular biology of axon guidance. *Science* 274:1123–1133.

Van der Merwe, P. A., Brown, M. H., Davis, S. J., and Barclay, A. N. (1993) Affinity and kinetic analysis of the interaction of the cell adhesion molecules rat CD2 and CD48. *EMBO J.* 12:4945–4954.

Walcheck, B., Kahn, J., Fisher, J. M., Wang, B. B., Fisk, R. S., Payan, D. G., Feehan, C., Betageri, R., Darlak, K., Spatola, A. F., and Kishimoto, T. K. (1996) Neutrophil rolling altered by inhibition of L-selectin shedding in vitro *Nature (Lond.)* 380:720–723.

Wellicome, S. M., Kapahi, P., Mason, J. C., Lebranchu, Y., Yarwood, H., and Haskard, D. O. (1993) Detection of a ciruculating form of vascular cell adhesion molecule-1: paired levels in rheumatoid arthritis and systemic lupus erythematosus. *Clin. Exp. Immunol.* 92:412–418.

Wenzel, K., Ernst, M., Rohde, K., Baumann, G., Speer, A. (1996) DNA polymorphisms in adhesion molecules genes—a new risk factor for early atherosclerosis *Hum. Genet.* 97:15–20.

Werb, Z. (1997) ECM and cell surface proteolysis: regulating cellular ecology. *Cell* 91:439–442.

Werb, Z., and Yang, Y. (1998) A cellular striptease act. *Science* 282:1279–1280.

Wolfsberg, T. G., Primakoff, P., Myles, D. G., and White, J. M. (1995) ADAM, a novel family of membrane proteins containing *a d*isintegrin *a*nd *m*etalloprotease domain: multipotential functions in cell–cell and cell–Matrix interactions. *J. Cell Biol.* 131:275–278.

16

Leukocyte Recruitment as Seen by Intravital Microscopy

KLAUS LEY

The term *leukocyte recruitment* encompasses all events that bring circulating leukocytes into inflamed tissues. Recruitment is thought to proceed in a cascade-like fashion (Ley, 1989; Butcher, 1991; Springer, 1995; Fig. 16.1). This cascade has many rocks, nooks, and dead-water zones because there are parallel pathways and many decision points along the way. In inflammation, neutrophils, eosinophils, monocytes, T-lymphocytes, and even basophils and B-lymphocytes can be recruited. Intravital microscopy is limited in its ability to distinguish leukocyte subpopulations. In most tissues and most models of inflammation, the neutrophil is the most prevalent cell. Therefore, this chapter uses neutrophil recruitment as an example to illustrate the determinants, parameters, models, and physiology of leukocyte recruitment.

Factors Determining Leukocyte Recruitment

Physiological parameters modulate and even determine successful leukocyte recruitment under in vivo conditions. Such parameters include fluid shear stress at the vessel wall, interactions of leukocytes with other blood elements, adhesion molecule expression, properties of the endothelium, regulatory mechanisms, and the availability of leukocytes as reflected by systemic leukocyte counts.

Wall Shear Stress

Leukocyte adhesion requires an initial binding event between the flowing leukocyte and the stationary endothelium, which is called *capture* or *tethering* (Lorant et al., 1993). The rate of flow is of critical importance in whether this initial interaction is successful. The rate of flow is the volume passing through a tube or blood vessel per unit of time, which is equal to the cross-sectional area multiplied by the average fluid velocity. Blood flow velocity can be measured in essentially all microvessels, and many excellent methods have been described (Wayland and Johnson, 1967; Intaglietta et al., 1970;

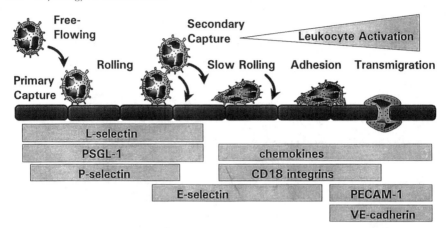

Fig.16.1. Leukocyte adhesion cascade (adapted from Jung et al, 1998a): Free-flowing leukocytes attach by primary or secondary capture and start to roll. During slow rolling, leukocytes are progressively activated (widening triangle) until they become adherent and transmigrate. L-selectin and P-selectin glycoprotein ligand-1 (PSGL-1) mediate primary and secondary capture and rolling. P-selectin mediates primary capture and rolling, but not secondary capture. E-selectin mediates slow rolling. CD18 integrins become increasingly important as leukocyte activation progresses. Chemokines and other chemoattractants activate rolling leukocytes and provide chemotactic gradients for transmigration. Platelet–endothelial cell adhesion molecule-1 (PECAM-1) and vascular endothelium (VE)–cadherin bonds between endothelial cells may have to release for transmigration to occur.

Baker and Wayland, 1974; Lipowsky and Zweifach, 1978; Tangelder et al., 1982; Pittman and Ellsworth, 1986; Pries, 1988). One of the oldest and still most popular ways to measure blood flow velocity is the dual-slit or optical Doppler method (Wayland and Johnson, 1967; Intaglietta et al., 1970; Baker and Wayland, 1974; Pittman and Ellsworth, 1986). The image of the microvessel is projected on two photodiodes that are aligned in the axis of the vessel and have a distance that corresponds to about one erythrocyte length in the projected image, or about 5μm. As a consequence of this arrangement, the downstream photodiode sees a light-and-dark pattern corresponding to the passing erythrocytes that is similar to, but delayed with respect to, that seen by the upstream photodiode. The two signals are multiplied with each other, and the upstream signal is incrementally delayed until the product reaches a maximum. This process of autotracking cross-correlation was first developed in the 1960s (Wayland and Johnson, 1967) and later implemented in commercial systems (Intaglietta et al., 1970). The velocity measured in this way is called the *centerline velocity*. It is higher than the average blood flow velocity because the flow velocity is higher in the center of the vessel than closer to the wall (Baker and Wayland, 1974; Lipowsky and Zweifach, 1978; Pittman and Ellsworth, 1986). Many theoretical and experimental studies have been devoted to determining the relationship between centerline and mean blood flow velocities. For most applications, the mean blood flow velocity is approximately equal to the centerline velocity divided by 1.6 (Baker and Wayland, 1974; Lipowsky and Zweifach, 1978; Pittman and Ellsworth, 1986).

Blood flow velocity and vessel diameter determine the wall shear rate, which is defined as the rate of change of the velocity near the vessel wall. The dimension of wall shear rate is therefore that of a velocity (mm/s) divided by a distance (mm), resulting in s^{-1}(Chien et al, 1984). The relation between blood flow velocity and wall shear rate is not simple in vivo. Many parameters, including the concentration of red blood cells (hematocrit), the vessel diameter, and the flow rate itself, influence the shape of the velocity profile. However, in microvessels between 20 and 40 μ in diameter, the wall shear rate can be estimated as approximately 17 multiplied by mean blood flow velocity divided by vessel diameter. This is based on empirical studies of velocity profiles in vivo (Reneman et al., 1992). In other vessels including capillaries and large vessels of the systemic circulation, this relationship must be modified (Chien et al., 1984).

Wall shear rate is directly related to the force that acts on the vessel wall. This force is usually normalized by the area over which it is applied, and is expressed as wall shear stress (Chien et al., 1984). Shear stress can be calculated from shear rate using the viscosity of the fluid in the area under consideration. Since blood-perfused vessels have a red cell-free area close to the vessel wall (Tangelder et al., 1982; Reneman et al., 1992), the wall shear stress in vivo can be calculated by multiplying the wall shear rate with plasma viscosity, which is about one centipoise, or 0.01 dyn.s/cm^2. Forces on adhering leukocytes in venules in vivo range between 10 piconewtons and 10 nanonewtons (10^{-11} to 10^{-8}newtons; House and Lipowsky, 1988), resulting from wall shear rates of less than 10 to more than 3000 s^{-1} (Damiano et al., 1996), and wall shear stresses of 0.01 to 3 pascals, (or 0.1 to 30 dyn/cm^{-2}). Although the force on each individual cell is exceedingly small, it is important to realize that these forces are balanced by the binding of one or a handful of adhesion molecules. In general, leukocyte adhesion and rolling are reduced with increasing wall shear stress (House and Lipowsky, 1988; Ley and Gaehtgens, 1991; Damiano et al., 1996). However, at least one class of adhesion molecules, the selectins, requires shear stress in order to support adhesion. The optimal shear stress for rolling adhesions mediated through L-selectin is about 0.8 dyn/cm^2, and for P-and E-selectin about 0.5 dyn/cm^2 (Finger et al., 1996; Lawrence et al., 1997).

Interactions with Other Blood Elements

Initial leukocyte adhesion or capture is promoted by the presence of red blood cells. Several phenomena including red cells pushing leukocytes to the vessel wall (Schmid-Schönbein et al., 1980), red cell aggregates occupying the center of the blood stream (Nobis et al., 1985), and hydrodynamic effects at confluent bifurcations (Bagge et al., 1983), contribute to a more efficient placement of free-flowing leukocytes next to the endothelium. Most of these mechanisms are operative in venules only, and thus contribute to preferential leukocyte adhesion in venules.

Leukocyte recruitment can also be amplified by free-flowing leukocytes interacting with already adherent leukocytes of the same or different type (Bargatze et al., 1994). This phenomenon is called *secondary capture* or *secondary tethering* (Alon et al., 1996) and requires L-selectin on the free-flowing leukocyte and L-selectin ligands on the adherent leukocytes (Bargatze et al., 1994; Alon et al, 1996). Although secondary capture does not appear to play an important role in neutrophil recruitment in acute inflammation (Kunkel et al., 1998), it may aid the recruitment of L-selectin positive leukocytes that cannot adhere to endothelial adhesion molecules, such as certain T-lymphocyte subsets. Because secondary capture was discovered in a large-bore perfusion system (Bargatze et al, 1994), it may be inferred that secondary capture could be involved in leukocyte recruitment in larger vessels, although this has not been investigated.

Platelets can also support leukocyte rolling (Buttrum et al., 1993) and adhesion (Zwaginga et al., 1999). Activated platelets express large amounts of P-selectin, which is crucial for initiating leukocyte–platelet interaction. Leukocyte–platelet adhesion is important for the recruitment of leukocytes into forming thrombi (Palabrica et al., 1992) and for leukocyte adhesion to areas of vascular injury (Zwaginga et al., 1999). In the microcirculation, platelets have also been observed to roll using a P-selectin–dependent mechanism (Frenette et al., 1995), but the physiological significance of this is not known. Activated platelets can bind to lymphocytes and direct their recruitment to secondary lymphatic organs (Diacovo et al., 1996), but activated platelets are normally not available in the circulation. However, platelet-dependent leukocyte recruitment could be significant in certain pathological conditions including sepsis, which can cause inappropriate activation of the hemostatic system. (chapter 20)

Adhesion Molecule Expression

The expression of the adhesion molecules relevant to inflammatory cell recruitment is exquisitely regulated at several levels, including transcription, translation, surface expression, proteolytic modification, glycosylation, sulfation, and conformational changes. Most known endothelial leukocyte adhesion molecules are preferentially or exclusively expressed on the venular endothelium (Klein et al., 1989; Fries et al., 1993; Gotsch et al., 1994; Jung and Ley, 1997). Adhesion molecule expression is the single most important determinant of leukocyte recruitment. Many of the mouse strains with null mutations in leukocyte–endothelial adhesion molecules have a defect in inflammatory cell recruitment. As examples, absence of P-selectin results in a lack of leukocyte rolling following acute tissue trauma (Mayadas et al., 1993), and absence of CD18 integrins results in an inability of rolling leukocytes to become firmly adherent (Scharffetter-Kochanek et al., 1998).

Properties of the Endothelium

Endothelial cells differ among organs (Gerritsen, 1987; Karasek, 1989) and, within one organ, among cells derived from arterioles, capillaries, or venules (Ley et al., 1992). In vivo, inflammatory adhesion molecules including P-selectin, E-selectin, intercellular adhesion molecule-1 (ICAM-1), and vascular cell adhesion molecule-1 (VCAM-1) are preferentially expressed on venular endothelium (Klein et al., 1989; Fries et al., 1993; Gotsch et al., 1994; Jung and Ley, 1997). In addition, the wall shear rate and hence wall shear stress is generally lower in venules than in arterioles of equal size (Zweifach and Lipowsky, 1984), which also tends to promote leukocyte adhesion in venules. Endothelial cells have other specializations like fenestrae, surface processes, a more cuboidal or more flattened phenotype, all of which may impact on leukocyte adhesion. Endothelial cells express and release pro- and anti-adhesive soluble factors, including interleukin-8 (Huber et al, 1991), prostacyclin (Grabowski et al., 1985), nitric oxide (Ignarro, 1990), and others. Regional and local differences in the secretion of such factors have not been explored systematically, but are likely to contribute to the ability of organs and tissues to recruit leukocytes in inflammation.

Systemic Leukocyte Counts

Leukocyte recruitment depends on the availability of circulating leukocytes (Fig. 16.2). In the presence of all inflammatory adhesion molecules and strong chemokines, no leukocyte recruitment will result when no circulating leukocytes are available. Even though this statement appears trivial, it is important, because many investigators have been misled into perceiving anti-inflammatory effects of certain interventions when in reality these interventions lowered the availability of circulating leukocytes. Under normal conditions, systemic leukocyte counts vary between about 3000 and 10 000 cells per microliter of blood. In a mouse with 8000 circulating leukocytes per microliter, about twice as many leukocytes roll and adhere in a postcapillary venule under otherwise equal inflammatory conditions than in a mouse with 4000 circulating leukocytes per microliter. This was experimentally shown by measuring the number of rolling leukocytes in many venules and many mice under similar conditions, and correlating the findings with systemic leukocyte counts (Ley et al., 1995a). The systemic leukocyte count is as stringent a predictor of rolling and adhesion as are blood flow velocity, microvessel diameter, and wall shear rate. Therefore, it is essential that the systemic leukocyte count is monitored in all experiments aimed at studying inflammation. Some mutant mice (Bullard et al., 1996; Frenette et al, 1996; Scharffetter-Kochanek et al., 1998) have very high systemic leukocyte counts. This is likely to impact leukocyte recruitment. It is not known whether leukocyte recruitment varies as a linear function of elevated leukocyte counts.

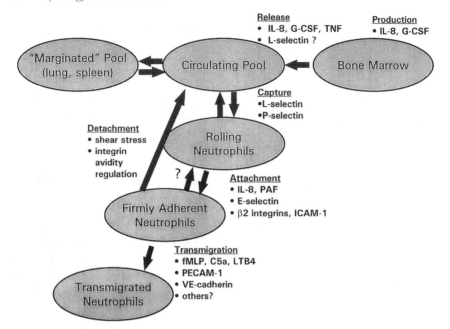

Fig.16.2. Model of neutrophil homeostasis: Successful recruitment of transmigrated neutrophils (bottom) requires many steps, starting with production in and release from the bone marrow (top right). The circulating pool of neutrophils is in dynamic equilibrium with a marginated pool. Some free-flowing leukocytes start to roll (rolling leukocyte flux fraction). Some detach, others become firmly adherent through slow rolling (adhesion efficiency). Some adherent neutrophils detach, others transmigrate. Major molecular and biomechanical factors indicated at each step.

Parameters of Leukocyte Rolling and Adhesion

It is impressive how leukocytes are invisible in the rapidly flowing blood of an intact arteriole; how they suddenly appear in capillaries where they may have to deform to negotiate vascular passages smaller than their own diameter (Bagge et al, 1980); how they cause a pileup of red blood cells behind them, called a *train*, as long as the vessel diameter is too small for the red cells to pass the leukocyte (Gaehtgens et al, 1984); how they start rolling immediately upon entering a postcapillary venule (Atherton and Born, 1972); how they deform while rolling (Damiano et al, 1996; Firrell and Lipowsky, 1989); how they become adherent in inflammation (Waller, 1846); and finally, how they transmigrate through the endothelium to reach the extravascular space (Metchnikoff, 1893). This brief description of the intravital microscopic observation of inflammation could have been given more than a century ago by Wagner, Virchow, Metchnikoff, or Cohnheim. However, in order to understand inflammation, these processes must be measured and described in quantitative terms. It is through these quantitative parameters that some of the functions of individual molecules can be understood.

Rolling Leukocyte Flux

Rolling leukocyte flux is defined as the number of rolling leukocytes per unit of time. It can easily be measured by counting the number of leukocytes rolling through a microvessel during 1 minute. This method takes advantage of the fortuitous fact that red blood cells usually travel too fast to be seen as individual cells at the shutter speed (1/60 sec) of common video cameras. It is simple and reasonably accurate in many, but not all, experimental situations. Table 16.1 lists several other parameters that have been proposed to characterize leukocyte rolling.

To identify rolling leukocytes precisely, a "critical velocity" can be defined, which separates the rolling from the free-flowing leukocytes (Ley and Gaehtgens, 1991). Experimentally, both types of leukocytes can be visualized by using stroboscopic epifluorescence microscopy (Ley and Gaehtgens, 1991). Since blood cell dimensions are of the same order of magnitude as the diameter of the microvessels through which they pass, the minimum or critical velocity a free-flowing leukocyte can assume in the absence of adhesive interactions is not zero (Gaehtgens et al, 1985). The minimum distance between the center of a blood cell and the vessel wall is dictated by the cell radius. The problem of a spherical particle (the leukocyte) flowing close to the wall of a blood vessel has been solved theoretically by Goldman et al. (1967). The value of calculated critical velocity depends on mean blood flow velocity, the cell-to-microvessel diameter ratio, and the clearance between the sphere and the wall. For a distance of 18 nanometers, which corresponds to the approximate length of some relevant adhesion molecules, the critical velocity can be estimated as the product of mean blood flow velocity and ε $(2 - \varepsilon)$, where ε is the ratio of leukocyte diameter to vessel diameter (Ley and Gaehtgens, 1991). This estimate of critical velocity is only an approximation, because leukocytes are not perfect spheres, the microvessel is not a smooth cylinder, the velocity profile is not parabolic, and experimental uncertainties exist in determining diameters and velocities. Nevertheless, the critical velocity estimated in this way separates rolling or transiently interacting (tethering) leukocytes remarkably well from freely flowing leukocytes. The concept of critical velocity is also applicable in the parallel plate flow chamber in vitro (Lawrence and Springer, 1991).

Leukocyte Rolling Velocity

Leukocyte rolling velocity is operationally defined as the distance traveled by a rolling leukocyte divided by the time it took to travel this distance. Time averages of rolling velocities for one leukocyte (Zhao et al., 1995) and population averages of the velocities of many rolling leukocytes (Ley and Gaehtgens, 1991) are sensitive to the details of the sampling procedure, which can

Table 16.1. Parameters Used to Characterize Leukocyte Rolling in Vivo (Adapted from Ley, 1997)

Parameter	Unit	Definition	Characteristics	Examples for Use
Rolling leukocyte flux	s^{-1}	Number of rolling leukocytes passing per unit of time	Varies with systemic leukocyte concentration, dependent on microvessel diameter, flow velocity (shear stress), independent of rolling velocity.	Firrell and Lipowsky, 1989
Rolling leukocyte flux fraction	%	Number of rolling leukocytes as fraction of all passing leukocytes (total leukocyte flux)	Independent of rolling velocity and systemic leukocyte concentration. Total leukocyte flux determined by stroboscopic fluorescence video microscopy or estimated from systemic leukocyte concentration and microvessel flow rate. Dependent on microvessel diameter and velocity (shear stress).	Ley and Gaehtgens, 1991
Normalized rolling leukocyte flux fraction	%	Rolling leukocyte flux fraction, empirically normalized for microvessel diameter and velocity	Independent of systemic leukocyte concentration, largely independent of microvessel diameter and blood flow velocity. Used to identify changes of adhesive properties between leukocytes and endothelium (as opposed to alterations of rolling caused by hemodynamics).	Ley et al, 1995a

Leukocyte rolling velocity distribution	μm/s	Histogram of velocities of individual rolling leukocytes	Represents population of rolling leukocytes. Sensitive to blood flow velocity (shear stress) and temporal variations of leukocyte rolling velocity. Labor-intensive interactive measurement.	Ley and Gaehtgens, 1991
Mean leukocyte rolling velocity	μm/s	Average velocity of all rolling leukocytes passing a point of observation	Sensitive to actual distribution of rolling velocities. Average rolling velocity of all leukocytes contained in a microvessel segment is lower (harmonic mean) than average velocity of all cells rolling past a point of observation (arithmetic mean).	Kubes et al., 1994
Rolling leukocytes per 100 μm venule	$(100 \ \mu m)^{-1}$	Number of rolling leukocytes present in a defined segment of venule	Varies with microvessel geometry (diameter), flow velocity, systemic leukocyte concentration, and leukocyte rolling velocity. "Composite" parameter reflecting "attendance" of microvessel segment by rolling leukocytes. Shares problems with rolling leukocyte flux.	Zimmerman et al., 1994
Rolling leukocyte volume fraction	%	Rolling leukocytes present in microvessel segment as % of all leukocytes present	Independent of systemic leukocyte concentration, but sensitive to rolling velocity. Similar to rolling leukocytes per 100 μm venule, it reflects "attendance" of microvessel segment by rolling leukocytes.	Fiebig et al., 1991

significantly skew experimental results. Here, the focus is on biological differences of rolling velocities under different experimental conditions. In a systematic fluorescence microscopic study using the critical velocity to identify all rolling leukocytes in rat mesenteric venules stimulated only by the surgical trauma associated with tissue preparation, the most frequent velocity range of rolling leukocytes was found to be between 20 to 40 $\mu m/s$ in different shear rate classes covering the physiological range (Ley and Gaehtgens, 1991). This type of rolling is largely P-selectin dependent (Bienvenu and Granger, 1993; Dore et al., 1993; Ley et al., 1995a). Other intravital microscopic studies in a variety of tissues have yielded essentially similar results (Atherton and Born, 1973; Schmidt et al., 1990; Perry and Granger, 1991; Mayiovitz, 1992; Bienvenu and Granger, 1993; Gaboury et al., 1994; Johnson et al., 1995). After induction of inflammation by injection of a pro-inflammatory cytokine like TNF-α, leukocyte rolling velocity drops dramatically to an average of 5 to 10 $\mu m/s$ (Kunkel and Ley, 1996; Jung et al., 1998a; Jung and Ley, 1999). This rolling requires the expression of E-selectin on endothelial cells (Kunkel and Ley, 1996; Jung and Ley, 1999) and CD18 integrins on the rolling leukocytes (Jung et al., 1998a; Kunkel et al., 2000), and has been termed *slow rolling* to distinguish it from the much faster rolling without cytokine stimulation. Slow rolling can be reproduced in vitro on substrates of E-selectin (Lawrence and Springer, 1993) and, at equivalent site densities, P-selectin (Lawrence and Springer, 1991). This suggests that slow rolling is not based on a unique property of E-selectin, but the expression of E-selectin and/or its ligands appears to be sufficiently high in vivo to support slow rolling. Current estimates of typical rolling velocities under different conditions in vivo are presented in Table 16.2.

Rolling velocity is relatively invariant with increasing shear stress. Although fewer cells roll, those that do maintain velocities below 50 $\mu m/s$ at wall shear stresses up to 30 dyn/cm^2 (Ley and Gaehtgens, 1991; Damiano et al., 1996). The velocity of E-selectin–dependent slow rolling is almost totally independent of wall shear stress (E. J. Kunkel and K. Ley, unpublished results, 1997). The invariance of rolling velocity with shear stress suggests that the rate-

Table 16.2. Estimates of Typical Leukocyte Rolling Velocities in Mouse Cremaster Venules ($\mu m/s$) (Based on Jung et al., 1996, Kunkel and Ley, 1996, Jung et al., 1998b, Jung and Ley, 1999)

Adhesion Molecule	Mouse Type	Trauma	TNF-α 2 hours	6 hours
L-selectin	E/P$^{-/-}$	120	No rolling	19
P-selectin	L/E$^{-/-}$	40	15	16
E-selectin	L/P$^{-/-}$	No rolling	4	5
α_4 integrin	E/L/P$^{-/-}$	No rolling	No rolling	14
L, P, E, α_4	Wild-type	43	5	12

limiting step of rolling may be found in the detachment of the molecular bonds causing rolling. This finding can be accommodated by models assuming that bonds with a short lifetime continuously form and break between leukocytes and endothelial cells (Hammer and Apte, 1992; Tözeren and Ley, 1992). Consistent with the notion of the rolling bond being strong but short-lived, investigation of the shapes of rolling leukocytes in vivo suggests that only the most deformable cells are able to roll at higher shear rates (Firrell and Lipowsky, 1989). Deformation of rolling leukocytes continues to increase throughout the physiological range up to the highest wall shear stress values observed in venules (Damiano et al., 1996).

Leukocyte Transit Time

Rolling leukocytes accumulate along microvessel walls. Even though they are not firmly adherent, their low velocity generates an increase in transit or residence time in the microvessel (Fiebig et al., 1991; Jung et al., 1998a). At a given rate of leukocyte flux (cells passing per unit of time), slowly moving leukocytes are more likely to be present in any given segment of microvessel than fast-moving ones. This is reflected by an increased microvascular concentration of leukocytes, which, in the absence of firm adhesion, can be shown to be proportional to the fraction of rolling leukocytes (Fiebig et al., 1991). Although the transit time of each individual leukocyte is inversely proportional to its rolling velocity, the average transit time of a leukocyte population is not equal to the inverse of the average rolling velocity, but depends strongly on the distribution of rolling velocities.

Reporting the transit time of rolling leukocytes in addition to their rolling velocities has provided important insights into the physiology of inflammation. A correlative study has shown that transit time through the microcirculation appears to be a key parameter in determining the success of the recruitment process as reflected in firm adhesion (Jung et al., 1998a). The important role of leukocyte transit time appears to be related to chemokines like interleukin-8 that are presented on the endothelial surface and are likely to be accessible to the leukocyte as long as it rolls. This is supported by tracking studies, in which individual rolling leukocytes were found to slow down systematically before becoming firmly adherent (Kunkel et al., 2000. More detailed, interventional studies will be needed to understand fully the impact of transit time on the activation process of the rolling leukocyte in vivo. It is possible that the time of endothelial contact is a better predictor of outcome than transit time, if rolling leukocytes are mainly activated by surface-bound chemoattractants and through adhesion molecule-based signaling. It is also possible that the velocity of rolling may have an effect independent of transit time, because secondary binding events (e.g., β_2 integrin-mediated) may not be able to form unless the leukocyte spends a certain amount of time in a position favorable for bond formation. Although slow rolling makes leukocyte recruitment much more efficient, it is not strictly required, because high concentrations of chemoattractants can also arrest fast-rolling leukocytes (Scharffetter-Kochanek et al., 1998).

Density of Adherent Leukocytes

In many studies, leukocyte adhesion is reported as the number of adherent leukocytes. However, because this number is always relative to a certain area of endothelial surface, this area should serve as the denominator so that leukocyte adhesion density has the dimension of cells per square millimeter. Alternatively, leukocyte adhesion can also be expressed as a concentration by dividing the number of adherent cells by the volume of the microvessel under investigation, yielding a dimension of cells per cubic millimeter.

When investigating adhesion parameters, it is important to keep their dynamic nature in mind. Leukocyte adhesion density is the net result of leukocytes arriving at the site of inflammation and leukocytes leaving the blood vessel. Hence, leukocyte adhesion density depends on rates of adhesion, detachment, and transmigration. These rates are not easy to measure, whereas leukocyte adhesion density is. Often, adhesion densities are reported under nonequilibrium conditions, that is, while more leukocytes are still accumulating. The most common interpretation of a reduced leukocyte adhesion density is that adhesion may be impaired. However, it is also possible that the rate of detachment or transmigration could be increased such that more leukocytes disappear from the adherent pool per unit of time. Like other leukocyte adhesion parameters, leukocyte adhesion density is sensitive to systemic leukocyte counts. For example, if systemic neutrophil counts are reduced by 50% in an experimental animal, and all rates remain the same, it can be expected that the leukocyte adhesion density is also reduced by 50%. In this case, a change in leukocyte adhesion density may not reflect a true change in adhesion behavior.

Transmigration Parameters

Leukocyte transmigration encompasses the processes starting with an adherent leukocyte and ending with a leukocyte in the interstitial tissue. Hence, the term includes transendothelial migration and passage through the subendothelial basement membrane. In intravital microscopic experiments, the number of transmigrated cells next to a venule is often reported. This is justified when the transmigration in response to microinjection of a chemoattractant is investigated, when the time course is relatively short (<30 min), and when the tissue is under continuous observation. In other situations, like cytokine-induced or immunological inflammation, the number of transmigrated cells reflects a steady-state balance between arrival of new cells from the vascular compartment, leukocytes migrating out of the reference volume, leukocytes leaving the tissue to enter the superfusion solution, and apoptosis, the process by which neutrophils rapidly die in the interstitial space. Similar to the adhesion parameters, the number of transmigrated cells can be reported per unit tissue area (cells per mm^2) or per unit tissue volume (cells/mm^3). The latter parameter is preferable, because it can easily be converted into cells per gram of tissue, which can also be measured by global methods such as density of radiolabeled neutrophils or myeloperoxidase activity (Lundberg and Arfors, 1983).

Efficiency Parameters

Owing to the fact that most measures of leukocyte recruitment reflect the net result of several processes occurring at the same time, and that leukocyte recruitment proceeds in an ordered sequence of events, it is reasonable to define efficiency parameters that relate each step to the preceding step (Jung et al., 1998a). This can aid the understanding of the dynamic nature of such seemingly static parameters as number of adherent or transmigrated neutrophils. Because the efficiency parameters as proposed (Table 16.3) consider only the preceding, and not the following, step in the cascade, they do not account for neutrophil disappearance into the downstream steps of the cascade. As an example, rolling leukocyte flux has been defined as the number of rolling leukocytes per minute, divided by the total number of leukocytes passing the same microvessel per minute. This parameter accurately accounts for the effects of flow rate and systemic leukocyte counts on the number of rolling leukocytes. However, leukocyte rolling flux fraction is still susceptible to an altered rate of leukocyte disappearance into downstream steps. This is illustrated by the elevated leukocyte rolling flux fraction seen in E-selectin–deficient mice (Kunkel and Ley, 1996) and wild-type mice treated with a blocking monoclonal antibody to E-selectin (Kunkel and Ley, 1996). Because the neutrophils cannot become adherent as efficiently (Ley et al, 1998; Milstone et al., 1998), they spend more time rolling.

Adhesion efficiency has been defined as the number of adherent leukocytes found per square millimeter of vascular surface, divided by the number of rolling leukocytes per minute (Jung et al., 1998a). Although this parameter accurately accounts for secondary effects on leukocyte adhesion due to altered leukocyte rolling, it does not consider altered rates of transmigration. Leukocyte adhesion efficiency could appear to be increased, because leu-

Table 16.3. Parameters Aimed at Characterizing Rolling, Adhesion, and Transmigration Efficiency

Parameter	Unit	Definition
Leukocyte rolling flux fraction	%	Number of rolling leukocytes as fraction of all passing leukocytes during same time
Adhesion efficiency	min/mm^2	Adherent leukocytes per mm^2 divided by number of rolling leukocytes per minute
Transmigration efficiency	—	Transmigrated leukocytes per mm^2 divided by adherent leukocytes per mm^2
Overall efficiency	mm	Transmigrated leukocytes per mm^2 divided by circulating leukocytes per mm^3

kocytes may not transmigrate fast enough, although adhesion itself is truly unaltered.

Currently, no comprehensive model of leukocyte recruitment exists that would quantitatively account for all steps of the recruitment cascade. Importantly, even under the simplest of conditions, many of the rate constants are unknown. Alternatively, and similar to the idea of efficiency parameters, neutrophils can be thought of as existing in pools such as the bone marrow pool, the blood pool, the marginated pool, the rolling pool, the adherent pool, and the tissue pool. The idea of pools of neutrophils was introduced by Metcalf et al, (1995). Both the pool idea and the idea of efficiency parameters can only be viewed as preliminary steps in the direction of a quantitative understanding of inflammation.

Intravital Microscopic Models of Inflammation

The purpose of this section is to review very briefly the different models suitable for intravital microscopy. Essentially, any tissue accessible to intravital microscopy can be used for inflammation studies. Amphibians are used for permeability studies, including inflammatory permeability (Nguyen et al, 1995). Mouse models are generally most suitable for genetic manipulations (Ley, 1995). Other rodents like hamsters and rats are used for pharmacological studies in inflammation. Rabbit models can often use monoclonal antibodies directed against human antigens because of widespread cross-reactivity (Arfors et al, 1987). Primate models may mimic some of the human characteristics (Mori et al, 1992). Dogs (Dore et al., 1993) are used for intravital microscopy when the goal is to characterize a process like myocardial infarction that is generally studied in this species. Intravital microscopy in humans is also possible (Bollinger et al, 1995).

The traditional use of intravital microscopy is limited to thin, transparent membranes such as the mesentery (Ley and Gaehtgens, 1991), cheek pouch (Duling, 1973), cremaster muscle (Baez, 1973), other thin muscles (Ley et al., 1988), the bat wing (Mayrovitz et al., 1980), and chronic skin chambers (Lehr et al., 1993). These tissues can be transilluminated, and rolling and adherent leukocytes can be seen without contrast-enhancing methods. Vessel dimensions can be measured by simple image processing, and flow velocity can be measured by dual-window based photometry and tracking cross-correlation (Intaglietta et al., 1970; Baker and Wayland, 1974; Pittman and Ellsworth, 1986), by spatial cross-correlation (Pries, 1988), and by particle-tracking methods (Tangelder et al., 1982; Ley and Gaehtgens, 1991). The degree of spatial resolution depends on the quality of the objective used. High numerical apertures can be achieved with salt water immersion objectives. To view leukocytes, it is often helpful to reduce the contrast of the red blood cells by inserting a red filter, preferably at an isosbestic wavelength, such that the red blood appears transparent. Using such a filter allows the investigator to see rolling and adherent leukocytes even at the far wall of a large (~80 μm) venule.

Nontransparent organs and tissues are suitable for studies of inflammation when epifluorescence is used. Epifluorescence requires a special adapter in the microscope. In most cases, the excitation light is filtered and reflected into the back aperture of the objective lens by a dichroic mirror mounted at a 45° angle to the light path. The light is focused on the object by the objective lens. Fluorescent light of longer wavelength emitted from the object passes through the dichroic mirror (i.e., is not reflected), is further filtered by a long-pass filter, and detected by a suitable video camera. With epifluorescence, the surfaces of almost all organs become accessible to intravital microscopy. Models to study the microcirculation of the lung (Lien et al., 1991), liver (Vollmar et al., 1995), spleen (Schmidt et al., 1990), brain (Lorenzl et al., 1993), kidney (Buhrle et al., 1986), lymph node (von Andrian and Mrini, 1998), intestinal wall (Kaminski and Proctor, 1989), Peyer's patch (Bargatze and Butcher, 1993), and many other organs have been described. A limitation common to all these approaches is that only the surface can be observed, so the interpretation of the data must rely on some known relation (often assumed to be identity) between the properties of the superficial layers and the bulk of the organ under study.

Epifluorescence microscopy is particularly useful for studies of leukocyte rolling and adhesion, and is even used in thin tissues accessible to transillumination. This is because circulating leukocytes can be labeled by simple intravenous injection of suitable intravital dyes (Ley and Gaehtgens, 1991), some with no noticeable side effects (Saetzler et al., 1997). In other cases, populations of leukocytes or transfected cells are labeled ex vivo and introduced by intravenous injection (Lien et al., 1991) or by intraarterial injection next to the organ of interest (Ley et al., 1993c Ley, et al., 1995b). This method allows the investigation of several cell types at a time by using different fluorochromes, but has the disadvantages associated with cell isolation prior to injection. Recently, transgenic mice have been developed that express a reporter gene, green fluorescent protein, under a cell-type specific promoter, for example, only in T lymphocytes (Manjunath, et al., 1999; Singbartl, et al., 2000). Epifluorescence microscopy is greatly enhanced by using stroboscopic (rapid flash) illumination for two reasons. First, the shortness of the flash allows the fluorochrome to recover and thus avoids photobleaching and the production of oxygen free radicals in the tissue (Saetzler et al., 1997). Second, it freezes the image such that even rapidly moving objects can be seen clearly. For example, the velocities of free-flowing leukocytes can routinely be measured using stroboscopic epifluorescence (Ley and Gaehtgens, 1991; Ley, et al., 1993b). Unfortunately, none of the microscope manufacturers offers a stroboscopic system off the shelf, so the investigator must be resourceful in finding the right instrumentation.

Chemoattractant-Induced Leukocyte Recruitment

Chemoattractants are small soluble molecules that bind to receptors on leukocytes and cause the target cell to migrate toward higher concentrations of the chemoattractant. All known chemoattractants bind to heptahelical,

G-protein–coupled receptors. The largest class of chemoattractants are chemokines. Other classes include lipid mediators, complement factors, and other peptides, which are discussed in other chapters. Leukocytes respond to chemoattractants by rapid activation. When used in vivo, chemoattractants cause leukocyte adhesion within a few seconds of application (Björk et al., 1982; Ley et al., 1993a; Morgan et al., 1997). Quantitative leukocyte accumulation can be measured as early as a few minutes after injection of chemoattractants (Cybulsky et al., 1989). Since chemoattractants can be specific for several leukocyte subclasses, each one produces a characteristic pattern of leukocyte recruitment.

In intravital microscopic experiments, chemoattractants can be applied by superfusion (Björk et al., 1982; House and Lipowsky, 1987), interstitial microinjection (Ley et al., 1993; Morgan et al., 1997) or intravenous injection (Ley et al., 1993a). The outcomes of these different modes of application are very different. Microinjection produces a local increase in the number of adherent leukocytes, followed by local transmigration. This response is straightforward and easy to understand, because the delivery of leukocytes to the site of inflammation is essentially unaltered. Superfusion of a chemoattractant produces leukocyte adhesion throughout the superfused tissue. This can be a problem when a small segment of tissue is viewed, as is common in intravital microscopy. In the window under observation, leukocyte adhesion usually increases, and leukocyte rolling flux usually decreases, because rolling leukocytes are rapidly arrested. However, it is possible to get a reduction in leukocyte adhesion in response to superfusion of chemoattractant if leukocytes are massively recruited at sites upstream from the site of observation. Intravenous injection of chemoattractant produces a paradoxical inhibition of leukocyte recruitment in response to the same or another chemoattractant (Ley et al., 1993a). Although the mechanism of this response is not fully understood, homotypic and heterotypic desensitization of leukocyte receptors and signaling pathways probably play a role (Foxman et al., 1997).

Cytokine-Induced Leukocyte Recruitment

Many cytokines can elicit an inflammatory response. The most commonly used cytokines in intravital microscopy are TNF-α (Ley et al., 1995a) and IL-1β (Olofsson et al., 1994). The action of inflammatory cytokines is fundamentally different from that of chemoattractants. Most inflammatory cytokines have their main effect on the endothelial cells, causing up-regulation of adhesion molecules (Pober, 1987), expression of genes for endogenous chemoattractants (Selvan et al., 1998), and shape and other changes (Kaplanski et al., 1994). Leukocyte recruitment in response to inflammatory cytokines is much slower than recruitment in response to chemoattractants, and sustained for a longer time (Cybulsky et al., 1989). Cytokine-induced inflammation shares many of the characteristics of acute inflammation by natural causes, the hallmark of which is endothelial activation. Leukocyte activation is mostly indirect, through endogenously produced chemokines

(Selvan et al., 1998), but some inflammatory cytokines, for example, TNF-α, have direct chemotactic effects on some leukocytes.

During cytokine-induced inflammation, leukocyte rolling slows down dramatically (Kunkel and Ley, 1996), a process that requires E-selectin and CD18 integrins (Kunkel and Ley, 1996; Jung et al, 1998a). Leukocyte rolling flux is usually unchanged or only slightly altered. In response to sustained inflammation, the bone marrow will produce more neutrophils. However, leukocyte adhesion and transmigration also increase. On balance, a reduction of systemic leukocyte counts with a relative increase of the neutrophil fraction results (Kunkel and Ley, 1996). If the tissue area exposed to inflammatory cytokines is large, the experimental animal will show systemic effects such as fever and signs of catabolic metabolism.

Models of Acute Inflammation

The simplest model of acute inflammation is realized in almost all intravital microscopic preparations. The surgery necessary for preparation of all but a few (Mayrovitz et al., 1980; Mayrovitz, 1992) tissues causes mast cell degranulation (Ley, 1994; Gaboury et al., 1995), leading to increased expression of P-selectin on the endothelial surface (Jung and Ley, 1997) and induction of leukocyte rolling (Fiebig et al., 1991; Ley, 1994; Gaboury et al., 1995). The inflammatory reaction in response to tissue trauma is reduced with time (Gaboury et al., 1995; Ley et al., 1995a), but does not disappear completely. This inflammatory response is very mild, leading to a transient increase in the number of intravascular leukocytes due to rolling and (some) firm adhesion (Fiebig et al., 1991). Usually, very few leukocytes transmigrate. In some tissues like the skin, leukocyte rolling is a constitutive property of venules (Mayrovitz, 1992; Nolte et al., 1994) and occurs even without tissue trauma (Janssen, et al., 1994).

A very popular model of acute inflammation is induced by tissue ischemia followed by reperfusion (Kubes et al., 1990; Kubes, 1993). This response is characterized by endothelial dysfunction, such as reduction of production of endothelium-derived nitric oxide (Kubes, 1993). Indeed, inhibition of nitric oxide biosynthesis causes an inflammatory response (Kubes, 1993; Armstead et al., 1997). Other currently used models of acute inflammation include those induced by application of a chemoattractant or an inflammatory cytokine. Although these models share many of the characteristics of "natural" acute inflammation, the response to a foreign body in the tissue or to invading microorganisms is much more complex than the response to chemoattractant or cytokine application. Complex intravital microscopic models of acute inflammation other than ischemia and reperfusion are not well developed at this time.

Models of Chronic Inflammation

Chronic inflammation can conveniently be elicited by using the immune system to drive the inflammatory response. Clinically relevant models include arthritis (Finkenauer et al., 1999), experimental allergic encephalomyelitis (EAE); (Koh et al., 1992), inflammatory bowel disease (Sartor, 1992), atherosclerosis (Zhang et al., 1992), and others. Very few of these models allow access by intravital microscopy. Notable exceptions include a delayed-type hypersensitivity to ovalbumin that can be induced in the mouse cremaster muscle (Kanwar et al., 1997), a model of arthritis in the knee (Finkenauer et al., 1999), and chronic uveitis with iriditis (Miyamoto et al., 1998). Because the chronic inflammatory response is quite different from the acute one, and also likely to differ between different organ systems, the development of more and improved intravital microscopic models of chronic inflammation is called for.

Physiology of Leukocyte Rolling, Adhesion, and Transmigration in Vivo

Based on intravital microscopic experiments using blocking monoclonal antibodies, transgenic and gene-targeted mice, and pharmacological interventions, investigators have constructed a model describing the physiology of inflammatory cell recruitment in vivo. Much more is known about the molecular mechanisms of leukocyte rolling and adhesion than about transmigration. Most studies investigate recruitment of neutrophils, although some intravital microscopic investigations into the recruitment of eosinophils (Sriramarao et al., 1994) and mononuclear cells (Xie et al., 1997) have been reported. It is generally believed that the concept of the leukocyte adhesion cascade as elaborated for neutrophil recruitment can, *mutandis mutatis*, be applied to other inflammatory cells.

In most review articles, leukocyte recruitment is described as a sequence of steps that follow each other in a cascade-like fashion. These steps usually include capture or tethering, rolling, activation, adhesion, and transmigration (Butcher, 1991; Springer, 1995). As a first approximation, capture and rolling can be thought of as being mediated by selectins and their ligands, and firm adhesion can be thought of as being mediated by leukocyte integrins and their ligands. However, a more precise analysis of these molecular mechanisms is possible based on recent data obtained in many experimental systems.

Role of Selectins and Their Ligands

The selectins are generally credited with being the "professional rolling molecules," although α_4 integrins also have been shown to mediate leukocyte rolling in vitro (Jones et al., 1994) and in vivo (Sriramarao et al., 1994). Even though all three selectins participate in mediating leukocyte rolling (Ley et al., 1991b; Dore et al., 1993; Kunkel and Ley, 1996), intravital microscopic investigations have clearly established that the functions of the three selectins are only partially overlapping.

P-selectin is rapidly expressed on the endothelial surface in response even to minimal tissue trauma (Ley, 1994; Gaboury et al., 1995; Jung and Ley,

1997), causing rapid induction of leukocyte rolling in all internal organs that have been investigated by intravital microscopy. In skin microvessels, P-selectin appears to be constitutively expressed, so that rolling is present even under baseline conditions (Mayrovitz, 1992). P-selectin–deficient mice have a defect in leukocyte rolling immediately following tissue exteriorization, and recruitment of neutrophils into inflammatory lesions is delayed by about 2 hours (Mayadas et al., 1993). In all other aspects including hemostasis (Subramaniam et al., 1996), neutrophil margination (Johnson et al., 1995), and the delayed-type hypersensitivity response (Staite et al., 1996), P-selectin–deficient mice are close to normal. Remarkably, these animals show moderate (Johnson et al., 1997) to substantial (Collins et al., 2000) protection from the development of atherosclerotic lesions, dependent on the model used. In TNF-α induced inflammation, P-selectin function is partially redundant with the functions of E-and L-selectin, so that the inflammatory defect is unremarkable (Kunkel and Ley, 1996). In allergic inflammation (Kanwar et al., 1997) and in ischemia followed by reperfusion (Weyrich et al., 1993; Winn et al., 1993; Naka et al., 1997), P-selectin appears to play a crucial role as shown by both antibody studies and use of P-selectin–deficient mice. A low level of P-selectin is expressed in cytokine-stimulated arterioles, supporting some leukocyte rolling (Kunkel et al., 1997). In atherosclerotic vessels (Johnson-Tidey et al., 1994), P-selectin is expressed near the shoulder region of the lesions and appears to be involved in monocyte recruitment into the vessel wall (Collins et al., 2000). P-selectin is also expressed on the surface of activated platelets and appears to participate in recruiting leukocytes into vascular defects and thrombi (Palabrica et al., 1992; Zwaginga et al., 1999).

Almost all P-selectin–dependent interactions require a specific glycoprotein on the leukocyte, called P-selectin glycoprotein ligand-1 (PSGL-1; Norgard et al, 1993). PSGL-1 is a sialylated, fucosylated, cell-surface mucin and contains one or more sulfated tyrosine residues toward the N-terminus (Pouyani and Seed, 1995). PSGL-1 antibodies inhibit 80%–90% of P-selectin–dependent leukocyte rolling in vivo (Norman et al., 1995; Borges et al., 1997). Homozygous mice lacking both alleles for PSGL-1 have a phenotype very similar to P-selectin–deficient mice (Yang et al., 1999). Although PSGL-1 has been suggested to function as an E-selectin ligand by biochemical studies (Lenter et al., 1994; Asa et al., 1995), no defect in E-selectin–dependent leukocyte rolling was found in PSGL-1–deficient mice (Yang et al., 1999). Other ligands of P-selectin are likely to exist, accounting for the remaining 10%–20% of leukocyte rolling. Intravital microscopy has shown that CD24 on cancer cells can serve as a P-selectin ligand (Aigner et al., 1998), but the functional significance of this finding for leukocyte rolling is unclear.

P-selectin–PSGL-1 interactions lead to rolling velocities of 20 to 50 μm/s in venules of tissues that have not been intentionally stimulated (Borges et al., 1997; Jung and Ley, 1999). After cytokine stimulation, P-selectin mediated rolling can be as slow as 15 μm/s (Kanwar et al., 1995; Kunkel and Ley, 1996), but usually not below 10 μm/s. P-selectin–dependent rolling shows a modest increase of rolling velocity with wall shear rate (Ley and Gaehtgens, 1991). These findings are consistent with the rolling behavior of leukocytes in flow chambers at P-selectin site densities between 50 and 200 μ^{-2} (Lawrence and Springer, 1991). Although the site density of P-selectin in vivo is not known, it is reasonable to assume that similar site densities may exist in venules in vivo. Of note, endothelial P-selectin expression is induced by cytokine treatment in mice, but not in humans (Pan et al., 1998). P-selectin can also mediate leukocyte capture, thus initiating the first contact between a free-flowing leukocyte and the endothelium. This is evident in mice lacking L-selectin, the other major capture molecule. They show only a limited defect of leukocyte capture as long as P-selectin is functional, but a severe defect when P-selectin is blocked or removed in addition to L-selectin (Kunkel and Ley, 1996; Jung and Ley, 1999).

E-selectin is expressed on inflamed endothelial cells in response to treatment with inflammatory cytokines (Bevilacqua et al., 1989). Intravital microscopic experiments have shown that its function in mediating leukocyte rolling is largely redundant with that of P-selectin (Bullard et al., 1996; Kunkel and Ley, 1996; Hickey et al., 1999). Consequently, E-selectin–deficient mice have only a subtle defect in leukocyte rolling as shown by much faster rolling velocities (Kunkel and Ley, 1996). E- and P-selectin double-deficient mice show no rolling in acute inflammation (Bullard et al., 1996), but mount a substantial inflammatory response at later times that relies on L-selectin and α_4 integrins for rolling (Jung et al., 1998; Jung and Ley, 1999). In addition to mediating leukocyte rolling, E-selectin participates in the conversion of rolling to firm adhesion. E-selectin–deficient mice have a reduced number of firmly adherent leukocytes in response to local chemoattractant (Ley et al., 1998) or cytokine stimulation (Milstone et al., 1998). This defect may be related to the more rapid rolling velocities in the absence of E-selectin. E-selectin is expressed in skin microvessels under baseline conditions (Keelan et al., 1994), and there is some evidence that E-selectin is of particular importance in skin inflammation, because it supports the recruitment of skin-specific T-lymphocytes (Picker et al., 1991a). There is no evidence that E-selectin can mediate capture of free-flowing leukocytes and initiate rolling. Parallel plate flow chamber experiments are inconclusive in this respect, because much of the capture is secondary in nature, caused by free-flowing cells first interacting with already adherent cells, and then rolling (Lawrence et al., 1994; Bargatze et al., 1994).

The ligand for E-selectin that is responsible for the rolling interaction is unknown. Two candidate ligands, PSGL-1 (Lenter et al., 1994; Asa et al., 1995) and E-selectin ligand-1 (ESL-1; Steegmaier et al., 1995) have not been shown to be required for E-selectin mediated leukocyte rolling under any condition. It is not clear whether the physiological ligand for E-selectin is a glycoprotein. Some glycolipids can support E-selectin–dependent rolling in vitro (Alon et al., 1995a).

E-selectin mediates much slower rolling than P-selectin. Dependent on the level of expression of E-selectin, rolling velocities range from less than 5 μm/ s (Kunkel and Ley, 1996; Jung et al., 1998a) to about 15 μm/s (Ley et al., 1998). As the dissociation rate or off-rate of E-selectin is very similar to that of P-selectin (Smith et al., 1999), it is very likely that E-selectin or its ligand or both are expressed at much higher site densities than P-selectin and PSGL-1. The velocity of E-selectin mediated rolling is remarkably invariant with wall shear rate (E. J. Kunkel and K. Ley, unpublished observations 1997). Based on the finding that E-selectin also participates in firm adhesion (Ley et al., 1998), mice deficient for both E-selectin and CD18, the common beta chain of the β_2 integrins were generated. These mice show a severe inflammatory defect leading to early lethality (Forlow et al., 1999), suggesting that E-selectin operates "downstream" from P-selectin, more toward the firm adhesion step of the cascade.

L-selectin is expressed on most circulating leukocytes. Although the requirement for L-selectin in leukocyte rolling in vivo was the first to be discovered (Ley et al., 1991; von Andrian et al., 1991b), the details of its involvement have remained elusive the longest. L-selectin participates in leukocyte rolling after tissue trauma (Ley et al., 1995a), but L-selectin alone mediates only a transient, intermittent rolling at high velocities (about 100 $\mu m/s$) under these conditions (Jung et al., 1996). More robust L-selectin–dependent rolling is seen after long-term cytokine stimulation of microvascular endothelial cells in vitro (Zakrzewicz et al., 1997) and in vivo (Jung et al., 1998b; Jung and Ley, 1999). L-selectin–deficient mice have a significant, but not complete impairment of inflammation for extended periods of time (Arbones et al., 1994; Tedder et al., 1995). They also have defects in lymphocyte homing (Arbones et al., 1994). Under many experimental conditions, blocking L-selectin has anti-inflammatory consequences (Watson et al., 1991; Kanwar et al., 1999), suggesting that L-selectin is required for efficient inflammation. L-selectin appears to be sufficient to mediate some leukocyte rolling and significant adhesion, as shown in E- and P-selectin double-mutant mice (Jung et al., 1998b).

The endothelial ligand(s) for L-selectin remain(s) elusive. None of the L-selectin ligands found in high endothelial venules of peripheral lymph nodes are expressed in inflamed venules. An early candidate ligand for L-selectin, E-selectin (Picker et al., 1991b), was not confirmed as being important in subsequent studies (Ley et al., 1993c; Varki, 1994; Kansas, 1996). There is some evidence that certain glycosylation patterns of endothelial cells are necessary for L-selectin ligand activity (Majuri et al., 1994), but it is unclear which molecule(s) bear(s) those modifications. Functional L-selectin ligands on inflamed endothelium appear to require sulfation (Zakrzewicz et al., 1997). There is a remarkable interaction between L-selectin and ICAM-1, such that L-selectin mediated rolling does not appear to function when ICAM-1 is absent (Kunkel et al., 1996; Steeber et al., 1998). However, these findings do not mean that ICAM-1 is a ligand for L-selectin.

Rolling leukocytes can be slowed down considerably by blocking L-selectin shedding in vitro (Walcheck et al., 1996a) or in vivo (Hafezi-Moghadam and Ley, 1999). L-selectin is continuously cleaved from the cell surface by a metalloproteinase possibly identical to the TNF-converting enzyme, TACE (Peschon et al., 1998). After cytokine treatment, L-selectin–dependent rolling is much slower (10–20 $\mu m/s$; Jung and Ley, 1999), and can be further reduced by blocking L-selectin shedding (A. Hafezi-Moghadam and K. Ley, unpublished observations, 2000). L-selectin appears to be very effective at initiating leukocyte capture. It does so by initiating direct leukocyte–endothelial inter-action and by secondary capture through already adherent leukocytes. In secondary capture, L-selectin transiently interacts with PSGL-1 (Alon et al., 1996; Walcheck et al., 1996b) and at least one other ligand that has not yet been identified (Alon et al., 1996; Ramos et al., 1998). The role of secondary capture for acute inflammation seems to be small (Kunkel et al., 1998), but this mechanism could be important in leukocyte recruitment in large vessels.

Role of Integrins and Their Ligands

The first adhesion molecule investigated by intravital microscopy was CD18 (Arfors et al., 1987), the beta chain common to all four β_2 integrins. Rabbits treated with a monoclonal antibody to CD18 were unable to recruit leuko-cytes in response to exogenous chemoattractant (Arfors et al., 1987), which was later confirmed in gene-targeted mice homozygous for a disrupted CD18 gene (Scharffetter-Kochanek et al., 1998). Interfering with CD18 function is one of the most efficient ways to curb leukocyte recruitment in many forms of experimental inflammation.

Although the response to exogenous chemoattractant is drastically reduced when CD18 is absent or not functional (Arfors et al., 1987; Scharffetter-Kochanek et al., 1998), cytokine treatment still yields a robust inflammatory response in gene-targeted mice lacking CD18 (Jung et al., 1998a). This sug-gests that CD18 integrins participate in leukocyte arrest, but are not always required. Neutrophils express small amounts of other integrins, including $\alpha_4\beta_1$ (Kubes et al., 1995), which may be important in these alternative path-ways. However, CD18-deficient mice have severe inflammatory defects in-cluding skin ulcerations, elevated neutrophil counts and immunoglobulin levels, increased susceptibility to *Streptococcus pneumoniae*, and a severe defect in leukocyte adhesion and T-cell activation (Scharffetter-Kochanek et al., 1998), a defect in leukocyte recruitment to peritonitis (Walzog et al., 1999), and a lack of neutrophil recruitment to the skin (Mizgerd et al., 1997). Pa-tients lacking CD18 expression suffer from leukocyte adhesion deficiency type 1 (LAD-1). When CD18 is totally absent, LAD-1 is a very severe disease that can lead to early lethality (Anderson and Springer, 1987).

Surprisingly, CD18 integrins also participate in leukocyte rolling under inflammatory conditions. This was first discovered as a change in leukocyte rolling flux in response to CD18 antibodies (Perry and Granger, 1991) and increased rolling velocity in CD18-deficient mice (Jung et al., 1998a). Later, the role of CD18 integrins in rolling was confirmed by direct tracking of individual leukocytes in CD18 null mice and in mice injected with a CD18 antibody (Kunkel et al., 2000). Among the β_2 integrins, only LFA-1 and Mac-1 have been investigated in vivo. Intravital microscopic studies suggest that LFA-1 is the most important β_2 integrin in firm leukocyte adhesion (Schmits et al., 1996), whereas Mac-1 has no apparent role in adhesion, but seems to be important in neutrophil activation and phagocytosis (Lu et al.,

1997). Nothing is known about the role of the α_x and α_d chains (CD11c and CD11d) in leukocyte adhesion or recruitment in vivo.

LFA-1 and Mac-1 both can bind to ICAM-1 and ICAM-2 (Dustin and Springer, 1988; Staunton et al., 1989; Diamond et al., 1990; Xie et al., 1995). A role for ICAM-2 in leukocyte recruitment has not been demonstrated so far. ICAM-2–deficient mice show a prolonged eosinophilic infiltrate in a model of allergic lung inflammation, but have no inflammatory defect (Gerwin et al., 1999). ICAM-1–deficient mice have a mild inflammatory defect (Sligh et al., 1993), not comparable with that seen in CD18-deficient mice. Although it has been argued that alternatively spliced forms of ICAM-1 found in these mice (King et al., 1995) may allow for residual leukocyte binding, these isoforms are only found in thymus and spleen and not in inflamed organs. Recently, an ICAM-1 null mouse has been produced that should bring definitive answers with respect to the role of ICAM-1 in inflammation. Leukocytes rolling in resting inflamed venules require ICAM-1 to stop in response to a chemoattractant (Argenbright et al., 1991). However, ICAM-1 is no longer required after activation with inflammatory cytokines (Ley et al., 1998; Foy and Ley, 1999), suggesting that other, unknown endothelial ligands for β_2 integrins must exist.

Monocytes, eosinophils, and many lymphocytes express $\alpha_4\beta_1$ integrin (Hynes, 1992), and neutrophils also express small amounts (Kubes et al., 1995). When other adhesion molecules are unavailable, $\alpha_4\beta_1$ integrin can mediate both leukocyte rolling (Sriramarao et al., 1994; Alon et al., 1995; Berlin et al., 1995) and firm adhesion. The $\alpha_4\beta_1$ integrin binds to endothelial VCAM-1 (Luscinskas et al., 1995) and alternatively spliced fibronectin (Guan and Hynes, 1990). Intravital microscopic evidence available to date suggests that most α_4-dependent binding is through VCAM-1, because antibodies to VCAM-1 applied in the microcirculation (U. Jung and K. Ley, unpublished observations, 1998) and in atherosclerotic arteries (Ramos et al., 1999) block leukocyte rolling and adhesion to a similar extent as α_4 antibodies. Since homozygous α_4 (Yang et al., 1995) or VCAM-1 (Gurtner et al., 1995) deficient mice die before birth due to morphogenetic failure unrelated to the inflammatory function of these molecules, definitive answers for the roles of these two adhesion molecules await the generation of tissue-specific and/or inducible null mutants.

Role of Chemoattractants and Their Receptors

Chemoattractants are treated in detail in Chapters 6 through 9. Here, only the effects of chemoattractants on leukocyte adhesion as observed by intravital microscopy are discussed. When a large dose of chemoattractant is applied to an uninflamed tissue locally, rapid leukocyte adhesion results (Arfors et al., 1987; Argenbright et al., 1991; Ley et al., 1993a). These adherent leukocytes are all recruited from the rolling pool. Adhesion requires CD18 integrins (Scharffetter-Kochanek et al., 1998) and, in resting venules, ICAM-1 (Argenbright et al., 1991; Foy and Ley, 1999). Most likely, LFA-1 is rapidly activated through a signaling cascade that starts with the chemoattractant bindings to its heptahelical receptor, which causes dissociation of a hetero-trimeric G-protein of the inhibitory (Gi) class, results in activation of phos-pholipase C, and a transient increase in intracellular free calcium. The down-stream events are less well defined, but intracellular changes are thought to result in a conformational change in the extracellular domain of LFA-1 and other integrins (Hynes, 1992), capacitating the hetorodimer for interaction with endothelial ligands.

In inflammation, cells in the interstitial space, in the vessel wall, and en-dothelial cells all elaborate chemoattractants. A prototype chemoattractant of this type is interleukin-8 (IL-8; Middleton et al., 1997). Mice lacking the interleukin-8 receptor homologue have substantial inflammatory defects (Ca-calano et al., 1994). Microinjection of MIP-2, a murine homologue of IL-8, does not lead to leukocyte adhesion in these mice (Morgan et al., 1997), but fMLP, a chemoattractant binding to a different receptor, functions normally. Conspicuously, leukocyte rolling proceeds at a faster velocity in IL-8 receptor-deficient mice (Morgan et al., 1997). These findings suggest that the IL-8 receptor homologue is required for slow leukocyte rolling during inflam-mation. IL-8 appears to be in a particularly suitable location to activate roll-ing leukocytes in inflammation, because it is presented on the luminal surface of endothelial cells by cell surface proteoglycans (Middleton et al., 1997).

In cytokine-induced inflammation, slow-rolling leukocytes do not stop abruptly, but show a gradual decrease of their rolling velocity before becom-ing adherent (Kunkel et al., 2000). This deceleration is strictly dependent on CD18 integrins (Kunkel et al., 2000). Because rolling leukocytes show a graded elevation of intracellular free calcium while rolling more and more slowly, it appears that they are partially activated before arrest. This process seems to take about 1 minute or more. Although IL-8 receptor is known to be involved, signaling through adhesion receptors, for example, L-selectin (Steeber et al., 1997), may also contribute to this process of physiological leukocyte recruitment.

Candidate Molecules Regulating Transmigration

Intravital microscopic evidence for the molecular mechanisms involved in leukocyte transmigration is very limited. In vitro studies have suggested that platelet–endothelial cell adhesion molecule-1 (PECAM-1 or CD31; Muller et al., 1993) and vascular endothelial (VE)-cadherin (Allport et al., 1997) may be involved in leukocyte transmigration. PECAM-1 has been investigated by intravital microscopy, using monoclonal antibody blockade (Wakelin et al., 1996) and gene-targeted mice lacking PECAM-1 expression (Duncan et al., 1999). These studies suggest that PECAM-1 is involved in transmigration, but not strictly required. The defect in cell movement appears to be at the level of traversing the basement membrane rather than the endothelial monolayer (Wakelin et al., 1996; Duncan et al., 1999). Very limited in vivo information is available on VE-cadherin (Gotsch et al., 1997). A VE-cadherin antibody seems to accelerate leukocyte transmigration in response to exogenous che-moattractant in an intravital microscopic rat model (C. Burns and K. Ley, unpublished observations, 1998), but the mechanism remains unclear.

In vitro cell culture assays have shown that CD18 integrins are involved in leukocyte transmigration through inflamed endothelial monolayers (Furie et al., 1991). Endothelia in vivo appear to be different enough from endothelial cells grown in culture to raise doubts as to whether this same mechanism is important in vivo. The only intravital microscopic study that attempted to measure transmigration separate from any effects on adhesion failed to dem-onstrate a specific transmigration defect in CD18 null mice (Jung et al., 1998a). In that study, it appeared that the reason for reduced leukocyte accumulation in the absence of CD18 integrins could be found in an adhe-sion defect, and that the number of transmigrated leukocytes was reduced as a consequence. Further intravital microscopic studies are necessary to address the role of CD18 and other adhesion molecules in transmigration in vivo.

Conclusion

This chapter summarizes methods used for, and results obtained by, intravital microscopic investigation of the inflammatory response in vivo. An attempt was made to present the certainties and, more importantly, uncertainties of the molecular basis of these events. In vitro model systems and in vivo ex-periments in which the microcirculation is treated as a "black box" to deliver leukocytes to sites of inflammation have yielded valuable insights. Mechanis-tic understanding requires molecule-based investigations at the intravital mi-croscopic level. The roles of selectins, β_2 and α_4 integrins, ICAM-1 and VCAM-1, IL-8, and its receptor have begun to be clarified. However, major molecular pathways including alternative β_2 integrin ligands and L-selectin ligands on inflamed endothelium remain to be discovered. Insights into the mechanisms of inflammation will continue to refine our understanding of this part of physiology.

References

Aigner, S., Ramos, C. L., Hafezi-Moghadam, A., Lawrence, M. B., Altevogt, P., and Ley, K. (1998) CD24 mediates rolling of breast carcinoma cells on P-selectin. *FASEB J.* 12:1241–1251.

Allport, J. R., Ding, H., Collins, T., Gerritsen, M. E., and Luscinskas, F. W. (1997) Endothelial-dependent mechanisms regulate leukocyte transmigration—a process involving the protea-some and disruption of the vascular endothelial–cadherin complex at endothelial cell-to-cell junctions. *J. Exp. Med.* 186:517–527.

Alon, R., Feizi, T., Yuen, C.-T., Fuhlbrigge, R. C., and Springer, T. A. (1995a) Glycolipid ligands for selectins support leukocyte tethering and rolling under physiologic flow conditions. *J. Immunol.* 154:5356–5366.

Alon, R., Kassner, P. D., Carr, M. W., Finger, E. B., Hemler, M. E., and Springer, T. A. (1995b) The integrin VLA-4 supports tethering and rolling in flow on VCAM-1. *J. Cell Biol.* 128:1243–1254.

Alon, R., Fuhlbrigge, R. C., Finger, E. B., and Springer, T. A. (1996) Interactions through L-selectin between leukocytes and adherent leukocytes nucleate rolling adhesions on selectins and VCAM-1 in shear flow. *J. Cell Biol.* 135:849–865.

Anderson, D. C., and Springer, T. A. (1987) Leukocyte adhesion deficiency: An inherited defect in the Mac-1, LFA-1 and p150,95 glycoproteins. *Annu. Rev. Med.* 38:175–194.

Arbones, M. L., Ord, D. C., Ley, K., Ratech, H., Maynard-Curry, C., Otten, G., Capon, D. J., and Tedder, T. F. (1994) Lymphocyte homing and leukocyte rolling and migration are impaired in L-selectin-deficient mice. *Immun.* 1:247–260.

Arfors, K.-E., Lundberg, C., Lindbom, L., Lundberg, K., Beatty, P. G., and Harlan, J. M. (1987) A monoclonal antibody to the membrane glycoprotein complex CD18 inhibits polymorphonuclear leukocyte accumulation and plasma leakage in vivo. *Blood* 69:338–340.

Argenbright, L. W., Letts, L. G., and Rothlein, R. (1991) Monoclonal antibodies to the leukocyte membrane CD18 glycoprotein complex and to Intercellular Adhesion Molecule-1 inhibit leukocyte–endothelial adhesion in rabbits. *J. Leukoc. Biol.* 49:253–257.

Armstead, V. E., Minchenko, A. G., Schuhl, R. A., Hayward, R., Nossull, T. O., and Lefer, A. M. (1997) Regulation of P-selectin expression in human endothelial cells by nitric oxide. *Am. J. Physiol.* 273:H740–H746.

Asa, D., Raycroft, L., Ma, L., Aeed, P. A., Kaytes, P. S., Elhammer, Å. P., and Geng, J.-G (1995) The P-selectin glycoprotein ligand functions as a common human leukocyte ligand for P- and E-selectins. *J. Biol. Chem.* 270:11662–11670.

Atherton, A., and Born, G.V.R. (1972) Quantitative investigations of the adhesiveness of circulating polymorphonuclear leukocytes to blood vessels. *J. Physiol. (Lond.)* 222:447–474.

Atherton, A., and Born, G.V.R. (1973) Relationship between the velocity of rolling granulocytes and that of the blood flow in venules. *J. Physiol. (Lond.)* 233:157–165.

Baez, S. (1973) An open cremaster muscle preparation for the study of blood vessels by in vivo microscopy. *Microvasc. Res.* 5:384–394.

Bagge, U., Amundson, B., and Lauritzen, C. (1980) White blood cell deformability and plugging of skeletal muscle capillaries in hemorrhagic shock. *Acta Physiol. Scand.* 180:159–163.

Bagge, U., Blixt, A., and Strid, K. G. (1983) The initiation of post-capillary margination of leukocytes: Studies in vitro on the influence of erythrocyte concentration and flow velocity. *Int. J. Microcirc: Clin. Exp.* 2:215–227.

Baker, M., and Wayland, H. (1974) On-line volume flow rate and velocity profile measurement for blood in microvessels. *Microvasc. Res.* 7:131–143.

Bargatze, R. F., and Butcher, E. C. (1993) Rapid G-protein–regulated activation event involved in lymphocyte binding to high endothelial venules. *J. Exp. Med.* 178:367–372.

Bargatze, R. F., Kurk, S., Butcher, E. C., and Jutila, M. A. (1994) Neutrophils roll on adherent neutrophils bound to cytokine-induced endothelial cells via L-selectin on the rolling cells. *J. Exp. Med.* 180:1785–1792.

Berlin, C., Bargatze, R. F., Campbell, J. J., von Andrian, U. H., Szabo, M. C., Hasslen, S. R., Nelson, R. D., Berg, E. L., Eriandsen, S. L., and Butcher, E. C. (1995) α_4 Integrins mediate lymphocyte attachment and rolling under physiologic flow. *Cell* 80:413–422.

Bevilacqua, M. P., Stengelin, S., Gimbrone, M. A., Jr., and Seed, B. (1989) Endothelial leukocyte adhesion molecule-1: An inducible receptor for neutrophils related to complement regulatory proteins and lectins. *Science* 243:1160–1165.

Bienvenu, K., and Granger, D. N. (1993) Molecular determinants of shear rate-dependent leukocyte adhesion in postcapillary venules. *Am. J. Physiol.* 264, H1504–H1508.

Björk, J., Hedqvist, P., and Arfors, K.-E. (1982) Increase in vascular permeability induced by leukotriene B4 and the role of polymorphonuclear leukocytes. *Inflamm.* 6:189–200.

Bollinger, A., Herrig, I., Fischer, M., Hoffmann, U., and Franzeck, U. K. (1995) Intravital capillaroscopy in patients with chronic venous insufficiency and lymphoedema—relevance to daflon 500 mg. *Int. J. Microcirc. Clini. Exp.* 15(1):41–44.

Borges, E., Eytner, R., Moll, T., Steegmaler, M., Campbell, M. A., Ley, K., Mossmann, H., and Vestweber, D. (1997) The P-selectin glycoprotein ligand-1 is important for recruitment of neutrophils into inflamed mouse peritoneum. *Blood* 90:1934–1942.

Buhrie, C. P., Hackenthal, E., Helmchen, U., Lackner, K., Nobiling, R., Steinhausen, M., and

Taugner, R. (1986) The hydronephrotic kidney of the mouse as a tool for intravital microscopy and in vitro electrophysiological studies of renin-containing cells. *Lab. Invest.* 54:462–472.

Bullard, D. C., Kunkel, E. J., Kubo, H., Hicks, M. J., Lorenzo, I., Doyle, N. A., Doerschuk, C. M., Ley, K., and Beaudet, A. L. (1996) Infectious susceptibility and severe deficiency of leukocyte rolling and recruitment in E-selectin and P-selectin double mutant mice. *J. Exp. Med.* 183: 2329–2336.

Butcher, E. C. (1991) Leukocyte–endothelial cell recognition—three (or more) steps to specificity and diversity. *Cell* 67:1033–1036.

Buttrum, S. M., Hatton, R., and Nash, G. B. (1993) Selectin-mediated rolling of neutrophils on immoblized platelets. *Blood* 82:1165–1174.

Cacalano, G., Lee, J., Kikly, K., Ryan, A. M., Pitts-Meek, S., Hultgren, B., Wood, W. I., and Moore, M. W. (1994) Neutrophil and B-cell expansion in mice that lack the murine IL-8 receptor homolog. *Science* 265:682–684.

Chien, S., Usami, S., and Skalak, R. (1984) Blood flow in small tubes. In: *Handbook of Physiology: The Cardiovascular System: Microcirculation.* E. M. Renkin and C. C. Michel, eds. Bethesda, MD: American Physiological Society, pp. 217–249.

Collins, R. G., Velji, R., Guevara, N. V., Hicks, M. J., Chan, L., and Beaudet, A. L. (2000) P-selectin or ICAM-1 deficiency substantially protects against atherosclerosis in apo E-deficient mice. *J. Exp. Med.* 191:189–194.

Cybulsky, M. I., McComb, D. J., and Movat, H. Z. (1989) Protein synthesis dependent and independent mechanisms of neutrophil emigration. *Am. J. Pathol.* 135:227–237.

Damiano, E. R., Westheider, J., Tözeren, A., and Ley, K. (1996) Variation in the velocity, deformation, and adhesion energy density of leukocytes rolling within venules. *Circ. Res.* 79:1122–1130.

Diacovo, T. G., Puri, K. D., Warnock, R. A., Springer, T. A., and von Andrian, U. H. (1996) Platelet-mediated lymphocyte delivery to high endothelial venules. *Science* 273:252–255.

Diamond, M. S., Staunton, D. E., de Fougerolles, A. R., Stacker, S. A., Garcia-Aguilar, J., Hibbs, M. L., and Springer, T. A. (1990) ICAM-1 (CD54): A counter-receptor for Mac-1 (CD11b/CD18). *J. Cell Biol.* 111:3129–3139.

Doré, M., Korthuis, R. J., Granger, D. N., Entman, M. L., and Smith, C. W. (1993) P-selectin mediates spontaneous leukocyte rolling in vivo. *Blood* 82:1308–1316.

Duling, B. R. (1973) The preparation and use of the hamster cheek pouch for studies of the microcirculation. *Microvasc. Res.* 5:423–429.

Duncan, G. S., Andrew, D. P., Takimoto, H., Kaufman, S. A., Yoshida, H., Spellberg, J., de la Pompa, J. L., Elia, A., Wakeham, A., Karan-Tamir, B., et al. (1999) Genetic evidence for functional redundancy of platelet/endothelial cell adhesion molecule-1 (PECAM-1): CD31-deficient mice reveal PECAM-1–dependent and PECAM-1–independent functions. *J. Immunol.* 162:3022–3030.

Dustin, M. L., and Springer, T. A. (1988) Lymphocyte function-associated antigen-1 (LFA-1) interaction with intercellular adhesion molecule-1 (ICAM-1) is one of at least three mechanisms for lymphocyte adhesion to cultured endothelial cells. *J. Cell Biol.* 107:321–331.

Fiebig, E., Ley, K., and Arfors, K.-E. (1991) Rapid leukocyte accumulation by "spontaneous" rolling and adhesion in the exteriorized rabbit mesentery. *Int. J. Microcirc: Clin. Exp.* 10:127–144.

Finger, E. B., Puri, K. D., Alon, R., Lawrence, M. B., von Andrian, U. H., and Springer, T. A. (1996) Adhesion through L-selectin requires a threshold hydrodynamic shear. *Nature* 379: 266–269.

Finkenauer, V., Bissinger, T., Funk, R.H.W., Karbowski, A., and Seiffge, D. (1999) Confocal laser scanning microscopy of leukocyte adhesion in the microcirculation of the inflamed rat knee joint capsule. *Microcirc.* 6:141–152.

Firrell, J. C., and Lipowsky, H. H. (1989) Leukocyte margination and deformation in mesenteric venules of rat. *Am. J. Physiol.* 256:H1667–H1674.

Forlow, S. B., Bullard, D. C., Lu, H. F., Beaudet, A. L., and Ley, K. (1999) Absence of slow leukocyte rolling and severe leukocyte recruitment defect in mice lacking E-selectin and CD18. *FASEB J.* 13:A311 (Abs).

Foxman, E. F., Campbell, J. J., and Butcher, E. C. (1997) Multistep navigation and the combinatorial control of leukocyte chemotaxis. *J. Cell Biol.* 139:1349–1360.

Frenette, P. S., Johnson, R. C., Hynes, M. R., and Wagner, D. D. (1995) Platelets roll on stimulated endothelium in vivo: an interaction mediated by endothelial P-selectin. *Proc. Natl. Acad. Sci. USA* 92:7450–7454.

Frenette, P. S., Mayadas, T. N., Rayburn, H., Hynes, R. O., and Wagner, D. D. (1996) Susceptibility to infection and altered hematopoiesis in mice deficient in both P- and E-selectins. *Cell* 84:563–574.

Fries, J.W.U., Williams, A. J., Atkins, R. C., Newman, W., Lipscomb, M. F., and Collins, T. (1993) Expression of VCAM-1 and E-selectin in an in vivo model of endothelial activation. *Am. J. Pathol.* 143:725–737.

Furie, M. B., Tancinco, M. C., and Smith, C. W. (1991) Monoclonal antibodies to leukocyte integrin CD11a/CD18 and integrin CD11b/CD18 or intercellular adhesion molecule-1 inhibit chemoattractant-stimulated neutrophil transendothelial migration in vitro. *Blood* 78:2089–2097.

Gaboury, J. P., Anderson, D. C., and Kubes, P. (1994) Molecular mechanisms involved in superoxide-induced leukocyte–endothelial cell interactions in vivo. *Am. J. Physiol.* 266:H637–H642.

Gaboury, J. P., Johnston, B., Niu, X.-F., and Kubes, P. (1995) Mechanisms underlying acute mast cell-induced leukocyte rolling and adhesion in vivo. *J. Immunol.* 154:804–813.

Gaehtgens, P., Pries, A. R., and Nobis, U. (1984) Flow behaviour of white cells in capillaries. In: *White Cell Mechanics: Basic Science and Clinical Aspects.* H. J. Meiselman, M. A. Lichtman, and P. L. LaCelle, eds. New York: A. R. Liss, pp. 147–157.

Gaehtgens, P., Ley, K., Pries, A. R., and Müller, R. (1985) Mutual interaction between leukocytes and microvascular blood flow. In: *White Cell Rheology and Inflammation*, K. Messmer and F. Hammersen, eds. Basel: Karger (Progress in Applied Microcirculation Series), volume 7, pp. 15–28.

Gerritsen, M. E. (1987) Functional heterogeneity of vascular endothelial cells. *Biochem. Pharmacol.* 36:2701–2711.

Gerwin, N., Gonzalo, J. A., Lloyd, C., Coyle, A. J., Reiss, Y., Banu, N., Wang, B. P., Xu, H., Avraham, H., Engelhardt, B., et al. (1999) Prolonged eosinophil accumulation in allergic lung interstitium of ICAM-2–deficient mice results in extended hyperresponsiveness. *Immun* 10:9–19.

Goldman, A. J., Cox, R. G., and Brenner, H. (1967) Slow viscous motion of a sphere parallel to a plane wall. II. Couette flow. *Chem. Eng. Sci.* 22:653–660.

Gotsch, U., Jäger, U., Dominis, M., and Vestweber, D. (1994) Expression of P-selectin on endothelial cells is upregulated by LPS and TNF-α in vivo. *Cell Adhesion and Commun.* 2:7–14.

Gotsch, U., Borges, E., Bosse, R., Boggemeyer, E., Simon, M., Mossmann, H., and Vestweber, D. (1997) VE-cadherin antibody accelerates neutrophil recruitment in vivo. *J. Cell Sci.* 110:583–588.

Grabowski, E. F., Jaffe, E. A., and Weksler, B. B. (1985) Prostacyclin production by cultured endothelial cell monolayers exposed to step increases in shear stress. *J. Lab. Clin. Med.* 105:36–43.

Guan, J.-L., and Hynes, R. O. (1990) Lymphoid cells recognize an alternatively spliced segment of fibronectin via the integrin receptor $\alpha_4\beta_1$. *Cell* 60:53–61.

Gurtner, G. C., Davis, V., Li, H., McCoy, M. J., Sharpe, A., and Cybulsky, M. I. (1995) Targeted disruption of the murine VCAM-1 gene: essential role of VCAM-1 in chorioallantoic fusion and placentation. *Genes Dev.* 9:1–14.

Hafezi-Moghadam, A., and Ley, K. (1999) Relevance of L-selectin shedding for leukocyte rolling in vivo. *J. Exp. Med.* 189:939–948.

Hammer, D. A., and Apte, S. M. (1992) Simulation of cell rolling and adhesion on surfaces in shear flow: general results and analysis of selectin-mediated neutrophil adhesion. *Biophys. J.* 63:35–57.

Hickey, M. J., Kanwar, S., McCafferty, D. M., Granger, D. N., Eppihimer, M. J., and Kubes, P. (1999) Varying roles of E-selectin and P-selectin in different microvascular beds in response to antigen. *J. Immunol.* 162:1137–1143.

House, S. D., and Lipowsky, H. H. (1987) Leukocyte–endothelium adhesion: Microhemodynamics in mesentery of the cat. *Microvaso. Res.* 34:363–379.

House, S. D., and Lipowsky, H. H. (1988) In vivo determination of the force of leukocyte–endothelium adhesion in the mesenteric microvasculature of the cat. *Circ. Res.* 63:658–668.

Huber, A. R., Kunkel, S. L., Todd, R. F., and Weiss, S. J. (1991) Regulation of transendothelial neutrophil migration by endogenous interleukin-8. *Science* 254:99–102.

Hynes, R. O. (1992) Integrins: Versatility, modulation, and signaling in cell adhesion. *Cell* 69:11–25.

Ignarro, L. J. (1990) Biosynthesis and metabolism of endothelium-derived nitric oxide. *Annu. Rev. Pharmacol. Toxicol.* 30:535–560.

Intaglietta, M., Tompkins, W. R., and Richardson, D. R. (1970) Velocity measurements in the microvasculature of the cat omentum by on-line method. *Microvasc. Res.* 2:462–473.

Janssen, G.H.G.W., Tangelder, G. J., oude Egbrink, M.G.A., and Reneman, R. S. (1994) Spontaneous leukocyte rolling in venules in untraumatized skin of conscious and anesthetized animals. *Am. J. Physiol.* 267:H1199–H1204.

Johnson, R. C., Mayadas, T. N., Frenette, P. S., Mebius, R. E., Subramaniam, M., Lacasce, A., Hynes, R. O., and Wagner, D. D. (1995) Blood cell dynamics in P-selectin deficient mice. *Blood* 86:1106–1114.

Johnson, R. C., Chapman, S. M., Dong, Z. M., Ordovas, J. M., Mayadas, T. N., Herz, J., Hynes, R. O., Schaefer, E. J., and Wagner, D. D. (1997) Absence of P-selectin delays fatty streak formation in mice. *J. Clin. Invest.* 99:1037–1043.

Johnson-Tidey, R. R., McGregor, J. L., Taylor, P. R., and Poston, R. N. (1994) Increase in the adhesion molecule P-selectin in endothelium overlying atherosclerotic plaques: Coexpression with intercellular adhesion molecule-1. *Am. J. Pathol.* 144:952–961.

Jones, D. A., McIntire, L. V., Smith, C. W., and Picker, L. J. (1994) A two-step adhesion cascade for T-cell/endothelial cell interactions under flow conditions. *J. Clin. Invest.* 94:2443–2450.

Jung, U., Bullard, D. C., Tedder, T. F., and Ley, K. (1996) Velocity difference between L-selectin and P-selectin dependent neutrophil rolling in venules of the mouse cremaster muscle in vivo. *Am. J. Physiol.* 271:H2740–H2747.

Jung, U., and Ley, K. (1997) Regulation of E-selectin, P-selectin and ICAM-1 expression in mouse cremaster muscle vasculature. *Microcirc.* 4:311–319.

Jung, U., Norman, K. E., Ramos, C. L., Scharffetter-Kochanek, K., Beaudet, A. L., and Ley, K. (1998a) Transit time of leukocytes rolling through venules controls cytokine-induced inflammatory cell recruitment in vivo. *J. Clin. Invest.* 102:1526–1533.

Jung, U., Ramos, C. L., Bullard, D. C., and Ley, K. (1998b) Gene-targeted mice reveal the importance of L-selectin–dependent rolling for neutrophil adhesion. *Am. J. Physiol.* 274:H1785–H1791.

Jung, U., and Ley, K. (1999) Mice lacking two or all three selectins demonstrate overlapping and distinct functions of each selectin. *J. Immunol.* 162:6755–6762.

Kaminski, P. M., and Proctor, K. G. (1989) Attenuation of no-reflow phenomenon, neutrophil activation, and reperfusion injury in intestinal microcirculation by topical adenosine. *Circ. Res.* 65:426–435.

Kansas, G. S. (1996) Selectins and their ligands: current concepts and controversies. *Blood* 88:3259–3287.

Kanwar, S., Johnston, B., and Kubes, P. (1995) Leukotriene C_4/D_4 induces P-selectin and sialyl Lewis^x-dependent alterations in leukocyte kinetics in vivo. *Circ. Res.* 77:879–887.

Kanwar, S., Bullard, D. C., Hickey, M. J., Smith, C. W., Beaudet, A. L., Wolitzky, B. A., and Kubes, P. (1997) The association between α_4-integrin, P-selectin, and E-selectin in an allergic model of inflammation. *J. Exp. Med.* 185:1077–1087.

Kanwar, S., Steeber, D. A., Tedder, T. F., Hickey, M. J., and Kubes, P. (1999) Overlapping roles for L-selectin and P-selectin in antigen-induced immune responses in the microvasculature. *J. Immunol.* 162:2709–2716.

Kaplanski, G., Farnarier, C., Benoliel, A.-M., Foa, C., Kaplanski, S., and Bongrand, P. (1994) A novel role for E- and P-selectins: Shape control of endothelial cell monolayers. *J. Cell Sci.* 107:2449–2457.

Karasek, M. A. (1989) Microvascular endothelial cell culture. *J. Invest. Dermatol.* 93 (Suppl.):33S–38S.

Keelan, E. T., Licence, S. T., Peters, A. M., Binns, R. M., and Haskard, D. O. (1994) Characterization of E-selectin expression in vivo with use of a radiolabeled monoclonal antibody. *Am. J. Physiol.* 266:H278–H290.

King, P. D., Sandberg, E. T., Selvakumar, A., Fang, P., Beaudet, A. L., and Dupont, B. (1995) Novel isoforms of murine intercellular adhesion molecule-1 generated by alternative RNA splicing. *J. Immunol.* 154:6080–6093.

Klein, L. M., Lavker, R. M., Matis, W. L., and Murphy, G. F. (1989) Degranulation of human mast cells induces an endothelial antigen central to leukocyte adhesion. *Proc. Natl. Acad. Sci. USA* 86:8972–8976.

Koh, D. R., Fung-Leung, W. P., Ho, A., Gray, D., Acha-Orbea, H., and Mak, T. W. (1992) Less mortality but more relapses in experimental allergic encephalomyelitis in CD8$^{-/-}$ mice. *Science* 256:1210–1213.

Kubes, P., Ibbotson, G., Russell, J. M., Wallace, J. L., and Granger, D. N. (1990) Role of platelet-activating factor in ischemia/reperfusion-induced leukocyte adherence. *Am. J. Physiol.* 259: G300–G305.

Kubes, P. (1993) Ischemia-reperfusion in feline small intestine: a role for nitric oxide. *Am. J. Physiol.* 264:G143–G149.

Kubes, P., Kurose, I., and Granger, D. N. (1994) NO donors prevent integrin-induced leukocyte adhesion but not P-selectin–dependent rolling in postischemic venules. *Am. J. Physiol.* 267: H931–H937.

Kubes, P., Niu, K., Smith, C. W., Kehrli, M. E., Reinhardt, P. H., and Woodman, R. C. (1995) A novel β_1-dependent adhesion pathway on neutrophils: a mechanism invoked by dihydrocytochalasin B or endothelial transmigration. *FASEB J.* 9:1103–1111.

Kunkel, E. J., Jung, U., Bullard, D. C., Norman, K. E., Wolitzky, B. A., Vestweber, D., Beaudet, A. L., and Ley, K. (1996) Absence of trauma-induced leukocyte rolling in mice deficient in both P-selectin and intercellular adhesion molecule-1 (ICAM-1). *J. Exp. Med.* 183:57–65.

Kunkel, E. J., and Ley, K. (1996) Distinct phenotype of E-selectin deficient mice: E-selectin is required for slow leukocyte rolling in vivo. *Circ. Res.* 79:1196–1204.

Kunkel, E. J., Jung, U., and Ley, K. (1997) TNF-α induces selectin-dependent leukocyte rolling in mouse cremaster muscle arterioles. *Am. J. Physiol.* 272:H1391–H1400.

Kunkel, E. J., Chomas, J. E., and Ley, K. (1998) Role of primary and secondary capture for leukocyte accumulation in vivo. *Circ. Res.* 82:30–38.

Kunkel, E. J., Dunne, J. L., and Ley, K. (2000) Leukocyte arrest during cytokine-dependent inflammation in vivo. *J. Immunol.* 164:3301–3308.

Lawrence, M. B., and Springer, T. A. (1991) Leukocytes roll on a selectin at physiologic flow rates: Distinction from and prerequisite for adhesion through integrins. *Cell* 65:859–873.

Lawrence, M. B., and Springer, T. A. (1993) Neutrophils roll on E-selectin. *J. Immunol.* 151:6338–6346.

Lawrence, M. B., Bainton, D. F., and Springer, T. A. (1994) Neutrophil tethering to and rolling on E-selectin are separable by requirement for L-selectin. *Immun.* 1:137–145.

Lawrence, M. B., Kansas, G. S., Ghosh, S., Kunkel, E. J., and Ley, K. (1997) Threshold levels of fluid shear promote leukocyte adhesion through selectins (CD62L, P, E). *J. Cell Biol.* 136: 717–727.

Lehr, H. A., Leunig, M., Menger, M. D., Nolte, D., and Messmer, K. (1993) Dorsal skinfold chamber technique for intravital microscopy in nude mice. *Am. J. Pathol.* 143:1055–1062.

Lenter, M., Levinovitz, A., Isenmann, S., and Vestweber, D. (1994) Monospecific and common glycoprotein ligands for E- and P-selectin in myeloid cells. *J. Cell. Biol.* 125:471–481.

Ley, K., Lindbom, L., and Arfors, K.-E. (1988) Hematocrit distribution in rabbit tenuissimus muscle. *Acta Physiol. Scand.* 132:373–383.

Ley, K. (1989) Granulocyte adhesion to microvascular and cultured endothelium. *Studia Biophys.* 134:179–184.

Ley, K., Cerrito, M., and Arfors, K.-E. (1991a) Sulfated polysaccharides inhibit leukocyte rolling in rabbit mesentery venules. *Am. J. Physiol.* 260:H1667–H1673.

Ley, K., and Gaehtgens, P. (1991) Endothelial, not hemodynamic differences are responsible for preferential leukocyte rolling in venules. *Circ. Res.* 69:1034–1041.

Ley, K., Gaehtgens, P., Fennie, C., Singer, M. S., Lasky, L. A., and Rosen, S. D. (1991b) Lectin-like cell adhesion molecule-1 mediates leukocyte rolling in mesenteric venules in vivo. *Blood* 77:2553–2555.

Ley, K., Gaehtgens, P., and Spanel-Borowski, K. (1992) Differential adhesion of granulocytes to five distinct phenotypes of cultured microvascular endothelial cells. *Microvasc. Res.* 43:119–133.

Ley, K., Baker, J. B., Cybulsky, M. I., Gimbrone, M. A. Jr., and Luscinskas, F. W. (1993a) Intravenous interleukin-8 inhibits granulocyte emigration from rabbit mesenteric venules without altering L-selectin expression or leukocyte rolling. *J. Immunol.* 151:6347–6357.

Ley, K., Linnemann, G., Meinen, M., Stoolman, L. M., and Gaehtgens, P. (1993b) Fucoidin, but not yeast polyphosphomannan PPME inhibits leukocyte rolling in venules of the rat mesentery. *Blood* 81:177–185.

Ley, K., Tedder, T. F., and Kansas, G. S. (1993c) L-selectin can mediate leukocyte rolling in untreated mesenteric venules in vivo independent of E- or P-selectin. *Blood* 82:1632–1638.

Ley, K. (1994) Histamine can induce leukocyte rolling in rat mesenteric venules. *Am. J. Physiol.* 267:H1017–H1023.

Ley, K. (1995) Gene-targeted mice in leukocyte adhesion research. *Microcirc.* 2:141–150.

Ley, K., Bullard, D. C., Arbones, M. L., Bosse, R., Vestweber, D., Tedder, T. F., and Beaudet, A. L. (1995a) Sequential contribution of L- and P-selectin to leukocyte rolling in vivo. *J. Exp. Med.* 181:669–675.

Ley, K., Zakrzewicz, A., Hanski, C., Stoolman, L. M., and Kansas, G. S. (1995b) Sialylated O-glycans and L-selectin sequentially mediate myeloid cell rolling in vivo. *Blood* 85:3727–3735.

Ley, K. (1997) The selectins as rolling receptors. In *The Selectins: Initiators of Leukocyte Endothelial Adhesion.* D. Vestweber, ed. Amsterdam, The Netherlands: Harwood Academic, pp. 63–104.

Ley, K., Allietta, M., Bullard, D. C., and Morgan, S. J. (1998) The importance of E-selectin for firm leukocyte adhesion in vivo. *Circ. Res.* 83:287–294.

Lien, D. C., Henson, P. M., Capen, R. L., Henson, J. E., Hanson, W. L., Wagner, W. W., and Worthen, G. S. (1991) Neutrophil kinetics in the pulmonary microcirculation during acute inflammation. *Lab. invest.* 65:145–159.

Lipowsky, H. H., and Zweifach, B. W. (1978) Application of the "two-slit" photometric technique to the measurement of microvascular volumetric flow rates. *Microvasc. Res.* 15:93–101.

Lorant, D. E., Topham, M. K., Whatley, R. E., McEver, R. P., McIntyre, T. M., Prescott, S. M., and Zimmerman, G. A. (1993) Inflammatory roles of P-selectin. *J. Clin. Invest.* 92:559–570.

Lorenzi, S., Koedel, U., Dimagi, U., Ruckdeschel, G., and Pfister, H. W. (1993) Imaging of leukocyte–endothelium interaction using in vivo confocal laser scanning microscopy during the early phase of experimental pneumococcal meningitis. *J. Infect. Dis.* 168:927–933.

Lu, H. F., Smith, C. W., Perrard, J., Bullard, D., Tang, L. P., Shappell, S. B., Entman, M. L., Beaudet, A. L., and Ballantyne, C. M. (1997) LFA-1 is sufficient in mediating neutrophil emigration in Mac-1 deficient mice. *J. Clin. Invest.* 99:1340–1350.

Lundberg, C., and Arfors, K. -E. (1983) Polymorphonuclear leukocyte accumulation in inflammatory dermal sites as measured by ^{51}Cr-labelled cells and myeloperoxidase. *Inflamm.* 7:247–255.

Luscinskas. F. W., Ding, H., and Lichtman, A. H. (1995) P-selectin and vascular cell adhesion molecule 1 mediate rolling and arrest, respectively, of CD4[+] T lymphocytes on tumor necrosis factor α-activated vascular endothelium under flow. *J. Exp. Med.* 181:1179–1186.

Majuri, M. L., Pinola, M., Niemelä, R., Tiisala, S., Natunen, J., Renkonen, O., and Renkonen, R. (1994) α2,3-Sialyl and α1,3-fucosyltransferase-dependent synthesis of sialyl Lewis x, an essential oligosaccharide present on L-selectin counterreceptors, in cultured endothelial cells. *Eur. J. Immunol.* 24:3205–3210.

Manjunath N., Shankar, P., Stockton, B., Dubey, P. D., Lieberman, J., and von Andrian, U. H. (1999) A transgenic mouse model to analyze CD8[+] effector T cell differentiation in vivo. *Proc. Natl. Acad. Sci. U.S.A.* 96:13932–13937.

Mayadas, T. N., Johnson, R. C., Rayburn, H., Hynes, R. O., and Wagner, D. D. (1993) Leukocyte rolling and extravasation are severely compromised in P-selectin-deficient mice. *Cell* 74:541–554.

Mayrovitz, H. N., Tuma, R. F., and Wiedeman, M. P. (1980) Leukocyte adherence in arterioles following extravascular tissue trauma. *Microvasc. Res.* 20:264–274.

Mayrovitz, H. N. (1992) Leukocyte rolling: A prominent feature of venules in intact skin of anesthetized hairless mice. *Am. J. Physiol.* 262:H157–H161.

Metcalf, D., Lindeman, G. J., and Nicola, N. A. (1995) Analysis of hematopolesis in max 41 transgenic mice that exhibit sustained elevations of blood granulocytes and monocytes. *Blood* 85:2364–2370.

Metchnikoff, M. E. (1893) *Lectures on the Comparative Pathology of Inflammation.* London, Kegan Paul, Trench & Truebner.

Middleton, J., Neil, S., Wintle, J., Clarklewis, I., Moore, H., Lam, C., Auer, M., Hub, E., and Rot, A. (1997) Transcytosis and surface presentation of IL-8 by venular endothelial cells. *Cell* 91: 385–395.

Milstone, D. S., Fukumura, D., Padgett, R. C., O'Donnell, P. E., Davis, V. M., Benavidez, O. J., Monsky, W. L., Melder, R. J., Jain, R. K., and Gimbrone, M. A. (1998) Mice lacking E-selectin show normal numbers of rolling leukocytes but reduced leukocyte stable arrest on cytokine-activated microvascular endothelium. *Microcirc.* 5:153–171.

Miyamoto, K., Ogura, Y., Hamada, M., Nishiwaki, H., Hiroshiba, N., Tsujikawa, A., Mandai, M., Suzuma, K., Tojo, S. J., and Honda, Y. (1998) In vivo neutralization of P-selectin inhibits leukocyte–endothelial interactions in retinal microcirculation during ocular inflammation. *Microvasc. Res.* 55:230–240.

Mizgerd, J. P., Kubo, H., Kutkoski, G. J., Bhagwan, S. D., Scharffetter-Kochanek, K., Beaudet, A. L., and Doerschuk, C. M. (1997) Neutrophil emigration in the skin, lungs, and peritoneum—different requirements for CD11/CD18 revealed by CD18-deficient mice. *J. Exp. Med.* 186:1357–1364.

Morgan, S. J., Moore, M. W., Cacalano, G., and Ley, K. (1997) Reduced leukocyte adhesion response and absence of slow leukocyte rolling in interleukin-8 (IL-8) receptor deficient mice. *Microvasc. Res.* 54:188–191.

Mori, E., Del Zoppo, G. J., Chambers, J. D., Copeland, B. R., and Arfors, K. E. (1992) inhibition of polymorphonuclear leukocyte adherence suppresses no-reflow after focal cerebral ischemia in baboons. *Stroke* 23:712–718.

Muller, W. A., Weigl, S. A., Deng, X., and Phillips, D. M. (1993) PECAM-1 is required for transendothelial migration of leukocytes. *J. Exp. Med.* 178:449–460.

Naka, Y., Toda, K., Kayano, K., Oz, M. C., and Pinsky, D. J. (1997) Failure to express the P-selectin gene or P-selectin blockade confers early pulmonary protection after lung ischemia or transplantation. *Proc. Natl. Acad. Sci. USA* 94:757–761.

Nguyen, L. S., Villablanca, A. C., and Rutledge, J. C. (1995) Substance P increases microvascular permeability via nitric oxide-mediated convective pathways. *Am. J. Physiol.* 268:R1060–R1068.

Nobis, U., Pries, A. R., Cokelet, G. R., and Gaehtgens, P. (1985) Radial distribution of white cells during blood flow in small tubes. *Microvasc. Res.* 29:295–304.

Nolte, D., Schmid, P., Jäger, U., Botzlar, A., Roesken, F., Hecht, R., Uhl, E., Messmer, K., and Vestweber, D. (1994) Leukocyte rolling in venules of striated muscle and skin is mediated by P-selectin, not by L-selectin. *Am. J. Physiol.* 267:H1637–H1642.

Norgard, K. E., Moore, K. L., Diaz, S., Stults, N. L., Ushiyama, S., McEver, R. P., Cummings, R. D., and Varki, A. (1993) Characterization of a specific ligand for P-selectin on myeloid cells. A minor glycoprotein with sialylated O-linked oligosaccharides. *J. Biol. Chem.* 268:12764–12774.

Norman, K. E., Moore, K. L., McEver, R. P., and Ley, K. (1995) Leukocyte rolling in vivo is mediated by P-selectin glycoprotein ligand-1. *Blood* 86:4417–4421.

Olofsson, A. M., Arfors, K. -E., Ramezani, L., Wolitzky, B. A., Butcher, E. C., and von Andrian, U. H. (1994) E-selectin mediates leukocyte rolling in interleukin-1–treated rabbit mesentery venules. *Blood* 84:2749–2758.

Palabrica, T., Lobb, R., Furie, B. C., Aronovitz, M., Benjamin, C., Hsu, Y.-M., Sajer, S. A., and Furie, B. (1992) Leukocyte accumulation promoting fibrin deposition is mediated in vivo by P-selectin on adherent platelets. *Nature* 359:848–851.

Pan, J. L., Xia, L. J., and McEver, R. P. (1998) Comparison of promoters for the murine and human P-selectin genes suggests species–specific and conserved mechanisms for transcriptional regulation in endothelial cells. *J. Biol. Chem.* 273:10058–10067.

Perry, M. A., and Granger, D. N. (1991) Role of CD11/CD18 in shear rate-dependent leukocyte–endothelial cell interactions in cat mesenteric venules. *J. Clin. Invest.* 87:1798–1804.

Peschon, J. J., Slack, J. L., Reddy, P., Stocking, K. L., Sunnarborg, S. W., Lee, D. C., Russell, W. E., Castner, B. J., Johnson, R. S., Fitzner, J. N., et al. (1998) An essential role for ectodomain shedding in mammalian development. *Science* 282:1281–1284.

Picker, L. J., Kishimoto, T. K., Smith, C. W., Warnock, R. A., and Butcher, E. C. (1991a) ELAM-1 is an adhesion molecule for skin-homing T cells. *Nature* 349:796–799.

Picker, L. J., Warnock, R. A., Burns, A. R., Doerschuk, C. M., Berg, E. L., and Butcher, E. C. (1991b) The neutrophil selectin LECAM-1 presents carbohydrate ligands to the vascular selectins ELAM-1 and GMP-140. *Cell* 66:921–933.

Pittman, R. N., and Ellsworth, M. L. (1986) Estimation of red cell flow in microvessels: Consequences of the Baker-Wayland spatial averaging model. *Microvasc. Res.* 32:371–388.

Pober, J. S. (1987) Effects of tumor necrosis factor and related cytokines on vascular endothelial cells. *Ciba Found. Symp.* 131:170–184.

Pouyani, T., and Seed, B. (1995) PSGL-1 recognition of P-selectin is controlled by a tyrosine sulfation consensus at the PSGL-1 amino terminus. *Cell* 83:333–343.

Pries, A. R. (1988) A versatile video image analysis system for microcirculatory research. *Int. J. Microcirc. Clin. Exp.* 7:327–345.

Ramos, C. L., Smith, M. J., Snapp, K. R., Kansas, G. S., Stickney, G. W., Ley, K., and Lawrence, M. B. (1998) Functional characterization of L-selectin ligands on human neutrophils and leukemia cell lines: Evidence for mucin-like ligand activity distinct from P-selectin Glycoprotein Ligand-1. *Blood* 91:1067–1075.

Ramos, C. L., Huo, Y., Jung, U., Ghosh, S., Manka, D. R., Sarembock, I. J., and Ley, K, (1999) Direct demonstration of P-selectin and VCAM-1-dependent mononuclear cell rolling in early atherosclerotic lesions of apolipoprotein E-deficient mice. *Circ. Res.* 84:1237–1244.

Reneman, R. S., Woldhuis, B., oude Egbrink, M.G.A., Slaaf, D. W., and Tangelder, G. J. (1992) Concentration and velocity profiles of blood cells in the microcirculation. In: *Advances in Cardiovascular Engineering.* N.H.C. Hwang, V. T. Turitto, and M.R.T. Yen, eds. New York: Plenum Press, pp. 25–40.

Saetzler, R. K., Jallo, J., Lehr, H. A., Philips, C. M., Vasthare, U., Arfors, K. E., and Tuma, R. F. (1997) Intravital fluorescence microscopy—impact of light-induced phototoxicity on adhesion of fluorescently labeled leukocytes. *J. Histochem. Cytochem.* 45:505–513.

Sartor, R. B. (1992) Animal models of intestinal inflammation. In: *Inflammatory Bowel Disease.* R. P. McDermott, and W. F. Stenson, eds. New York; Elsevier, pp. 337–353.

Scharffetter-Kochanek, K., Lu, H., Norman, K. E., van Nood, N., Munoz, F., Grabbe, S., McArthur, M., Lorenzo, I., Kaplan, S., Ley, K., Smith, C. W., et al. (1998) Spontaneous skin ulceration and defective T-cell function in CD18 null mice. *J. Exp. Med.* 188:119–131.

Schmid-Schönbein, G. W., Usami, S., Skalak, R., and Chien, S. (1980) The interaction of leukocytes and erythrocytes in capillary and postcapillary vessels. *Microvasc. Res.* 19:45–70.

Schmidt, E. E., MacDonald, I. C., and Groom, A. C. (1990) Interactions of leukocytes with vessel walls and with other blood cells, studied by high-resolution intravital videomicroscopy of spleen. *Microvasc. Res.* 40:99–117.

Schmits, R., Kündig, T. M., Baker, D. M., Shumaker, G., Simard, J.J.L., Duncan, G., Wakeham, A., Shahinian, A., van der Heiden, A., Bachmann, M. F., et al. (1996) LFA-1 deficient mice show normal CTL responses to virus but fail to reject immunogenic tumor. *J. Exp. Med.* 183: 1415–1426.

Selvan, R. S., Kapadia, H. B., and Platt, J. L. (1998) Complement-induced expression of chemokine genes in endothelium: regulation by IL-1-dependent and- independent mechanisms. *J. Immunol.* 161:4388–4395.

Singbartl, K., Day, K., and Ley, K. (2000) Development of a CD2-Enhanced Green Fluorescent Protein (CD2-EGFP) transgenic mouse for studying lymphocyte trafficking in inflammation. *FASEB J.* 14, A704.

Sligh, J. E., Jr., Ballantyne, C. M., Rich, S. S., Hawkins, H. K., Smith, C. W., Bradley, A., and

Beaudet, A. L. (1993) Inflammatory and immune responses are impaired in mice deficient in intercellular adhesion molecule-1. *Proc. Natl. Acad. Sci. USA* 90:8529–8533.

Smith, M. J., Berg, E. L., and Lawrence, M. B. (1999) A direct comparison of selectin-mediated transient adhesive events using high temporal resolution. *Biophys. J.* 77:3371–3383.

Springer, T. A. (1995) Traffic signals on endothelium for lymphocyte recirculation and leukocyte emigration. *Annu. Rev. Physiol.* 57:827–872.

Sriramarao, P., von Andrian, U. H., Butcher, E. C., Bourdon, M. A., and Broide, D. H. (1994) L-selectin and very late antigen-4 integrin promote eosinophil rolling at physiological shear rates in vivo. *J. Immunol.* 153:4238–4246.

Staite, N. D., Justen, J. M., Sly, L. M., Beaudet, A. L., and Bullard, D. C. (1996) Inhibition of delayed-type contact hypersensitivity in mice deficient in both E-selectin and P-selectin. *Blood* 88:2973–2979.

Staunton, D. E., Dustin, M. L., and Springer, T. A. (1989) Functional cloning of ICAM-2, a cell adhesion ligand for LFA-1 homologous to ICAM-1. *Nature* 339:61–64.

Steeber, D. A., Engel, P., Miller, A. S., Sheetz, M. P., and Tedder, T. F. (1997) Ligation of L-selectin through conserved regions within the lectin domain activates signal transduction pathways and integrin function in human, mouse, and rat leukocytes. *J. Immunol.* 159:952–963.

Steeber, D. A., Campbell, M. A., Basit, A., Ley, K., and Tedder, T. F. (1998) Optimal selectin-mediated rolling of leukocytes during inflammation in vivo requires intercellular adhesion molecule-1 expression. *Proc. Natl. Acad. Sci. USA* 95:7562–7567.

Steegmaier, M., Levinovitz, A., Isenmann, S., Borges, E., Lenter, M., Kocher, H. P., Kleuser, B., and Vestweber, D. (1995) The E-selectin-ligand ESL-1 is a variant of a receptor for fibroblast growth factor. *Nature* 373:615–620.

Subramaniam, M., Frenette, P. S., Saffaripour, S., Johnson, R. C., Hynes, R. O., and Wagner, D. D. (1996) Defects in hemostasis in P-selectin–deficient mice. *Blood* 87:1238–1242.

Tangelder, G. J., Slaaf, D. W., Teirlinck, H. C., Alewijnse, R., and Reneman, R. S. (1982) Localization within a thin optical section of fluorescent blood platelets flowing in a microvessel. *Microvasc. Res.* 23:214–230.

Tedder, T. F., Steeber, D. A., and Pizcueta, P. (1995) L-selectin deficient mice have impaired leukocyte recruitment into inflammatory sites. *J. Exp. Med.* 181:2259–2264.

Tözeren, A., and Ley, K. (1992) How do selectins mediate leukocyte rolling in venules? *Biophys. J.* 63:700–709.

Varki, A. (1994) Selectin ligands. *Proc. Natl. Acad. Sci. USA* 91:7390–7397.

Vollmar, B., Glasz, J., Menger, M. D., and Messmer, K. (1995) Leukocytes contribute to hepatic ischemia/reperfusion injury via intercellular adhesion molecule-1-mediated venular adherence. *Surgery* 117:195–200.

von Andrian, U. H., Chambers, J. D., McEvoy, L. M., Bargatze, R. F., Arfors, K.-E., and Butcher, E. C. (1991) Two-step model of leukocyte–endothelial cell interaction in inflammation: Distinct roles for LECAM-1 and the leukocyte β_2 integrins in vivo. *Proc. Natl. Acad. Sci. USA* 88:7538–7542.

von Andrian, U. H., and Mrini, C. (1998) In situ analysis of lymphocyte migration to lymph nodes. *Cell Adhesion Commun.* 6:85–96.

Wakelin, M. W., Sanz, M. -J., Dewar, A., Albelda, S. M., Larkin, S. W., Boughton-Smith, N., Williams, T. J., and Nourshargh, S. (1996) An anti-platelet–endothelial cell adhesion molecule-1 antibody inhibits leukocyte extravasation from mesenteric microvessels in vivo by blocking the passage thorugh the basement membrane. *J. Exp. Med.* 184:229–239.

Walcheck, B., Kahn, J., Fisher, J. M.,Wang, B. B., Fisk, R. S., Payan, D. G., Feehan, C., Betageri, R., Dariak, K., Spatola, A. F., and Kishimoto, T. K. (1996a) Neutrophil rolling altered by inhibition of L-selectin shedding in vitro. *Nature* 380:720–723.

Walcheck, B., Moore, K. L., McEver, R. P., and Kishimoto, T. K. (1996b) Neutrophil–neutrophil interactions under hydrodynamic shear stress involve L-selectin and PSGL-1—A mechanism that amplifies initial leukocyte accumulation on P-selectin in vitro. *J. Clin. Invest.* 98:1081–1087.

Waller, A. (1846) Microscopic examination of some of the principal tissues of the animal frame, as observed in the tongue of the living frog, toad, etc. *Phil. Mag.* 29:271–287.

Walzog, B., Scharffetter-Kochanek, K., and Gaehtgens, P. (1999) Impairment of neutrophil emigration in CD18 null mice. *Am. J. Physiol.* 276:G1125–G1130.

Watson, S. R., Fennie, C., and Lasky, L. A. (1991) Neutrophil influx into an inflammatory site inhibited by soluble homing receptor-IgG chimaera. *Nature* 349:164–167.

Wayland, H., and Johnson, P. C. (1967) Erythrocyte velocity measurement in microvessels by two-slit photometric method. *J. Appl. Physiol.* 22:333–337.

Weyrich, A. S., Ma, X., Lefer, D. J., Albertine, K. H., and Lefer, A. M. (1993) In vivo neutralization of P-selectin protects feline heart and endothelium in myocardial ischemia and reperfusion injury. *J. Clin. Invest.* 91:2620–2629.

Winn, R. K., Liggitt, D., Vedder, N. B., Paulson, J. C., and Harlan, J. M. (1993) Anti-P-selectin monoclonal antibody attenuates reperfusion injury to the rabbit ear. *J. Clin. Invest.* 92:2042–2047.

Xie, J. L., Li, R., Kotovuori, P., Vermot-Desroches, C., Wijdenes, J., Arnaout, M. A., Nortamo, P., and Gahmberg, C. G. (1995) Intercellular adhesion molecule-2 (CD102) binds to the leukocyte integrin CD11b/CD18 through the A domain. *J. Immunol.* 155:3619–3628.

Xie, X., Raud, J., Hedqvist, P., and Lindborn, L. (1997) In vivo rolling and endothelial selectin binding of mononuclear leukocytes is distinct from that of polymorphonuclear cells. *Eur. J. Immunol.* 27:2935–2941.

Yang, J., Hirata, T., Croce, K., Merrill-Skoloff, G., Tchernychev, B., Williams, E., Flaumenhaft, R., Furie, B. C., and Furie, B. (1999) Targeted gene disruption demonstrates that P-selectin glycoprotein ligand 1 (PSGL-1) is required for P-selectin-mediated but not E-selectin-mediated neutrophil rolling and migration. *J. Exp. Med.* 190:1769–1782.

Yang, Y. T., Rayburn, H., and Hynes, R. O. (1995) Cell adhesion events mediated by α_4 integrins are essential in placental and cardiac development. *Development* 121:549–560.

Zakrzewicz, A., Grafe, M., Terbeek, D., Bongrazio, M., Auch-Schwelk, W., Walzog, B., Graf, K., Fleck, E., Ley, K., and Gaehtgens, P. (1997) L-selectin-dependent leukocyte adhesion to microvascular but not to macrovascular endothelial cells of the human coronary system. *Blood* 89:3228–3235.

Zhang, S. H., Reddick, R. L., Piedrahita, J. A., and Maeda, N. (1992) Spontaneous hypercholesterolemia and arterial lesions in mice lacking apolipoprotein E. *Science* 258:468–471.

Zhao, Y. H., Chien, S., and Skalak, R. (1995) A stochastic model of leukocyte rolling. *Biophys. J.* 69:1309–1320.

Zimmerman, B. J., Paulson, J. C., Arrhenius, T. S., Gaeta, F.C.A., and Granger, D. N. (1994) Thrombin receptor peptide-mediated leukocyte rolling in rat mesenteric venules: Roles of P-selectin and sialyl Lewis X. *Am. J. Physiol.* 267:H1049–H1053.

Zwaginga, J. J., Torres, H.I.G., Lammers, J.W.J., Sixma, J. J., Koenderman, L., and Kuijper, P.H.M. (1999) Minimal platelet deposition and activation in models of injured vessel wall ensure optimal neutrophil adhesion under flow conditions. *Arterioscl. Thromb. Vasc. Biol.* 19:1549–1554.

Zweifach, B. W., and Lipowsky, H. H. (1984) Pressure-flow relations in blood and lymph microcirculation. In: *Handbook of Physiology. The Cardiovascular System: Microcirculation.* E. M. Renkin, and C. C. Michel, eds. Bethesda, MD: American Physiological Society, pp. 251–307.

17

Transmigration of Leukocytes

BRIAN STEIN, YEESIM KHEW-GOODALL, and MATHEW VADAS

Migration of cells through a vascular endothelial monolayer is an essential step in inflammation, and thus in host defense and healing. Migration of neutrophils is the most studied form, providing basis for understanding the migration of other cell types. Of the series of events involved in transmigration, this chapter will limit its scope to the process of moving across the endothelial monolayer, and refer briefly to events immediately surrounding that process. Other events and mediators, such as endothelial activation and firm adhesion and the selectins, integrins, and chemoattractants, are dealt with elsewhere in this volume.

The Normal Endothelium

The endothelium normally exists in a resting state, without adherent or transmigrating cells (Grant, 1973). This is consistently reproduced in vitro, where neutrophil migration across unstimulated endothelium is insignificant (Furie et al. 1987, 1989; Moser et al., 1989). Lymphocyte transmigration is part of recirculation, an aspect of immune surveillance that can occur without perturbation through specialized endothelia characterized by their morphology (high endothelia). This specialized aspect of transmigration (De Bruyn and Cho, 1990; Imhoff et al., 1995) will not be considered in this chapter.

Two Types of Transmigration

Neutrophils in vitro migrate across resting or unactivated endothelium if an exogenous chemoattractant is present (Furie et al., 1989, 1991; Huang and Silverstein, 1992). For example, addition of a gradient of IL-8 or n-formyl-leucinyl-phenylalanine (fMLP) results in transmigration, which is dose-dependent and can cause 50%–90% of the neutrophils to transmigrate (Furie et al., 1991; Smith et al., 1991, 1994). This has been termed *leukocyte-driven transmigration* (Huang et al., 1992), but because the leukocytes are responding to exogenous chemoattractants, we believe that *chemotactic transmigration* is a more accurate description.

Table 17.1. Classes of Chemoattractants Produced by the Endothelium

Class	Example	Example Target Cell
Arachidonic acid metabolites	LTB_4	neutrophils, eosinophils
Ether lipids	PAF	neutrophils, eosinophils
CXC chemokines	IL-8	neutrophils
CC chemokines	MCP-1	monocytes, T-cells, eosinophils

The pathophysiological hallmark of the established inflammatory reaction is endothelial activation, an event requiring transcription and protein synthesis. As a result, adhesion molecules are up-regulated, inflammatory mediators are produced, and the endothelium secretes chemoattractants, all of which contribute to transmigration. Endothelial chemoattractants [summarized in Table 17.1] are critical for transmigration. They are secreted in significant amounts: concentrations in vitro reach those producing maximal chemotactic responses (Smith 1994). The stimulus for endothelial activation in vivo is probably local production of cytokines and other inflammatory mediators released on tissue injury.

Table 17.2. Chemotactic and Cytokine-activated Transmigration: Overview

	Chemotactic	Cytokine-activated
synonyms	leucocyte dependent transmigration	endothelial dependent transmigration
time for activation	minutes	hours
duration of action	hours	days
stimulus	exogenous chemoattractants	activation of the endothelium e.g., by cytokines

	Chemotactic	Cytokine-activated
chemoattractants	exogenous	local (endothelial production)
requires protein synthesis	no	yes
upregulation of endothelial adhesion molecules	?	yes
PECAM-1 dependent	no	yes
Endothelial IAP	not required	required
CD18 dependent	yes	yes
ICAM-1 dependent	yes	yes
dependent on endothelial $[Ca^{++}]_i$	yes	yes
in vivo correlate	early response	established inflammatory focus

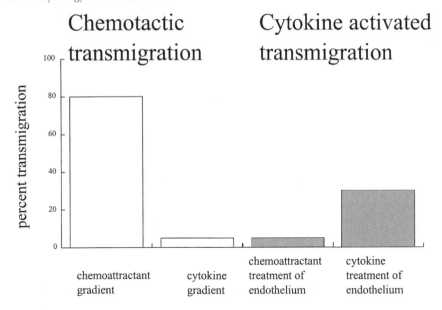

Figure 17.1. A schematic illustrating the difference between chemotactic and cytokine-activated transmigration. The graph illustrates that, in an in vitro transmigration model, chemoattractants drive transmigration by being present as a gradient during the experiment. In contrast, cytokines drive transmigration by activating the endothelium, which requires pretreatment.

To differentiate these two types of transmigration clearly, we will refer to them as chemotactic and cytokine-activated transmigration. These differences are summarized in Table 17.2 and Figure 17.1. Both mechanisms are important pathophysiological events. Chemotactic transmigration is probably the mechanism by which early responses to tissue injury are generated, and cytokine-activated transmigration enables the generation of later, more prolonged responses. Chemotactic transmigration has been studied less than cytokine-activated transmigration, and as summarized in Table 17.2, there may be differences in mechanism.

An Overview of Transmigration in Vivo

Transmigration has been conceptualised as involving three steps: (a) rolling, (b) activation or triggering resulting in firm adhesion, and (c) migration across the endothelium and into the tissues (Butcher, 1991; Springer, 1994). This is based on direct views of transmigration, for example, by intravital microscopy of the exteriorized mesentery. On exposure, the postcapillary venules contain a number of leukocytes that are peripheral to the central stream of blood flow, and moving more slowly. They are in contact with the vessel wall, along which they roll. The experimental preparation provides sufficient stimulation to the endothelium to induce rolling (Smith, 1992). Rolling consists of adhesive interactions sufficient to slow the leukocyte, but not enough to overcome blood flow and stop the leukocyte. If a chemoattractant or an inflammatory stimulus is then applied, large numbers of leukocytes will become firmly adherent to the side of the vessel, forming a layer like pebbles in a stream. In contrast to the adhesion involved in rolling, firm adhesion is associated with sufficient strength of adhesion to overcome blood flow. Firm adhesion is usually rapidly followed by migration across the endothelial monolayer. After transmigration there is often a hold-up of cells at the basement membrane (Grant, 1973; Huber and Weiss, 1989). Leukocytes remain adherent to the basal aspect of the endothelium and may form a temporary sheath around the vessel before moving into the tissues (Grant, 1973).

The molecular mediators of these three steps are discussed at length elsewhere in this volume, and some of the critical molecules in transmigration and their endothelial distribution are outlined in Table 17.3 and Figure 17.2. In a nutshell, rolling slows the leukocyte, allowing it to come into greater contact with the endothelium. With increased endothelial contact it appears that receptors on the leukocyte bind chemoattractants produced or presented by the endothelium (Rainger et al., 1997; outlined in Table 17.1). Chemoattractant stimulation together with signaling generated by binding to adhesion molecules results in activation of members of the integrin class of adhesion molecules on the leukocyte, particularly the β_2 integrins (Crockett-Torabi et al., 1995; Gopalan et al., 1997); it is not yet clear if these two mechanisms are redundant. Integrins on the activated leukocyte are able to interact with

Table 17.3. Some Important Molecules in Transmigration

Molecule	Synonyms	Location
Platelet-endothelial cell adhesion molecule-1 (PECAM-1)	CD31	neutrophils, monocytes, some T-cell subtypes, eosinophils & endothelium
β_2-integrin	CD18	all leucocytes
$\alpha_L\beta_2$ chain of β_2-integrin	CD11a, LFA-1	all leucocytes
$\alpha_M\beta_2$ chain of β_2-integrin	CD11b, Mac-1	NK cells, neutrophils, monocytes, eosinophils
$\alpha_4\beta_1$-integrin	CD49d/CD29, VLA-4	lymphocytes, monocytes, eosinophils
Intercellular adhesion molecule-1 (ICAM-1)	CD54	endothelium, monocytes, some T cells
Integrin associated protein (IAP)	CD47	all leucocytes & endothelium
Vascular cell adhesion molecule-1 (VCAM-1)	CD106	cytokine activated endothelium

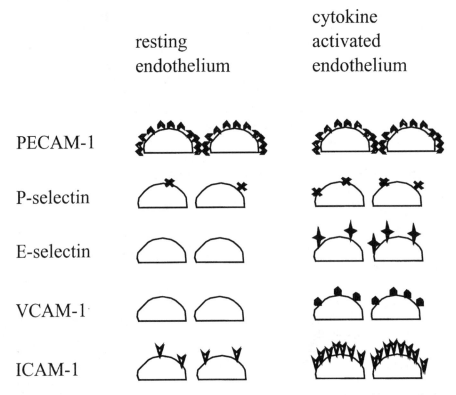

Figure 17.2. A schematic illustrating the relative abundance and cytokine regulation of certain endothelial adhesion molecules that are pertinent to transmigration.

their ligands on the endothelium, members of the immunoglobulin super-family of adhesion molecules, and form a strong adhesive bond, bringing the cell to a halt. This second step is then followed by migration across the endothelial cell monolayer (Butcher, 1991; Springer, 1994).

Transmigration Is a Final Result of Many Factors

A number of interactions occur between the leukocyte and the endothelium during transit from the blood stream to the tissues. Abolition of interactions that precede transit across the endothelium may reduce the number of cells that transmigrate, without affecting the mechanism by which cells move across the endothelium. For example, inhibition of selectin binding significantly reduces transmigration. This does not imply selectins are involved in passage across the monolayer. It reflects the requirement for selectin-mediated slowing of leukocyte flow velocity, which, in turn, is required for firm adhesion (Lawrence et al., 1990). Similarly, blocking firm adhesion by inhibiting integrins like CD-18 may prevent transmigration without necessarily altering passage across the monolayer. This can make it difficult to define the role of a particular molecule in the transmigration process.

We will concentrate on mechanisms that specifically operate after firm binding has occurred and, generally, will not discuss alterations in steps leading up to firm adhesion that result in decreased transmigration.

The Experimental Study of Transmigration

In Vitro Systems

These systems have the major advantage of being easily manipulable, and are relatively well defined. They are not simple systems. There are five basic variables in in vitro systems of transmigration: the leukocyte subtype, the presence of shear stress from fluid flow, the source of the cellular barrier, the support the cells are grown on, and the stimulus to transmigration.

Leukocyte Subtype
Neutrophils, monocytes, eosinophils, NK, and T cells can all be isolated in relatively pure preparations from human blood and used; preparation of neutrophils is the simplest procedure, and this may contribute to their popularity as experimental models. Although closest to the physiological situation, the requirement for fresh preparation prior to each experiment is a disadvantage. The isolation process may lead to some activation of the cells: neutrophils, for example, show some phenotypic changes after purification reflecting activation, and it is likely that the small background transmigration of neutrophils across unactivated endothelial cells (EC) reflects this. Cell lines have also been used: HL-60 can be differentiated toward a neutrophil or monocytoid phenotype, and U937 have also been used as monocyte surrogates. The ability to transfect these cells is a significant advantage and has been used to good effect in studying chemoattractant receptor function (Hsu et al., 1997; Kew et al., 1997).

The Presence of Shear Stress
In general, flow chambers have been used to investigate adhesive interactions between leukocytes and endothelial cells; they are difficult experiments to set up, and their use in transmigration is hampered by the difficulty in counting the number of cells migrating. Systems using fluid flow have the advantage of being more physiological; however, transmigration is the final result of many factors, thus flow systems may be limited in their ability to dissect out features essential in passage across the endothelial monolayer. In view of these problems, the majority of in vitro experiments are performed as static assays.

The Cellular Barrier and Culture Substrate
The cellular barrier is an important variable. The majority of studies use primary endothelial cells. Although cultured EC do provide a good model,

there are differences between EC in vivo and in vitro, between microvascular and large vessel endothelium, and between endothelia from different organs (reviewed in Kvietys and Granger, 1997), hence results in vitro generally require in vivo correlation.

Endothelial cells from large vessels, for example, bovine aortic endothelium or human umbilical vein endothelium are relatively easy to harvest and support transmigration. Much of the molecular understanding of transmigration has come from studies using these cells. They do have a weakness: transmigration in vivo occurs in the microvasculature, not large vessels, thus some features of the process may be missed by using these cells. Microvascular endothelial cells have been used in studies of transmigration, but harvesting these cells in sufficient numbers is more difficult. Endothelial cells change with passage, for example, losing their responses to inflammatory cytokine stimuli, and thus should be used in early passages.

Cell lines have the advantage of less line-to-line variation in their responses and avoid problems of harvesting primary cells. The potential cost is being a further step removed from the physiological situation. This has led to limited use. Recombinant "endothelial cells," mesenchymal cells such as fibroblasts transfected with a molecule of interest and used as a monolayer (Zocchi et al., 1996), are yet a further step removed from physiological systems. Although attractive from a mechanistic viewpoint, interpretation of results from such systems must be made with great care: there are significant differences between transmigration across endothelia and other cell types, for example, epithelia (Parkos, 1997) or synovial fibroblasts (Shang et al., 1998b).

To form a monolayer, the endothelial cells must be grown on a supportive substrate. The choices are between a simpler system, glass or a polycarbonate porous support coated with an adhesion molecule such as fibronectin (Smith et al., 1989), or a complex structure, amniotic membrane (Furie et al., 1989), or thick, denatured collagen gels (Luscinskas et al., 1991). Whereas transmigration in vivo will expose leukocytes to basement membrane and extracellular matrix molecules, in vitro, the situation may differ because it may take up to 3 weeks for the basement membrane secreted by endothelial cells to resemble the basement membrane in vivo (Huber and Weiss, 1989). Whether the matrix secreted by endothelial cells used in most transmigration systems is sufficient to trigger all the changes generated in vivo is uncertain. It is thus possible that some conflicting results may reflect differences in the extracellular matrix that leukocytes are exposed to as they transmigrate across human umbilical vein endothelial cells (HUVEC) growing on amniotic membrane and those growing on fibronectin-coated surfaces.

The Stimulus to Transmigration

Finally, a choice must be made about which stimulus will be used. Monocytes may exhibit significant levels of transmigration across unstimulated EC, but in general, eosinophils, neutrophils, and T cells require activation for significant numbers to migrate. Both cytokine activation of endothelial cells or the presence of an exogenous chemoattractant gradient (the choice of chemoattractant depending on the cell type used) across the monolayer result in transmigration; however, the mechanisms may differ significantly.

In Vivo Systems

These systems have the advantage of being closer to the pathophysiology of inflammation, although this is balanced by the increase in complexity involved in using whole animals. There are two major in vivo models of transmigration. The first involves direct viewing of the vasculature and its contents with intravital microscopy (discussed elsewhere in this volume), and the second involves counting the number and type of leukocytes migrating into a tissue after a period of time. Typical examples are: the use of subcutaneous air pouches and the peritoneal cavity; and transmigration stimulated by injection of chemoattractants or substances designed to elicit an inflammatory reaction. The critical variables are the species of animal, the stimulus to transmigration, the organ system used, and the manipulation. The importance of species will not be dealt with at any length: it is clear there are important interspecies differences. There are significant differences in the response of different organ systems illustrated by the various models of CD18-independent transmigration. Stimuli to transmigration are far more complex in whole animal models: secondary effects, for example, activation of tissue macrophages and mast cells, can occur even with the simplest manipulation. Furthermore, in vivo migration of monocytes and lymphocytes is relatively late in comparison to neutrophils. As a result, evaluating migration of these cell types outside the context of a chronic inflammatory stimulus is difficult. Manipulation of transmigration predominantly involves use of relatively specific reagents such as monoclonal antibodies. Knock out animals lacking adhesion molecules have also been a valuable tool, although there are suggestions that compensation for a missing molecule can occur (Doerschuk et al., 1996).

The Problem of Endothelial Heterogeneity

It is clear that the high endothelial venules in lymph nodes are specialized for lymphocyte transmigration (Mebius et al., 1993), and specific mechanisms may exist in such regions of habitual transmigration. There are significant variations in endothelial morphology (Palade, 1988), responses to growth factors (Brindle, 1993), expression of adhesion molecules and gap junctions (Pepper et al., 1992; Brindle, 1993), and transmigration (Grant, 1973) between different parts of the circulation. These differences between vascular beds are not extensively addressed by current in vitro experimental models. These variations appear important. For example, platelet–endothelial cell adhesion molecule-1 (PECAM-1) appears necessary for migration into the peritoneum but not into the liver (Chosay et al., 1998). The effect of endothelial heterogeneity is an important area where current understanding, particularly of migration across the endothelium, needs to be extended.

The Process of Transmigration

A global overview is provided in Figure 17.3. The process begins with firm adhesion, triggered by leukocyte activation from endogenous or exogenous chemoattractants. This is followed by signaling from the leukocyte to the endothelium. In vitro models suggest that firm adhesion is followed by leukocyte migration toward the interendothelial junction. It seems likely the endothelial signaling pathways alter the junction and endothelial cytoskeleton to allow passage of the leukocyte across the endothelial monolayer. This is then followed by migration into the tissues.

Firm Adhesion Is Necessary, But Not Sufficient, For Transmigration

Only Firmly Adherent Cells Transmigrate
Firm adhesion is a prerequisite for transmigration. Both in vivo (reviewed in Grant, 1973) and in vitro experiments (Furie et al., 1987; Smith, 1992) clearly show that only firmly adherent cells can transmigrate.

Firm Adhesion Is Separate from Transmigration
Three lines of evidence support the idea that firm adhesion per se is necessary, but not sufficient, for transmigration.

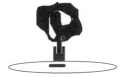

1. Endothelium to leukocyte signalling
via chemoattractants

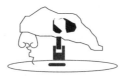

2. Leukocyte activation and firm adhesion

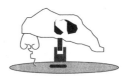

3. Leukocyte to endothelial signalling

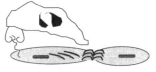

4. Downstream signals
Cytoskeletal changes.
? Junctional changes
? Signalling between endothelial cells
Crawling to the junction

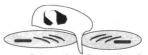

5. Insertion of pseudopod
Formation of endothelial tunnel
Interaction between leukocyte and endothelial junctional molecules

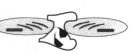

6. Transmigration

Figure 17.3. A drawing illustrating the model of transmigration: The initial stippling indicates the initial signaling flux, for example, elevations in intracellular calcium. This results in changes in the endothelial cells that are presumed to be important in facilitating transmigration.

Leukocyte Adhesion Alone Does Not Trigger Transmigration. Firm adhesion per se is not enough to promote transmigration: treating neutrophils with TNF, for example, induces firm adhesion to resting HUVEC, but does not promote transmigration. Similarly, binding induced by other mechanisms, for example, via immunoglobulin Fc receptors does not induce transmigration (Moser et al., 1989). Thus, leukocytes do not have an inherent migratory mechanism that is triggered on binding and results in transmigration. This suggests an event separate from firm adhesion is required for transmigration. Cytokine-activated transmigration can be blocked without decreasing firm adhesion. Endothelial and exogenous chemoattractants are critical in transmigration. As chemoattractant inhibitors may decrease transmigration without altering firm adhesion, this provides another argument that adhesion and transmigration are separate events. Although there are disagreements, a number of results show dissociation of adhesion and transmigration using chemoattractant inhibition. Kuijpers et al. (1992a) found that IL-1 pretreatment of HUVEC induced both neutrophil adherence and transmigration. Transmigration was inhibited in a dose-dependent manner by the platelet-activating factor (PAF) antagonist WEB 2086, but adhesion was unaffected. This has been confirmed by others (Hill et al., 1994) in vivo: firm adhesion resulting from IL-1 activation of rat mesenteric vessels was not affected, but transmigration was reduced by 60% by pretreatment with either of two PAF antagonists (Nourshargh et al., 1995). Kuijpers et al. (1992a) also reported that IL-8 antisera reduced transmigration, without altering firm adhesion. Smith et al. (1993) confirmed this finding by inhibiting IL-8 effects through desensitization of neutrophils. Not all groups have confirmed the importance of PAF: Smith et al. (1993), among others (Bevario et al., 1988; Smart and Casale, 1994), found that PAF antagonism had little effect on neutrophil transmigration across TNF-activated HUVEC. Huber et al. (1991) reported inhibition of both adhesion and transmigration with IL-8 antibodies. These differences remain unreconciled, but may reflect differences in the in vitro models that the various groups have used.

Perturbation of Intracellular Signaling Can Inhibit Transmigration Without Altering Firm Adhesion. Probably the strongest argument in favor of adhesion and transmigration being separate events comes from direct alteration of second messengers in intracellular signaling pathways: blockade of intracellular signaling pathways, such as calcium fluxes, in the endothelium strongly inhibits transmigration across both cytokine-activated endothelium, and toward a chemoattractant gradient (Huang et al., 1993). This argues strongly for an extra endothelial step after binding, which requires signaling.

Are Leukocytes Limited in Their Capacity to Transmigrate?

In chemotactic transmigration (exogenous chemoattractant and resting HUVEC) in vitro, the majority of neutrophils will migrate (Smith et al., 1991, 1993). When PAF or IL-8 is used as a stimulus, almost all the neutrophils can be induced to transmigrate (Smith et al., 1991, 1993). This suggests that there are few inherently immotile or unresponsive neutrophils. Chemoattractants do vary in potency (Casale et al., 1992), which might explain some differences between chemotactic transmigration systems. For example, in contrast to IL-8, fMLP generally induces only 40% of neutrophils to transmigrate (Casale et al., 1992). Given the similarities in receptors, signaling, and other functional activation (Baggiolini et al., 1993), it is unclear why this difference exists.

In contrast to chemotactic transmigration, only 25%–50% of neutrophils transmigrate across cytokine-activated endothelium (Furie et al., 1987, 1989; Moser et al 1989). The origin of this limitation is not clear. It seems unlikely to be a limit in chemoattractant production because activated endothelium in vitro can generate concentrations of IL-8 close to those providing optimal migratory stimulus in chemotactic transmigration. Furthermore, addition of exogenous chemoattractants to cytokine-activated endothelium only increases transmigration by approximately 10% (Moser et al., 1989; Furie et al., 1989, 1992). The limitation may be leukocyte mediated because the proportion of neutrophils migrating is independent of the number of cells added (Furie et al., 1987, 1989). A possible mechanism might be that cytokine activation results in secretion of chemoattractants bidirectionally; without flow, there will be accumulation of chemoattractant in the lumen. In this latter state, desensitization may occur (Smith et al., 1993), down-regulating leukocyte responses to the agent.

Firm Adhesion Signals to the Endothelium

Signaling as a result of adhesion molecules binding to their ligands (reviewed in Hynes, 1992) clearly occurs in the context of transmigration, in both leukocytes and in the endothelium. The detection of signals in the endothelium on interaction with the leukocyte suggests that these signals play a role in transmigration, and that modulation of signaling pathways can inhibit transmigration is an idea in keeping with this hypothesis. At present, signaling pathways are being mapped out; their eventual targets are not known, but it seems reasonable to speculate that they may modulate the junction or cytoskeleton.

Calcium

Adhesion of neutrophils and monocytic U937 cells induces a rise in endothelial cell intracellular calcium ($[Ca^{2+}]_i$; Huang et al., 1993; Ziegelstein et al., 1994). This is specific as it is not seen after binding of red cells or inert microspheres (Ziegelstein et al., 1994). These effects appear functionally important in transmigration because buffering endothelial intracellular calcium decreased transmigration of neutrophils to either an fMLP gradient or across IL-1–activated HUVEC by over 85%, but neutrophil adhesion was unaltered (Huang et al., 1993). It is not entirely clear what the signal transduction mechanism is. Several reports implicate CD18 and intercellular adhesion molecule-1 (ICAM 1; Ziegelstein et al., 1994; Pfau et al., 1995; Clayton et al., 1998). Other investigators have suggested that this effect is mediated by alternate adhesion molecules (P-and E-selectin and vascular cell adhesion molecule, VCAM-1) (Lorenzon et al., 1998). Endothelial calcium release is probably mediated through release from intracellular stores, as thapsigargin can inhibit calcium fluxes (Ziegelstein et al., 1994). Hence, the signaling pathway is likely to involve generation of inositol 1,4,5-trisphosphate: how adhesion to ICAM-1 or VCAM-1 triggers release of inositol 1,4,5-trisphosphate remains to be seen.

Leukocytes also respond to binding to endothelium; for example, binding to endothelium induces an increase in neutrophil $[Ca^{2+}]_i$. If this increase is prevented by calcium chelators, CD-11b up-regulation is impaired (Kuijpers et al., 1992b). This may indicate cross-talk between the leukocyte and the endothelium. For example, on firm adhesion of NK cells to endothelium, there was an initial change in NK cell $[Ca^{2+}]_i$, and an oscillatory change in endothelial $[Ca^{2+}]_i$ that occurred after strong adhesion. If the NK cell $[Ca^{2+}]_i$ changes were prevented, the endothelial $[Ca^{2+}]_i$ changes did not occur. Antibodies to ICAM-1 or LFA-1 could prevent the changes in endothelial $[Ca^{2+}]_i$, suggesting that these adhesion molecules are necessary (Pfau et al., 1995).

Downstream of Calcium

The downstream pathways from calcium are not completely elucidated. Endothelial myosin light chain phosphorylation appears important because inhibitors of myosin light chain kinase (MLCK) partially inhibit transmigration (Garcia et al., 1998), and inhibition of phosphatases that can regulate MLCK increases transmigration (Garcia et al., 1998). MLCK appears to be downstream of $[Ca^{2+}]_i$, because calcium/calmodulin antagonists inhibit myosin light chain phosphorylation (Garcia et al., 1998).

A mechanism by which MLCK may act is opening of the endothelial junction through mechanical retraction. Increased endothelial myosin light chain phosphorylation, which is induced by addition of activated neutrophils (Garcia et al., 1998; Saito et al., 1998), is correlated with increases in isometric tension in the monolayer (Hixenbaugh et al., 1997). Increased tension has been suggested to open the interendothelial junction and reduce the endothelial barrier. Endothelial retraction is seen with soluble agents like histamine that also induce myosin light chain phosphorylation (Garcia et al., 1995); however, gross endothelial retraction is not a feature of transmigration, suggesting that the process is finely tuned.

Cyclic Adenosine Monophosphate

It is possible that cyclic adenosine monophosphate (cAMP), another classical second messenger, is activated and important in regulating transmigration. Oppenheimer-Marks et al., (1994) reported treatment of endothelial cells with prostaglandin E_2 (PGE_2) decreased T-lymphocyte transmigration. This effect may be mediated by cAMP as transmigration was increased by increasing cAMP through adding dibutryl cAMP or by inhibition of phosphodiesterase activity (Oppenheimer Marks et al., 1994). Decreased transmigration was correlated with decreased endothelial permeability to macromolecules. It is not clear if signaling via cAMP is induced by leukocytes; some endothelial activators (e.g., IL-1) do appear to up-regulate endothelial adhesiveness via cAMP-dependent pathways. The time course of inhibition of transmigration does suggest that these inhibitors are not directly altering IL-1 signaling.

Gap Junctions

Another possible mechanism of communication is through gap junctions, as these aqueous channels allow direct communication between adjacent cells. The channels are made up of six protein subunits, the connexins. There is significant heterogeneity in the tissue distribution of gap junctions, and in the connexins comprising them (reviewed in Beyer, 1993). During firm adhesion, extensive contact occurs between leukocyte and endothelium, with areas of close apposition. Gap junctions could form in such areas and would allow rapid communication between the cells, providing a good mechanism for modulation of the endothelial barrier. Although endothelial cells have gap junctions on EM (Palade, 1988) and express connexins (Reed et al., 1993), their relevance to transmigration is unclear. Dye transfer has been found between lymphocytes and endothelium (Guinan et al., 1988), strongly suggesting functional gap junctions, but others have not found dye transfer between monocytes and endothelium (Polacek et al., 1993). A further problem may be provided by the requirement for homophilic connexin expression on both cells for gap junction pore formation, although this is not an absolute requirement. For example, HUVEC express connexin 43 (Reed et al., 1993), but unstimulated leukocytes do not (Bruzzone et al., 1993; Jara et al., 1995). This might be altered by stimulation, as in vivo and in vitro models have demonstrated up-regulation of connexin 43 in neutrophils and monocytes (Jara et al., 1995). Thus, it is not clear if gap junctions are important in transmigration, although they would provide a mechanism for rapid communication between leukocyte and endothelium.

Soluble Signaling Molecules

Soluble factors produced by leukocytes can provide signals to the endothelium, and the close proximity between the transmigrating leukocyte and endothelium should prevent soluble mediators from being removed by blood flow. As yet, these signals have no established role in transmigration, but some reported effects are suggestive. For example, endothelial cells produce soluble IL-6, release of soluble IL-6 receptor α chain from activated neutrophils for IL-6 signaling to occur in the endothelium. This signaling results in endothelial activation (Modur et al., 1997). Similarly, it has been noted that neutrophils can produce leukotrienes like LTA_4 that endothelial cells can metabolize to potent chemoattractants like LTB_4 (Maclouf, 1993; Brady et al., 1995). Perhaps more importantly, neutrophil soluble factors can up-regulate endothelial production of matrix metalloproteinase-2 (MMP-2, Schwartz et al., 1998). This might be important in passage across the basement membrane.

Moving to the Junction

Furie et al., (1987) observed that initial adherence to the endothelium was random and not predisposed to the interendothelial junctions. Because the leukocyte transmigrates through the interendothelial junction, there must be some means to locate it. A mechanism for this is suggested by in vivo observations (Grant, 1973; Harlan et al., 1992) that adherent leukocytes crawl over the endothelial surface, seeming to probe for an opening, before transmigrating. This suggests that two components are operating: motility, for which adhesion is required, and guidance.

Crawling involves a series of attachments and detachments from the substrate, development of tension through the cytoskeleton (Harris, 1994), and active remodeling of the cytoskeleton (Devreotes, 1988; Stossel, 1993). Without adhesion, crawling and all the subsequent movement-dependent steps in transmigration will be inhibited. Agents that affect the cytoskeleton, like paclitaxel (Taxol; Oppenheimer Marks et al., 1994), inhibit transmigration, presumably by preventing crawling. Less obviously, interference with detachment from the substrate, as is seen with up-regulation of β_1 integrin function, may prevent crawling, the leukocyte being "glued" to one spot (Kuijpers et al., 1993; Harris, 1994). Some of the molecules involved in transmigration may act during this phase of transmigration as well as passage through the junction.

Finding the Junction

Adherent leukocytes move toward the interendothelial junction with speed and apparent purpose (Muller and Weigl, 1992). This argues against a chemoattractant-stimulated random walk as a mechanism for finding the junction, and argues for the existence of directional information.

Physical Guidance Mechanisms

Physical features of the cellular environment can give directional information in vitro. These mechanisms include contact guidance (directional information from differences in geometry), and haptotaxis (directional information from gradients of adhesion). The role these mechanisms play in vivo is not clear.

In vitro, many cells including neutrophils (Wilkinson and Lackie, 1983), can use topographical information as a guide to migration (Clark et al., 1990). For the transmigrating leukocyte, the geometry of the endothelial cell may contain directional information. Endothelial cells exposed to shear align themselves in the direction of the force (Davies, 1995), and are ridged (Barbee et al., 1994), with the ridges aligned in the direction of flow. Structures of this order of magnitude can give guidance clues (Clark et al., 1992); this ridging may then provide directional information. Neutrophils also readily align themselves along grooves (Wilkinson et al., 1982) such as may occur at the intercellular junction. In a fibrin matrix under tension, neutrophils prefer to move parallel to the fiber axes (Wilkinson et al., 1982). In this system there are clearly geometrical cues, but there may well be cues from differences in rigidity, as fibers subject to a tensile strain will be more rigid, and this may provide contact guidance (Lackie, 1986).

In addition to contact guidance, guidance can come from gradients of adhesiveness (haptotaxis; Carter, 1965). Haptotaxis has been shown to induce cell migration in vitro (Lackie, 1986): E-selectin is haptotactic to neutrophils (Lo et al 1991); thrombospondin is haptotactic to monocytes and neutrophils (Mansfield and Suchard, 1993, 1994); and fibronectin, vitronectin, and collagen IV are haptotactic for activated T cells (Hauzenberger et al., 1994). Evidence for in vivo relevance of haptotaxis has been provided in embryological systems, but has not conclusively been demonstrated for transmigration. In vitro, there may be a gradient of E-selectin adhesiveness directed toward the periphery of the endothelial cell, as the force required to remove HL-60 cells from activated endothelium (measured directly with atomic force microscopy) increased toward the periphery, and was abolished by E-selectin antibodies (Sung et al., 1994). In keeping with a haptotactic gradient, P-selectin up-regulation in response to histamine or thrombin appears to be preferentially at intercellular borders, and results in preferential capture at these regions (Burns et al., 1999). The extracellular matrix proteins in the junction may also provide a haptotactic gradient. Similarly, the distribution of PECAM-1, maximal in the interendothelial junctional region, suggests a potential for haptotactic guidance, although this has not been directly examined.

Chemical Guidance

Gradients of chemical substances give directional information in vitro. Furthermore, complex directional information can come from combinations of chemical gradients: neutrophils can move from a chemotactic gradient of one substance to a gradient of another substance, for example, from the chemokine IL-8 to the classical chemoattractant fMLP (Foxman et al., 1998). This would allow complex navigational information to be presented. Because a stable gradient is required for chemotaxis (Zigmond, 1978), a problem arises from blood flow.

Blood flow might remove chemoattractants, making a gradient of soluble material unstable. In contrast, as endothelial cells secrete some chemoattractants in both directions, blood flow might disperse the component secreted into the lumen, maintaining a gradient of chemoattractant. Furthermore, it has been debated whether chemoattractants can act in the blood stream or are diluted by blood flow and are relatively ineffective. This problem might be solved if chemoattractants could bind to a surface, as this would ensure a concentration gradient immune to the effects of flow. Many chemoattractants have anionic or hydrophobic sites that are potential areas for surface binding (Miller and Kraugel, 1992). PAF, for example, is predominantly inserted in the endothelial cell membrane (Kuijpers et al., 1992a), and IL-8 can bind to extracellular matrix or basement membrane and to endothelial cells (Schonbeck et al., 1995), where it is presented on the tips of the microvilli (Middleton et al., 1997). Surface-bound chemokines may also have other modes of action: for example, IL-8 and C5a, but not fMLP, are haptotactic in vitro (Rot, 1992). Whereas chemotactic gradients exist across the endothelium, the extent to which they provide guidance to the junction is uncertain. We are unaware of any demonstration of gradients of surface-bound chemokines leading to the junction, nor of a gradient extending through the junction. However, it seems likely that chemoattractants play an important role not just in triggering firm adhesion, but also in providing directional information leading the transmigrating leukocyte through the intracellular junction.

Transmigration Is Paracellular, Occurring Through the Interendothelial Junction

Movement through the monolayer is rapid, occurring within 30 seconds (Beesley et al., 1978); however, the route through the endothelium is debated. There have been reports suggesting transcellular transmigration in vivo (Feng et al., 1998). These studies have used reconstruction of serial electron microscopic sections to determine this route. This methodology is technically demanding, and can be subject to artifactual distortions. In contrast, ultrastructural studies in vivo (Grant, 1973) and in vitro (Furie et al., 1987; Smith, 1992) show that adherent neutrophils extrude pseudopodia that indent the surface of the endothelium, and extrude between neighboring cells. Confocal microscopy reveals formation of a tunnel between endothelial cells through which a monocyte pseudopod extends (Sandig et al., 1997), and others localize transmigration to the tricorner area among three adjacent endothelial cells (Burns et al., 1997). At present the contribution of a transcellular route is unclear in vivo; in vitro, it seems that the paracellular route is central. This being the case, the migrating leukocyte must first locate and then traverse a potentially formidable barrier formed by the multiple adhesion systems in the interendothelial junction.

The Structure of the Junction

Endothelial cells are polygonal and extend in the direction of blood flow, along the long axis of the vessel (Adamson, 1993). The interendothelial cell junction is little longer than a straight line joining the surface to the basement membrane (Adamson, 1993), between 0.12 and 0.64 microns in length (Adamson, 1990, 1993), although it is often tortuous in the apico-basal direction (Franke et al., 1988). Endothelial cells are strongly adherent to the basement membrane, and adhere to each other via adherens, and tight and gap junctions (Franke et al., 1988; Caveda et al., 1994). The intercellular junctions, especially adherens junctions, form a continuous belt around the cell (Franke et al., 1988). Intracellular actin and myosin are close to the junction in vivo and in vitro, and may regulate junction opening through endothelial contraction (Goeckeler and Wysolmerski, 1995). The principal molecules in the extracellular space of the junction appear to be $\alpha_2\beta_1$, $\alpha_3\beta_1$, and $\alpha_5\beta_1$ integrins, PECAM-1, VE-cadherin (also known as cadherin-5; Albelda et al., 1991, Lampugnani et al., 1991, 1992, 1995; Ayalon et al., 1994), and the recently described junctional adhesion molecule (JAM; Huang et al., 1998).

Integrins and Associated Proteins. Immunofluorescence studies (Lampugnani et al., 1991) initially revealed two integrins, $\alpha_2\beta_1$ and $\alpha_5\beta_1$ in the junction, more recently $\alpha_3\beta_1$ integrin has also been found (Yanez-Mo et al., 1998). Their ligands are unclear: collagen, laminin, thrombospondin, and fibronectin are all produced by endothelial cells and found in the cell–cell interaction rims (Volker et al., 1991; Kowalczyk et al., 1990; Kowalczyk and McKeown-Longo, 1992; Lampugnani et al., 1995). The $\alpha_5\beta_1$ integrin may bind to endothelial cells as aggregation in suspension can be inhibited by specific antibodies (Lampugnani et al., 1991). The integrins appear to modulate monolayer permeability because antibodies to $\alpha_2\beta_1$ or $\alpha_5\beta_1$ integrins increase endothelial permeability (Lampugnani et al., 1991) as do arginine-glycine-aspartic acid (RGD) peptides (Qiao et al., 1995). In contrast, antibodies to the various matrix components do not alter permeability. The integrins appear to be associated with other molecules: $\alpha_3\beta_1$ integrin co-localizes with CD9, CD81, and CD151 (Yanez-Mo et al., 1998); $\alpha_5\beta_1$ integrin also appears to co-localize with CD151 (Sincock et al., 1997). CD9, CD81, and CD151 are members of the tetraspan superfamily, which appear to regulate integrin function (Maecker et al., 1997). Antibody blockade of CD81 and CD151 decreased endothelial cell motility, and increased adhesion of endothelial cells to extracellular matrix (ECM) proteins (Yanez-Mo et al., 1998).

Cadherins. Cadherins are a family of adhesion molecules (reviewed in (Takeichi, 1990) that bind homophilically and heterophilically in a cation-dependent and protease-sensitive manner. Endothelial cells express three cadherins: N-, P-, and VE-cadherin: the first is diffusely spread across the cell (Salomon et al. 1992); the second is present in trace amounts (Liaw et al. 1990); and the third is specifically localized to the interendothelial cell junction (Lampugnani et al., 1992). VE-cadherin seems important in maintaining endothelial permeability, as monolayers of transfected cells show calcium-dependent reductions in permeability (Lampugnani et al. 1992). Inhibition of VE-cadherin by antibodies increases both permeability and neutrophil transmigration in vivo (Gotsch et al. 1997). This is in keeping with the idea that regulation of the interendothelial junction is an important component in the control of transmigration. A new cadherin, VE-cadherin 2, has recently been described; it appears to be able to modulate homotypic adhesion, but unlike VE-cadherin, does not seem to play a role in endothelial permeability (Telo et. al., 1998).

Immunoglobulin Superfamily of Adhesion Molecules. Platelet–endothelial cell adhesion molecule-1 (PECAM-1, CD31) is a member of the immunoglobulin superfamily of adhesion molecules (reviewed in DeLisser et al., 1993; Muller, 1995). It is concentrated at the interendothelial junction in monolayers (Lampugnani et al., 1991). PECAM-1 expression is widespread, with highest levels seen on endothelial cells and platelets, but significant expression is also seen on myeloid and lymphoid lineages (Shaw, 1994). The PECAM-1 molecule is a single-chain membrane-spanning glycoprotein of 130 kD molecular weight with six extracellular Ig-like domains of the C_2 subclass (Newman et al., 1990). Homophilic interactions appear to require all six Ig domains, as loss of one domain disables binding (Piali et al., 1995). Active binding sites are proposed to reside in domains 2 to 3 & 5 to 6 (Fawcett et al., 1995). Heterophilic binding is cation-dependent and is impaired by sulfated glycosaminoglycans. The second Ig domain contains a heparin-binding consensus sequence and appears necessary for heterophilic interactions. The $\alpha_v \beta_3$ integrin has been shown to be a ligand for PECAM-1 on lymphokine-activated killer cells (Piali et al., 1995).

Unlike many other endothelial cell adhesion molecules, PECAM-1 expression is not significantly up-regulated by activation with TNF or interferon (IFN)-γ in usual doses (Romer et al., 1995). Furthermore, PECAM-1 does not appear to be redistributed during cytokine or chemotactic transmigration (Allport et al., 1997). PECAM-1 association with the cytoskeleton might be altered by activation, one group demonstrating a reduction (Romer et al., 1995), which could not be confirmed by others (Lampugnani et al., 1995). The PECAM-1 cytoplasmic tail has five potential phosphorylation sites (Muller, 1995), suggesting another mechanism for regulation. Phosphorylation of PECAM-1 has been reported after platelet activation and is associated with reduced mobility on the membrane. Phosphorylation is also seen after endothelial activation, and this suggests that this is a likely mechanism for regulating PECAM-1 function (Muller, 1995).

Junctional Adhesion Molecule (JAM). A new molecule has recently been described as having a functional role in the junction: Junctional Adhesion Molecule (JAM: Huang et al., 1998). This 49 kD transmembrane protein has two V type immunoglobulin domains. It is concentrated at the junctions, and distributed predominantly at the apex of the junction, where it codistributes with components of tight junctions such as ZO-1 (Huang et al. 1998).

Organisation of Molecular Systems. Ultrastructural and confocal microscopic studies (Ayalon et al., 1994) show PECAM-1 to be located more basally in the junction than VE-cadherin. PECAM-1 is not associated with electron microscopic adherens junctions, in contrast to VE-cadherin. In newly plated monolayers of endothelial cells, PECAM-1 appears in the junction some hours after VE-cadherin, but unlike the cadherin, cation chelation does not lead to its redistribution. JAM appears specifically localized to tight junctions (Huang et al., 1998), which are predominantly apical; the time course of its appearance in the junction is unknown.

Negotiating the Interendothelial Cell Junction
At present we do not have a coordinated picture of transit through the junction. It does seem that the endothelium plays a role; there are probably dynamic arrangements of the endothelial cytoskeleton and junctional adhe-

sion molecules occurring during the process. This probably facilitates a component of mechanical force from the motile leukocyte that allows movement through the junction.

The endothelium is clearly active in cytokine-activated transmigration in vitro, producing chemoattractants and altering expression of adhesion molecules. In contrast, the endothelium has been hypothesized to have no active role in chemotactic transmigration in vitro (Huang et al., 1992), because unstimulated neutrophils do not migrate across resting endothelium. As inhibition of endothelial cytoskeletal rearrangement and intracellular signaling interferes with transmigration, there is clearly an endothelial component in vitro. We would predict that similar events are required in transmigration of unstimulated T cells and monocytes across resting endothelium.

The Endothelial Cytoskeleton. Endothelial cytoskeleton function appears important in transmigration. Transmigrating monocytes move through a tunnel formed by two endothelial cells; this tunnel is rich in filamentous actin, suggesting F-actin plays a role in transmigration (Sandig et al., 1997). In keeping with this, direct interference with the cytoskeleton has been reported to alter transmigration, although some of the effects reported have been contradictory. Doukas et al., (1987) have shown that phalloidin (which abolishes actin rearrangement) decreases transmigration, and cytochalasin (which disintegrates the actin cytoskeleton) increases transmigration. In contrast, Kielbassa et al. (1998) noted that treating the endothelium with cytochalasin or latrunculin A decreased monocyte transmigration. If these actin-depolymerizing agents were not adequately removed, they would alter monocyte motility, which might explain the difference between the two results. There are also correlations between cytoskeletal rearrangements and agents that promote or inhibit transmigration. For example, increases in cAMP and decreases in $[Ca^{2+}]_i$ in endothelium increase peripheral actin density and reduce chemotactic transmigration (Huang et al., 1933). There is also indirect evidence supporting an active role of the actin cytoskeleton. For example, neutrophil transmigration has been associated with increases in F-actin, phosphorylation of myosin light chain, and formation of actin filaments (Sandig et al., 1997); inhibition of MLCK reduces transmigration and supports the idea that these changes are relevant. Other indirect modulators of cytoskeletal function like norepinephrine and serotonin both significantly decrease migration across bovine aortic endothelial cells induced by fMLP, as well as basal neutrophil migration, without altering firm adhesion (Doukas et al., 1987). This suggests that modulation of the cytoskeleton is the important event. In addition, the microtubule network may be important: preventing microtubule reorganization with paclitaxel decreased transmigration, whereas dissolving the microtubule skeleton with nocodazole increased it (Kielbassa et al., 1998).

Thus, it seems probable that the endothelial cytoskeleton alters during transmigration, and that these alterations are a necessary part of the mechanisms regulating transmigration. It is tempting to speculate that alterations in the cytoskeleton that increase endothelial rigidity prevent movement of the endothelium, which prevents cells transmigrating through the interendothelial junction.

Proteolysis of the Endothelial Barrier is Probably Not Important. Direct evidence using HUVEC on complex supports shows that inhibition of elastase does not prevent transmigration (Furie et al., 1984) 1987; Huber et al., 1989), although when HUVEC on simpler supports are used, elastase inhibitors can reduce transmigration. In vivo elastase appears necessary (Kvietys and Granger 1997), although this may well be in passage across the basement membrane. Inhibition of urokinase or depletion of plasmin or plasminogen does not inhibit transmigration (Huang and Silverstein, 1992). Inhibitors of many enzyme systems did not affect neutrophil penetration in a model using HUVEC on a complex substrate (Huber et al., 1989). Although it seems unlikely, other enzymes may be important. Indiscriminant release of granule enzymes, such as cathepsin G (Huang and Silverstein, 1992), are associated with endothelial cell injury, which is not seen in vitro. This suggests that if granule enzymes are involved, they are regulated in some way, and not released indiscriminately.

The Extracellular Matrix in the Junction. As outlined previously, the matrix may function as a guidance source, directly through haptotaxis and contact guidance, and may provide a stable chemotactic gradient through chemoattractants bound to it. The extracellular matrix in the junction may also provide a substrate for the transmigrating cell to use for traction. This may be direct by adhesion of the cell to the matrix. For example, fibronectin in the junction might be a ligand for leukocyte $\alpha_4\beta_1$ integrin. There is some indirect evidence for this as antibodies to VCAM-1 plus blockade of fibronectin binding are required to give the same inhibition of transmigration as VLA-4 blockade (Bianchi et al., 1993; Meerschaert and Furie, 1994). Alternatively, this might be independent of adhesion. Cells crawling in a three-dimensional matrix might use the geometrical characteristics of a mesh for traction: protruding a pseudopod through a narrow region and allowing it to expand distally to provide a source of traction that does not require specific adhesion molecules (Lackie, 1986). Although T cells can penetrate a three-dimensional matrix despite inhibition of adhesion to a two-dimensional surface of the same material (Friedl et al., 1995), suggesting that such a mechanism may be involved, there is no proof that meshwork effects are important in transmigration.

Intercellular Adhesion Molecules in the Junction. In view of the role of PECAM-1, a molecule enriched in the junction in transmigration, it seems logical to hypothesize that modulation of other junctional adhesion molecules could be important in transmigration. In keeping with this, adhesion of neutrophils to endothelium was reported to cause dissociation of VE-cadherin from the junction and from the cytoskeleton, which correlated with transmigration (Del Maschio et al., 1996; Allport et al., 1997). This dissociation appears to be an in vitro artifact caused by release of neutrophil proteases

(Moll et al., 1998); this is in keeping with dynamic studies suggesting little change in VE-cadherin during transmigration (Sandig et al., 1997). It is not clear how transmigrating cells traverse the junctional molecules, but to some extent they may avoid the problem. In vitro, the region joining three cells is preferred; this area has low densities of VE-cadherin (Burns et al., 1997). No information is yet available on alterations in JAM or VE-cadherin 2 during transmigration.

Molecules Critical in Passage Through the Junction

PECAM-1 Is Critical in Passage Through the Junction in Cytokine-Activated Transmigration

PECAM-1 is clearly important in the passage of monocytes and neutrophils through the junction. Anti–PECAM-1 antibodies reduce monocyte transmigration through resting endothelium, and both monocyte and neutrophil transmigration through cytokine-activated endothelium by 70%–90% (Muller et al., 1993; Muller, 1995); binding to endothelium is not affected. If endothelial cells or leukocytes or both are treated with antibodies, effects last at least 48 hours (Bogen et al., 1994; Muller, 1995). The efficacy of PECAM-1 antibodies in vivo has been confirmed in other inflammatory models (Vaporciyan et al., 1993; Muller, 1995). The neutrophils and monocytes that are blocked in transmigration accumulate at the junction (Muller et al., 1993), where they remain firmly adherent. Electron microscopy of the monocytes showed that most had at least a small pseudopod inserted into the junction (Muller et al., 1993). In vivo, the mesenteric vessels of treated animals contain an excess of adherent neutrophils (Bogen et al., 1994). Collectively, these observations strongly suggest a role for PECAM-1 in passage through the interendothelial junction. Monoclonal antibodies mapped to domain 1 and 2 inhibit transmigration, but other monoclonal antibodies are not inhibitory(Liao et al., 1995). Although $\alpha_v\beta_3$ integrin is a lymphokine-activated, killer cell ligand for PECAM-1 (Piali et al., 1995), and monocytes lacking β_3 integrin transmigrate poorly, this appears to be due to modulation of CD11a/CD18 rather than to an interaction with PECAM-1.

Lymphocyte transmigration has not been examined using the standard transmigration system. Using changes in the proportion of PECAM-1–expressing cells after transmigration as a surrogate measure of PECAM-1 dependence, Bird et al. (1993) were not able to show a role for PECAM-1 in lymphocyte transmigration. This finding is important, but needs confirmation in a standard assay.

PECAM-1–Independent Transmigration

In contrast to cytokine-activated transmigration, PECAM-1 seems to have little role in chemotactic transmigration. PECAM-1 antibodies do not decrease chemotactic transmigration in vivo (Wakelin et al., 1996), nor do they decrease transmigration triggered by thrombin (Scalia et al., 1998). In addition, there is often a significant residual transmigration (~10%–30%) after

PECAM-1 inhibition, that suggests that other mechanisms may operate in passage through the junction in cytokine-activated transmigration. These observations suggest that the mechanisms operating in cytokine-activated and chemotactic transmigration overlap to only a small degree. The mechanism of PECAM-1–independent transmigration is unknown. Neutrophils and monocytes from CD11a knockout mice do not require PECAM-1 for transmigration (Andrew et al., 1998), suggesting that CD11a and PECAM-1 somehow operate in a similar pathway of migration. ICAM-1 seems particularly important in transmigration, but there is insufficient evidence to place it in context on PECAM-1–independent transmigration, and although JAM seems to have a role solely in passage through the interendothelial junction, little is known about its role in comparison to PECAM-1.

Junctional Adhesion Molecule

The role of this molecule is still being clarified: blocking antibodies prevented spontaneous, cytokine-activated, and chemotactic transmigration of monocytes (Huang et al., 1998) in vitro. Whether it is important in transmigration of other leukocytes, or whether it plays a role in vivo remains to be seen. Its location at the apex of the intercellular junction (Huang et al., 1998) does suggest that its role is limited to passage across the junction.

Other Molecules Required for Transmigration

Adhesion molecules probably provide the adherence mechanism for most leukocyte movement (Table 17.3 outlines some of the critical molecules). In contrast to PECAM-1, which seems particularly important in migration through the interendothelial junction, there are several adhesion molecules whose roles are not definitively associated with a particular step. These molecules may act in adhesive interactions required for crawling to the interendothelial junction, or they may function in passage through the interendothelial junction. Many of these molecules are reviewed in greater depth elsewhere in this volume.

Intercellular Adhesion Molecule-1

ICAM-1 (CD54) is a member of the immunoglobulin superfamily of adhesion molecules, and contains five Ig-like domains. It is one of the principal ligands for the leukocyte β_2 integrin CD11a/CD18 (LFA-1) and CD11b/CD18 (Mac-1; Diamond et al., 1991), although in the context of transmigration, it seems that CD11a predominantly binds to ICAM-1, whereas CD11b is more promiscuous (Shang and Issekutz, 1998). ICAM-1 is constitutively expressed on endothelial cells, and is significantly up-regulated by cytokine stimulation (Dustin et al., 1986). The time course of cytokine-induced up-regulation is prolonged. Expression gradually increases, peaking at 12 hours, but remaining significantly elevated until 72 hours (Carlos and Harlan, 1994).

In vivo, ICAM-1 knockout mice show significantly impaired neutrophil migration into an inflamed peritoneum (Bullard et al., 1995; Sligh et al., 1993), and ICAM-1 antibodies reduce acute and chronic inflammation in a number of animal models (Carlos and Harlan, 1994). ICAM-1 antibodies reduce cytokine-activated transmigration of neutrophils in vitro, by over 85% (Smith et al., 1988; Luscinskas et al., 1991). ICAM-1 is also important in chemotactic transmigration. Antibodies inhibit neutrophil chemotactic transmigration by nearly 55% (Furie et al., 1991). ICAM-1 seems more important in flow situations: antibodies do not inhibit neutrophil adhesion, but do reduce transmigration by more than 85% (Lawrence et al., 1990).

ICAM-1 is involved in transmigration of many leukocyte subtypes. As well as reducing neutrophil transmigration, antibodies reduce transmigration of resting and activated T cells across resting HUVEC by 50%, and across cytokine-activated HUVEC by about 40% (Oppenheimer Marks et al., 1991). Although their efficacy individually was not reported, a combination of ICAM-1 and CD18 antibodies reduced migration of monocytes in a combination chemotactic and inflammatory transmigration model by 50%–75% (Chuluyan and Issekutz, 1993; Chuluyan et al., 1995). This combination did not alter spontaneous monocyte transmigration (Chuluyan and Issekutz, 1993).

In T-cell and monocyte transmigration, ICAM-1 is localized to the interendothelial junction and to the regions of T-cell or monocyte–endothelium contact (Oppenheimer Marks et al., 1991; Sandig et al., 1997). The localization of ICAM-1 in T-cell transmigration (Oppenheimer Marks et al., 1991) suggests that ICAM-1 is involved in passage through the interendothelial junction. As blocking ICAM-1 function is not associated with accumulation of leukocytes at the interendothelial junction, as seen with PECAM-1, it suggests that its role is not limited to passage through the interendothelial junction. ICAM-1 is probably also required for crawling across the endothelium to the interendothelial junction because it is predominantly located on the apical surface of resting endothelial cells (Almenar-Queralt et al., 1995; Bradley et al., 1995) and during cytokine activation, it is up-regulated on the apical surface (Almenar-Queralt et al., 1995).

β_2 Integrins

Four different alpha chains, α_L(CD11a), α_M(CD11b), α_X(CD11c), and α_d(CD11d) can form heterodimers with the common β_2 integrin chain (CD18), which is expressed on all leukocytes. The CD11/CD18 complex is one of the critical determinants of neutrophil transmigration, and plays an important role in transmigration of other leukocyte subsets. The functional importance of CD18 is exemplified by a congenital deficiency syndrome: leukocyte adhesion deficiency syndrome type I (LAD-1; Anderson and Springer, 1987). Afflicted individuals cannot resolve infections and have impaired wound healing. Histologically there is no neutrophil influx, although monocyte, eosinophil, and lymphocyte responses are relatively preserved. In vitro, LAD-1 neutrophils adhere and transmigrate poorly. There are some situations in vivo in which some transmigration does occur. Inflammation in the lung can generate some neutrophil influx, suggesting that a CD18-

Table 17.4a. Chemotactic Transmigration: Inhibition by Blocking Antibodies

Molecule	Neutrophils	Monocytes	T-cells	Eosinophils
CD18	+++	++		
ICAM-1	+++			
CD11a				
CD11b		− (in vivo)		
VLA-4		+ (in vivo)		+− (in vivo)

independent mechanism of neutrophil transmigration exists (Anderson and Springer, 1987).

Use of β_2-integrin antibodies in animal models generally confirms a phenotype similar to that of patients with LAD-1 syndrome. As in LAD-1, in some circumstances neutrophil transmigration can still occur (Doerschuck et al., 1990). CD18 antibodies are also effective inhibitors of transmigration in vitro (Tables 17.4a and 17.4b); however, the degree of inhibition seen in neutrophils is consistently greater than other leukocyte populations. This appears related to the ability of monocytes, eosinophils, and lymphocytes to use alternative adhesive systems, primarily mediated through VLA-4. The mechanism of inhibition of transmigration is not settled: in vivo the effects may be predominantly indirect through abolition of firm adhesion, rather than on passage across the monolayer (Jung et al., 1998).

Where their effects have been examined, combinations of CD11a and CD11b antibodies are very similar to CD18 antibodies (Smith et al., 1989; Anderson et al., 1990; Furie et al., 1991; Issekutz and Issekutz, 1992), suggesting that these are the most important alpha chains. Antibodies to the CD11a and CD11b subunits alone are not as potent as antibodies to CD18.

Table 17.4b. Cytokine-activated Transmigration: Inhibition by Blocking Antibodies

Molecule	Neutrophils	Monocytes	T-cells	Eosinophils	NK cells
CD18	+++	+ to ++	+++	+++	++
ICAM-1	+++		++	+	
CD11a	+++	+ (in vivo)	+++	+	
CD11b	+	− (in vivo)	+++	++	
VLA-4	−	+ to ++	++ (resting) − (activated)	− (resting) ++ (primed)	++

In contrast, CD11c does not appear to be necessary for transmigration because blocking antibodies do not reduce neutrophil or NK cell transmigration (Luscinskas et al., 1991; Bianchi et al., 1993), nor do antibodies reduce monocyte adhesion to endothelial cells (Hakkert et al., 1991). CD11d has recently been described. Whereas antibody studies suggest it is involved in inflammatory lung injury, a role in transmigration has not been evaluated (Jones et al., 1998). The $\alpha_L\beta_2$ integrin (LFA-1, CD11a/CD18) is expressed on all leukocytes. Its ligands are ICAM-1 and ICAM-2 on the endothelium. It is involved in a broad array of adhesive functions (Kishimoto and Anderson, 1992). Circulating leukocytes constitutively express LFA-1 in an inactive conformation.

Activation is required for ligand binding (Dustin and Springer, 1989). This activation can be generated by intracellular signals (inside out signaling). In addition, cross-linking of LFA-1 can induce signals (outside-in) signaling (Hynes, 1992; Arroyo et al., 1994). Blocking antibodies to CD11a do inhibit transmigration of neutrophils, T lymphocytes, and to a lesser degree, eosinophils (Table 17.4a and 17.4b). Blockade is generally less potent and more variable than antibodies to CD18. Monoclonal antibodies can reduce inflammation in vivo, but their efficacy depends on the model. For example, monoclonal antibodies reduce IgG immune-complex lung injury, but not IgG immune-complex glomerulonephritis in the rat (Albelda et al., 1994). LFA-1 knockout mice show significant impairment in transmigration of neutrophils, lymphocytes, and to a lesser degree monocytes. The $\alpha_M\beta_2$ integrin (Mac-1, CD11b/CD18, CR3) is expressed on neutrophils, monocytes, and NK cells. It is expressed on the cell surface, and is stored in secondary and tertiary granules (Jones et al., 1990; Edwards, 1994). Inflammatory mediators cause increases in cell surface expression, although functional up-regulation does not require quantitative up-regulation. Ligands are relatively widespread including fibrinogen, C3bi, some microbial determinants, coagulation factor X, and ICAM-1 (Diamond et al., 1990). As well as contributing toward phagocytosis, binding to surfaces through CD11b leads to massive activation of the respiratory burst in primed neutrophils. Monoclonal antibody studies have shown several different functional epitopes, some antibodies inhibiting adhesion more than aggregation and vice versa (Diamond et al., 1989). Despite the significant inhibition of such functions as chemotaxis in vitro, in general, antibodies to CD11b are not particularly effective in inhibiting transmigration in vitro (Tables 17.4a and 17.4b), nor do CD11b knockout mice show defective transmigration (Lu et al., 1997). CD11b monoclonal antibodies can inhibit inflammation in vivo, but in contrast to CD11a antibodies, CD11b antibodies reduce IgG immune-complex glomerulonephritis, but not IgG immune-complex lung injury (Albelda et al., 1994).

CD11a is thus critical in neutrophil transmigration, and important in transmigration of other leukocyte subtypes. CD11b antibodies alone are not potent inhibitors of neutrophil transmigration in vitro, but add significantly to the effect of CD11a antibodies in vitro. In vivo, both CD11a and CD11b monoclonal antibodies can reduce inflammation, suggesting both a redundancy and a dependence on the inflammatory stimulus and organ involved.

Very Late Antigen-4

VLA-4 ($\alpha_4 \beta_1$ integrin, CD49d/CD29) is expressed by most leukocytes but is observed on neutrophils only under special conditions. It binds to fibronectin and the immunoglobulin superfamily member VCAM-1. VCAM-1 binding occurs with approximately four times greater affinity than binding to fibronectin. The involvement of VLA-4 in transmigration in vitro is variable. It is likely that this reflects redundancy with β_2 integrins, as well as the degree of VCAM-1 expression on endothelium, which in turn reflects the state of endothelial activation. It appears unimportant in neutrophil transmigration in vitro (Hakkert et al., 1991), and in transmigration of activated T cells (Oppenheimer Marks et al., 1991). VLA-4 antibodies do not reduce transmigration of resting T cells across resting endothelium, nor do they reduce transmigration of monocytes across resting endothelium (Oppenheimer Marks et al., 1991; Meerschaert and Furie, 1994, 1995; Chuluyan et al., 1995). Resting T-cell and NK cell cytokine-activated transmigration are reduced by 40% and 30%, respectively (Oppenheimer Marks et al., 1991; Bianchi et al., 1993). As firm adhesion is reduced to a similar extent, it is unclear whether this is a specific effect on passage across the endothelium. Eosinophil adhesion to cytokine-activated endothelial cells also involves VLA-4 adhesion to VCAM-1 (Bochner et al., 1991; Schleimer et al., 1992). Cytokine-activated migration in vitro was not significantly inhibited by VLA-4 antibodies alone (Ebisawa et al., 1992; Moser et al., 1992b), but after IL-4 priming, VLA-4 antibodies significantly reduced transmigration (Moser et al., 1992a). VLA-4 probably provides a secondary system in cytokine-activated transmigration of monocytes. When used in vitro with CD18 antibodies, antibodies to VLA-4 decrease transmigration (Hakkert et al., 1991; Meerschaert and Furie, 1994; Lub et al., 1995; Shang et al., 1998), although the inhibition varies from 20% to nearly 100%. When used alone, several groups report little effect of VLA-4 blockade on transmigration (Meerschaert and Furie, 1994; Chuluyan et al., 1995), suggesting redundancy with CD18. The precise role of VLA-4 is not clearly limited to movement across the monolayer, as inhibition of adhesion is seen; thus, it might be as important for firm adhesion or movement to the junction. VLA-4 may play a role in chemotactic transmigration of monocytes as monoclonal antibodies are able to inhibit migration to injected dermal chemoattractants by 20%– 30% (Issekutz, 1995).

Of the two VLA-4 ligands, antibodies to VCAM-1 alone do not inhibit transmigration of T cells (Oppenheimer Marks et al., 1991), nor of monocytes (Chuluyan and Issekutz, 1993), but adding VCAM-1 antibodies and CS-1 peptide to CD18 antibodies does increase the blockade of adhesion to levels similar to that of VLA-4 and CD18 antibodies in combination (Bianchi et al., 1993; Meerschaert and Furie, 1994), suggesting both $\alpha_4 \beta_1$ ligands are used by NK cells and monocytes.

Integrin-Associated Protein

Integrin-associated protein (IAP, CD47) is a single-chain glycoprotein that, on the basis of its primary structure, has five potential membrane-spanning regions and a large extracytoplasmic amino-terminal with homology to the IgV domain of the immunoglobulin superfamily (Lindberg et al., 1993, 1994). It is expressed widely and appears to be associated with β_3 integrins (Brown et al., 1990), but its expression is not limited to cells expressing integrins (Rosales et al., 1992). Blocking antibodies have suggested a variety of functions, for example, elevations in intracellular calcium due to endothelial cell binding to extracellular matrix components, and neutrophil chemotaxis and adhesion to entactin are IAP and β_3-integrin dependent (Senior et al., 1992; Zhou and Brown, 1993). Not all β_3 integrins are functionally associated with IAP: platelet GpIIb/IIIa-dependent functions are not IAP dependent (Fujimoto et al., 1995). These observations have led to suggestions that IAP functions as a calcium channel (Schwartz et al., 1993) or as a signal transduction unit, modulating the effect of integrin function (Zhou and Brown, 1993), possibly through interaction with the cytoplasmic tail of the β_3 integrin (Blystone et al., 1995). Cooper et al., (1995) have shown the critical dependence of transmigration on IAP function. Treatment of neutrophils with blocking antibodies inhibited chemotactic and cytokine-activated transmigration by more than 80% and inhibited neutrophil chemotaxis. This appears to be the case with monocyte transmigration (Weerasinghe et al., 1998); in this case, it seems IAP acts as a regulator of β_3 integrin, which in turn modulates LFA-1 and presumably inhibits transmigration by inhibiting leukocyte motility. This is in keeping with the slowing of inflammatory responses seen in IAP knockout mice (Lindberg et al., 1996), and is reminiscent of the $\alpha_v \beta_3$-integrin–mediated modulation of $\alpha_8 \beta_1$-integrin–dependent phagocytosis, which depends on IAP (Blystone et al., 1994, 1995). The exact mechanism by which this modulation occurs is unclear. In contrast, when the endothelium alone is treated with IAP-blocking antibodies, only cytokine-activated transmigration is inhibited (Cooper et al., 1995). Although there is no data to link it specifically to passage through the junction, and the mechanism of action on the endothelium is unclear, the lack of inhibition of adhesion and its effects on $[Ca^{2+}]_i$ provide some suggestion that it may be critical in this phase of migration.

Other Molecules

There are other adhesion molecules of potential importance in transmigration, and some relevant candidates that appear to play no role.

β_3 Integrin and Integrin Modulators. Modulation of integrins can alter their function and thus inhibit migration. The α_v and β_3 integrins appear to act in this way by modulating the function of LFA-1 (Weerasinghe et al., 1998). Molecules of the tetraspan family associate with integrins and can modulate their function (Maecker et al., 1997); members of this class such as CD151 and CD81 have been reported to modulate cellular motility (Yanez-

Mo et al., 1998). It is unclear whether these molecules play a role in transmigration.

CD44. CD44 is expressed on neutrophils, monocytes, NK, and T cells. It binds to hyaluronan, a component of many extracellular matrices, as well as other ligands. It has been implicated in many migratory processes including metastasis, with some isoforms conferring greater metastatic potential (Sleeman et al., 1995). CD44 has been implicated in migration of activated but not resting T cells across cytokine-activated HUVEC (Oppenheimer Marks et al., 1990), and blocking antibodies have been reported to reduce lymphocytic infiltration in a murine arthritis model (Mikecz et al., 1995), but its role in transmigration of other leukocyte types is not clear.

CD43. Sialophorin (CD43) is a large, heavily sialylated, cell surface glycoprotein present only on hematopoietic cells. It has been reported to be a counter receptor for ICAM-1 (Rosenstein et al., 1991), and may function as a signaling molecule because ligation can induce cell activation (Mentzer et al., 1987). Antibodies trigger neutrophil aggregation via a β_2-integrin–dependent pathway (Rosekrantz et al., 1993) and decrease monocyte adhesion to endothelium (McEvoy et al., 1997). These observations suggest a potential role as an inhibitor of adhesion, and that CD43 needs to be lost or downregulated to allow maximal adhesion to develop.

CD10. CD10 is a surface endopeptidase found in a number of myeloid lineage cells. It may have a specific and limited role: inhibitors increase transmigration across epithelia only toward bacterial peptides like fMLP (Hofman et al., 1998). It has not been evaluated in transendothelial migration.

VLA-5 ($\alpha_5\beta_1$ integrin CD49e/CD29). In view of its up-regulation by chemokines (slower onset but more prolonged than VLA-4; Weber et al., 1996), VLA-5 has been evaluated in monocyte transmigration, where blocking antibodies were not inhibitory, suggesting that its role in transmigration, if any, may be after passage through the endothelium (Shang and Isserkutz, 1998; Shang et al., 1998). This work also suggested that blockade of monocyte but not endothelial β_1 integrins contributed to decreased transmigration.

β_2 Integrin–Independent Transmigration of Neutrophils

Observations on patients with LAD-1 suggested that in some circumstances their neutrophils could transmigrate. In vivo models of this process have been developed (Doerschuk et al., 1990; Gao et al., 1994; Burns and Doerschuk, 1994; Burns et al., 1994); like the situation in LAD-1, there seems to be a specific set of circumstances required to elicit the phenomenon that varies with the stimulus, the vascular bed involved, and the species of experimental animal used. Its importance lies in the possibility of pointing to novel molecular mechanisms in transmigration.

An in vitro model of this process has been developed (Issekutz et al., 1995).

The phenomenon was seen only when CD18-antibody-treated neutrophils were induced to transmigrate across cytokine-activated HUVEC, which also had a chemotactic gradient of C5a or LTB4, but not IL-8 or fMLP. The mechanism remains unknown; the logical candidates—$\alpha_4 \beta_1$, β_3 integrins, PECAM-1, ICAM-1, and VCAM-1—appear to be excluded because blocking antibodies did not alter transmigration. The models of β_2-integrin–independent transmigration may also be useful in examining PECAM-1–independent neutrophil transmigration.

Events After Transmigration

Consequences of Migration Across the Endothelial Monolayer

Effects on Leukocytes. Leukocytes exhibit a number of functional changes in response to transmigration. Some of these are identical to those induced by exposure to chemoattractants. For example, PAF induces neutrophil degranulation, shedding of L-selectin, and up-regulation of CD11b (Edwards, 1994). In contrast, investigators have found a number of changes in varying leukocyte types that could not be reproduced merely by exposure to chemoattractants; in some cases these changes appear to specifically require transmigration (Kubes et al., 1995; Romanic et al., 1997; Roussel and Gringras, 1997). For example, transmigration of neutrophils induces expression of cell surface β_1 integrin, particularly $\alpha_4\beta_1$ integrin (Kubes et al., 1995); others have found up-regulation of VLA-6 (Roussel and Gringras, 1997) and down-regulation of PECAM-1 (Christofidou-Solomidou et al., 1997). Transmigration of T cells can decrease expression of LFA-1 and VLA-4 and up-regulate VLA-5 expression and function (Romanic et al., 1997). Transmigration of eosinophils up-regulated CD11b, and CD35, and primed the eosinophil respiratory burst (Walker et al., 1993). These changes may be functionally important: up-regulation of neutrophil VLA-6 appears to promote migration across fibroblast monolayers in vitro (Roussel and Gringras, 1997); migration through extracellular matrix might be enhanced by altering the repertoire of surface integrins (Weber et al., 1996); and up-regulated production of monocyte MMP-9 after binding to endothelium (Amorino and Hoover, 1998) might be important in passage across the basement membrane and into the tissues.

The stimulus for these changes may involve signaling from adhesion to HUVEC. In the eosinophil, up-regulation of CD11b occurred on exposure to membrane fragments of IL-1 activated HUVEC, and similar changes occurred after adhesion to intact HUVEC. The adhesion molecule responsible for this has not been identified: the changes were not inhibited by antibodies to E-selectin, VCAM-1, or ICAM-1, nor by PAF antagonists (Walker et al., 1993). Another signaling stimulus may come from adhesion of leukocytes to extracellular matrix components in the interendothelial junction or basement membrane. Extracellular matrix components have been reported to induce a variety of functional changes (reviewed in Pakianathan, 1995), for example, up-regulation of cytokine synthesis by neutrophils and monocytes. Of note, exposure of neutrophils to the basement membrane component entactin can induce expression of $\beta_3$integrin (Senior et al., 1992), and induce CD18-independent migration.

Effects on the Endothelium. It is less clear if the endothelium is altered by transmigration. Spontaneous migration of monocytes across resting endothelium does increase migration by subsequent monocytes and T cells 4 to 6 hours later (de Jong et al., 1996). The mechanism appears to be paracrine: transmigrating monocytes are stimulated to produce TNF which then activates the endothelium. Although adhesion to ICAM-1 results in increases in expression of mRNA for ICAM-1 and VCAM-1 (Clayton et al., 1998), this does not appear to require transmigration per se. Activation of endothelial phospholipase D (an enzyme involved in intracellular signaling) has been cited as a specific consequence of transmigration (Saito et al., 1998); however, it was only seen when the stimulus to migration was provided by LTB_4, which has been suggested to activate endothelium (Nohgawa et al., 1997). Further investigation of this phenomenon might help explain the transition from initial neutrophil influx to other cell types later.

Migration Across the Basement Membrane

After transmigration, intravital microscopic studies show that leukocytes pause at the basement membrane, and further migration is delayed until the basement membrane is penetrated (Grant, 1973; Huber et al., 1989). Neutrophils remain adherent to the basal aspect of the endothelium and in some species may form a temporary sheath around the vessel before moving into the tissues (Grant, 1973). In contrast to adhesion and earlier steps in transmigration, relatively little is known about penetration of the basement membrane.

Huber et al., (1989) used prolonged HUVEC culture to generate an in vitro model of basement membrane passage to test these observations. They noted that transmigration of large numbers of neutrophils did not result in morphological alterations of the basement membrane, but did increase its permeability. The permeability defect was repaired within 4 hours in a process dependent on transcription and protein synthesis by endothelial cells. Neutrophil penetration of the basement membrane was not dependent on protein synthesis. Using a series of inhibitors, they were unable to implicate a number of metalloproteinases, other proteases, or heparanase in passage across the endothelium-basement membrane complex. In contrast, migration across basement membrane-like barriers without endothelium requires matrix metalloproteases. For example, migration of resting and IL-2–activated T cells across a Matrigel barrier required gelatinase B (92 kD type IV collagenase, matrix metalloproteinase-9), which is constitutively expressed by T cells (Leppert et al., 1995). The structurally related gelatinase A (72 kD type IV collagenase, matrix metalloproteinase-2), may also be involved in basement membrane degradation (Simon et al., 1991; Leppert et al., 1995). Increasing the complexity of the problem, in vivo data show that inhibition of elastase can inhibit transmigration (Kvietys and Granger, 1997), although this is not unequivocally at the level of migration across the basement membrane.

The specifics of passage across the basement membrane are also unclear. Antibodies against PECAM-1 can prevent migration across the basement membrane in vivo (Wakelin et al., 1996). Migration of T cells through basement membrane constructs does not occur randomly, but cells tend to migrate through an area where a previous cell had passed (Leppert et al., 1995). Whether this represents a focal loss of resistance to migration, generation of a chemohaptotactic gradient from release of matrix-bound factors, or a combination of these remains to be seen, but may be an important model of directional clues in tissues.

Migration into the Tissues

Although the specific molecular details are not yet well understood, PECAM-1 is important in monocyte migration into the extracellular matrix after transmigration. Unlike passage through the junction, which is inhibited by antibodies to domain 1 and 2, but not by antibodies to domain 6, heparin and antibodies to domain 6 inhibit migration through the extracellular matrix (Liao et al., 1995). The β_2 integrins also play an important role (Saltzman et al., 1999). Migration through three-dimensional matrices is increased by the presence of hyaluronan, a CD44 ligand. Monoclonal antibodies that activate CD44 (Friedl et al., 1995) have a similar effect, and it is likely that CD44 has a role in migration through the extracellular matrix. Although not specifically examined, it is likely that VLA-4 will be important in this process. ICAM-1 is expressed on fibroblasts and epithelium (Shaw, 1994) and appears to be involved in leukocyte migration through tissues (Parkos, 1997). In the case of neutrophils, CD11b appears to be the predominant integrin involved (Parkos, 1997), in contrast to the situation in transendothelial migration where CD11a is dominant.

Negative Regulators of Transmigration

The resting endothelium appears to provide a barrier to transmigration. There are clearly active promigratory processes such as up-regulation of adhesion molecules, and synthesis of chemoattractants. There is evidence to suggest that there are antimigratory mechanism, which may either require down-regulation to allow transmigration, or may act to limit the duration of transmigration and restore the status quo. As transmigration is the final result of many factors, inhibition of rolling or firm adhesion will decrease leukocyte efflux. Several adhesion molecules are produced in soluble form (Ohno et al., 1997; Kusterer et al., 1998), and these may decrease transmigration through competitive inhibition. For example, soluble ICAM-1 has been shown to decrease adhesion in in vivo models. Similarly, substances like transforming growth factor-β (TGF-β) may limit transmigration by down-regulating the effects of inflammatory cytokines: decreasing surface adhesion molecule expression and IL-8 production (Smith et al., 1996).

Migration may be limited by substances like the eicosanoids lipoxin A_4 and B_4. They are generated by neutrophils and inhibit both neutrophil and endothelial components of adhesion and transmigration stimulated by LTB_4

(Papayianni et al., 1996). Specific mechanisms limiting the passage across the endothelial monolayer have not yet been detected; however, the importance of endothelial signaling suggests that alteration of signaling pathways might effectively decrease transmigration. A final mechanism limiting tissue infiltration would be induction of apoptosis in the transmigrating cell. Activation of vascular endothelium with TNF is associated with down-regulation of Fas ligand on the endothelial cell surface; constitutive up-regulation of Fas ligand was associated with increased monocyte apoptosis and decreased tissue infiltration (Sata and Walsh, 1998).

Questions in Transmigration Research

Several major questions remain before our understanding of transmigration becomes more complete. One major area relates to the process of transmigration. First, what is the role of transcellular transmigration in vivo? What is its quantitative contribution? In what circumstances is it important? How does it differ from paracellular transmigration? Second, in paracellular transmigration, what are the nature and consequences of the endothelial signaling event(s)? How is the junction regulated? What other molecules are involved in passage through the junction? How do they interact with the transmigrating leukocyte? As no interaction is known to be entirely specific for transmigration, this is a significant set of questions. Third, is regulation of passage across the endothelial monolayer an important part in regulating the inflammatory infiltrate, either in determining its cellular specificity, or duration? Another area relates to endothelial heterogeneity. Vascular beds differ significantly in other aspects, this raises the question whether the mechanisms of transmigration and its regulation are likewise varied. If, as seems probable, there are differences among vascular beds, how do they differ and can these differences be turned to therapeutic advantage?

References

Adamson, R. H. (1990) Permeability of frog mesenteric capillaries after partial pronase digestion of the endothelial glycocalyx. *J. Physiol. (Lond.)* 428:1–13.

Adamson, R. H. (1993) Microvscular endothelial cell shape and size in situ. *Microvasc. Res.* 46: 77–88.

Albelda, S. M., Muller, W. A., Buck, C. A., and Newman, P. J. (1991) Molecular and cellular properties of PECAM-1 (endoCAM/CD31): a novel vascular cell–cell adhesion molecule. *J. Cell Biol.* 114:1059–1068.

Albelda, S. M., Smith, C. W., and Ward, P. A. (1994) Adhesion molecules and inflammatory injury. *FASEB J.* 8:504–512.

Allport, J. R., Ding, H., Collins, T., Gerritsen, M. E., and Luscinskas, F. W. (1997) Endothelial-dependent mechanisms regulate leukocyte transmigration: a process involving the proteasome and disruption of the vascular endothelial–cadherin complex at endothelial cell-to-cell junctions. *J. Exp. Med.* 186:517–527.

Almenar-Queralt, A., Duperray, A., Miles, L., Felez, J., and Altieri, D.C. (1995) Apical topography and modulation of ICAM-1 expression on activated endothelium. *Am. J. Pathol.* 147:1278–1288.

Amorino, G. P., and Hoover, R. L. (1998) Interactions of monocytic cells with human endothelial cells stimulate monocytic metalloproteinase production. *Am. J. Pathol.* 152:199–207.

Anderson, D. C., and Springer, T. A. (1987) Leukocyte adhesion deficency: An inherited defect in the Mac-1, LFA-1, and p150, 95 glycoproteins. *Ann. Rev. Med.* 38:175–194.

Anderson, D. C., Rothlein, R., Marlin, S. D., Krater, S. S., and Smith, C. W. (1990) Impaired transendothelial migration by neonatal neutrophils: abnormalities of Mac-1 (CD11b/CD18)-dependent adherence reactions. *Blood* 76:2613–2621.

Andrew, D. P., Spellberg, J. P., Takimoto, H., Schmits, R., Mak, T. W., and Zukowski, M. M. (1998) Transendothelial migration and trafficking of leukocytes in LFA-1–deficient mice. *Eur. J. Immunol.* 28:1959–1969.

Arroyo, A. G., Campanero, M. R., Sanchez-Mateos, P., Zapata, J. M., Ursa, M. A., and del Pozo, M. A. (1994) Induction of tyorosine phosphrylaion during ICAM-3 and LFA-1 mediated intercellular adhesion and its regulation by the CD-45 tyrosine phosphatase. *J. Cell Biol.* 126: 1277–1286.

Ayalon, O., Sabanai, H., Lampugnani, M. G., Dejana, E., and Geiger, B. (1994) Spatial and temporal relationships between cadherins and PECAM-1 in cell–cell junctions of human endothelial cells. *J. Cell Biol.* 126:247–258.

Baggiolini, M., Boulay, F., Badwey, J. A., and Curnutte, J. T. (1993) Activation of neutrophil leukocytes: chemoattractant receptors and respiratory burst. *FASEB J.* 7:1004–1010.

Barbee, K. A., Davies, P. F., and Lal, R. (1994) Shear stress-induced reorganisation of surface topography of living endothelial cells imaged by atomic microscopy. *Cir. Res.* 74: 163–171.

Beesley, J. E., Pearson, J. D., Hutchings, A., Carleton, J. S., and Gordon, J. L. (1978) Interaction of leukocytes with vascular cells in culture. *J. Cell Sci.* 33:85–101.

Bevario, F., Bertocchi, F., Dejana, E., and Bussolino, F. (1988) IL-1 induced adhesion of polymorphonuclear leukocytes to cultured endothelial cells: role for platelet-activating factor. *J. Immunol.* 141:3391–3397.

Beyer, E. C. (1993) Gap junctions. *Int. Rev. Cytol.* 137:1–38.

Bianchi, G., Sironi, M., Ghibaudi, E., Selvaggini, C., Elices, M., Allavena, P., and Mantovani, A. (1993) Migration of natural killer cells across endothelial cell monolayers. *J. Immunol.* 151: 5135–5144.

Bird, I. N., Spragg, J. H., Ager, A., and Matthews, N. (1993) Studies of lymphocyte transendothelial migration: analysis of migrated cell phenotypes with regard to CD31 (PECAM-1), CD45RA and CD45RO. *Immunol.* 80:553–560.

Blystone, S. D., Graham, I. L., Lindberg, F. P., and Brown, E. J. (1994) Integrin $a_v b_3$ differentially regulates adhesive and phagocytic functions of the fibronectin receptor $a_5 b_1$ *J. Cell Biol.* 127: 1129–1137.

Blystone, S. D., Lindberg, F. P., LaFlamme, S. E., and Brown, E. J. (1995) Integrin b_3 cytoplasmic tail is necessary and sufficient for regulation of $a_5 b_1$ phagocytosis by $a_v b_3$ and integrin-associated protein. *J. Cell Biol.* 130:745–754.

Bochner, B. S., Luscinskas, F. W., Gimbrone, M. A. Jr., Newman, W., Sterbinsky, S. A., Derse-Anthony, C. P., Klunk, D., and Schleimer, R. P. (1991) Adhesion of human basophils, eosinophils, and neutrophils to interleukin 1-activated human vascular endothelial cells: contributions of endothelial cell adhesion molecules. *J. Exp. Med.* 173:1553–1557.

Bogen, S., Pak, J., Garifallou, M., Deng, X., and Muller, W. A. (1994) Monoclonal antibody to murine PECAM-1 (CD-31) blocks acute inflammation in vivo. *J. Exp. Med.* 17, 1059: 1064.

Bradley, J. R., Thiru, S., and Pober, J. S. (1995) Hydrogen peroxide-induced endothelial retraction is accompanied by a loss of the normal spatial organization of endothelial cell adhesion molecules. *Am. J. Pathol.* 147:627–641.

Brady, H. R., Lamas, S., Papayianni, A., Takata, S., Matsubara, M., and Marsden, P. A. (1995) Lipoxygenase product formation and cell adhesion during neutrophil–glomerular endothelial cell interaction. *Am. J. Physiol.* 268:F1–F12.

Brindle, N.P.J. (1993) Growth factors in endothelial regeneration. *Cardiovasc. Res.* 27:1162–1172.

Brown, E., Hooper, L., Ho, T., and Gresham, H. (1990) Integrin-associated protein: a 50-kD plasma membrane antigen physically and functionally associated with integrins. *J. Cell Biol.* 111:2785–2794.

Bruzzone, R., Haefliger, J. A., Gimlich, R. L., and Paul, D. L. (1993) Connexin40, a component of gap junctions in vascular endothelium, is restricted in its ability to interact with other connexins. *Mol. Biol. Cell* 4:7–20.

Bullard, D. C., Qin, L., Lorenzo, I., Quinlin, W. M., Doyle, N. A., Bosse, R., Vestweber, D., Doerschuk, C. M., and Beaudet, A. L. (1995) P-selectin/ICAM-1 double mutant mice: acute emigration of neutrophils into the peritoneum is completely absent but is normal into pulmonary alveoli. *J. Clin. Invest.* 95:1782–1788.

Burns, A. R., and Doerschuk, C. M. (1994) Quantitation of L-selectin and CD18 expression on rabbit neutrophils during CD18-independent and CD18-dependent emigration in the lung. *J. Immunol.* 153:3177–3188

Burns, A. R., Takei, F., and Doerschuk, C. M. (1994) Quantitation of ICAM-1 expression in mouse lung during pneumonia. *J. Immunol.* 153:3189–3198.

Burns, A. R., Walker, D. C., Brown, E. S., Thurmon, L. T., Bowden, R. A., Keese, C. R., Simon, S. I., Entman, M. L., and Smith, C. W. (1997) Neutrophil transendothelial migration is independent of tight junctions and occurs preferentially at tricellular corners. *J. Immunol.* 159: 2893–2903.

Burns, A. R., Bowden, R. A., Abe, Y., Walker, D. C., Simon, S. I., Entman, M. L., and Smith, C. W. (1999) P-selectin mediates neutrophil adhesion to endothelial cell borders. *J. Leuk. Biol.* 65: 299–306.

Butcher, E. C. (1991) Leukocyte–endothelial cell recognition: three (or more) steps to specificity and diversity. *Cell* 67:1033–1036.

Carlos, T. M., and Harlan, J. M. (1994) Leukocyte–endothelial adhesion molecules. *Blood* 84: 2068–2101.

Carter, S. B. (1965) Principles of cell motility: the direction of cell movement and cancer invasion. *Nature* 208:1183–1187.

Casale, T. B., Abbas, M. K., and Carolan, E. J. (1992) Degree of neutrophil chemotaxis is dependent upon the chemoattractant and barrier. *Am. J. Respir. Cell Mol. Biol.* 7:112–117.

Caveda, L., Corada, M., Padura, I. M., Del Mascio, A., Brevario, F., Lampugnani, M. G., and Dejana, E. (1994) Structural characteristics and functional role of endothelial cell to cell junctions. *Endothelium* 2:1–10.

Chosay, J. G., Fisher, M. A., Farhood, A., Ready, K. A., Dunn, C. J., and Jaeschke, H. (1998) Role of PECAM-1 (CD31) in neutrophil transmigration in murine models of liver and peritoneal inflammation. *Am. J. Physiol.* 274:G776–G782.

Christofidou-Solomidou, M., Nakada, M. T., Williams, J., Muller, W. A. and DeLisser, H. M. (1997) Neutrophil platelet endothelial cell adhesion molecule-1 participates in neutrophil recruitment at inflammatory sites and is down-regulated after leukocyte extravasation. *J. Immunol.* 158:4872–4878.

Chuluyan, H. E., and Issekutz, A. C. (1993) VLA-4 integrin can mediate CD11/CD18-independent transendothelial migration of human monocytes. *J. Clin. Invest.* 92:2768–2777.

Chuluyan, H. E., Osborn, L., Lobb, R., and Issekutz, A. C. (1995) Domains 1 and 4 of vascular cell adhesion molecule-1 (CD-106) both support very late activation antigen-4 (CD-49d/CD-29)-dependent monocyte transendothelial migration. *J. Immunol.* 155:3135–3144.

Clark, P., Connolly, P., Curtis, A.S.G., Dow, J.A.T., and Wilkinson, C.D.W. (1990) Topographic control of cell behaviour: II. multiple grooved substrata. *Development* 108:635–644.

Clark, P., Connolly, P., and Moores, G. R. (1992) Cell guidance by micropatterned adhesiveness in vitro. *J. Cell Sci.* 103:287–292.

Clayton, A., Evans, R. A., Pettit, E., Hallett, M., Williams, J. D., and Steadman, R. (1998) Cellular activation through the ligation of intercellular adhesion molecule-1. *J. Cell Sci.* 111:443–453.

Cooper, D., Lindberg, F. P., Gamble, J. R., Brown, E. J., and Vadas, M. A. (1995) Transendothelial migration of neutrophils involves integrin-associated protein (CD47). *Proc. Natl. Acad. Sci USA* 92:3978–3982.

Crockett-Torabi, E., Sulenbarger, B., Smith, C. W., and Fantone, J. C. (1995) Activation of human neutrophils through L-selectin and Mac-1 molecules. *J. Immunol.* 154:2291–2302.

Davies, P. F. (1995) Flow-mediated endothelial mechanotransduction. *Physiol. Rev.* 75:519–560.

De Bruyn, P.P.H., and Cho, Y. (1990) Structure and function of high endothelial postcapillary venules in lymphocyte circulation. *Curr. Topics Pathol.* 84:85–101.

de Jong, A. L., Green, D. M., Trial, J. A., and Birdsall, H. H. (1996) Focal effects of mononuclear leukocyte transendothelial migration: TNF-alpha production by migrating monocytes promotes subsequent migration of lymphocytes. *J. Leukoc. Biol.* 60:129–136.

DeLisser, H. M., Newman, P. J., and Albelda, S. M. (1993) Platelet endothelial cell adhesion molecule (CD31). *Curr. Top. Microbiol. Immunol.* 184:37–45.

Del Maschio, A., Zanetti, A., Corada, M., Rival, Y., Ruco, L., Lampugnani, M. G., and Dejana, E. (1996) Polymorphonuclear leukocyte adhesion triggers the disorganization of endothelial cell-to-cell adherens junctions. *J. Cell Biol.* 135:497–510.

Devreotes, P. N. (1988) Chemotaxis in eukaryotic cells: a focus on leukocytes and Dictyostelium. *Annu. Rev. Cell Biol.* 4:649–686.

Diamond, M. S., Johnson, S. C., Dustin, M. L., McCaffery, P., and Springer, T. A. (1989) Differential effects on leukocyte functions of CD-11a, CD-11b, and CD-18 monoclonal antibodies. In *Leukocyte Typing* W. Knapp, B. Dorken, W. R. Gilks, and S. Shaw, ed. London: Oxford University Press, vol. 4, p. 570–574.

Diamond, M. S., Staunton, D. E., de Fougerolles, A. R., Stacker, S. A., Garcia Aguilar, J., Hibbs, M. L., and Springer, T. A. (1990) ICAM-1 (CD54): a counter-receptor for Mac-1 (CD11b/CD18). *J. Cell Biol.* 111:3129–3139.

Diamond, M. S., Staunton, D. E., Marlin, S. D., and Springer, T. A., (1991) Binding of the integrin Mac-1 (CD-11b/CD-18) to the third immunoglobulin like domain of ICAM-1 (CD-54) and its regulation by glycosylation. *Cell* 65:961–971.

Doerschuk, C. M., Winn, R. K., Coxson, H. O., and Harlan, J. M. (1990) CD-18–dependent and independent mechanisms of neutrophil emigration in the pulmonary and systemic microcirculation of rabbits. *J. Immunol.* 144:2327–2333.

Doerschuk, C. M., Quinlan, W. M., Doyle, N. A., Bullard, D. C., Vestweber, D., Jones, M. L., Takei, F., Ward, P. A., and Beaudet, A. L. (1996) The role of P-selectin and ICAM-1 in lung injury as determined by blocking antibodies and mutant mice. *J. Immunol.* 157:4609–4614.

Doukas, J., Shepro, D., and Hechtman, H. (1987) Vasoactive amines directly modify endothelial cells to affect polymorphonuclear leukocyte diapedesis in vitro. *Blood* 69:1563–1569.

Dustin, M. L., Rothlein, R., Bhan, A. K., Dinarello, C. A., and Springer, T. A. (1986) Induction by IL-1 and interferon-gamma: tissue distribution, biochemistry, and function of a natural adherence molecule (ICAM-1). *J. Immunol.* 137:245–254.

Dustin, M. L., and Springer, T. A. (1989) T-cell receptor cross-linking transiently stimulates adhesiveness through LFA-1. *Nature* 341:619–624.

Ebisawa, M., Bochner, B. S., Georas, S. N., and Schleimer, R. P. (1992) Eosinophil transendothelial migration induced by cytokines. I. Role of endothelial and eosinophil adhesion molecules in IL-1 beta-induced transendothelial migration. *J. Immunol.* 149:4021–4028.

Edwards, S. W. (1994) *Biochemistry and Physiology of the Neutrophil.* Cambridge: Cambridge University Press.

Fawcett, J., Buckley, C., Holness, C. L., I. N. Bird, J. H. Spragg, J. Saunders, A. Harris, and D. L. Simmons. (1995) Mapping the homotypic binding sites in CD31 and the role of CD31 adhesion in the formation of interendothelial cell contacts. *J. Cell Biol.* 128:1229–1241.

Feng, D., Nagy, J. A., Pyne, K., Dvorak, H. F., and Dvorak, A. M. (1998) Neutrophils emigrate from venules by a transendothelial cell pathway in response to FMLP. *J. Exp. Med.* 187:903–915.

Foxman, E. F., Campbell, J. J., and Butcher, E. C. (1998) Multistep navigation and the combinatorial control of leukocyte chemotaxis. *J. Cell Biol.* 139:1349–1369.

Franke, W. W., Cowin, P., Grund, C., Kuhn, C., and Kapprell, H-P. (1988) The endothelial junction: the plaque and its components. In *Endothelial Cell Biology in Health and Disease*, N. Simionescu and M. Simionescu, eds. New York: Plenum, 147–166.

Friedl, P., Noble, P. B., and Zanker, K. S. (1995) T lymphocyte locomotion in a three-dimensional collagen matrix. Expression and function of cell adhesion molecules. *J. Immunol.* 154:4973–4985.

Fujimoto, T., Fujimura, K., Noda, M., Takafuta, T., Shimomura, T., and Kuramoto, A. (1995)

50-kD Integrin-associated protein does not detectably influence several functions of glycoprotein IIb–IIIa complex in human platelets. *Blood* 86:2174–2182.

Furie, M. B., Cramer, E. B., Naprstek, B. L., and Silverstein, S. C. (1984) Cultured endothelial cell monolayers that restrict the transendothelial passage of macromolecules and electrical current. *J. Cell Biol.* 98:1033–1042.

Furie, M. B., Naprstek, B. L., and Silverstein, S. C. (1987) Migration of neutrophils across monolayers of cultured microvascular endothelial cells. *J. Cell Sci.* 88:161–175.

Furie, M. B., and McHugh, D. D. (1989) Migration of neutrophils across endothelial monolayers is stimulated by treatment of the monolayers with interleukin-1 or tumor necrosis factor-alpha. *J. Immunol.* 143:3309–3317.

Furie, M. B., Tancinco, M. C., and Smith, C. W. (1991) Monoclonal antibodies to leukocyte integrins CD11a/CD18 and CD11b/CD18 or intercellular adhesion molecule-1 inhibit chemoattractant-stimulated neutrophil transendothelial migration in vitro. *Blood* 78:2089–2097.

Furie, M. B., Burns, M. J., Tancinco, M. C., Benjamin, C. D., and Lobb, R. R. (1992) E-selectin (endothelial–leukocyte adhesion molecule-1) is not required for the migration of neutrophils across IL-1–stimulated endothelium in vitro. *J. Immunol* 148:2395–2404.

Gao, J. X., Issekutz, A. C., and Issekutz, T. B., (1994) Neutrophils migrate to delayed-type hypersensitivity reactions in joints, but not in skin. Mechanism is leukocyte function-associated antigen-1-/Mac-1-independent. *J. Immunol.* 153:5689–5697.

Garcia, J.G.N., Davis, H. W., and Patterson, C. E. (1995) Regulation of endothelial cell gap formation and barrier dysfunction: role of myosin light chain phosphorylation. *J. Cell. Physiol.* 163:510–522.

Garcia, J.G.N., Verin, A. D., Herenyiova, M., and English, D. (1998) Adherent neutrophils activate endothelial myosin light chain kinase: role in transendothelial migration. *J. Appl. Physiol.* 84: 1817–1821.

Goeckeler, Z. M., and Wysolmerski, R. B. (1995) Myosin light chain kinase-regulated endothelial cell contraction: the relationship between isometric tension, actin polymerization, and myosin phosphorylation. *J. Cell Biol.* 130:613–627.

Gopalan, P. K., Smith, C. W., Lu, H., Berg, E. L., McIntyre, L. V., and Simon, S. I. (1997) Neutrophil CD18-dependent arrest on intracellular adhesion molecule 1 (ICAM-1) in shear dependent flow can be activated through L-selectin. *Immunol.* 158:367–375.

Gotsch, U., Borges, E., Bosse, R., Boggenmeyer, E., Simon, M., Mossmann, H., and Vestweber, D. VE-cadherin antibody accelerates neutrophil recruitment in vivo. *J. Cell Sci.* 110: 583–588.

Grant, L. (1973) The sticking and emigration of white blood cells in inflammation. In *The Inflammatory Process.* B. Zweifach, L. Grant, and L. McCluskey, New York: Academic Press, pp. 205–249.

Guinan, E. C., Smith, B., Davies, P. F., and Pober, J. S. (1988) Cytoplasmic transfer between endothelium and lymphocytes. *Am. J. Pathol.* 132:406–409.

Hakkert, B. C., Kuijpers, T. W., Leeuwenberg, J. F., van Mourik, J. A. and Roos, D. (1991) Neutrophil and monocyte adherence to and migration across monolayers of cytokine-activated endothelial cells; the contribution of CD18, ELAM-1, and VLA-4. *Blood* 78:2721–2726.

Harlan, J. M., Winn, R. K., Vedder, N. B., Doerschuk, C. M., and Rice, C. L. (1992) In vivo models of leukocyte adherence to endothelium. In *Adhesion: Its Role in Inflammatory Disease*, J. M. Harlan and D. Y. Liu, eds. New York: Freeman, pp. 117–150.

Harris, A. K. (1994) Locomotion of tissue culture cells considered in relation to ameboid locomotion. *Int. Rev. Cytol.* 150:35–68.

Hauzenberger, D., Klominek, J., and Sundqvist, K. G. (1994) Functional specialization of fibronectin-binding beta 1-integrins in T lymphocyte migration. *J. Immunol.* 153:960–971.

Hill, M. E., Bird, I. N., Daniels, R. H., Elmore, M. A., and Finnen, M. J. (1994) Endothelial cell-associated platelet-activating factor primes neutrophils for enhanced superoxide production and arachidonic acid release during adhesion to but not transmigration across IL-1 beta-treated endothelial monolayers. *J. Immunol.* 153:3673–3683.

Hixenbaugh, E. A., Goeckeler, Z. M., Papaiya, N. N., Wysolmerski, R. B., Silverstein, S. C., and

Huang, A. J. (1997) Stimulated neutrophils induce myosin light chain phosphorylation and isometric tension in endothelial cells. *Am. J. Physiol.* 273: H981–H988.

Hofman, P., Selva, E., LeNegrate, G., d'Andrea L., Guerin, S., Rossi, B., and Auberger, P. (1998) CDIC inhibitors increase f-Met-Leu-Phe-induced neutrophil transmigration. *J. Leuk. Biol.* 63: 1998, pp 312–320.

Hsu, M. H., Chiang, S. C., Ye, R. D., and Prossnitz, E. R. (1997) Phosphorylation of the N-formyl peptide receptor is required for receptor internalization but not chemotaxis. *J. Biol. Chem.* 272: 29426–29429.

Huang, A. J., and Silverstein, S. C. (1992) Mechanisms of neutrophil migration across the endothelium. In *Endothelial cell dysfunctions*, N. Simionescu and M. Simionescu, eds. New York: Plenum Press, pp. 201–232.

Huang, A. J., Manning, J. E., Bandak, T. M., Ratau, M. C., Hanser, K. R., and Silverstein, S. C. (1993) Endothelial cell cytosolic free calcium regulates neutrophil migration across monolayers of endothelial cells. *J. Cell. Biol.* 120:1371–1380.

Huang, C., Friend, D. S., Qiu, W. T., Wong, G. W., Morales, G., Hunt, J., and Stevens, R. L. (1998) Induction of a selective and persistent extravasation of neutophils into the peritoneal cavity by tryptase mouse mast cell protease 6, *J. Immunol.* 160:1910–1919.

Huber, A. R., and Weiss, S. J., (1989) Disruption of the subendothelial basement membrane during neutrophil diapedesis in an in vitro construct of a blood vessel wall. *J. Clin. Invest.* 83: 1122–1136.

Huber, A. R., Kunkel, S. L., Todd, R. F., and Weiss, S. J., (1991) Regulation of transendothelial neutrophil migration by endogenous interleukin-8. *Science* 254:99–102. [published errata appear in *Science* 1991 (Nov 1) 254 (5032):631 and 1991 (Dec 6 254 (5037): 1435].

Hynes, R. O. (1992) Integrins: versatility, modulation, and signaling in cell adhesion. *Cell* 69:11–25.

Imhoff, B. A., and Dunon, D. (1995) Leukocyte migration and adhesion. *Advances Immunol.* 58: 345–416.

Issekutz, A. C., and Issekutz, T. B. (1992) The contribution of LFA-1 (CD11a/CD18) and MAC-1 (CD11b/CD18) to the in vivo migration of polymorphonuclear leucocytes to inflammatory reactions in the rat. *Immunol.* 76:655–661.

Issekutz, A. C., Chuluyan, H. E., and Lopes, N. (1995) CD11/CD18-independent transendothelial migration of human polymorphonuclear leukocytes and monocytes: involvement of distinct and unique mechanisms. *J.Leukoc Biol.* 57:553–561.

Issekutz, T. B. (1995) In vivo monocyte migration to acute inflammatory reactions, IL-1alpha, TNF-alpha, IFN-gamma, and C5a utilizes LFA-1, Mac-1, and VLA-4 *J. Immunol.* 154:6533–6540.

Jara, P. I., Boric, M. P., and Saez, J. C. (1995) Leukocytes express connexin 43 after activation with lipopolysaccharide and appear to form gap junctions with endothelial cells after ischemia-reperfusion. *Proc. Natl. Acad. Sci USA* 92:7011–7015.

Jones, D. H., Schmalstieg, F. C., Dempsey, K., Krater, S. S., Nannen, D. D., Smith, C. W., and Anderson, D. C. Subcellular distribution and mobilization of MAC-1 (CD11b/CD18) in neonatal neutrophils. *Blood* 75:488–498.

Jones, S. L., Knaus, U. G., Bokoch, G. M., and Brown, E. J. (1998) Two signaling mechanisms for activation of alphaM beta2 avidity in polymorphonuclear neutrophils. *J. Biol. Chem.* 273: 10556–10566.

Jung, U., Norman, K. E., Ramos, C. L., Scharffetter-Kochanek, K., Beaudet, A. L., and Ley, K. (1998) Transit time of leukocytes rolling through venules controls cytokine-induced inflammatory cell recruitment in vivo. *J. Clin. Invest.* 102:1526–1533.

Kew, R. R., Peng, T., DiMartino, S. J., Madhavan, D., Weinman, S. J., Cheng, D., and Prossnitz, E. R. (1999) Undifferentiated U937 cells transfected with chemoattractant receptors: a model system to investigate chemotactic mechanisms and receptor structure/function relationships. *J. Leuk. Biol.* 61:329–337.

Kielbassa, K., Schmitz, C., and Gerke, V. (1998) Disruption of endothelial microfilaments selectively reduces the transendothelial migration of monocytes. *Exp. Cell Res.* 243:129–141.

Kishimoto, T. K., and Anderson, D. C. (1992) The role of integrins in inflammation. In *Inflammation. Basic Principles and Clinical Correlates*, J. I. Gallin, I. M. Goldstein, and R. Snyderman, eds. New York: Raven Press, New York 1992 pp. 353–406.

Kowalczyk, A. P., Tullch, R. H., and McKeown-Longo, P. J. (1990) Polarized fibronectin eecretion and localised matrix assembly sites correlate with subendothelial matrix formation. *Blood* 75: 2335–2342.

Kowalczyk, A. P., and McKeown-Longo, P. J. (1992) Basolateral distribution of fibronectin matrix assembly sites on vascular endothelial monolayers is regulated by substratum fibronection. *J. Cell. Physiol.* 152:126–134.

Kubes, P., Niu, X., Smith, C. W., Kehrli, M. E., Reinhardt, P. H., and Woodman, R. C. (1995) A novel betal-dependent adhesion pathway on neutrophils: a mechanism invoked by dihydro-cytochalsin B or endothelial transmigration. *FASEB J.* 9:1103–1111.

Kuijpers, T. W., Hakkert, B. C., Hart, M. H., and Roos, D. (1992a) Neutrophil migration across monolayers of cytokine-prestimulated endothelial cells: a role for platelet-activating factor and IL-8. *J. Cell Biol.* 117:565–577. 1992a, pp. 565–572

Kuijpers, T. W., Hoogerwerf, M., and Roos, D. (1992b) Neutrophil migration across monolayers of resting or cytokine-activated endothelial cells. Role of intracellular calcium changes and fusion of specific granules with the plasma membrane. *J. Immunol.* 148: 72–77.

Kuijpers, T. W., Mul, E. P., Blom, M., Kovach, N. L., Gaeta, F. C., Tollefson, V., Elices, M. J., and Harlan, J. M. (1993) Freezing adhesion molecules in a state of high-avidity binding blocks eosinophil migration. *J. Exp. Med.* 178:279–284.

Kusterer, K., Bojunga, J., Enghofer, M., Heidenthal, E., Usadel, K. H., Kolb, H., and Martin, S. (1998) Soluble ICAM-1 reduces leukocyte adhesion to vascular endothelium in ischemia–reperfusion injury in mice. *Am. J. Physiol.* 275:G377–G380.

Kvietys, P. R., and Granger, D. N. (1997) Endothelial cell monolayers as a tool for studying microvascular pathophysiology. *Am. J. Physiol.* 273: G1189–G1199.

Lackie, J. M. (1984) *Cell Movement and Cell Behavior.* London: Unwin & Allen.

Lampugnani, M. G., Resnati, M., Dejana, E., and Marchisio, P. C. (1991) The role of integrins in the maintenance of endothelial monolayer integrity. *J. Cell Biol.* 112:479–490.

Lampugnani, M. G., Resnati, M., Raiteri, M., Lampugnani, M. G., Resnati, M., Raiteri, M., Pigott, R., Pisacane, A., Houen, G., Ruco, L. P., and Dejana, E. (1992) A novel endothelial-specific membrane protein is a marker of cell–cell contacts. *J. Cell Biol.* 118:1511–1522.

Lampugnani, M. G., Corada, M., Caveda, L., Breviario, F., Ayalon, O., Geiger, B., and Dejana, E. The molecular organization of endothelial cell to cell junctions: differential association of plakoglobin, beta-catenin, and alpha-catenin with vascular endothelial cadherin (VE-cadherin). *J. Cell Biol.* 129:203–217.

Lawrence, M. B., Smith, C. W., Eskin, S. G., and McIntire, L. V. (1990) Effect of venous shear stress on CD18-mediated neutrophil adhesion to cultured endothelium. *Blood* 75: 227–237.

Leppert, D., Waubant, E., Galardy, R., Bunnett, N. W., and Hauser, S. L. (1995) T-cell gelatinases mediate basement membrane transmigration in vitro. *J. Immunol.* 154: 4379–4389.

Liao, F., Huynh, H. K., Eiroa, A., Greene, T., Polizzi, E., and Muller, W. A. (1995) Migration of monocytes across endothelium and passage through extra-cellular matrix involve separate molecular domains of PECAM-1. *J. Exp. Med.* 182:1337–1343.

Liaw, C. W., Cannon, C., Power, M. D., Kiboneta, P. K., and Rubin, L. L. (1990) Identification and cloning of two species of cadherins in bovine endothelial cells. *Eur. Mol. Biol. Org. J.* 9: 2701–2708.

Lindberg, F. P., Gresham, H. D., Schwarz, E., and Brown, E. J. (1993) Molecular cloning of integrin-associated protein: an immunoglobulin family member with multiple membrane spanning domains implicated in alphavbeta3-dependent ligand binding. *J. Cell Biol.* 123: 1993, 485–496.

Lindberg, F. P., Lublin, D. M., Telen, M. J., et al. (1994) Rh-related antigen CD-47 is the signal-transducer integrin-associated protein. *J. Biol. Chem.* 269:1567–1570.

Lindberg, F. P., Bullard, D. C., Caver, T. E., Gresham, H. D., Beaudet, A. L., and Brown, E. J. (1996) Decreased resistance to bacterial infection and granulocyte defects in IAP-deficient mice. *Science* 274:795–798.

Lorenzon, P., Vecile, E., Nardon, E., Ferrero, E., Harlan, J. M., Tedesco, F., and Dobrina, A. (1998) Endothelial cell E-and P-selectin and vascular cell adhesion molecule-1 function as signalling receptors. *J. Cell Biol.* 142: 1381–1391.

Lu, H., Smith, C. W., Perrard, J., Bullard, D., Tang, L., Shappell, S. B., Entman, M. L., Beaudet, A. L., and Ballantyne, C. M. (1997) LFA-1 is sufficient in mediating neutrophil emigration in Mac-1-deficient mice. *J. Clin. Invest.* 99:1340–1350.

Lub, M., Van Kooyk, Y., and Figdor, C. G. (1995) Ins and outs of LFA-1. *Immunol. Today* 16:479–483.

Luscinskas, F. W., Cybulsky, M. I., Kiely, J. M., Peckins, C. S., Davis, V. M. and Gimbrone, M.A.J. (1991) Cytokine-activated human endothelial monolayers support enhanced neutrophil transmigration via a mechanism involving both endothelial-leukocyte adhesion molecule-1 and intercellular adhesion molecule-1. *J. Immunol.* 146:1617–1625.

Maclouf, J. (1993) Transcellular biosynthesis of arachidonic acid metabolites: from in vitro investigations to in vivo reality. *Ballieres Clin. Haematol.* 6:593–608.

Maecker, H. T., Todd, S. C., and Levy, S. (1997) The tetraspanin superfamily: molecular facilitators. *FASEB J.* 11:428–442.

Mansfield, P. J., and Suchard, S. J. (1993) Thrombospondin promotes both chemotaxis and haptotaxis in neutrophil-like HL-60 cells. *J. Immunol.* 150:1959–1970.

Mansfield, P. J., and Suchard, S. J. (1994) Thrombospondin promotes chemotaxis and haptotaxis of human peripheral blood monocytes. *J. Immunol.* 153:4219–4229.

McEvoy, L. M., Jutila, M. A., Teao, P. S., Cooke, J. P., and Butcher, E. C. (1997) Anti-CD43 inhibits monocyte–endothelial adhesion in inflammation and atherogenesis. *Blood* 90:3587–3594.

Mebius, R. E., Watson, S., and Kraal, G. (1993) High endothelial venules: regulation of activity and specificity. *Behring. Inst. Mitt.* 92:8–14.

Meerschaert, J., and Furie, M. B. (1994) Monocytes use either CD11/CD18 or VLA-4 to migrate across human endothelium in vitro. *J. Immunol.* 152:1915–1926.

Meerschaert, J., and Furie, M. B. (1995) The adhesion molecules used by monocytes for migration across endothelium include CD11a/CD18, CD11b; shCD18, and VLA-4 on monocytes and ICAM-1, VCAM-1, and other ligands on endothelium. *J. Immunol.* 154:4099–4112.

Mentzer, S. J., Remopld-O'Donnell, E., Crimmins, M.A.V., Bierer, B. E., Rosen, F. S., and Burakoff, S. J. (1987) Sialophorin, a surface glycoprotein defective in Wiskott–Aldrich syndrome, is involved in human T-lymphocyte proliferation. *J. Exp. Med.* 165: 1383–1392.

Middleton, J., Neil, S., Wintle, J., Clarke-Lewis, I., Moore, H., Lam, C., Auer, M., Hub, E., and Rot, A. Transcytosis and surface presentation of IL-8 by venular endothelial cells. *Cell* 91:385–395.

Mikecz, K., Brennon, F. R., Kim, J. H., and Glant, T. T. (1995) Anti-CD44 treatment abrogates tissue oedema and leukocyte infiltration in murine arthritis. *Nat. Med.* 1:558–563.

Miller, M. D., and Krangel, M. S. (1992) Biology and biochemistry of the chemokines: a family of chemotactic and inflammatory cytokines. *Crit. Rev. Immunol.* 12:17–46.

Modur, V., Li, Y., Zimmerman, G. A., Prescott, S. M., and McIntyre, T. M. (1997) Retrograde inflammatory signaling from neutrophils to endothelial cells by soluble interleukin-6 receptor alpha. *J. Clin. Invest.* 100:2752–2756.

Moll, T., Dejana, E., and Vestweber, D. (1998) In vitro degradation of endothelial catenins by a neutrophil protease. *J. Cell. Biol.* 140:403–407.

Moser, R., Schleiffenbaum, B., Groscurth, P., and Fehr, J. (1989) Interleukin-1 and tumor necrosis factor stimulate human vascular endothelial cells to promote transendothelial neutrophil passage. *J. Clin. Invest.* 83:444–455.

Moser, R., Fehr, J., and Bruijnzeel, P. L. (1992a) IL-4 controls the selective endothelium-driven transmigration of eosinophils from allergic individuals. *J. Immunol.* 149: 1432–1438.

Moser, R., Fehr, J., Olgiati, L., and Bruijnzeel, P. L. (1992b) Migration of primed human eosinophils across cytokine-activated endothelial cell monolayers. *Blood* 79:2937–2945.

Muller, W. A., and Weigl, S. A. (1992) Monocyte-selective transendothelial migration: dissection of the binding and transmigration phases by an in vitro assay. *J. Exp. Med.* 176:819–828.

Muller, W. A., Weigl, S. A., Deng, X., and Phillips, D. M. (1993) PECAM-1 is required for transendothelial migration of leukocytes. *J. Exp. Med.* 178:449–460.

Muller, W. A. (1995) The role of PECAM-1 (CD31) in leukocyte emigration: studies in vitro and in vivo. *J. Leukoc. Biol.* 57:523–528.

Newman, P. J., Berndt, M. C., Gorski, J., White, G. C., Lyman S., Paddock, C., and Muller, W. A.

(1990) PECAM-1 (CD31) cloning and relation to adhesion molecules of the immunoglobulin gene superfamily. *Science* 247:1219–1222.

Nohgawa, M., Sasada, M., Maeda, A., et al. (1997) Leukotriene B4-activated human endothelial cells promote transendothelial neutrophil migration. *J. Leukoc. Biol.* 62:203–209.

Nourshargh, S., Larkin, S. W., Das, A., and Williams, T. J. (1995) Interleukin-1–induced leukocyte extravasation across rat mesenteric microvessels is mediated by platelet-activating factor. *Blood* 85:2553–2558.

Ohno, N., Ichikawa, H., Coe, L., Kvietys, P. R., Granger, D. N., and Alexander, J. S. (1997) Soluble selectins and ICAM-1 modulate neutrophil–endothelial adhesion and diapedesis in vitro. *Inflammation* 21:313–324.

Oppenheimer Marks, N., Davis, L. S., and Lipsky, P. E. (1990) Human T lymphocyte adhesion to endothelial cells and transendothelial migration. Alteration of receptor use relates to the activation status of both the T cell and the endothelial cell. *J. Immunol.* 145:140–148.

Oppenheimer Marks, N., Davis, L. S., Bogue, D. T., Ramberg, J., and Lipsky, P. E. (1991) Differential utilization of ICAM-1 and VCAM-1 during the adhesion and transendothelial migration of human T lymphocytes. *J. Immunol.* 147:2913–2921.

Oppenheimer Marks, N., Kavanaugh, A. F., and Lipsky, P. E. (1994) Inhibition of the transendothelial migration of human T lymphocytes by prostaglandin *J. Immunol.* 152:5703–5713.

Pakianathan, D. R. (1995) Extracellular matrix proteins and leukocyte function. *J. Leukoc. Biol.* 57:699–702.

Palade, G. E. (1988) The microvascular endothelium revisited. In *Endothelial Cell Biology in Health and Disease*, eds. N. Simionescu and M. Simionescu, New York: Plenum, 3–22.

Papayianni, A., Serhan, C. N., and Brady, H. R. (1996) Lipoxin A4 and B4 inhibit leukotriene-stimulated interactions of human neutrophils and endothelial cells. *J. Immunol.* 156:2264–2272.

Parkos, C. A. (1997) Molecular events in neutrophil transepithelial migration. *BioEssays* 19:865–873.

Pepper, M. S., Montesano, R., el Aoumari, A., Gros, D., Orci, L., and Meda, P. (1992) Coupling and connexin 43 expression in microvacsular and large vessel endothelial cells. *Am. J. Physiol.* 262: C1246–C1257.

Pfau, S., Leitenberg, D., Rinder, H., Smith, B. R., Pardi, R., and Bender, J. R. (1995) Lymphocyte adhesion-dependent calcium signaling in human endothelial cells. *J. Cell Biol.* 128:969–978.

Piali, L., Hammel. P., Uherek, C., Bachmann, F., Gisler, R. H., Dunon, D., and Imhoff, B. A. (1995) CD-31/PECAM-1 is a ligand for alphavbeta3 integrin involved in adhesion of leucocytes to entothelium. *J. Cell Biol.* 130:451–460.

Polacek, D., Lal, R., Volin, M. V., and Davies, P. F. (1993) Gap junctional communication between vascular cells. Induction of connexin43 messenger RNA in macrophage foam cells of atherosclerotic lesions. *Am. J. Pathol.* 142:593–606.

Qiao, R., Yan, W., Lum, H., and Malik, A. B. (1995) Arg-gly-asp peptide increase endothelial hydraulic conductivity: comparison with thrombin response. *Am. J. Physiol.* 269: C110–C117.

Rainger, G. E., Fisher, A. C., and Nash, G. B. (1997) Endothelial-borne platelet-activating factor and interleukin-8 rapidly immobilize rolling neutrophils. *Am. J. Physiol*, 272: H114–H122.

Reed, K. E., Westphale, E. M., Larson, D. M., Wang, H. Z., Veenstra, R. D., and Beyer, E. C. (1993) Molecular cloning and functional expression of human connexin37, an endothelial cell gap junction protein. *J. Clin. Invest.* 91:997–1004.

Romanic, A. M., Graesser, D., Baron, J. L., Visintin, I., Janeway, C. A. Jr., and Madri, J. A. (1997) T-cell adhesion to endothelial cells and extracellular matrix is modulated upon transendothelial cell migration. *Lab. Invest.* 76:11–23.

Romer, L. H., McLean, M. V., Yan, H. C., Daise, M., Sun, J., and DeLisser, H. M. (1995) IFN-gamma and TNF-alpha induce redistribution of PECAM-1 (CD-31) on human endothelial cells. *J. Immunol.* 154:6582–6592.

Rosales, C., Gresham, H. D., and Brown, E. J. (1992) Expression of the 50-kDa integrin-associated protein on myeloid cells and erythrocytes. *J. Immunol.* 149:2759–2764.

Rosenkrantz, A. R., Majdic, O., Stščkl, J., Pickl, W., Stockinger, H., and Knapp, W. (1993) Induction of neutrophil homotypic adhesion via sialophorin (CD-43), a surface sialoglycoprotein restricted to haematopoietic cells. *Immunol.* 80:431–438.

Rosenstein, Y., Park, J. K., Hahn, W. C., Rosen, F. S., Bierer, B. E., and Burakoff, S. J. (1991) CD43, a molecule defective in Wiskott–Aldrich syndrome, binds ICAM-1. *Nature* 354:233–235.

Rot, A. (1992) Endothelial cell binding of NAP-1/IL-8: role in neutrophil emigration. *Immunol. Today* 13:291–294.

Roussel, E., and Gingras, M. C. (1997) Transendothelial migration induces rapid expression on neutrophils of granule-release VLA6 used for tissue infiltration. *J. Leuk. Biol.* 62:356–362.

Saito, H., Minamiya, Y., Kitamura, M., Saito, S., Enomoto, K., Terada, K., and Ogawa, J. (1998) Endothelial myosin light chain kinase regulates neutrophil migration across human umbilical vein endothelial cell monolayer. *J. Immunol.* 161:1533–1540.

Salomon, D., Ayalon, O., Patel King, R., Hynes, R. O., and Geiger, B. (1992) Extrajunctional distribution of N-cadherin in cultured human endothelial cells. *J. Cell Sci.* 102:7–17.

Saltzman, W. M., Livingston, T. L., and Parkhurst, M. R. (1999) Antibodies to CD18 influence neutrophil migration through extracellular matrix. *J. Leuk. Biol.* 65:356–363.

Sandig, M., Negrou, E., and Rogers, K. A. (1997) Changes in the distribution of LFA-1, catenins, and F-actin during transendothelial migration of monocytes in culture. *J. Cell Sci.* 110:2807–2818.

Sata, M., and Walsh, K. (1998) TNF-alpha regulation of Fas ligand expression on the vascular endothelium modulates leukocyte extravasation. *Nat. Med.* 4:415–420.

Scalia, R., and Lefer, A. M. (1998) In vivo regulation of PECAM-1 activity during acute endothelial dysfunction in the rat mesenteric microvasculature. *J. Leukoc. Biol.* 64:163–169.

Schleimer, R. P., Sterbinsky, S. A., Kaiser, J., Bickel, C. A., Klunk, D. A., Tomioka, K., Newman, W., Luscinskas, Jr. F. W., Gimbrone, M. A., McIntyre, B. W. (1992) IL-4 induces adherence of human eosinophils and basophils but not neutrophils to endothelium. Association with expression of VCAM-1. *J. Immunol.* 148:1086–1092.

Schwartz, J. D., Monea, S., Marcus, S. G., Patel, S., Eng, K., Galloway, A. C., Mignatti, P., and Shamamian, P. (1998) Soluble factor(s) released from neutrophils activates endothelial cell matrix metalloproteinase-2. *J. Surg. Res.* 76:79–85.

Schwartz, M. A., Brown, E. J., and Fazeli, B. (1993) A 50-kD integrin-associated protein is required for integrin-regulated calcium entry in endothelial cells. *J. Biol. Chem.* 268:19931–19934.

Schonbeck, U., Brandt, E., Petersen, F., Flad, H-D., and Loppnow, H. (1995) IL-8 specifically binds to endothelial but not to smooth muscle cells. *J. Immunol.* 154:2375–2383.

Senior, R. M., Gresham, H. D., Griffin, G. L., Brown, E. J., and Chung, A. E. (1992) Entactin stimulates neutrophil adhesion and chemotaxis through interactions between its arg-gly-asp (RGD) domain and the leukocyte response integrin. *J. Clin. Invest.* 90:2251–2257.

Shang, X. Z., and Issekutz, A. C. (1998) "Contribution of CD11a/CD18, CD11b/CD18, ICAM-1 (CD54), and- 2 (CD102) to human monocyte migration through endothelium and connective tissue fibroblast barriers, *Eur. J. Immunol.* 28: 1970–1979.

Shang, X. Z., Lang, B. J., and Issekutz, A. C. (1998) Adhesion molecule mechanisms mediating monocyte migration through synovial fibroblast and endothelium barriers: role for CD11/CD18, very late antigen-4 (CD49d/CD29), very late antigen-5 (CD49e/CD29), and vascular cell adhesion molecule-1 (CD106). *J. Immunol.* 160: 467–474.

Shaw, S. (1994) Leukocyte differentiation antigen database [database]. (International workshop on leukocyte differentiation antigens: Available from S. Shaw, National Institutes of Health on disk; NIH ftp site balrog.nci.nih.gov, Bethesda.

Simon, M. M., Kramer, M. D., Prester, M., and Gay, S. (1991) Mouse T-cell associated serine proteinase 1 degrades collagen type IV: a structural basis for the migration of lymphocytes through vascular basement membranes. *Immunol.* 73: 117–119.

Sincock, P. M., Mayrhofer, G., and Ashman, L. K. (1997) Localisation of the transmembrane 4 superfamily (TM4SF) member PETA-3 (CD151) in normal human tissues: comparison with CD9, CD63, and alpha5beta1 integrin. *Histochem. Cytochem.* 45: 515–525.

Sleeman, J., Moll, J., Sherman, L., Dall, P., Pals, S. T., and Ponta, H. (1995) The role of CD-44 splice variants in human metastatic cancer. In *Ciba Foundation Symposium 189: Cell Adhesion and Human Disease,* J. Marsh and J. A. Goode, eds. Chichester: Wiley, pp. 142–151.

Sligh, J. E., Ballantyne, C. M., Rich, S. S., Hawkins, H. K., Smith, C. W., Bradley, A., and Beaudet, A. L. (1993) Inflammatory and immune responses are impaired in ICAM-1 deficient mice. *Proc. Natl. Acad. Sci USA* 90: 8529–8533.

Smart, S. J., and Casale, T. B. (1994) TNF-alpha-induced transendothelial neutrophil migration is IL-8 dependent. *Am. J. Physiol.* 266: L238–L245.

Smith, C. W., Rothlein, R., Hughes, B. J., Mariscalco, M. M., Rudloff, H. E., Schmalstieg, F. C., and Anderson, D. C. (1988) Recognition of an endothelial determinent for CD-18 dependent human neutrophil adherence and transendothelial migration. *J. Clin. Invest.* 82: 1746–1756.

Smith, C. W., Marlin, S. D., Rothlein, R., Toman, C., and Anderson, D. C. (1989) Cooperative interactions of LFA-1 and Mac-1 with intercellular adhesion molecule-1 in facilitating adherence and transendothelial migration of human neutrophils in vitro. *J. Clin. Invest.* 83: 2008–2017.

Smith, C. W. (1992) Transendothelial migration. In *Adhesion: Its Role in Inflammatory Disease,* J. M. Harlan and D. Y. Liu, eds. New York: Freeman, pp. 83–116.

Smith, W. B., Gamble, J. R., Clark Lewis, I., and Vadas, M. A. (1991) Interleukin-8 induces neutrophil transendothelial migration. *Immunol.* 72: 65–72.

Smith, W. B., Gamble, J. R., Clark Lewis, I., and Vadas, M. A. (1993) Chemotactic desensitization of neutrophils demonstrates interleukin-8 (IL-8)–dependent and IL-8–independent mechanisms of transmigration through cytokine-activated endothelium. *Immunol.* 78: 491–497.

Smith, W. B. (1994) *The Mechanisms and Regulation of Neutrophil Transendothelial Migration* [Ph.D. thesis]. Adelaide: University of Adelaide.

Smith, W. B., Gamble, J. R., and Vadas, M. A. (1994) The role of granulocyte-macrophage and granulocyte colony-stimulating factors in neutrophil transendothelial migration: comparison with interleukin-8 [see comments]. *Exp. Hematol.* 22: 329–334.

Smith, W. B., Noack, L., Khew-Goodall, Y., Isenmann, S., Vadas, M. A., and Gamble, J. R. (1996) Transforming growth factor-betal inhibits the production of IL-8 and the transmigration of neutrophils through activated endothelium. *J. Immunol.* 157:360–368.

Springer, T. A. (1994) Traffic signals for lymphocyte recirculation and leukocyte emigration: the multistep paradigm. *Cell* 76: 301–314.

Stossel, T. P. (1993) On the crawling of animal cells. *Science* 260: 1086–1094.

Sung, K. L., Saldivar, E., and Phillips, L. (1994) Interleukin-1 betainduces differential adhesiveness on human endothelial cell surfaces. *Biochem. Biophys, Res. Commun.* 202: 866–872.

Takeichi, M. (1990) Cadherins: a molecular family important in selective cell-cell adhesion. *Annu. Rev. Biochem.* 59: 237–252.

Telo, P., Brevario, F., Huber, P., Panzeri, C., and Dejana, E. (1998) Identification of a novel cadherin (vascular endothelial cadherin 2) located at intercellular junctions in endothelial cells. *J. Biol. Chem.* 273: 17565–17572.

Vaporciyan, A. A., DeLisser, H. M., Yan, H. C., Mendiguren, I. I., Thom, S. R., Jones, M. L., Ward, P. A., and Albelda, S. M. (1993) Involvement of platelet–endothelial cell adhesion molecule-1 in neutrophil recruitment in vivo. *Science* 262: 1580–1582.

Volker, W., Schon, P., and Vischer, P. (1991) Binding and endocytosis of thrombospondin and thrombospondin fragments in endothelial cell cultures analysed by cuprolinic blue staining, colloidal gold labeling, and silver enhancement techniques. *J. Histochem. Cytochem.* 39: 1385–1394.

Wakelin, M. W., Sanz, M. J., Dewar, A., Albelda, S. M., Larkin, S. W., Boughton-Smith, N., Williams, T. J., and Nourshargh, S. (1996) An anti-platelet–endothelial cell adhesion molecule-1 antibody inhibits leukocyte extravasation from mensenteric microvessels in vivo by blocking the passage through the basement membrane. *J. Exp. Med* 184: 229–239.

Walker, C., Rihs, S., Braun, R. K., Betz, S., and Bruijnzeel, P. L. (1993) Increased expression of CD11b and functional changes in eosinophils after migration across endothelial cell monolayers. *J. Immunol.* 150: 4061–4071.

Weber, C., Alon, R., Moser, B., and Springer, T. A. (1996) Sequential regulation of alpha4 betal and alpha5betal integrin avidity by CC chemokines in monocytes: implications for transendothelial chemotaxis. *J. Cell, Biol.* 134: 1063–1073.

Weerasinghe, D., McHugh, K. P., Ross, F. P., Brown, E. J., Gisler, R. H., and Imhof, B. A. (1998) A role for the alphavbeta3 integrin in the transmigration of monocytes. *J. Cell Biol.* 142: 595–607.

Wilkinson, P. C., Shields, J. M., and Haston, W. S. (1982) Contact guidance of human neutrophil leucocytes. *Exp. Cell Res.* 140: 55–62.

Wilkinson, P. C., and Lackie, J. M. (1983) The influence of contact guidance on chemotaxis of human neutrophil leukocytes. *Exp. Cell Res.* 145: 255–264.

Yanez-Mo, M., Alfranca, A., Cabanas, C., Marazuela, M., Tejedor, R., Ursa, M. A., Ashman, L. K., de Landazuri, M. O., and Sanchez-Madrid, F. (1998) Regulation of endothelial cell motility by complexes of tetraspan molecules CD81/TAPA-1 and CD151/PETA-3 with alpha3beta1 integrin localized at endothelial lateral junctions. *J. Cell Biol.* 141: 791–804.

Zhou, M., and Brown, E. J. (1993) Leukocyte response integrin and Integrin-associated protein act as a signal transduction unit in generation of a phagocyte respiratory burst. *J. Exp. Med.* 178: 1165–1174.

Ziegelstein, R. C., Corda, S., Pili, R., et al. (1994) Initial contact and subsequent adhesion of human neutrophils or monocytes to human aortic endothelial cells releases an endothelial intracellular calcium store. *Circulation* 90: 1899–1907.

Zigmond, S. (1998) Chemotaxis by polymorphonuclear leukocytes. *J. Cell Biol.* 77: 269–287.

Zocchi, M. R., Ferrero, E., Leone, B. E., et al. (1996) CD31/PECAM-1–driven chemokine-independent transmigration of human T lymphocytes. *Eur. J. Immunol.* 26: 759–767.

18

Knockout Mice in Inflammation Research

DANIEL C. BULLARD

The study of mutations has tremendously aided the identification of genes and their functions in many different experimental organisms. In the past, researchers working in mammalian systems relied on naturally occurring mutations or those induced by chemicals or radiation to study the different biological roles of a gene. These efforts were tremendously aided by the development of strategies during the 1980s that allowed the generation of mice carrying specific gene mutations (Capecchi, 1989; Joyner, 1993). This technique was referred to as *gene targeting* and has been widely used to study the functions of many different mammalian genes in physiologic processes. More recently, gene targeting has been applied to genes that mediate inflammation.

There are several advantages in using gene targeted mutations or "knockout mice" for research. Analyses of mice containing heterozygous or homozygous mutations allow investigators to look at the function of a specific gene during the organism's entire lifetime. This has led to the discovery of previously unknown roles for some genes. For example, VCAM—1/VLA-4 interactions had been formerly shown to be important for a wide variety of immune and inflammatory functions including lymphocyte rolling and adhesion, and lymphocyte stimulation (Berlin et al., 1995). Surprisingly, mice homozygous for null mutations in either VCAM-1 or VLA-4 died during midgestation (Gurtner et al., 1995; Kwee et al., 1995; Yang et al., 1995). This important role for both genes in embryonic development had not been predicted from previous studies. Another advantage of knockouts is their specificity, which may not be achieved with other inhibitors. For example, monoclonal antibodies have been used extensively to inhibit receptor–ligand interactions between leukocytes and endothelial cells. However, these reagents can cross-react with other proteins and may bind to Fc receptors on leukocytes. Often, these nonspecific effects are difficult to identify.

Knockout mice have also been used to investigate genes that cannot be easily inhibited by antibodies or other means, or genes where no specific inhibitor is available. This is the case for many chemokine proteins and their receptors. Studies of the roles of different proteins in both chronic inflammation and inflammatory diseases have also benefited from the availability of knockout mice. Gene targeted mutations allow the assessment of a particular protein in both the initiation and progression phases of chronic inflammation. This obviates the need to continually maintain sufficient circulating concentrations of inhibitors, which is usually very difficult.

Some of the potential problems that can be encountered when using gene targeted mice include embryonic lethality, decreased reproductive fitness, and sterility. In addition, several knockout mutations lead to early postnatal lethality, increased infectious susceptibility, or spontaneous inflammatory organ disease (Table 18.1). These phenotypes, although interesting, can prevent or make it more difficult to study the specific effects of a gene mutation in an inflammatory model.

Table 18.1. Gene Targeted Mutations in Inflammatory Proteins

Mutant Strain	Major Inflammatory Phenotype(s)	References
P-selectin	Inhibition of acute leukocyte rolling, inhibition of acute peritoneal neutrophil emigration	Mayadas et al., 1993 Bullard et al., 1995 Ley et al., 1995
	Inhibition of atherosclerotic lesion formation	Johnson et al., 1997 Nageh et al., 1997
	Reduced neutrophil adhesion and/ or injury during ischemia–reperfusion	Horie et al., 1997 Naka et al., 1997 Sun et al., 1997 Kanwar et al., 1998 Zibari et al., 1998 Scalia et al., 1999
	Increased severity of immune complex-mediated glomerulonephritis	Rosenkranz et al., 1999
E-selectin	Absence of slow leukocyte rolling, reduced firm adhesion	Kunkel & Ley, 1996 Ley et al., 1998 Milstone et al., 1998
	Increased susceptibility to systemic *Streptococcus pneumoniae* infection	Munoz et al., 1997
L-selectin	Inhibition of acute leukocyte rolling and emigration, impaired lymphocyte homing	Arbones et al., 1994 Ley et al., 1995 Tedder et al., 1995
	Decreased mortality following LPS administration	Tedder et al., 1995
	Reduced delayed-type contact hypersesitivity response (DTH)	Tedder et al., 1995 Catalina et al., 1996 Xu et al., 1996
E-/P-selectin	Increased susceptibility to mucocutaneous infections, absence of acute leukocyte rolling and emigration	Bullard et al., 1996 Frenette et al., 1996
	Reduced DTH response	Staite et al., 1996

(continued)

Table 18.1.—Continued

Mutant Strain	Major Inflammatory Phenotype(s)	References
	Inhibition of atherosclerotic lesion formation	Dong et al., 1998
	Impaired wound healing	Subramaniam et al., 1997
ICAM-1	Inhibition of acute peritoneal neutrophil emigration, reduced DTH response	Sligh et al., 1993 Xu et al., 1994
	Decreased mortality following lipopolysaccharide (LPS) administration	Xu et al., 1994
	Reduced neutrophil adhesion and/or injury during ischemia–reperfusion	Connolly et al., 1996 Kelly et al., 1996 Soriano et al., 1996 Horie et al., 1997 Kitagawa et al., 1998
	Reduced incidence of collagen-induced arthritis	Bullard et al., 1996a
	Inhibition of atherosclerotic lesion formation	Nageh et al., 1997
	Inhibition of glomerulonephritis and vasculitis during murine lupus	Bullard et al., 1997 Lloyd et al., 1997
	Increased severity of disease during experimental allergic encephalomyelitis (EAE)	Samoilova et al., 1998
ICAM-2	Reduced eosinophil transendothelial migration	Gerwin et al., 1999
PECAM-1	None reported	Duncan et al., 1999
CD18 Hypomorph	Inhibition of acute peritoneal neutrophil emigration, delayed cardiac transplant rejection	Wilson et al., 1993
	Spontaneous development of inflammatory skin disease in PL/J mice	Bullard et al., 1996c
	Inhibition of atherosclerotic lesion formation	Nageh et al., 1997
CD18 Null	Increased infectious susceptibility, inhibition of leukocyte firm adhesion	Jung et al., 1998 Scharffetter-Kochanek et al., 1998
	Inhibition of acute neutrophil emigration in skin	Mizgerd et al., 1997
CD11b (Mac-1)	Reduced phagocytosis and homotypic aggregation	Lu et al., 1997 Coxon et al., 1996
	Reduced leukocyte firm adhesion	Coxon et al., 1996
	Reduced ischemia–reperfusion injury	Soriano et al., 1999
CD11a (LFA-1)	Inhibition of acute peritoneal neutrophil emigration	Schmits et al., 1996

(continued)

Table 18.1. Gene Targeted Mutations in Inflammatory Proteins—Continued

Mutant Strain	Major Inflammatory Phenotype(s)	References
	Inhibition of transendothelial migration	Andrew et al., 1998
Fucosyl-transferase VII (FucTVII)	Inhibition of acute leukocyte rolling, inhibition of acute peritoneal neutrophil emigration, impaired lymphocyte homing	Maley et al., 1996
Core 2β1-6-N-acetylglucosaminyl transferase (C2 GlcNAcT)	Inhibition of acute peritoneal neutrophil emigration	Ellies et al., 1998
P-selectin/ICAM-1	Inhibition of acute neutrophil and eosinophil rolling and emigration	Bullard et al., 1995 Kunkel et al., 1996 Broide et al., 1998a, 1998b
	Inhibition of atherosclerotic lesion formation	Nageh et al., 1997
L-selectin/ICAM-1	Inhibition of acute rolling, inhibition of acute peritoneal neutrophil emigration	Steeber et al., 1998
E-selectin/ICAM-1	None reported	Mizgerd et al., 1998
E-selectin/P-selectin/ICAM-1	Inhibition of acute neutrophil emigration	Mizgerd et al., 1998 Mizgerd et al., 1999
CXC Chemokine Receptor 2 (CXCR2)	Inhibition of acute peritoneal neutrophil emigration, impaired neutrophil emigration in response to urate crystals	Calcalano et al., 1994 Terkeltaub et al., 1998
	Inhibition of leukocyte firm adhesion and absence of slow rolling	Morgan et al., 1997
	Inhibition of atherosclerotic lesion formation	Boisvert et al., 1998
CC Chemokine Receptor 1 (CCR1)	Inhibition of neutrophil chemotaxis, impaired granuloma formation	Gao et al., 1997
CC Chemokine Receptor 2 (CCR2)	Inhibition of monocyte/macrophage recruitment during peritonitis, impaired granuloma formation	Boring et al., 1997 Kuziel et al., 1997
	Inhibition of leukocyte firm adhesion	
	Inhibition of atherosclerotic lesion formation	Boring et al., 1998
Monocyte Chemoattractant Protein-1 (MCP-1)	Inhibition of monocyte/macrophage recruitment during peritonitis and skin DTH, impaired granuloma formation	Lu et al., 1998
	Inhibition of atherosclerotic lesion formation	Gu et al., 1998

(continued)

Table 18.1.—Continued

Mutant Strain	Major Inflammatory Phenotype(s)	References
Inducible Nitric Oxide Synthase (iNOS)	Enhanced acute leukocyte rolling and firm adhesion following endotoxin treatment	Hickey et al., 1997
	Inhibition of endotoxin-induced lung injury	Kristof et al., 1998
	Reduction in cerebrovascular infarct size during ischemic brain injury	Iadecola et al., 1997
	Reduced tissue injury during hemorrhagic shock	Hierholzer et al., 1998
	Increased incidence and mortality during the development of EAE	Sahrbacher et al., 1998 Fenyk-Melody et al., 1998
Endothelial Cell Nitric Oxide Synthase (ecNOS)	Increased myocardial ischemia–reperfusion injury following coronary artery occlusion	Jones et al., 1999
Cyclooxygenase-1 (COX-1)	Prolonged gestation period, reduced sensitivity to indomethacin, inhibition of platelet aggregation	Langenbach et al., 1995
Cyclooxygenase-2 (COX-2)	Decreased survival, renal dysplasia, cardiac fibrosis, reduced hepatic necrosis following endotoxin administration	Dinchuk et al., 1995 Morham et al., 1995
Complement Protein C1q	Decreased survival, autoantibody formation, immune complex glomerulonephritis	Botto et al., 1998
Complement Protein C3	Increased susceptibility to group B streptococcal infection	Wessels et al., 1995
	Increased sensitivity to endotoxic shock	Fischer et al., 1997
	Reduced tissue injury during ischemia–reperfusion	Weiser et al., 1996
	Inhibition of acid-induced lung injury	Weiser et al., 1997
Complement Protein C4	Increased susceptibility to group B Streptococcal infection	Wessels et al., 1995
	Increased sensitivity to endotoxic shock	Fischer et al., 1997
	Reduced tissue injury during ischemia–reperfusion	Weiser et al., 1996
Complement C5a Receptor	Defective clearance and increased mortality following intrapulmonary instillation of *Pseudomonas aeruginosa*	Hopken et al., 1996
	Inhibition of neutrophil emigration, cytokine production, and edema formation during the reverse passive Arthus reaction	Hopken et al., 1997

General Principles of Gene Targeting

In order to use knockout mice successfully, a general understanding of how they are produced is useful. Therefore, I will give a brief introduction of the general methods used in gene targeting and some of the experimental problems observed in the development and characterization of knockout mice. The key procedures involved in generating a mutation by gene targeting are diagrammed in Figure 18.1. In this chapter, mice produced by these methods are exclusively referred to as *gene targeted mutations* or *knockouts*. The term *transgenic* is also sometimes used, but more appropriately describes mice produced by injection of DNA into fertilized mouse eggs. In transgenic mice, the DNA construct integrates randomly in the genome, rather than at a specific region. During gene targeting, a DNA vector containing a mutated version of a gene is electroporated into a mouse embryonic stem (ES) cell line. At low frequency, the vector will homologously recombine with the endogenous gene and cause a mutation.

The initial step in any knockout experiment is the development of the targeting construct, designed to create a mutation in the gene of interest following homologous recombination. This requires at least some genomic information about the structure of the gene, such as a partial sequence of the coding regions, the exon/intron structure, and the positions of restriction enzyme sites. These data are used to generate a vector (using different cloning techniques) that contains homologous DNA from the target locus and a selection cassette. The selection cassette contains a gene, such as neomycin, driven by various promoters that are constitutively active in ES cells. Two different types of constructs, termed replacement and insertion vectors, have been described. A replacement construct is generally used to delete coding regions or exons from the gene (Fig. 18.2). In contrast, insertion vectors result in the integration of the entire construct, including plasmid sequences, at the target locus. This leads to the duplication of specific genomic regions. Both these strategies will result in mutating the gene and can cause null mutations if the construct is correctly designed. However, there are several published reports describing targeting constructs that failed to create null mutations. For example, two different lines of ICAM-1 mutant mice were developed using replacement constructs designed to integrate the neomycin gene into exon 5 or exon 4 (Sligh et al., 1993; Xu et al., 1994). Reverse transcription-polymerase chain reaction (RT-PCR) analyses revealed the presence of alternatively spliced isoforms of ICAM-1 in mutant mice (King et al., 1995). Immunohistochemical staining further

---

Fig. 18.1. Overview of gene targeting: The different experimental steps involved in creating a knockout mouse strain are outlined. Step 1 Electroporation and selection. Step 2 Identification of homologous recombinant clones (Southern or polymerase chain reaction [PCR]): expansion of correctly targeted clones. Step 3 Injection of mutated embryonic stem (ES) cells into blastocysts. Step 4 Implantation into pseudopregnant females. Step 5 Breeding of chimeric mice to nonmutants in order to determine whether the mutant ES cells have contributed to the germline.

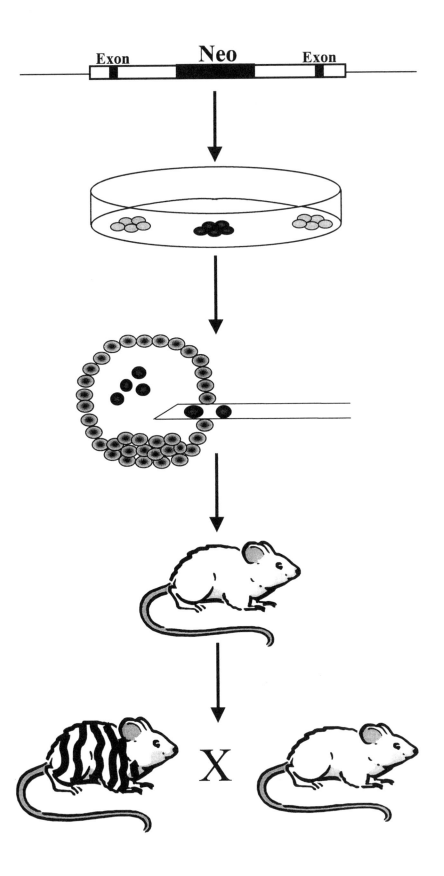

Exon Neo Exon

X

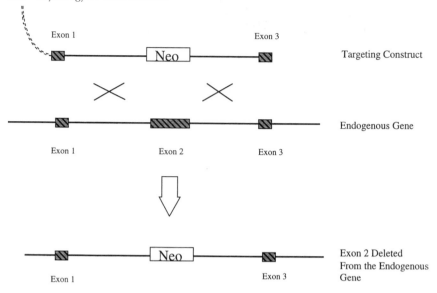

Fig. 18.2. Diagram of typical replacement targeting construct. Following homologous recombination, a specific deletion is generated at the target locus. Black lines represent genomic sequences and the dashed lines correspond to the plasmid vector; exons are indicated by hatched boxes (NEO = neomycin selectable gene).

identified the presence of ICAM-1 in the thymus and lung (King et al., 1995). These isoforms were also found in wild-type mice. Studies of these ICAM-1 mutants, however, have revealed a significant inhibition in inflammatory cell recruitment in several different models (Table 18.1), and the role of these variant forms of ICAM-1, if any, remains to be determined. Thus, the targeting construct must be carefully designed to completely knock out expression of the target gene following homologous recombination.

After the targeting construct is generated, it is transfected into an ES cell line by electroporation, and selection is applied (for neomycin selection, G418 is generally used). ES cells are pluripotent and derived from the inner cell mass of blastocyst-stage embryos (day 3.5 postfertilization). These cells have the capacity to form all tissues of the adult mouse including the germline. Most ES cell lines were originally derived from the mouse strain 129/Sv although lines from other strains are now also being used. Only ES cells that have incorporated the construct into their genome will survive selection. These cells then undergo several rounds of cell division and form a visible colony within 5 to 7 days. Colonies are then picked and replated for amplification and DNA analysis. The frequency of homologous recombination using a single selection system is generally low, and most of the colonies that survive will have the targeting construct integrated randomly in the genome. Therefore, it is necessary to analyze DNA from all ES cell colonies that survive (by Southern or polymerase chain reaction [PCR]) to identify homologous recombinants. Sometimes, both a positive and negative selection system (double selection) is used to increase the frequency of correctly targeted clones. This involves the use of another selectable gene, most often thymidine kinase (TK), which is cloned into the gene targeting vector outside the region of homology. This strategy takes advantage of the fact that random integration of the targeting construct, unlike homologous recombination, will result in the incorporation of the entire targeting vector into a chromosome (including the TK gene). Therefore, any cell that has a functional TK gene present will not survive following the addition of drugs such as gancyclovir.

Once correctly targeted ES cells have been identified and propagated, they are then injected into blastocysts (generally derived from C57BL/6 mice) and implanted into a pseudopregnant mouse. Generally, between 10 to 15 cells are injected into the blastocoele cavity where they can incorporate with the inner cell mass cells of the donor blastocyst. The mutant cells then divide and contribute to the various cell lineages of the embryo. All progeny are analyzed for their coat color pattern to identify mice that are highly chimeric. 129/Sv cells carry the agouti (brown) coat color gene, whereas the C57BL/6 strain contains the black coat color allele. Coat color is used as an indicator of the relative level of contribution of the 129/Sv cells in a mouse derived from ES cell injection. Highly chimeric mice are then bred to test whether the mutation is passed on to the progeny (and thus whether the chimer a carries the mutation in the germline). Heterozygotes are then mated together to establish a homozygous mutant line.

Most of the initial experiments performed on a new knockout mutation are done using mice from a mixed 129/Sv X C57BL/6 strain background. Inbred 129/Sv mutants are generally not used because of the poor breeding efficiency associated with this strain. Allelic variation in loci other than the targeted gene can alter the inflammatory response of individual mice and can also affect the phenotype of a particular knockout mutation. Therefore, it is necessary to use knockout mice and controls that have similar backgrounds in order to avoid nonspecific genetic effects. One of the best examples of how genetic background differences can influence the phenotype of a knockout mutation was revealed in studies of mice containing a gene-targeted mutation in the CD18 gene. These mice on a 129/Sv or 129/Sv X C57BL/6 mixed genetic background display an inflammatory phenotype characterized by impaired neutrophil emigration and leukocytosis (Wilson et al., 1993). However, when this mutation was backcrossed onto the PL/J strain background, all mice developed a noninfectious chronic skin disease characterized by erythema, alopecia, and scale and crust formation (Bullard et al., 1996c). This disease has several similarities to human psoriasis and has not been reported in CD18 mutant 129/Sv or C57BL/6 mice, or in humans with leukocyte adhesion deficiency type I, or LAD-I. This example also illustrates how studies of knockout mice can lead to the discovery of previously unknown functions of different genes involved in the inflammatory response.

Specific Examples of Gene-Targeted Mutations in Inflammatory Proteins

Table 18.1 presents a summary of some of the gene targeted mutations generated in inflammatory proteins. Background information on all of the genes and their previously known functions is given in other chapters. This is not intended to be a comprehensive review of all the studies published to date for each mutation; rather, some of the major functional findings made from these mice are highlighted.

Leukocyte–Endothelial Cell Adhesion Molecule Mutations

Leukocyte–endothelial cell adhesion molecules play essential roles in the development of inflammatory responses by mediating leukocyte emigration and activation (Springer, 1994). The development and analysis of adhesion molecule mutant mice has significantly advanced our understanding of the functions of these proteins. Multiple mutant strains containing single, double, or even triple mutations have now been reported. Much of the early work focused on the role of these proteins in the acute inflammatory response, especially their role in mediating early neutrophil emigration. These studies allowed the development of a more precise model of the leukocyte adhesion cascade (tethering and rolling → activation and firm adhesion → transendothelial migration). Many of the acute inflammatory phenotypes of these adhesion molecule knockout strains are listed in Table 18.1 and are further detailed in Chapter 16.

Analyses of these mice have identified several previously unknown roles for different adhesion molecules in inflammatory responses. For example, mice containing mutations in both P-selectin and ICAM-1, unlike P-selectin or ICAM-1 single mutant strains, showed a complete inhibition of trauma-induced rolling (0–2 hours) and peritoneal neutrophil emigration (0–4 hours) following intraperitoneal injection of *Streptococcus pneumoniae* (Bullard et al., 1995; Kunkel et al., 1996). These studies suggested that that ICAM-1 could influence neutrophil rolling under certain inflammatory conditions. Recent studies of L-selectin/ICAM-1 double mutant mice support this hypothesis and suggest that ICAM-1 may directly or indirectly affect L-selectin–dependent neutrophil rolling (Steeber et al., 1998). Further work is necessary to define the exact relationship between these two adhesion molecules. Another interesting or surprising finding was discovered following the generation of mice containing homozygous null mutations in both E-and P-selectin. These mice, unlike single selectin mutants, developed severe mucocutaneous infections and periodontitis over time (Bullard et al., 1996b; Frenette et al., 1996). This phenotype suggests that although there is significant redundancy among the selectins in mediating leukocyte rolling, L-selectin is not able to compensate for the loss of both E-and P-selectin.

Adhesion molecule expression has been reported in many chronic inflammatory diseases, including atherosclerosis, rheumatoid arthritis, and lupus erythematosus (McMurray, 1996; Price and Loscalzo, 1999). Gene targeted mice are now being used to elucidate the specific functions of different molecules in the initiation and progression of chronic tissue inflammation. The mouse is an excellent organism for studies of chronic inflammation with several well-characterized disease models available. Many of the reported studies have focused on determining the effects of adhesion molecule mutations on the development of atherosclerosis. P-selectin, ICAM-1, P-selectin/ICAM-1, and CD18 mutant mice were all shown to have a significant decrease in mean lesion size in the C57BL/6 high-fat diet model (Nageh et al., 1997). The P-selectin, E-selectin, and E-/P-selectin strains were also analyzed in the low-density lipoprotein receptor (LDLR) mutant model of atherosclerosis (Ishibashi et al., 1993). LDLR mutant mice were bred with each of these mutations and the development of aortic lesions was assessed. Both P-selectin/LDLR and E-selectin/P-selectin/LDLR mutants showed significant inhibition of lesion formation (Johnson et al., 1997; Dong et al., 1998). E-selectin/LDLR mutants, however, did not show any significant differences from LDLR mutant mice (Dong et al., 1998). These findings suggest that E-and P-selectin cooperatively mediate rolling on aortic vessels, although P-selectin plays a greater role in this process. All these studies, taken together, indicate that many different adhesion molecules are involved in the development of lesion formation, perhaps by mediating early monocyte recruitment to the vessel wall.

The effects of ICAM-1 or P-selectin deficiency have also been addressed in several other murine disease models, often with contrasting results. ICAM-1 mutant mice showed a significant reduction in the incidence of collagen-induced arthritis when compared to nonmutant mice, whereas P-selectin mutants showed an accelerated form of the disease with increased severity (Bullard et al., 1996a, Bullard et al., 1999). The ICAM-1 mutation was also bred into the MRL/MpJ-Fas[1pr] strain, a mouse model of human lupus erythematosus and immune complex-mediated diseases (Theofilopoulos & Dixon, 1985). ICAM-1 deficiency resulted in increased survival of MRL/MpJ-Fas[1pr] mice associated with both reduced severity of glomerulonephritis and a significant inhibition of the development of vasculitis (Bullard et al., 1997; Lloyd et al., 1997). Recent findings in our laboratory have shown that P-selectin deficiency in MRL/MpJ-Fas[1pr] mice leads to an acceleration of death, with all P-selectin mutant and nonmutant mice developing severe renal disease (D. C. Bullard, unpublished data, 2000). Finally, ICAM-1 mutant mice were analyzed in the experimental allergic encephalomyelitis (EAE), a model of multiple sclerosis (Zamvil & Steinman 1990). Interestingly, loss of ICAM-1 resulted in a more severe form of neurologic disease (Samoilova et al., 1998). The analysis of P-selectin mutant mice in the EAE model has not yet been reported. These findings, along with those reported in more acute inflammatory models, further illustrate how the function of a particular adhesion molecule can vary dramatically depending on the stimulus and tissue affected.

Cytokine Mutations

Cytokines are major regulators of both immune and inflammatory responses. Gene targeted mutations have now been reported in many different cytokine genes, including TNF-α, IL-1, IL-2, IL-4, and IL-10 (for reviews, see Ryffel, 1996; Durum and Muegge, 1998). Analyses of these mice have further established the important roles of these mediators in hematopoiesis, lymphocyte selection, and the development of immune responses. Studies of these mutants in inflammatory models have also elucidated the important roles of these mediators in both the promotion and suppression of the leukocyte recruitment and activation, as well as in the development of tissue damage.

Chemoattractant Knockouts

Chemokines and chemokine receptors regulate many different cellular functions including leukocyte chemotaxis, angiogenesis, and hematopoeisis (see Chapter 6). Specific inhibitors are not available for all these proteins and their receptors, and gene targeted mice are being used to define their functions during inflammatory responses. One of the first reported mutations in this group was in the mouse homologue of the IL-8 receptor, CXCR2 (Cacalano et al., 1994). IL-8 can mediate leukocyte activation and chemotaxis and is an important regulator of the inflammatory response. Mice containing a null mutation in CXCR2 do not spontaneously develop infections in pathogen-free conditions, but develop both lymphadenopathy and splenomegaly attributed to an increase in B cells and myeloid elements, respectively (Cacalano et al., 1994). Analysis of these mice in acute inflammatory models revealed a significant reduction in acute neutrophil emigration during both thioglycollate peritonitis and in response to urate crystals in a subcutaneous air pouch model, inhibition of leukocyte firm adhesion in cremaster venules, and an absence of slow leukocyte rolling (Cacalano et al., 1994; Morgan et al., 1997; Terkeltaub et al., 1998). CXCR2 bone marrow was transferred into LDLR-deficient mice to study the role of this receptor during the development of atherosclerosis. CXCR2/LDLR double deficient mice showed a significant reduction in mean atherosclerotic lesion area when compared to LDLR single mutants (Boisvert et al., 1998). Immunohistochemical staining of lesions also revealed fewer intimal macrophages in the CXCR2/LDLR mice.

MCP-1 is a CC chemokine that serves as a major attractant for monocytes as well as memory T cells and natural killer cells (Lu et al., 1998). The major receptor for MCP-1 is CCR2. Gene targeted mutations have now been reported in both of these genes. The inflammatory phenotypes are very similar, with both mutant strains showing significant impairment in monocyte/macrophage recruitment during thioglycollate peritonitis, and reduced ability to form granulomas in the lung and liver when compared to nonmutant mice (Boring et al., 1997; Kuziel et al., 1997; Lu et al., 1998). CCR2 mutant mice also displayed a significant reduction in the number of firmly adherent leukocytes in cremaster venules following MCP-1 administration (Kuziel et al., 1997). CCR2/ApoE double mutant mice were developed to assess the contribution of this chemokine receptor and MCP-1 during atherosclerotic lesion formation (Boring et al., 1998). CCR2/ApoE mutant mice showed a significant decrease in lesion formation compared to ApoE mutant mice. Thus, these studies provide evidence for the important roles of these receptors and their ligands in mediating monocyte recruitment during both acute and chronic inflammatory responses.

Nitric Oxide Synthases

Nitric oxide (NO) participates in many different physiological processes and is a key regulator of inflammation (see Chapter 22). Nitric oxide is synthesized by three distinct genes: neuronal nitric oxide synthase (nNOS), endothelial nitric oxide synthase (eNOS), and inducible nitric oxide synthase (iNOS). Mutations have now been reported for all three isozymes. The development of these mutant strains, unlike many of the previous studies of nitric oxide function that used pharmacological inhibitors, have allowed the analyses of individual nitric oxide synthase genes. The phenotypes of these mutant mice (especially iNOS) in different inflammatory models have been shown to vary dramatically, and these studies have further established the role of nitric oxide as both a pro-and anti-inflammatory mediator (for reviews, see Nathan, 1997; Huang 1998; Huang and Lo, 1998).

Cyclooxygenase 1 and 2

Prostaglandins are a diverse group of hormones that mediate many different physiologic processes, including inflammation (for review, see Hla *et al.*, 1999). Prostaglandin synthase is a key enzyme involved in prostaglandin production and occurs in two isoforms, cyclooxygenase 1 and 2 (COX-1 and COX-2). COX-1 is constitutively expressed and is thought to function in cytoprotection of the gastric mucosa, vascular homeostasis, regulation of renal blood flow, platelet aggregation, and several reproductive functions. COX-2 is normally not expressed in most tissues, but high expression can be induced in inflammatory cells by cytokines and other inflammatory mediators. Nonsteroidal anti-inflammatory drugs (NSAIDS) inhibit cyclooxygenase activity and thus reduce prostaglandin production. Mutations in both COX-1 and COX-2 genes were generated to study the individual contribution of these isoforms in physiological responses. COX-1 mutant mice did not show any obvious pathological abnormalities, although gestation length was prolonged in these mice resulting in mortality in some of the pups (Langenbach et al.,

1995). Surprisingly, these mice did not develop spontaneous gastric lesions and showed reduced sensitivity to indomethacin. Platelet aggregation was also inhibited in COX-1 mice when compared to wild-type.

In contrast to COX-1 mutant mice, COX-2 homozygous mutants show a progressive decrease in survival and female infertility (Dinchuk et al., 1995; Morham et al., 1995). All surviving adult homozygous mutant mice developed severe renal dysplasia, with some animals also showing cardiac fibrosis and increased susceptibility to peritonitis. COX-2 mutant and wild-type mice showed similar inflammatory responses in response to tetradecanoyl phorbol acetate (TPA) and arachidonic acid (AA) as nonmutant mice, but developed less extensive hepatocyte necrosis following administration of D-galactosamine and lipopolysaccharide (LPS; Dinchuk et al., 1995; Morham et al., 1995). Further studies of both COX-1 and COX-2 mice are necessary to evaluate the roles of these individual enzymes in other inflammatory models.

Complement Proteins

Over 30 different proteins have been associated with the complement system (see Chapter 8) and gene knockout mice are now being developed to define further the roles of these proteins during the development of inflammatory responses. Gene targeted mutations in a number of different genes encoding complement proteins, such as C1q, C3, C4, and the C5a receptor have now been reported (Table 18.1). Mice containing complete deficiency of C1q showed a high rate of mortality and autoantibody production (Botto et al., 1998). Pathological analyses of these mice revealed extensive glomerulonephritis, characterized by immune complex deposition and multiple apoptotic cell bodies. The phenotype of these mice suggests that C1q plays an important role in the clearance of apoptotic bodies, which may be important in preventing the development of autoimmunity. Analyses of both C3-and C4-deficient mice showed increased susceptibility to group B streptococcal infection, increased sensitivity to endotoxic shock, and reduced reperfusion injury in the hind limb following ischemia when compared to nonmutant mice (Wessels et al., 1995; Weiser et al., 1996; Fischer et al., 1997). C3 mutant mice, unlike C4 mutant mice, were also shown to be protected from acid-induced lung injury (Weiser et al., 1997).

The complement component C5a mediates a wide variety of inflammatory functions including leukocyte chemotaxis. C5a receptor-deficient mice displayed defective clearance of *Pseudomonas aeruginosa* and significant mortality from pneumonia following intrapulmonary instillation of this organism (Hopken et al., 1996). Loss of the C5a receptor, however, did not result in a decrease in neutrophil influx into the lung, suggesting other chemoattractants are important in this process. Studies of these mice in both skin and peritoneal reverse passive Arthus reaction models revealed a significant decrease in neutrophil emigration, cytokine production, and edema formation when compared to nonmutant mice (Hopken et al., 1997). However, the absence of the C5a receptor did not completely prevent mice from developing tissue injury in the skin or peritoneal cavity, suggesting that other neutrophil chemoattractants are also important in these models.

Summary and Future Directions

Studies of gene targeted mutant mice have significantly advanced our understanding of the functions of many different inflammatory proteins. In addition, analyses of these mice have identified previously unknown functions during embryonic development, reproduction, or other physiologic processes. The genetic approach has also uncovered the significant level of redundancy that exists among many of the different genes involved in the development of an inflammatory response. This information may be important for the design of future therapeutics, which may target different inflammatory proteins. Finally, the phenotypes of these mutations have further demonstrated that the function of a specific inflammatory gene can vary dramatically, depending on the stimulus and tissues affected.

Future genetic analyses of inflammatory genes in mice will focus on several areas. New gene-targeted mutants (from genes that have not yet been knocked out) will be generated, and additional double and triple mutations will also be made. Studies of combinatorial mutations have been extremely valuable for determining the level of functional redundancy between different proteins. In addition, they further define the specific genetic pathways that are used during an inflammatory response. Future studies should also focus more on identifying the roles of these different genes in the development of chronic inflammation. This information is critical for the understanding of how both genetic and environmental factors influence susceptibility to various diseases.

New gene targeting strategies have recently been developed that allow the investigator to mutate genes in specific cell types, eliminate expression at a defined time point, or create point mutations or other minor alterations of the gene (Orban et al., 1992; Gu et al., 1994; Rossant & McMahon, 1999). Many of these techniques involve the use of the bacterial (Cre/lox) or yeast (FLP) recombinases and/or inducible promoters that are regulated by compounds such as tetracycline, ecdysone, or synthetic steroids (Saez et al., 1997; Rossant & McMahon, 1999). Several experimental problems, however, have been encountered with these systems. These include the generation of hypomorphic mutations, "leakiness" of expression, and difficulties in finding cell-specific promoters. Despite these problems, these new techniques will eventually prove to be extremely valuable for future investigations of inflammatory gene function. For example, they can be used to circumvent embryonic lethality in order to study the function of a gene in the adult organism, or to analyze the effects of a mutation at a specific time period during the development of an inflammatory response.

References

Andrew, D. P., Spellberg, J. P., Takimoto, H., Schmits, R., Mak, T. W., and Zukowski, M. M. (1998) Transendothelial migration and trafficking of leukocytes in LFA-1–deficient mice. *Eur. J. Immunol.* 28:1959–1969.

Arbones, M. L., Ord, D. C., Ley, K., Ratech, H., Maynard-Curry, C., Otten, G., Capon, D. J., and Tedder, T. F. (1994) Lymphocyte homing and leukocyte rolling and migration are impaired in L-selectin–deficient mice. *Immun.* 1:247–260.

Berlin, C., Bargatze, R. F., Campbell, J. J., Andrian, U.V.H., Szabo, M. C., Hasslen, S. R., Nelson, R. D., Berg, E. L., Erlandsen, S. L. and Butcher, E. C. (1995) α_4 Integrins mediate lymphocyte attachment and rolling under physiologic flow. *Cell*, 80:413–422.

Boisvert, W. A., Santiago, R., Curtiss, L. K., and Terkeltaub, R. A. (1998) A leukocyte homologue of the IL-8 receptor CXCR-2 mediates the accumulation of macrophages in atherosclerotic lesions of LDL receptor-deficient mice. *J. Clin. Invest.* 101:353–63.

Boring, L., Gosling, J., Chensue, S. W., Kunkel, S. L., Farese, R. V., Broxmeyer, H. E., and Charo, I. F. (1997) Impaired monocyte migration and reduced type 1 (Th1) cytokine responses in C-C chemokine receptor 2 knockout mice. *J. Clin. Invest.* 100:2552–2561.

Boring, L., Gosling, J., Cleary, M., and Charo, I. F. (1998) Decreased lesion formation in CCR2$^{-/-}$ mice reveals a role for chemokines in the initiation of atherosclerosis. *Nature* 394: 894–897.

Botto M., Dell'Agnola C., Bygrave A. E., Thompson E. M., Cook H. T., Petry F., Loos M., Pandolfi P. P., and Walport M. J. (1998) Homozygous C1q deficiency causes glomerulonephritis associated with multiple apoptotic bodies. *Nat. Gen.* 19:56–59.

Broide, D. H., Humber, D., Sullivan, S., and Sriramarao, P. (1998a) Inhibition of eosinophil rolling and recruitment in P-selectin and intracellular adhesion molecule-1–deficient mice. *Blood* 91:2847–2856.

Broide, D. H., Sullivan, S., Gifford, T., and Sriramarao, P. (1998b) Inhibition of pulmonary eosinophilia in P-selectin and ICAM-1–deficient mice. *Amer. J. Resp. Cell Mol. Biol.* 18:218–225.

Bullard, D. C., Qin, L., Lorenzo, I., Quinlin, W. M., Doyle, N. A., Bosse, R., Vestweber, D., Doerschuk, C. M., and Beaudet, A. L. (1995) P-selectin/ICAM-1 double mutant mice: Acute emigration of neutrophils into the peritoneum is completely absent but is normal into pulmonary alveoli. *J. Clin. Invest.* 95:1782–1788.

Bullard, D. C., Hurley, L. A., Lorenzo, I., Sly, L. M., Beaudet, A. L., and Staite, N. D. (1996a) Reduced susceptibility to collagen-induced arthritis in mice deficient in intercellular adhesion molecule-1. *J. Immunol.* 157:3153–3158.

Bullard, D. C., Kunkel, E. J., Kubo, H., Hicks, M. J., Lorenzo, I., Doyle, N. A., Doerschuk, C. M., Ley, K., and Beaudet, A. L. (1996b) Infectious susceptibility and severe deficiency of leukocyte rolling and recruitment in E-selectin and P-selectin double mutant mice. *J. Exp. Med.* 183: 2329–2336.

Bullard, D. C., Scharffetter-Kochanek, K., McArthur, M. J., Chosay, J. G., McBride, M. E., Montgomery, C. A., and Beaudet, A. L. (1996c) A polygenic mouse model of psoriasiform skin disease in CD18-deficient mice. *Proc. Natl. Acad. Sci. USA* 93:2116–2121.

Bullard, D. C., King, P. D., Hicks, M. J., Dupont, B., Beaudet, A. L., and Elkon, K. B. (1997) Intercellular adhesion molecule-1 deficiency protects MRL/MpJ-*Fas*^lpr mice from early lethality. *J. Immunol.* 159:2058–2067.

Bullard, D. C., Mobley, J. M., Justen, J. M., Sly, L. M., Chosay, J. G., Dunn, C. J., Lindsey, J. R., Beudet, A. L., and Staite, N. D. (1999) Acceleration and increased severity of collagen-induced arthritis in P-selectin mutant mice. *J. Immunol.* 163:2844–2849.

Cacalano, G., Lee, J., Kikly, K., Ryan, A. M., Pitts-Meek, S., Hultgren, B., Wood, W. I., and Moore, M. W. (1994) Neutrophil and B-cell expansion in mice that lack the murine IL-8 receptor homolog. *Science* 265:682–684.

Capecchi, M. R. (1989) The new mouse genetics: Altering the genome by gene targeting. *Trends Genet.* 5:70–76.

Catalina, M. D., Carroll, M. C., Arizpe, H., Takashima, A., Estess, P., and Siegelman, M. H. (1996)

The route of antigen entry determines the requirement for L-selectin during immune responses. *J. Exp. Med.* 184:2341–2351.

Connolly, E. S. Jr., Winfree, C. J., Springer, T. A., Naka, Y., Liao, H., Yan, S. D., Stern, D. M., Solomon, R. A., Gutierrez-Ramos, J. C., and Pinksy, D. J. (1996) Cerebral protection in homozygous null ICAM-1 mice after middle cerebral artery occlusion. Role of neutrophil adhesion in the pathogenesis of stroke. *J. Clin. Invest.* 97:209–216.

Coxon, A., Rieu, P., Barkalow, F. J., Askari, S., Sharpe, A. H., Andrian, U.V.H., Arnaout, M. A., and Mayadas, T. N. (1996) A novel role for the beta 2 integrin CD11b/CD18 in neutrophil apoptosis: A homeostatic mechanism in inflammation. *Immun.* 5:653–666.

Dinchuk, J. E., Car, B. D., Focht, R. J., Johnston, J. J., Jaffee, B. D., Covington, M. B., Contel, N. R., Eng, V. M., Collins, R. J., Czerniak, P. M., et al. (1995) Renal abnormalities and an altered inflammatory response in mice lacking cyclooxygenase II. *Nature* 378:406–409.

Dong, Z. M., Chapman, S. M., Brown, A. A., Frenette, P. S., Hynes, R. O., and Wagner, D. D. (1998) The combined role of P- and E-selectins in atherosclerosis. *J. Clin. Invest.* 102:145–152.

Duncan, G. S., Andrew, D. P., Takimoto, M., Kaufman, S. A., Yoshida, H., Spellberg, J., Pompa, J. L.d.l., Elia, A., Wakeham, A., Karan-Tamir, B., et al. (1999) Genetic evidence for functional redundancy of platelet/endothelial cell adhesion molecule-1 (PECAM-1):CD31-deficient mice reveal PECAM-1–dependent and PECAM-1–dependent functions. *J. Immunol.* 162:3022–3030.

Durum, S. K., and Muegge, K., eds. (1998) *Cytokine Knockouts.* Totowa. NJ: Humana Press.

Ellies, L. G., Tsuboi, S., Petryniak, B., Lowe, J. B., Fukuda, M., and Marth, J. D. (1998) Core 2 oligosaccharide biosynthesis distinguishes between selectin ligands essential for leukocyte homing and inflammation. *Immun.* 9:881–890.

Fenyk-Melody, J. E., Garrison, A. E., Brunnert, S. R., Weidner J. R., Shen, F., Shelton, B. A., and Mudgett, J. S. (1998) Experimental autoimmune encephalomyelitis is exacerbated in mice lacking the NOS2 gene. *J. Immunol.* 160:2940–2946.

Fischer, M. B., Prodeus, A. P., Nicholson-Weller, A., Ma, M., Murrow, J., Reid, R. R., Warren, H. B., Lage, A. L., Moore, F. D. Jr., Rosen, F. S., and Carroll, M. C. (1997) Increased susceptibility to endotoxin shock in complement C3- and C4-deficient mice is corrected by C1 inhibitor replacement. *J. Immunol.* 159:976–982.

Frenette, P. S., Mayadas, T. N., Rayburn, H., Hynes, R. O., and Wagner, D. D. (1996) Susceptibility to infection and altered hematopoiesis in mice deficient in both P- and E-selectins. *Cell* 84:563–574.

Gao, J. L., Wynn, T. A., Chang, Y., Lee, E. J., Broxmeyer, H. E., Cooper, S., Tiffany, H. L., Westphal, H., Kwon-Chung, J., and Murphy, P. M. (1997) Impaired host defense, hematopoiesis, granulomatous inflammation and type 1–type 2 cytokine balance in mice lacking CC chemokine receptor 1. *J. Exp. Med.* 185:1959–1968.

Gerwin, N., Gonzalo, J. A., Lloyd, C., Coyle, A. J., Reiss, Y., Banu, N., Wang, B., Xu, H., Avraham, H., Engelhardt, B., et al. (1999) Prolonged eosinophil accumulation in allergic lung interstitium of ICAM-2 deficient mice results in extended hyperresponsiveness. *Immun.* 10:9–19.

Gu, H., Marth, J. D., Orban, P. C., Mossmann, H. and Rajewsky, K. (1994) Deletion of a DNA polymerase b gene segment in T cells using cell type-specific gene targeting. *Science* 265:103–106.

Gu, L., Okada, Y., Clinton, S. K., Gerard, C., Sukhova, G. K., Libby, P., and Rollins, B. J. (1998) Absence of monocyte chemoattractant protein-1 reduces atherosclerosis in low-density lipoprotein reeptor-deficient mice. *Mol. Cell.* 2: 275–281.

Gurtner, G. C., Davis, V., Li, H., McCoy, M. J., Sharpe, A., and Cybulsky, M. I. (1995) Targeted disruption of the murine VCAM-1 gene: Essential role of VCAM-1 in chorioallantoic fusion and placentation. *Genes Dev.* 9:1–14.

Hickey, M. J., Sharkey, K. A., Sihota, E. G., Reinhardt, P. H., Macmicking, J. D., Nathan, C., and Kubes, P. (1997) Inducible nitric oxide synthase-deficient mice have enhanced leukoycte–endothelium interactions in endotoxemia. *FASEB J.* 11:955–964.

Hierholzer, C., Harbrecht, B., Menezes, J. M., Kane, J., MacMicking, J., Nathan, C. F., Peitzman, A. B., Billiar, T. R., and Tweardy, D. J. (1998) Essential role of induced nitric oxide in the initiation of the inflammatory response after hemorrhagic shock. *J. Exp. Med.* 187:917–928.

Hla, T., Bishop-Bailey, D., Liu, C. H., Schaefers, H. J., and Trifan, O. C. (1999). Cyclooxygenase-1 and -2 isoenzymes. *Int. J. Biochem. Cell. Biol.* 31:551–557.

Hopken, U. E., Lu, B., Gerard, N. P., and Gerard, C. (1996) The C5a chemoattractant receptor mediates mucosal defence to infection. *Nature* 383:86–89.

Hopken, U. E., Lu, B., Gerard, N. P., and Gerard, C. (1997) Impaired inflammatory responses in the reverse Arthus reaction through genetic deletion of the C5a receptor. *J. Exp. Med.* 185: 749–756.

Horie, Y., Wolf, R., Anderson, D. C., and Granger, D. N. (1997) Hepatic leukostasis and hypoxic stress in adhesion molecule-deficient mice after gut ischemia/reperfusion. *J. Clin. Invest.* 99: 781–788.

Huang, P. L. (1998) Disruption of the endothelial nitric oxide synthase gene: effect on vascular response to injury. *Am. J. Cardiol.* 82: 57S–59S.

Huang, P. L., and Lo, E. H. (1998) Genetic analysis of NOS isoforms using nNOS and eNOS knockout animals. *Prog. Brain Res.* 118: 13–25.

Iadecola, C., Zhang, F., Casey, R., Nagayama, M., and Ross, M. E. (1997) Delayed reduction of ischemic brain injury and neurological deficits in mice lacking the inducible nitric oxide synthase gene. *J. Neurosci.* 17:9157–9164.

Ishibashi, S., Brown M. S., Goldstein J. L., Gerard R. D., Hammer R. E., and Herz J. (1993) Hypercholesterolemia in LDL receptor knockout mice and its reversal by adenovirus-mediated gene delivery. *J. Clin. Invest.* 92:883–893.

Johnson, R. C. Chapman, S. M., Dong, Z. M., Ordovas, J. M., Mayadas, T. N., Herz, J., Hynes, R. O., Schaefer, E. J., and Wagner, D. D. (1997) Absence of P-selectin delays fatty streak formation in mice. *J. Clin. Invest.* 99:1037–1043.

Jones, S. P., Girod, W. G., Palazzo, A. J., Granger, D. N., Grisham, M. B., Jourd'Heuil, D., Huang, P. L., and Lefer, D. J. (1999) Myocardial ischemia–reperfusion injury is exacerbated in the absence of endothelial cell nitric oxide synthase. *Am. J. Physiol.* 276:H1567–1573.

Joyner, A. L. (1993) *Gene Targeting: A Practical Approach.* New York: Oxford University Press.

Jung, U., Norman, K. E., Scharffetter-Kochanek, K., Beaudet, A. L., and Ley, K. (1998) Transit time of leukocytes rolling through venules controls cytokine-induced inflammatory cell recruitment in vivo. *J. Clin. Invest.* 102:1526–1533.

Kanwar, S., Smith, C. W., and Kubes, P. (1998) An absolute requirement for P-selectin in ischemia/reperfusion-induced leukocyte recruitment in cremaster muscle. *Microcir.* 5:281–287.

Kelly, K. J., Williams, W. W. Jr., Colvin, R. B., Meehan, S. M., Springer, T. A., Gutierrez-Ramos, J. C., and Bonventre, J. V. (1996) Intercellular adhesion molecule-1–deficient mice are protected against ischemic renal injury. *J. Clin. Invest.* 97:1056–1063.

King, P. D., Sandberg, E. T., Selvakumar, A., Fang, P., Beaudet, A. L., and Dupont, B. (1995) Novel isoforms of murine intercellular adhesion molecule-1 generated by alternative RNA splicing. *J. Immunol.* 154:6080–6093.

Kitagawa, K., Matsumoto, M., Mabuchi, T., Yagita, Y., Ohtsuki, T., Hori, M., and Yanagihara, T. (1998) Deficiency of intercellular adhesion molecule-1 attenuates microcirculatory disturbance and infarction size in focal cerebral ischemia. *J. Cereb. Blood Flow Metab.* 18:1336–1345.

Kristof, A. S., Goldberg, P., Laubach, V., and Hussain, S. N. (1998) Role of inducible nitric oxide synthase in endotoxin-induced acute lung injury. *Am. J. Respir. Crit. Care Med.* 158:1883–1889.

Kunkel, E. J., Jung, U., Bullard, D. C., Norman, K. E., Wolitzky, B. A., Vestweber, D., Beaudet, A. L., and Ley, K. (1996) Absence of trauma-induced leukocyte rolling in mice deficient in both P-selectin and intercellular adhesion molecule-1. *J. Exp. Med.* 183:57–65.

Kunkel, E. J., and Ley, K. (1996) Distinct phenotype of E-selectin–deficient mice: E-selectin is required for slow leukocyte rolling in vivo. *Circ. Res.* 79:1196–1204.

Kuziel, W. A., Morgan, S. J., Dawson, T. C., Griffin, S., Smithies, O., Ley, K., and Maeda, N. (1997) Severe reduction in leukocyte adhesion and monocyte extravasation in mice deficient in CC chemokine receptor 2. *Proc. Natl. Acad. Sci.* 94:12053–12058.

Kwee, L., Baldwin, H. S., Shen, H. M., Stewart, C. L., Buck, C., Buck, C. A., and Labow, M. A. (1995) Defective development of the embryonic and extraembryonic circulatory systems in vascular cell adhesion molecule (VCAM-1) deficient mice. *Development* 121:489–503.

Langenbach, R., Morham, S. G., Tiano, H. F., Loftin, C. D., Ghanayem, B. I., Chulada, P. C., Mahler, J. F., Lee, C. A., Goulding, E. H., Kluckman, K. D., et al. (1995) Prostaglandin synthase 1 gene disruption in mice reduces arachidonic acid-induced inflammation and indomethacin-induced gastric ulceration. *Cell* 83:483–492.

Ley, K., Allietta, M., Bullard, D. C., and Morgan, S. (1998) Importance of E-selectin for firm leukocyte adhesion in vivo. *Circ. Res.* 83:287–294.

Ley, K., Bullard, D., Arbones, M. L., Bosse, R., Vestweber, D., Tedder, T. F., and Beaudet, A. L. (1995) Sequential contribution of L- and P-selectin to leukocyte rolling in vivo. *J. Exp. Med.* 181:669–675.

Lloyd, C. M., Gonzalo, J.-A., Salant, D. J., Just, J., and Gutierrez-Ramos, J.-C. (1997) Intercellular adhesion molecule-1 deficiency prolongs survival and protects against the development of pulmonary inflammation during murine lupus. *J. Clin. Invest.* 100:963–971.

Lu, B., Rutledge, B. J., Gu, L., Fiorillo, J., Lukacs, N. W., Kunkel, S. L., North, R., Gerard, C., and Rollins, B. J. (1998) Abnormalities in monocyte recruitment and cytokine expression in monocyte chemoattractant protein 1-deficient mice. *J. Exp. Med.* 187:601–608.

Lu, H., Smith, C. W., Perrard, J., Bullard, D. C., Tang, L., Beaudet, A. L., Entman, M. L., and Ballantyne, C. M. (1997) LFA-1 is sufficient in mediating neutrophil transmigration in Mac-1 deficient mice. *J. Clin. Invest.* 99:1340–1350.

Maly, P., Thall, A., Petryniak, B., Rogers, C. E., Smith, P. L., Marks, R. M., Kelly, R. J., Gersten, K. M., Cheng, G., Saunders, T. L., et al. (1996) The alpha (1,3) fucosyltranferase Fuc-TVII controls leukocyte trafficking through an essential role in L-, E-, and P-selectin ligand biosynthesis. *Cell* 86:643–653.

Mayadas, T. N., Johnson, R. C., Rayburn, H., Hynes, R. O., and Wagner, D. D. (1993) Leukocyte rolling and extravasation are severely compromised in P-selectin-deficient mice. *Cell* 74:541–554.

McMurray, R. W. (1996) Adhesion molecules in autoimmune disease. *Sem. Arth. Rheum.* 25:215–233.

Milstone, D. S., Fukumura, D., Padgett, R. C., O'Donnell, P. E., Davis, V. M., Benavidez, O. J., Monsky, W. L., Melder, R. J., Jain, R. K., and Gimbrone, M. A. Jr. (1998) Mice lacking E-selectin show normal numbers of rolling leukocytes but reduced leukocyte stable arrest on cytokine-activated microvascular endothelium. *Microcirc.* 5:153–171.

Mizgerd, J. P., Kubo, H., Kutkoski, G. J., Bhagwan, S. D., Scharffetter-Kochanek, K., Beaudet, A. L., and Doerschuk, C. M. (1997) Neutrophil emigration in the skin, lungs, and peritoneum: different requirements for CD11/CD18 revealed by CD18-deficient mice. *J. Exp. Med.* 186:1357–1364.

Mizgerd, J. P., Quinlan, W. M., LeBlanc, B. W., Kutkoski, G. J., Bullard, D. C., Beaudet, A. L., and Doerschuk, C. M. (1998) Combinatorial requirements for adhesion molecules in mediating neutrophil emigration during bacterial peritonitis in mice. *J. Leuk. Biol.* 64:291–297.

Mizgerd, J. P., Bullard, D. C., Hicks, M. J., Beaudet, A. L., and Doerschuk, C. M. (1999) Endothelial adhesion molecules and acute neutrophil emigration in the skin. *J. Immunol.* 162:5444–5448.

Morgan, S. J., Moore, M. W., Cacalano, G., and Ley, K. (1997) Reduced leukocyte adhesion response and absence of slow leukocyte rolling in interleukin-8 receptor-deficient mice. *Microvasc. Res.* 54:188–91.

Morham, S. G., Langenbach, R., Loftin, C. D., Tiano, H. F., Vouloumanos, N., Jennette, J. C., Mahler, J. F., Kluckman, K. D., Ledford, A., Lee, C. A., et al. (1995) Prostaglandin synthase 2 gene disruption causes severe renal pathology in the mouse. *Cell* 83:473–482.

Munoz, F. M., Hawkins, E. P., Bullard, D. C., Beaudet, A. L., and Kaplan, S. L. (1997) Host defense against systemic infection with *Streptococcus pneumoniae* is impaired in E-, P-, and E-/P-selectin–deficient mice. *J. Clin. Invest.* 100:2099–2106.

Nageh, M., Sandberg, E. T., Marotti, K. R., Lin, A. H., Melchior, E. P., Bullard, D. C., and Beaudet, A. L. (1997) Deficiency of inflammatory cell adhesion molecules protects against atherosclerosis. *Arter. Thromb. Vasc. Biol.* 17:1517–1520.

Naka, Y., Toda, K., Kayano, K., Oz, M. C., and Pinsky, D. J. (1997) Failure to express the P-selectin gene or P-selectin blockade confers early pulmonary protection after lung ischemia or transplantation. *Proc. Natl. Acad. Sci USA* 94:757–761.

Nathan, C. (1997) Inducible nitric oxide synthase: What difference does it make? *J. Clin. Invest.* 100:2417–2423.

Orban, P. C., Chui, D., and Marth, J. D. (1992) Tissue- and site-specific DNA recombination in transgenic mice. *Proc. Natl. Acad. Sci. USA* 89:6861–6865.

Price, D. T., and Loscalzo, J. (1999) Cellular adhesion molecules and atherogenesis. *Am. J. Med.* 107:85–97.

Rossant, J., and McMahon, A. (1999) "Cre"-ating mouse mutants—a meeting review on conditional mouse genetics. *Genes Dev.* 13:142–145.

Rosenkranz, A. R., Mendrick, D. L., Cotran, R. S., and Mayadas. T. N. (1999) P-selectin deficiency exacerbates experimental glomerulonephritis: a protective role for endothelial P-selectin in inflammation. *J. Clin. Invest.* 103:649–659.

Ryffel, B. (1996) Gene knockout mice as investigative tools in pathophysiology. *Int. J. Exp. Path.* 77:125–141.

Saez, E., No, D., West, A., and Evans, R. M. (1997) Inducible gene expression in mammalian cells and transgenic mice. *Cur. Opin. Biotech.* 8:608–616.

Sahrbacher, U. C., Lechner, F., Eugster, H. P., Frei, K., Lassmann, H., and Fontana, A. (1998) Mice with an inactivation of the inducible nitric oxide synthase gene are susceptible to experimental autoimmune encephalomyelitis. *Eur. J. Immunol.* 28:1332–1338.

Samoilova, E. B., Horton, J. L., and Chen, Y. (1998) Experimental autoimmune encephalomyelitis in intercellular adhesion molecule-1-deficient mice. *Cell Immunol.* 190:83–89.

Scalia, R., Armstead, V. E., Minchenko, A. G., and Lefer, A. M. (1999) Essential role of P-selectin in the initiation of the inflammatory response induced by hemorrhage and reinfusion. *J. Exp. Med.* 189:931–938.

Scharffetter-Kochanek, K., Lu, H., Norman, K., Van Nood, N., Munoz, F., Grabbe, S., McArthur, M., Lorenzo, I., Kaplan, S., Ley, K., et al. (1998) Spontaneous skin ulceration and defective T-cell function in CD18 null mice. *J. Exp. Med.* 188:119–131.

Schmits, R., Kundig, T. M., Baker, D. M., Shumaker, G., Simard, J.J.L., Duncan, G., Wakeham, A., Shahinian, A., Heiden, A.V.D., Bachmann, M. F., et al. (1996) LFA-1–deficient mice show normal CTL responses to virus but fail to reject immunogenic tumor. *J. Exp. Med.* 183:1415–1426.

Sligh, J. E., Ballantyne, C. M., Rich, S. S., Hawkins, H. K., Smith, C. W., Bradley, A., and Beaudet, A. L. (1993) Inflammatory and immune responses are impaired in mice deficient in intercellular adhesion molecule 1. *Proc. Natl. Acad. Sci. USA* 90:8529–8533.

Soriano, S. G., Coxon, A., Wang, Y. F., Frosch, M. P., Lipton, S. A., Hickey, P. R., and Mayadas, T. N. (1999) Mice deficient in Mac-1 (CD11b; shCD18) are less susceptible to cerebral ischemia/reperfusion injury. *Stroke* 30:134–139.

Soriano, S. G., Lipton, S. A., Wang, Y. F., Xiao, M., Springer, T. A., Gutierrez-Ramos, J.-C., and Hickey, P. R. (1996) Intercellular adhesion molecule-1–deficient mice are less susceptible to cerebral ischemia–reperfusion injury. *Ann. Neurol.* 39:618–624.

Soriano, S. G., Coxon, A., Wang, Y. F., Frosch, M. P., Lipton, S. A., Hickey, P. R., and Mayadas, T. N. (1999) Mice deficient in Mac-1 (CD11b/CD18) are less susceptible to cerebral ischemia/reperfusion injury. *Stroke* 30:134–139.

Springer, T. A. (1994) Traffic signals for lymphocyte recirculation and leukocyte emigration: the multistep paradigm. *Cell* 76:301–314.

Staite, N. D., Justen, J. M., Sly, L. M., Beaudet, A. L., and Bullard, D. C. (1996) Inhibition of delayed-type contact hypersensitivity in mice deficient in both E-selectin and P-selectin. *Blood* 88:2973–2979.

Steeber, D. A., Campbell, M. A., Basit, A., Ley, K., and Tedder, T. F. (1998) Optimal selectin-mediated rolling of leukocytes during inflammation in vivo requires intercellular adhesion molecule-1 expression. *Proc. Natl. Acad. Sci. USA* 95:7562–7567.

Subramaniam, M., Saffaripour, S., Van de Water, L., Frenette, P. S., Mayadas, T. N., Hynes, R. O., and Wagner, D. D. (1997) Role of endothelial selectins in wound repair. *Am. J. Pathol.* 150:1701–1709.

Sun, X., Rozenfeld, R. A., Qu, X., Huang, W., Gonzalez-Crussi, F., and Hsueh, W. (1997) P-selectin–deficient mice are protected from PAF-induced shock, intestinal injury, and lethality. *Am. J. Physiol.* 273:G56–61.

Tedder, T. F., Steeber, D. A., and Pizcueta, P. (1995) L-selectin–deficient mice have impaired leukocyte recruitment into inflammatory sites. *J. Exp. Med.* 181:2259–2264.

Terkeltaub, R., Baird, S., Sears, P., Santiago, R., and Boisvert, W. (1998) The murine homolog of the interleukin-8 receptor CXCR-2 is essential for the occurrence of neutrophilic inflammation in the air pouch model of acute urate crystal-induced gouty synovitis. *Arth. Rheum.* 41: 900–909.

Theofilopoulos, A. N., and Dixon, F. J. (1985) Murine models of systemic lupus erythematosus. *Adv. Immunol.* 37:269–391.

Weiser, M. R., Pechet, T. T., Williams, J. P., Ma, M., Frenette, P. S., Moore, F. D., Kobzik, L., Hines, R. O., Wagner, D. D., Carroll, M. C., and Hechtman, H. B. (1997) Experimental murine acid aspiration injury is mediated by neutrophils and the alternative complement pathway. *J. Appl. Physiol.* 83:1090–1095.

Weiser, M. R., Williams, J. P., Moore, F. D., J. F., Kobzik, L., Ma, M., Hechtman, H. B., and Carroll, M. C. (1996) Reperfusion injury of ischemic skeletal muscle is mediated by natural antibody and complement. *J. Exp. Med.* 183:2343–2348.

Wessels, M. R., Butko, P., Ma, M., Warren, H. B., Lage, A. L., and Carroll, M. C. (1995) Studies of group B streptococcal infection in mice deficient in complement component C3 or C4 demonstrate an essential role for complement in both innate and acquired immunity. *Immunol.* 92:11490–11494.

Wilson, R. W., Ballantyne, C. M., Smith, C. W., Montgomery, C., Bradley, A., O'Brien, W. E., and Beaudet, A. L. (1993) Gene targeting yields a CD18-mutant mouse for study of inflammation. *J. Immunol.* 151:1571–1578.

Xu, H., Gonzalo, J. A., St. Pierre, Y., Williams, I. F., Kupper, T. S., Cotran, R. S., Springer, T. A., and Gutierrez-Ramos, J. C. (1994) Leukocytosis and resistance to specific shock in intercellular adhesion molecule 1-deficient mice. *J. Exp. Med.* 180:95–109.

Xu, J., Grewal, I. S., Geba, G. P., and Flavell, R. A. (1996) Impaired primary T–cell responses in L-selectin–deficient mice. *J. Exp. Med.* 183: 589–598.

Yang, J. T., Rayburn, H., and Hynes, R. O. (1995) Cell adhesion events mediated by alpha 4 integrins are essential in placental and cardiac development. *Development* 121:549–560.

Zamvil S. S., and Steinman, L. (1990) The T lymphocyte in experimental allergic encephalomyelitis. *Ann. Rev. Immunol.* 8:579–621.

Zibari, G. B., Brown, M. F., Burney, D. L., Granger, N., and McDonald, J. C. (1998) Role of P-selectin in the recruitment of leukocytes in mouse liver exposed to ischemia and reperfusion. *Transplant. Proc.* 30:2327–2330.

19

Interface Between Inflammation and Coagulation

DARIO C. ALTIERI

Blood coagulation maintains the homeostatic balance of internal body fluids against potentially life-threatening blood losses. Acquired or congenitally inherited aberrations of this process result in severe hemorrhagic or thrombotic disorders. Furthermore, dysregulation of coagulation invariably contributes to vascular and atherosclerotic disorders, cancer, infections, and immune-inflammatory diseases. Since coagulation was defined more than 30 years ago as a "waterfall" of sequential, limited proteolytic activation culminating in fibrin formation, our understanding of this process has progressed tremendously. The primary sequences of coagulation proteins have been elucidated at the cDNA and genomic level, the biochemical requirements of substrate recognition and catalysis have been defined, and, in many cases the tertiary structure of coagulation proteins and cofactors has been resolved by X-ray crystallography. What has also emerged is the pivotal role of vascular cells, and of leukocytes in particular, in coagulation. In addition to providing a surface of negatively charged phospholipids to promote assembly of coagulation, recent experimental evidence has also underscored a *nonhemostatic* function of vascular cells in coagulation. Through the recognition of specialized membrane receptors, the assembly of coagulation proteins on leukocytes and endothelial cells contributes to intracellular signal transduction, modulation of gene expression, synthesis and release of growth factors/cytokines, and regulation of cell-to-cell adhesion. The objective of this chapter is to focus on the ability of coagulation proteins/proteases to act as modulators of leukocyte effector functions, and their far-reaching implications in human diseases. As a unifying theme, coagulation will be proposed as a *response to injury*, integrating the preservation of the hemostatic balance with host defense and immune-inflammatory responses.

Fibrinogen

The first histopathological description of an association of fibrinogen with inflammatory cells was reported more than two decades ago and postulated to involve specialized membrane receptors (Sherman and Lee, 1977; Hogg, 1983). The main fibrinogen receptor on monocytes/macrophages, neutrophils, and natural killer cells was later identified as the β_2 integrin Mac-1 (CD11b/CD18, complement receptor type 3, $\alpha_M\beta_2$; Altieri et al., 1988; Trezzini et al., 1988; Wright et al., 1988; Gustafson et al., 1989). Similar to other integrins (Arnaout, 1990; Hynes, 1992), Mac-1 is a promiscuous receptor, binding several unrelated ligands, including fibrinogen, the complement fragment C3bi, the coagulation zymogen factor X, and membrane-associated counterreceptors of the Ig gene superfamily (Arnaout, 1990; Hynes, 1992). As first determined in quantitative ligand-binding studies (Altieri et al., 1988; Trezzini et al., 1988; Wright et al., 1988; Gustafson et al., 1989), binding of fibrinogen to Mac-1 is specific and saturable with a Kd = 0.1µM. At variance with fibrinogen receptors on platelets ($\alpha_{IIb}\beta_3$) or endothelial cells ($\alpha_V\beta_3$) (Hynes, 1992), this interaction is not mediated by Arg–Gly–Asp sequences in the γ chains or the Arg–Gly–Asp-like motif HHLGGAKQAGDV in the γ chain (Altieri et al., 1990a). Rather, a synthetic peptide Gly[190]-Val[202] in the fibrinogen γ chain was identified as a Mac-1 binding site (Altieri et al., 1993), whereas epitope-mapped monoclonal antibodies (mAbs) (Diamond et al., 1993) and direct binding studies (Zhou et al., 1994) identified a ~200 amino acid I-domain in the α-subunit of Mac-1 as the fibrinogen binding site.

The leukocyte–fibrinogen interaction is a regulated process that requires a transient state of receptor activation. This can be recapitulated by various inflammatory stimuli, including adenine nucleotides (Freyer et al., 1988; Altieri et al., 1990a; Balazovich and Boxer, 1990), chemoattractants, Ca^{2+} ionophores (Wright and Meyer, 1986; Altieri et al., 1990b), or by optimal engagement of the receptor divalent ion-binding site by Mn^{2+} ions (Altieri, 1991). Both mechanisms produce a qualitative state of receptor activation, without increased receptor expression at the cell surface. This activation state can be "marked" by mAbs to activation-dependent neo-antigenic epitopes on Mac-1. This was first suggested from the ability of mAb 7E3, which was originally raised against the platelet integrin $\alpha_{IIb}\beta_3$, to cross-react with the activated form of Mac-1 on monocytes (Altieri and Edgington, 1988) and Mac-1 transfectants (Simon et al., 1997). Consistent with a role of β_2 integrin I domains in conformational changes of receptor activation (Landis et al., 1993), the mAb 7E3 cross-reacting epitope was mapped to the Mac-1 I domain (Zhou et al., 1994), and localized to the most amino-terminal I domain sequence, Gly[127]–Phe[150] (Plescia et al., 1998). Several additional activation-dependent mAbs, and mAbs cross-reacting between leukocyte and platelet integrins, were identified and epitope-mapped to the I domain (Diamond and Springer, 1993; Elemer and Edgington, 1994; De Nichilo et al., 1996). Although inflammatory stimuli also induce a rapid translocation of a mobilizable subcellular pool of Mac-1 to the cell surface (Miller et al., 1987), it is unclear if these newly recruited Mac-1 molecules actually contribute to leukocyte adherence (Buyon et al., 1988; Vedder and Harlan, 1988).

The possibility that Mac-1-fibrinogen interactions could participate in inflammation has been intensely investigated. Using in vivo defibrinogenation, it became clear that fibrinogen was absolutely required for inflammatory responses during intraperitoneal bacterial infections (McRitchie et al., 1991), and immune-complex glomerulonephritis (Wu et al., 1994). This was further substantiated using an an in vivo model of inflammation in response to biomaterials, in which sponges of polyester terephthalate coated with fibrinogen and inserted in the rat peritoneal cavity became rapidly covered with activated monocytes and neutrophils (Tang and Eaton, 1993). This process was specific for fibrinogen, and unaffected by IgG adsorption or complement activation (Tang and Eaton, 1993). At the molecular level, inflammatory cell recruitment to biomaterials was entirely mediated by Mac-1–fibrinogen interaction (Tang et al., 1996), recapitulated by the γ chain peptide Gly[190]–Val[202] (Altieri et al., 1993), and critically involved infiltrating mast cells (Tang et al., 1998). In addition to chemotaxis and neutrophil recruitment mediated by fibrinogen (Skogen et al., 1988), it was postulated that Mac-1–fibrinogen interaction could trigger specialized inflammatory responses. In this context, Mac-1–dependent attachment of monocytes to immobilized fibrinogen resulted in a rapid oxidative burst (Trezzini et al., 1991), in agreement with the signaling role of β_2 integrins in tumor necrosis factor-α (TNF-α)–dependent production of oxidative radicals (Nathan et al., 1989). Similarly, Mac-1 binding of fibrinogen potentiated endotoxin or T-cell cytokines to induce a two-to-eight-fold enhancement of tissue factor-dependent monocyte procoagulant activity (Fan and Edgington, 1991), and a seven-fold upregulation of TNF-α mRNA in these cells (Fan and Edgington, 1993). Consistent with the concept of outside-in signaling, in which β_2 integrins transduce extracellular signals inside the cell, ligand binding to Mac-1 on mononuclear cells produced an early increase in cytosolic free Ca^{2+}, in a reaction regulated by the state of cell activation/differentiation (Ng-Sikorski et al., 1991; Altieri et al., 1992). This was followed by generation of second messengers, which required an intact protein Kinase C (PKC)-dependent pathway (Kreuzer et al., 1996), and culminated with downstream events of gene induction, as reflected in the increased transcription of the IL-1β gene and IL-1 release in fibrinogen adherent cells (Perez and Roman, 1995). Consistent with these findings, it was recently demonstrated that modulation of gene transcription by Mac-1–dependent adhesion to fibrinogen resulted in activation of the pleiotropic transcription factor, nuclear factor kappa-B (NF-κB; Sitrin et al., 1998).

The binding of fibrinogen to Mac-1 has also been implicated in leukocyte–endothelium interaction. This process is perceived as a stepwise adhesion cascade involving integrins, selectins, and Ig-like molecules (Kuijpers and Harlan, 1993; Carlos and Harlan, 1994; Springer, 1994), thus preserving leukocyte trafficking in immune-inflammatory responses. Among the cellular mediators of leukocyte–endothelium interaction, thus enabling leukocyte trafficking, intercellular adhesion molecule-1 (ICAM-1) has received considerable attention. ICAM-1 is a single membrane-spanning glycoprotein receptor expressed on monocytes, T- and B-lymphocytes, and various epithelial cell types (Springer, 1990). Structurally, ICAM-1 is a member of the Ig gene superfamily, with five disulfide-bonded Ig-like domains (Simmons et al.,

1988), and is prominently up-regulated on endothelial cells by cytokines and other inflammatory stimuli (Pober et al., 1986). ICAM-1 interacts with β_2 integrins, LFA-1, and Mac-1, in a receptor–counter receptor interaction, and mediates firm attachment of leukocytes to endothelial cell monolayers (Dustin and Springer, 1989; Springer, 1990). Several ICAM-1 ligands have also been identified, including antigenic determinants on rhinoviruses, coxsackieviruses (Greeve et al., 1989; Staunton et al., 1990), and *Plasmodium falciparum* (Berendt et al., 1989, 1992), thus facilitating viral and parasite entry. Additionally, ICAM-1 binds fibrinogen, as first-determined in affinity purification experiments, and further corroborated in direct binding studies to recombinant ICAM-1, and functional inhibition with anti–ICAM-1 mAbs (Languino et al., 1993). By peptidyl mimicry, it was found that a peptide duplicating the fibrinogen γ chain sequence 119–133, and designated γ3, contained the fibrinogen-binding site for ICAM-1 (Altieri et al., 1995). Conversely, the ICAM-1 binding site for fibrinogen was identified with a novel panel of functionally inhibitory anti–ICAM-1 mAbs, and mapped to Pro[70] and Arg[26] in the first Ig domain (Duperray et al., 1997). This panel of fibrinogen-blocking mAbs failed to diminish LFA-1–mediated T-cell binding to recombinant ICAM-1, thus demonstrating that the fibrinogen- and LFA-1–binding sites on the first Ig domain of ICAM-1 were structurally and spatially separate (Duperray et al., 1997).

The biological relevance of fibrinogen binding to ICAM-1 was demonstrated in cell-to-cell adhesion experiments. Through its simultaneous binding to Mac-1 and ICAM-1 on opposing cells, fibrinogen acted as a bridging molecule to enhance leukocyte attachment to endothelial cells (Languino et al., 1993). This mechanism of "intercellular bridging" occurred at physiologic concentrations of fibrinogen and in a normal plasma milieu, and was not reduced by Arg–Gly–Asp-containing antagonists, thus ruling out an involvement of $\alpha_v\beta_3$ integrin. By immunofluorescence and confocal microscopy, and independently confirmed by immuno-gold electron microscopy, ICAM-1 was exclusively localized to the apical surface of cytokine (TNF-α)–stimulated endothelial cells, and preferentially expressed on elongated cellular processes protruding from the endothelial cell surface (Almenar-Queralt et al., 1995; van de Stolpe et al., 1996). This preferential topography appeared ideal to facilitate an ICAM-1 interaction with Mac-1–bound fibrinogen or β_2 integrins on rolling leukocytes. Consistent with this view, the fibrinogen-dependent pathway of intercellular bridging mediated tight adhesion of monocytes to postcapillary venules of the exteriorized rabbit mesentery circulation at reduced shear forces, whereas no rolling was observed under these conditions (Sriramarao et al., 1996). Peptide- or mAb-dependent inhibition of fibrinogen–ICAM-1 interaction blocked leukocyte–endothelial cell bridging in vivo in a dose-dependent manner (Sriramarao et al., 1996). Altogether, these data suggested that intercellular bridging mediated by fibrinogen may provide a nonredundant pathway of leukocyte recruitment to endothelial cells, independently of (and potentially synergistically with) receptor–counterreceptor interactions maintained by β_2 integrins. A potential role of fibrinogen-dependent intercellular bridging in leukocyte transendothelial cell migration has been also proposed. After adhering to endothelium via fibrinogen, vitamin D_3-differentiated monocyte HL-60 cells were shown to migrate actively across the endothelial cell monolayer, independently of chemoattractant or cytokine stimulation (Languino et al., 1995). Finally, a similar paradigm of fibrinogen-dependent intercellular bridging has been suggested for mediating monocyte adhesion to mesothelioma cells (Shetty et al., 1996).

There are potentially important pathophysiological implications for the role of fibrinogen in leukocyte–endothelial bridging and transendothelial migration. First, this mechanism may provide a molecular basis for the increased risk of vascular diseases associated with high plasma concentrations of fibrinogen (Belch et al., 1998; Danesh et al., 1998). Typically, fibrin(ogen) is abundantly deposited on endothelial cells in atherosclerotic lesions (Bini et al., 1989), and ICAM-1 is prominently expressed in all forms of atherosclerotic lesions, except fibrous plaque, thus correlating with increased leukocyte recruitment (Poston et al., 1992; van der Wal et al., 1992). Accordingly, increased plasma fibrinogen concentrations correlated with increased monocyte adhesion to endothelium in patients with advanced atherosclerosis (Duplaa et al., 1993). In this context, increased monocyte adhesion to damaged endothelium followed by transendothelial migration and intimal accumulation constitutes some of the earliest pathogenetic events in atherosclerosis (Ross, 1993). The increased expression of fibrinogen and ICAM-1 on atherosclerosic endothelium in vivo may facilitate the mechanism of intercellular bridging, and promote increased monocyte recruitment at the site of vascular injury (Languino et al., 1993, 1995). Fibrinogen binding to vascular cell receptors has also been shown to enhance platelet–leukocyte interaction (Diacovo et al., 1996) and may participate in mixed thrombus formation in an $\alpha_{IIb}\beta_3$ integrin-dependent recognition (Weber and Springer, 1997). Not surprisingly, novel therapeutic approaches target the intercellular bridging pathway mediated by fibrinogen as a means to reduce leukocyte recruitment to acutely injured vessels. In recent studies, preincubation of monocyte THP-1 cells with mAb 7E3 (Altieri and Edgington, 1988; Simon et al., 1997) abolished the recruitment of these cells to balloon-injured iliofemoral arteries ex vivo (Plescia et al., 1998), a lesion associated with prominent deposition of fibrinogen (Frebelius et al., 1996; Hatton et al., 1996). Similar results were also obtained with another rabbit model of vascular injury, in which mAb prevention of monocyte–fibrinogen interaction suppressed intimal thickening after angioplasty or stent implantation in vivo (Rogers et al., 1998). Albeit preliminary, these studies suggest that targeting the Mac-1–fibrinogen interaction may prove beneficial at reducing aberrant leukocyte accumulation to injured vessel. A similar strategy may be also exploited to reduce platelet–leukocyte cooperation in mixed thrombus formation (Diacovo et al., 1996; Weber and Springer, 1997), thus targeting two of the most frequent and threatening complications of vascular diseases.

Thrombin

In addition to fibrinogen, several other coagulation/fibrinolytic proteases have been implicated in leukocyte activation and cellular effector functions. Thrombin, the effector protease of the coagulation cascade, has been one of the most intensely studied cofactors at the interface between inflammation and coagulation. The association of thrombin with platelets, monocytes/macrophages, endothelium, and various mesenchymal cells is mediated by a family of seven transmembrane domain G-protein–coupled receptors, designated protease activated receptors (PAR; Coughlin, 1994). Structurally, these molecules have two identifiable features. First, they function as membrane-associated substrates for limited proteolytic activation by thrombin (or other proteases); and second, they provide a new mechanism of cell activation in which the tethered new amino-terminus exposed by proteolytic cleavage binds to an extracellular site in the receptor and initiates signal transduction (Coughlin, 1994). Consistent with this model of proteolytic activation, short synthetic peptides duplicating the receptor's new amino-terminus act as agonists to initiate signal transduction (Vu et al., 1991).

It has been appreciated for the past two decades that thrombin stimulates far broader cellular responses than platelet activation and fibrinogen cleavage. One of the earliest characterized nonhemostatic functions of catalytically active thrombin was the ability to stimulate DNA synthesis and proliferation of fibroblasts and mesenchymal cells (Chen and Buchanan, 1975; Carney and Cunningham, 1978; Glenn and Cunningham, 1979). This was associated with stimulation of phosphatidic acid metabolism in endothelial cells, increase in cytosolic free Ca^{2+} (Garcia et al., 1992), and a three-to-five-fold increased expression of platelet-derived growth factor (Daniel et al., 1986). Similar results were also reported in vascular smooth muscle cells, which responded to thrombin or thrombin receptor-activating peptides with increased expression of the urokinase receptor, increased cell migration, and cell proliferation (McNamara et al., 1993; Noda-Heiny and Sobel, 1995). Thrombin stimulation of mesenchymal cell proliferation may contribute to vascular injury in atherosclerosis (Ross, 1993; Walters et al., 1994). This was suggested by the demonstration that antisense down-regulation of thrombin receptor inhibited thrombin-induced smooth muscle cell proliferation by 82%, as compared with control cultures with scrambled oligonucleotides (Chaikof et al., 1995).

The possibility that thrombin signaling could influence inflammatory cell functions has been experimentally addressed. In earlier studies, catalytically active thrombin-stimulated splenocyte proliferation (Chen et al., 1976), promoted monocyte chemotaxis (Bar-Shavit et al., 1983), and stimulated de novo proliferation of G_0/G_1-arrested murine J774 mouse macrophages (Bar-Shavit et al., 1986). These reponses were associated with thrombin-initiated signal transduction with synthesis and release of thromboxane in neutrophils (Bizios et al., 1987), and increase in cytosolic free Ca^{2+} and inositol triphosphate generation in T cells (Hoffman and Church, 1993; Tordai et al., 1993). In parallel studies, thrombin synergized with colony-stimulating factor 1 (CSF-

1) to stimulate proliferation in response to mitogens, superantigens, and an anti-CD3 mitogenic mAb, with increased production of IL-2 and IL-6 and increased expression of IL-2 receptor (Naldini et al., 1993). Moreover, monocyte stimulation with catalytically active thrombin-increased phagocytic activity for albumin-coated fluorescent beads and induced monocyte release of the chemotactic cytokine IL-8, but not IL-6 (Sower et al., 1996). In addition to cytokine gene induction in monocytes (Kranzhofer et al., 1996; Sower et al., 1996) thrombin stimulates a prominent release of IL-6 in fibroblasts, epithelial cells (Sower et al., 1995), and vascular smooth muscle cells (Kranzhofer et al., 1996). This response may have profound pathogenetic implications for the multiple inflammatory response syndrome, where released IL-6 has been recognized as a cornerstone mediator of both inflammation/ acute phase response and initiation of coagulation. Consistent with this concept, administration of neutralizing antibodies to IL-6 prevented consumption coagulopathy (Esmon et al., 1991), and significantly extended survival in a primate model of septic shock (van der Poll et al., 1994).

In addition to cytokine gene induction, thrombin plays a critical role in leukocyte migration/chemotaxis and leukocyte-endothelial cell interaction (Carlos and Harlan, 1994; MCP-1 Springer, 1994). The ability of thrombin to stimulate leukocyte chemotaxis directly (Bar-Shavit et al., 1983), or indirectly through the release of chemotactic cytokines IL-8 and Macrophage chemoattractant protein-1 (Colotta et al., 1994; Granddaliano et al., Uneo et al., 1996), may provide a critical mechanism to localize inflammatory cells at the site of vascular injury in vivo. Moreover, thrombin has been shown to induce immediate release and membrane association of the rolling adhesion receptor, P-selectin (Toothill et al., 1990 Sugama et al., 1992;), and to upregulate the expression of ICAM-1 (Sugama et al., 1992) and E-selectin (Shankar et al., 1994) on endothelium. As an additional endothelial cell adhesion-promoting pathway, thrombin induces release of platelet-activating factor (PAF; Zimmerman et al., 1985), which provides a tethered activator of neutrophil–endothelial cell interaction (Zimmerman et al., 1992). In rat models of acute inflammation, thrombin acted as a genuine inflammatory mediator, promoting recruitment and chemotaxis of activated and degranulated mast cells associated with increased vascular permeability in the rat paw (Cirino et al., 1996).

Factor Xa

Factor Xa is the product of limited proteolytic activation of factor X, and contributes to coagulation by promoting the conversion of prothrombin to thrombin (Davie et al., 1991; Furie and Furie, 1992). The regulated membrane assembly of factor Xa on platelets (Tracy et al., 1992), monocytes (Tracy et al., 1983, 1993), and endothelial cells (Rodgers and Shuman, 1983) contributes to the procoagulant activity of these cells. By analogy with thrombin, the interaction of factor Xa with vascular and nonvascular cell types has been shown to contribute to signal transduction and modulation of gene expression. In earlier studies, catalytically active factor Xa stimulated release of platelet-derived growth factor-like activity from endothelial cells (Gajdusek et al., 1986) in a pathway involving receptor-ligand recognition, internalization of membrane-bound factor Xa in clathrin-coated pits, and accumulation in a chloroquine-sensitive lysosomal compartment (Nawroth et al., 1985). Using function-blocking mAbs, a potential candidate factor Xa receptor was identified in monocytes (Altieri and Edgington, 1989) and designated effector cell protease receptor-1 (EPR-1; Altieri, 1994). At variance with the paradigm of PARs (Coughlin, 1994), binding of factor Xa to this receptor did not require a catalytic active site, and was instead mediated by a short inter-epidermal growth factor sequence Leu[82]-Leu[88] in factor Xa (Ambrosini et al., 1997). Expression and function of EPR-1 has been independently demonstrated on thrombin-stimulated platelets (Bouchard et al., 1997a) brain pericytes (Bouchard et al., 1997b, and endothelial cells (Nicholson et al., 1996; Bono et al., 1997).

Factor Xa stimulated oscillations of cytosolic Ca^{2+} in epithelial cells (Camera et al., 1996) and increased cytosolic Ca^{2+} and phosphoinositide turnover in endothelial cells (Bono et al., 1997). A downstream consequence of factor Xa-dependent signal transduction was cell proliferation. In earlier experiments, catalytically active factor Xa stimulated DNA synthesis and proliferation of rat aortic smooth muscle cells (Gasic et al., 1992), and a two-to-three-fold increased endothelial cell proliferation (Nicholson et al., 1996; Bono et al., 1997). In this context, factor Xa stimulated the release of platelet-derived growth factor (PDGF) from rat smooth muscle cells in vitro in a reaction associated with up-regulation of early genes c-*fos* and c-*jun*, and activation of Ras, Raf-1 42 and 44 kD MAP kinase, and tyrosine kinase phosphorylation (Ko et al., 1996). However, a potential cell surface receptor mediating the factor Xa induction of PDGF responses had not been investigated. Consistent with these mitogenic properties on mesenchymal cells, a potential role of factor Xa on inflammation and immune effector functions was investigated. In this context, factor Xa significantly enhanced proliferation of peripheral blood mononuclear cells by synergizing with submitogenic doses of phorbol ester or low doses of IL-2 (Altieri and Stamnes, 1994). Using an in vivo model of acute inflammation, it was also demonstrated that injection of factor Xa induced a rapid and concentration-dependent edema of the rat paw with accumulation of activated and degranulated mast cells (Cirino et al., 1997). In control experiments, the homologous clotting protease, factor IXa was ineffective (Cirino et al., 1997). Consistent with a role of factor Xa in the chronic and more sustained phase of inflammation, it was also demonstrated that factor Xa stimulated endothelial cell release of inflammatory cytokines IL-6 and IL-8, and up-regulated expression of endothelial cell adhesion molecules ICAM-1, VCAM-1, and E-selectin (Senden et al., 1998). This response required a catalytically active factor Xa, and potentially involved additional mediators of factor Xa-dependent signaling at the vascular cell surface (Senden et al., 1998). The role of factor Xa in endothelial cell activation was also corroborated in independent studies. Administration of catalytically active factor Xa resulted in rapid increase in nitric oxide generation by endothelial cells, which was also associated with prominent release of IL-6 and endothelial cell dependent vasorelaxation in vivo and in isolated vascular rings (Papapetropoulos et al., 1998). In summary, compelling experimental evidence supports a role of catalytically active factor Xa generated in a vascular microenvironment during activation of coagulation in both acute and chronic inflammation. Although reminiscent of thrombin-dependent signal transduction for cytokine activation, control of vasoregulation, acute inflammation, and modulation of surface adhesion molecules, this pathway occurs independently of thrombin and may potentially implicate more than one class of signal-transducing membrane receptors.

Urokinase

The main fibrinolytic pathway in humans is centered on the ability of the serine protease plasmin to proteolyze cross-linked fibrin. Plasmin is generated by limited proteolysis of the zymogen plasminogen by two distinct activators; urokinase-type plasminogen activator (uPA, or simply, urokinase), and tissue type plasminogen activator (tPA). When fibrinolysis occurs in a pericellular environment, local digestion of extracellular matrix proteins may facilitate cell motility, crawling, and migration. These observations led to the working hypothesis that various cell types may have the ability to concentrate components of the fibrinolytic pathway in a specific and receptor-mediated fashion, and that this mechanism could result in digestion of extracellular matrix components and modulation of cell motility.

A cDNA encoding a cell surface receptor for urokinase potentially mediating pericellular fibrinolysis was isolated and characterized (Roldan et al, 1990). The urokinase receptor has a very broad vascular cell distribution, being expressed on monocytes/macrophages, activated T cells, neutrophils, platelets, endothelial cells, and various tumor cells lines. A similarly broad tissue distribution has also been reported for another cellular receptor for the urokinase substrate, plasminogen (Miles and Plow, 1987), suggesting that assembly of the fibrinolytic cascade may occur in a regulated, receptor-mediated fashion, potentially relevant for cell migration (Plow et al., 1986). At variance with PARs, binding of urokinase to its receptor does not require an intact catalytic active site, and does not involve limited receptor proteolysis. Rather, synthetic peptidyl mimicry identified the amino-terminal EGF-like module in urokinase as containing the receptor-binding site (Appella et al., 1987), whereas the ligand-binding site on the urokinase receptor was localized to the first 90 amino-terminal residues using sequential receptor proteolysis (Pöllänen, 1993). As an additional ligand, the urokinase receptor has been shown to interact specifically with vitronectin, thus anticipating its role in modulation of leukocyte adhesion to substratum (Simon et al, 1996). The urokinase receptor undergoes extensive posttranslational modifications that change its membrane-anchoring moiety and produce a glycosylphosphatidylinositol (GPI) membrane anchor (Ploug et al., 1991). Neutrophil secretory granules contain a rapidly mobilizable pool of urokinase receptor, potentially modulating the fibrinolytic potential at the cell surface during inflammatory reactions (Plesner et al., 1994).

One of the proposed functions of membrane assembly of fibrinolysis is to facilitate cell migration and leukocyte chemotaxis in a gradient movement. Accordingly, urokinase and plasmin cleave not only plasminogen and fibrin, but also extracellular matrix proteins, laminin, and fibronectin (Chapman et al., 1984; Mochan and Keler, 1984), and activate latent collagenases and metalloproteinases (Salo et al.; 1982 Chen et al., 1984). A unique membrane topography of the receptor, which was polarized to the leading edge of migrating monocytes (Estreicher et al, 1990) appeared consistent with this model. During membrane assembly of the fibrinolytic cascade, it was shown that urokinase remained bound to its receptor for an extended period of time and was fully catalytically active at the cell surface. Perhaps not surprisingly, pericellular proteolysis was implicated in invasion of cancer cells through the natural barrier offered by interstitial and basement membrane proteins (Liotta et al., 1979; Dano et al., 1985; Ossowski, 1988). In this context, blockade of urokinase or its receptor by neutralizing mAbs or antisense oligonucleotides significantly reduced the invasive phenotype of cancer cells, in vitro and in vivo (Kook et al., 1994). Despite these results, urokinase receptor knockout animals did not display a dramatic defect of pericellular fibrinolysis or cell migration (Dewerchin et al., 1996).

Despite the results obtained with urokinase receptor-deficient animals (Dewerchin et al., 1996), the potential role of this molecule in leukocyte movement has been intensely investigated. Intriguingly, an activation-dependent monocyte surface molecule, designated as Mo3 (Todd et al., 1985; Liu and Todd, 1986); and functionally implicated in adhesion, was found to be identical to the urokinase receptor (Min et al., 1992). Moreover, expression of the urokinase receptor on T lymphocytes was dynamically regulated by cell activation and proliferation in response to phorbol ester, polyclonal lectins, anti-CD3 mitogenic mAbs or alloantigen (Nykjaer et al., 1994). Increased expression of the urokinase receptor was also observed after treatment with the inflammatory cytokines IL-2 and IL-7 (Nykjaer et al., 1994), or following TNF-α and/or interferon-γ monocyte stimulation (Kirchheimer et al., 1988).

The ability of the urokinase receptor to transduce intracellular signals relevant to gene induction and leukocyte migration has also been investigated. In this context, mAbs to the urokinase receptor inhibited induction of cathepsin B and the 92 kD gelatinase genes in phorbol ester-treated myeloid cells, whereas mAbs to other surface receptors, including GPI-linked molecules (i.e., CD14), were ineffective (Rao et al., 1995). Co-expression of the urokinase receptor and β_2 integrin Mac-1 also increased cytosolic free Ca^{2+} and enhanced superoxide production in response to fMLP stimulation (Cao et al., 1995). Consistent with its intrinsic intracellular signaling properties, targeting the urokinase receptor with inhibitory mAbs or antisense oligonucleotides significantly inhibited monocyte chemotaxis in response to formyl peptide, whereas catalytic inactivation or down-regulation of urokinase had no effect (Gyetko et al., 1994). Similar results were also reported in neutrophils, where mAb blockade of the urokinase receptor inhibited migration induced by fMLP (Gyetko et al., 1995). These results suggest that modulation of leukocyte migration by the urokinase receptor may not involve pericellular fibrinolysis, but receptor-initiated signal transduction. Consistent with this view, ligand binding to the urokinase receptor induced specific and reversible adhesion of cytokine-treated monocytic U937 cells, independently of the enzyme's catalytic activity (Waltz et al., 1993), and ligation of the urokinase receptor on monocytic THP-1 cells synergistically increased TNF-α release (Sitrin et al., 1996a). These pro-inflammatory properties of urokinase–urokinase receptor may play an important role in disease, at least under certain conditions in vivo. Using a mouse transgenic model, it was shown that expression of urokinase might contribute to acute pulmonary inflammation to *Cryptococcus neoformans* (Gyetko et al., 1996). In these experiments, urokinase-deficient mice had significantly fewer pulmonary inflammatory cells as compared with wild-type animals. This translated in a significantly increased mortality in the urokinase $^{-/-}$ group, with 15 of 19 animals succumbing to the infection as opposed to 3 of 19 animals that died in the control urokinase $^{+/+}$ group (Gyetko et al., 1996).

A close relationship between signaling through the urokinase receptor and leukocyte adhesion mediated by Mac-1 (Arnaout, 1990) has also been elucidated. First, it was found that both receptors were topographically concentrated on the ventral aspect of monocytes adhering to fibrinogen, and that mAb blockade of the urokinase receptor inhibited monocyte adhesion to fibrinogen but not to β_1 integrin ligands i.e., fibronectin (Sitrin et al., 1996b). Similarly, antisense down-regulation of urokinase receptor on monocytes blocked Mac-1–dependent adhesion in a pathway independent of receptor occupancy by urokinase (Sitrin et al., 1996). Consistent with the idea that Mac-1 and the urokinase receptor form a functional unit, immunofluorescence, co-capping, and resonance energy transfer studies, demonstrated that the urokinase receptor was physically associated with Mac-1 on neutrophils (Xue et al., 1994). Interestingly, this was a dynamic association, influenced by cell shape (Kindzelskii et al., 1996). Although linked together in resting cells, the urokinase receptor dissociated from Mac-1 during cell polarization and distributed to the lamellipodium, while Mac-1 formed a cluster at the uropod of the migrating cell (Kindzelskii et al., 1996). Consistent with a reciprocal modulation by these two receptors, it was shown that urokinase binding to its receptor blocked Mac-1 interaction with factor X and interfered with internalization of fibrinogen (Simon et al., 1996). Deactivating cytokines, including IL-4, IL-10, and IL-13, have also been shown to modulate Mac-1–urokinase receptor interaction, thus influencing cell adhesion to fibrinogen and vitronectin (Paysant et al., 1998).

The concept of a functional unit between integrins and the urokinase receptor has been recently extended to β_1 integrins (Wei et al., 1996). These experiments demonstrated that a physical interaction with β_1 integrins was mediated by the urokinase receptor's extracellular domain (Wei et al., 1996), and required a topographical co-localization of both molecules to caveolae

(Schwartz et al., 1995). Functionally, engagement of the urokinase receptor disrupted the active conformation of β_1 integrins and resulted in a profound inhibition of ligand binding and cell adherence (Wei et al., 1996). Consistent with these findings, immunofluorescence and electron microscopy studies demonstrated that expression of the urokinase receptor to caveolae resulted in enhanced assembly of fibrinolytic activity and increased pericellular proteolysis on a human melanoma cell line (Stahl and Mueller, 1995).

The ability of the urokinase receptor to form large supramolecular complexes contributing to inflammatory signal transduction was recently substantiated. In cell fractionation and immunoprecipitation experiments, both Mac-1 and LFA-1 were physically linked with the urokinase receptor in a large complex with numerous signaling molecules, including protein tyrosine kinases p60[fyn], p53–56[lyn], p58–64[hck], and p59[fgr] (Bohuslav et al., 1995). This supramolecular complex was specific for the urokinase receptor because other GPI-linked molecules did not associate with integrins or signaling molecules. Consistent with previous observations (Dumler et al., 1993), urokinase binding to its receptor stimulated tyrosine phosphorylation, thus confirming the functional link between urokinase receptor engagement and generation of intracellular signals (Bohuslav et al., 1995). The molecular basis of signal transduction through GPI-linked molecules, like the urokinase receptor, has not been completely elucidated. However, one potential model may involve the physical association of these molecules with membrane-spanning receptors, like β_1/β_2 integrins. Another possibility is that a topographical localization of the urokinase receptor in a specialized membrane compartment, like caveolae, may facilitate the interaction with signal-transducing molecules, thus modulating outside-in signaling after receptor engagement.

Conclusion

In summary, considerable experimental evidence accumulated in several laboratories points to a broad participation of coagulation proteins in various aspects of inflammation. As detailed previously, these run the gamut from intercellular adhesive reactions mediated by fibrinogen to elaborated pathways of gene regulation and cytokine gene induction mediated by thrombin, factor Xa, and urokinase. Several cell surface proteins potentially acting as receptors or binding proteins for coagulation proteins/proteases have been identified, but potentially more remain to be identified. The present challenge in the field is to dissect the molecular requirements of the various signaling pathways triggered by coagulation proteins and to define their actual participation in a pathophysiologic inflammatory setting. A formidable aid will be also provided by gene-targeting technology. Several knockout mice of various coagulation proteins and their receptors have been generated. In some cases (thrombin, tissue factor, factor V), these animals die during embryogenesis of massive hemorrhages. But in other cases (fibrinogen, factor X), the animals remain viable at birth, offering exciting opportunities for establishing a variety of in vivo models of inflammation and immune response.

References

Almenar-Queralt, A., Duperray, A., Miles, L. A., Felez, J., and Altieri, D. C., (1995). Apical topography and modulation of ICAM-1 expression on activated endothelium *Am. J. Pathol.* 147: 1278–1288.

Altieri, D. C., Mannucci, P. M., and Capitanio, A. M. (1986) Binding of fibrinogen to human monocytes. *J. Clin. Invest.* 78:968–976.

Altieri, D. C., Bader, R., Mannucci, P. M., and Edgington, P. M. (1988) Oligospecificity of the cellular adhesion receptor Mac-1 encompasses an inducible recognition for fibrinogen. *J. Cell Biol.* 107:1893–1900.

Altieri, D. C., and Edgington, T. S. (1988) A monoclonal antibody reacting with distinct adhesion molecules defines a transition in the functional state of the receptor CD11b/CD18 (Mac-1). *J. Immunol.* 141:2656–2660.

Altieri, D. C., and Edgington, T. S. (1989) Sequential receptor cascade for coagulation proteins on monocytes: Constitutive biosynthesis and functional prothrombinase activity of a membrane form of factor. V/Va. *J. Biol. Chem.* 264:2969–2972.

Altieri, D. C., Agbanyo, F. R., Plescia, J., Ginsberg, M. H., Edgington, T. S., and Plow, E. F. (1990a) A unique recognition site mediates the interaction of fibrinogen with the leukocyte integrin Mac-1 (CD11b/CD18) *J. Biol. Chem.* 265:12119–12122.

Altieri, D. C., Wiltse, W. L., and Edgington, T. S. (1990b) Signal transduction initiated by extracellular adenine nucleotides regulates the high affinity ligand recognition of the adhesive receptor CD11b/CD18. *J. Immunol.* 662–760.

Altieri, D. C. (1991) Occupancy of CD11b/CD18 (Mac-1) divalent ion binding site(s) induces leukocyte adhesion. *J. Immunol.* 147:1891–1898.

Altieri, D. C., Stamnes, S. J., and Gahmberg, C. G. (1992) Regulated Ca^{2+} signalling through leukocyte CD11b/CD18 integrin. *Biochem. J.* 288:465–473.

Altieri, D. C., Plescia, J., and Plow, E. F. (1993) The structural motif glycine 190-valine 202 of the fibrinogen γ chain interacts with CD11b/CD18 integrin ($\alpha_M\beta_2$, mac-1) and promotes leukocyte adhesion. *J. Biol. Chem.* 268:1847–1853.

Altieri, D. C. (1994) Molecular cloning of effector cell protease receptor-1, a novel cell surface receptor for the protease factor Xa. *J. Biol. Chem.* 269:3139–3142.

Altieri, D. C., and Stamnes, S. J. (1994) Protease-dependent T-cell activation: Ligation of effector cell protease receptor-1 (EPR-1) stimulates lymphocyte proliferation. *Cell Immunol.* 155:372–383.

Altieri, D. C., Duperray, A., Plescia, J., Thornton, G. B., and Languino, L. R. (1995) Structural recognition of a novel fibrinogen γ chain sequence (117–133) by intercellular adhesion molecule-1 mediates leukocyt–endothelium interaction. *J. Biol. Chem.* 270:696–699.

Ambrosini, G., Plescia, J., Chu, K. C., High, K. A., and Altieri, D. C. (1997) Activation-dependent exposure of the inter-EGF sequence Leu[83]-Leu[88] in factor Xa mediates ligand binding to effector cell protease receptor-1. *J. Biol. Chem.* 272:8340–8345.

Appella, E., Robinson, E. A., Ullrich, S. J., Stoppelli, M. P., Corti, A., Cassani, G., and Blasi, F. (1987) The receptor-binding sequence of urokinase: A biological function for the growth-factor module of proteases. *J. Biol. Chem.* 262: 4437–4440.

Arnaout, M. A. (1990) Structure and function of the leukocyte adhesion molecules CD11/CD18. *Blood.* 75:1037–1050.

Balazovich, K. J., and Boxer, L. A. (1990) Extracellular adenosine nucleotides stimulate protein kinase C activity and human neutrophil activation. *J. Immunol.* 144:631–637.

Bar-Shavit, R., Kahn, A., Wilner, G. D., and Fenton, J. W., II. (1983) Monocyte chemotaxis: stimulation by specific exosite region in thrombin. *Science* 220:728–731.

Bar-Shavit, R., Kahn, A. J., Mann, K. G., and Wilner, G. D. (1986) Identification of a thrombin sequence with growth factor activity on macrophages. *Proc. Natl. Acad. Sci. USA* 83:976–980.

Belch, J., McLaren, M., Hanslip, J., Hill, A., and Davidson, D. (1998) The white blood cell and plasma fibrinogen in thrombotic stroke. A significant correlation. *Int. Angiol.* 17:120–124.

Berendt, A. R., Simmons, D. L., Tansey, J., Newbold, C. I., and Marsh, K. (1989) Intercellular adhesion molecule-1 is an endothelial cell adhesion receptor for *Plasmodium Falciparum*. *Nature* 341:57–59.

Berendt, A. R., McDowall, A., Craig, A. G., Bates, P. A., Sterberg, M.J.E., Marsh, K., Newbold, C. I., and Hogg, N. (1992) The binding site on ICAM-1 for plasmodium falsciparum-infected erythrocytes overlaps, but is distinct from, the LFA-1 binding site. *Cell* 66:71–81.

Bini, A., Fenoglio, J., Jr., Mesa-Tejada, R., Kudryk, B., and Kaplan, K. L. (1989) Identification and distribution of fibrinogen, fibrin, and fibrin(ogen) degradation products in atherosclerosis. Use of monoclonal antibodies. *Arteriosclerosis* 9:109–121.

Bizios, R., Lai, L., Fenton, J. W., II, and Malik, A. B. (1987) Thrombin-induced thromboxane generation by neutrophils and lymphocytes: dependence on enzymic site. *J. Cell Physiol.* 132:359–362.

Bohushlav, J., Horejsí, V., Hansmann, C., Stöckl, J., Weidle, U. H. Majdic, O., Bartke, I., Knapp, W., and Stockinger, H. (1995) Urokinase plasminogen activator receptor, β_2-integrins, and Src-kinases within a single receptor complex of human monocytes. *J. Exp. Med.* 181:1381–1390.

Bono, F., Herault, J. P., Avril, C., Schaeffer, P., and Herbert, J. M. (1997) Human umbilical vein endothelial cells express high affinity receptors for factor Xa. *J. Cell. Physiol.* 172–777.

Bouchard, B. A., Catcher, C. S., Thrash, B. R., Adida, C., and Tracy, P. B. (1997) Effector cell protease receptor-1, a platelet activation-dependent membrane protein, regulates prothrombinase-catalyzed thrombin generation. *J. Biol. Chem.* 272:9244–9251.

Bouchard, B. A., Shatos, M. A., and Tracy, P. B. (1997b) Human brain pericytes differentially regulate expression of procoagulant enzyme complexes comprising the extrinsic pathway of blood coagulation. *Arterioscler. Thromb. Vasc. Biol.* 17:1–9.

Buyon, J. P., Abramson, S. B., Philips, M. R., Slade, S. G., Ross, G. D., Weissman, and Winchester, R. J. (1988) Dissociation between increased surface expression of Gp 165/95 and homotypic neutrophil aggregation. *J. Immunol.* 140:3156–3160.

Camerer, E., Rottingen, J. A., Iversen, J. G., and Prydz, H. (1996) Coagulation factors VII and X induce Ca^{2+} oscillations in Madin–Darby canine kidney cells only when proteolytically active. *J. Biol. Chem.* 271:29034–29042.

Cao, D., Mizukami, I. F., Garni-Wagner, B. A., Kindzelskii, A. L., Todd, R. F., III, Boxer, L. A., and Petty, H. R. (1995) Human urokinase-type plasminogen activator primes neutrophils for superoxide anion release. Possible roles of complement receptor type 3 and calcium. *J. Immunol.* 545:1817–1829.

Carlos, T. M., and Harlan, J. M. (1994) Leukocyte–endothelial adhesion molecules. *Blood.* 84:2068–2101.

Carney, D. H., and Cunningham, D. D. (1978) Role of specific cell surface receptors in thrombin-stimulated cell division. *Cell* 15:1341–1349.

Chaikof, E. L., Caban, R., Yan, C. N., Rao, G. N., and Runge, M. S. (1995) Growth-related responses in arterial smooth muscle cells are arrested by thrombin receptor antisense sequences. *J. Biol. Chem.* 7431–7436.

Chapman, H. A. Jr., Stone, O. L., and Vavrin, Z. (1984) Degradation of fibrin and elastin by intact human alveolar macrophages in vitro. Characterization of of a plaminogen activator and its role in matrix degradation. *J. Clin. Invest.* 73:806–815.

Chen, L. B., and Buchanan, J. M. (1975) Mitogenic activity of blood components I. Thrombin and prothrombin. *Proc. Natl. Acad. Sci. USA* 72:131–135.

Chen, L. B., Teng, N.N.H., and Buchanan, J. M. (1976) Mitogenicity of thrombin and surface alterations on mouse splenocytes. *Exp. Cell Res.* 60:219–230.

Chen, W.-T., Olden, K., Bernard, B. A., and Chu, F.-F. (1984) Expression of transformation-associated proteases that degrade fibronectin at cell contact sites. *J. Cell Biol.* 98:1546–1555.

Cirino, G., Cicala, C., Bucci, M., Sorrentino, L., Maragonore, J. M., and Stone, S. R. (1996) Thrombin functions as an inflammatory mediator through activation of its receptor. *J. Exp. Med.* 183:821–827.

Cirino, G., Cicala, C., Bucci, M., Sorrentino, L., Ambrosini, G., DeDominicis, G., and Altieri,

D. C. (1997) Factor Xa as an interface between inflammation and coagulation. Molecular mimicry of factor Xa interaction with effector cell protease receptor-1 induces acute inflammation in vivo. *J. Clin. Invest.* 99:2446–2451.

Clohisy, D. R., Erdmann, J. M., and Wilner, G. D. (1990) Thrombin binds to murine bone marrow-derived macrophages and enhances colony-stimulating factor-1-driven mitogenesis. *J. Biol. Chem.* 265:7729–7732.

Colotta, F., Sciacca, F. L., Sironi, M., Luini, W., Rabiet, M. J., and Mantovani, A. (1994) Expression of monocyte chemotactic protein-1 by monocytes and endothelial cells exposed to thrombin. *Am. J. Pathol.* 144:975–985.

Coughlin, S. R. (1994). Protease-activated receptors start a family. *Proc. Natl. Acad. Sci. USA* 91: 9200–9202.

Danesh, J., Collins, R., Appleby, P., and Peto, R. (1998) Association of fibrinogen, C-reactive protein, albumin, or leukocyte count with coronary heart disease: meta-analyses of prospective studies. *JAMA* 279:1477–1482.

Daniel, T. O., Gibbs, V. C., Milfay, D. F., Garovoy, M. R., and Williams, L. T. (1986) Thrombin stimulates c-sis gene expression in microvascular endothelial cells. *J. Biol. Chem.* 261:9579–9582.

Dano, K., Andreasen, P. A., Grondhal-Hansen, J., Kristensen, P. Nielsen, L. S., and Skriver, L. (1985) Plasminogen activators, tissue degradation, and cancer. *Adv. Cancer Res.* 44:139–266.

Davie, E. W., Fujikawa, K., and Kisiel, W. (1991) The coagulation cascade: Initiation, maintenance, and regulation. *Biochem.* 30: 10363–10370.

De Nichilo, M. O., Shafren, D. R., Carter, W. M., Berndt, M. C., Burns, G. F., and Boyd, A. W. (1996) A common epitope on platelet integrin $\alpha_{IIb}\beta_3$ (glycoprotein IIbIIIa; CD41b/CD61) and $\alpha_M\beta_2$ (Mac-1; CD11b/CD18) detected by a monoclonal antibody. *J. Immunol.* 156:284–288.

Dewerchin, M, Van Nuffelen, A., Wallays, G., Bouché, A., Moons, L., Carmeliet, P., Mulligan, R. C., and Collen, D. (1996) Generation and characterization of urokinase receptor-deficient mice. *J. Clin. Invest.* 97:870–878

Diacovo, T. G., Roth, S. J., Buccola, J. M., Bainton, D. F., and Springer, T. A. (1996) Neutrophil rolling, arrest, and transmigration across activated, surface-adherent platelets via sequential action of P-selectin and β_2 integrin CD11b/CD18. *Blood* 88:146–157.

Diamond, M. S., Garcia-Aguilar, J., Bickford, J. K., Corbi, A. L., and Springer, T. A. (1993) The I domain is a major recognition site on the leukocyte integrin Mac-1 (CD11b/CD18) for four distinct adhesion ligands. *J. Cell Biol.* 120:1031–1043.

Diamond, M. S., and Springer, T. A. (1993) A subpopulation of Mac-1 (CD11b/CD18) molecules mediates neutrophil adhesion to ICAM-1 and fibrinogen. *J. Cell Biol.* 120:545–556.

Dumler, I., T. Petri, and Schkeuning, W. D. (1993) Interaction of urokinase-type plasminogen activator (u-PA) with its cellular receptor (uPAR) induces phosphorylation on tyrosine of a 38 kDA protein. *Fed. Eur. Biochem. Soc. Lett.* 322:37–40.

Duperray, A., Languino, L. R., Plescia, J., McDowall, A., Hogg, N., Craig, A. G., Berendt, A. R., and Altieri, D. C. (1997) Molecular identification of a novel fibrinogen binding site on the first domain of ICAM-1 regulating leukocyte-endothelium bridging *J. Biol. Chem.* 272:435–441.

Duplaa, C., Couffinhal, T., Labat, L., Fawaz, J., Moreau, C., Bietz, I., and Bonnet, J, (1993) Monocyte adherence to endothelial cells in patients with atherosclerosis: relationships with risk factors. *Eur. J. Clin. Invest.* 23:474–479.

Dustin, M. L., and Springer, T. A. (1989) T-cell receptor cross-linking transiently stimulates adhesiveness through LFA-1. *Nature* 341:619–624.

Elemer, G. S., and Edgington, T. S. (1994) Monoclonal antibody to an activation neoepitope of $\alpha_M\beta_2$ inhibits multiple $\alpha_M\beta_2$ functions. *J. Immunol.* 152:5836–5844.

Esmon, C. T., Taylor, F. B., and Snow, T. R. (1991) Inflammation and coagulation: Linked processes potentially regulated through a common pathway mediated by protein C *Thromb. Haemost.* 66:160–165.

Estreicher, A., Muhlhauser, J., Carpentier, J.-L., Orci, L., and Vassalli, J.-D. (1990) The receptor for urokinase type plasminogen activator polarizes expression of the protease to the leading edge of migrating monocytes and promotes degradation of enzyme inhibitor complexes. *J. Cell Biol.* 111:783–792.

Fan, S.-T., and Edgington, T. S. (1991) Coupling of the adhesive receptor CD11b/CD18 to functional enhancement of effector macrophage tissue factor response. *J. Clin. Invest.* 87:50–57.

Fan, S.-T., and Edgington, T. S. (1993) Integrin regulation of leukocyte inflammatory functions. CD11b/CD18 enhancement of the tumor necrosis factor-alpha responses of monocytes. *J. Immunol.* 150:2972–2980.

Frebelius, S., Isaksson, S., and Swedenborg, J. (1996) Thrombin inhibition by antithrombin III on the subendothelium is explained by the isoform AT beta. *Arterioscler. Thromb. Vasc. Biol.* 16:1292–1297.

Freyer, D. R., Boxer, L. A., Axtell, R. A., and Todd, R. F., III (1988) Stimulation of human neutrophil adhesive properties by adenine nucleotides. *J. Immunol.* 141:580–586.

Furie, B., and Furie, B. C. (1992) Molecular and cellular biology of blood coagulation. *N. Engl. J. Med.* 326:800–806.

Gajdusek, C., Carbon, S., Ross, R., Nawroth, P., and Stern, D. (1986) Activation of coagulation releases endothelial cell mitogens. *J. Cell Biol.* 103:419–428.

Garcia, J. G., Fenton, J. W., II, and Natarajan, V. (1992) Thrombin stimulation of human endothelial cell phospholipase D activity. Regulation by phospholipase C, protein kinase C, and cyclic adenosine 3'5'-monophosphate. *Blood* 79:2056–2067.

Gasic, G. P., Arenas, C. P., Gasic, T. B., and Gasic, G. J. (1992) Coagulation factors X, Xa, and protein S as potent mitogens of cultured aortic smooth muscle cells. *Proc. Natl. Acad. Sci. USA* 89:2317–2320.

Glenn, K. C., and Cunningham, D. D. (1979) Thrombin-stimulated cell division involves proteolysis of its own cell surface receptor. *Nature* 278:711–718.

Grandaliano, G., Valente, A. J., and Abboud, H. E. (1994) A novel biologic activity of thrombin: Stimulation of monocyte chemotactic protein production. *J. Exp. Med.* 179:1737–1741.

Greeve, J. M., Davis, G., Meyer, A. M., Forte, C. P., Yost, S. C., Marlor, C. W., Kamarck, M. E., and McClelland, A. (1989) The major human rhinovirus receptor is ICAM-1. *Cell* 56:839–847.

Gustafson, E. J., Lukasiewicz, H., Wachtfogel, Y. T., Norton, K. J., Schmaier, A. H., Niewiarowski, S., and Colman, R. W. (1989) High molecular weight kininogen inhibits fibrinogen binding to cytoadhesins of neutrophils and platelets. *J. Cell Biol.* 109:377–387.

Gyetko, M. R., Chen, G.-H., McDonald, R. A., Goodman, R., Huffnagle, G. B., Wilkinson, C. C., Fuller, J. A., and Toews, G. B. (1996) Urokinase is required for the pulmonary inflammatory response to *Cryptococcus neoformans*. A murine transgenic model. *J. Clin. Invest.* 97:1818–1826.

Gyetko, M. R., Sitrin, R. G., Fuller, J. A., Todd, R. F., III, Petty, H., and Standiford, T. J. (1995) Function of urokinase receptor (CD87) in neutrophil chemotaxis. *J. Leukoc Biol.* 58:533–538.

Gyetko, M. R., Todd, R. F., III, Wilkinson, C. C., and Sitrin, R. G. (1994) The urokinase receptor is required for human monocyte chemotaxis in vitro. *J. Clin. Invest.* 93:1380–1387.

Hatton, M. W., Southward, S. M., Ross-Ouellet, B., DeReske, M., Blajchman, M. A., and Richardson, M. (1996) An increased uptake of prothrombin, antithrombin, and fibrinogen by the rabbit balloon-deendothelialized aorta surface in vivo is maintained until reendothelialization is complete. *Arterioscler. Thromb. Vasc. Biol.* 16:1147–1155.

Hoffman, M., and F. C. Church (1993) Response of blood leukocytes to thrombin receptor peptides. *J. Leukoc. Biol.* 54:145–151.

Hogg, N. (1983) Human monocytes are associated with the formation of fibrin. *J. Exp. Med.* 157:473–485.

Hynes, R. O. (1992) Integrins: Versatility, modulation, and signaling in cell adhesion. *Cell* 69:11–25.

Kindzelskii, A. L, Laska, Z. O., Todd, R. F., III, and Petty, H. R. (1996) Urokinase-type plasminogen activator receptor reversibly dissociates from complement receptor type 3 ($\alpha_M\beta_2$ CD11b/CD18) during neutrophil polarization. *J. Immunol* 156:297–309.

Kirchheimer, J. C., Nong, Y.-H., and Remold, H. G. (1988) IFN-γ, tumor necrosis factor-α, and urokinase regulate the expression of urokinase receptors on human monocytes. *J. Immunol.* 141:4229–4234.

Ko, F. N., Yang, Y. C., Huang, S. C., and Ou, J. T. (1996) Coagulation factor Xa stimulates platelet-derived growth factor release and mitogenesis in cultured vascular smooth muscle cells of rat. *J. Clin. Invest.* 98:1493–1501.

Kook, Y. H., Adamski, J., Zelent, A., and Ossowski, L. (1994) The effect of antisense inhibition of urokinase receptor in human squamous cell carcinoma on malignancy. *EMBO J.* 13:3983–3991.

Kranzhofer, R., Clinton, S. K., Ishii, K., Coughlin, S. R., Fenton, J. W. and Libby, P. (1996) Thrombin potently stimulates cytokine production in human vascular smooth muscle cells but not in mononuclear phagocytes. *Circ. Res.* 79:286–294.

Kreuzer, J., Denger, S., Schmidts, A., Jahn, L., Merten, M., and von Hodenberg, E. (1996) Fibrinogen promotes monocyte adhesion via a protein kinase C-dependent mechanism. *J. Mol. Med.* 74:161–165.

Kuijpers, T. W., and Harlan, J. M. (1993) Monocyte–endothelial interactions: Insights and questions. *J. Lab. Clin. Med* 122:641–651.

Landis, R. C., Bennet, R. I., and Hogg, N. (1993) A novel LFA-1 activation epitope maps to the I domain. *J. Cell Biol.* 120:1519–1527.

Languino, L. R., Plescia, J., Duperray, A., Brian, A. A., Plow, E. F., Geltosky, J. E., and Altieri D. C. (1993) Fibrinogen mediates leukocyte adhesion to vascular endothelium through an ICAM-1–dependent pathway. *Cell* 73:1423–1434.

Languino, L. R., Duperray, A., Joganic, K. J., Fornaro, M., Thornton, G. B., and Altieri, D. C. (1995) Regulation of leukocyte–endothelium interaction and leukocyte transendothelial migration by intercellular adhesion molecule 1-fibrinogen recognition. *Proc. Natl. Acad. Sci. USA* 92:1505–1509.

Liotta, L. A., Shigeto, A., Robey, P. G., and Martin, G. R. (1979). Preferential digestion of basement membrane collagen by an enzyme derived from a metastatic murine tumor. *Proc. Natl. Acad. Sci. USA* 76:2268–2272.

Liu, D. Y., and Todd, R. F., III (1986) A monoclonal antibody specific for a monocyte-macrophage membrane component blocks the human monocyte response to migration inhibitory factor. *J. Immunol.* 137:448–455.

McNamara, C. A., Sarembock, I. J., Gimple, L. W., Fenton, J. W., Coughlin, S. R., and Owens, G. K. (1993) Thrombin stimulates proliferation of cultured rat aortic smooth muscle cells by a proteolytically activated receptor. *J. Clin. Invest.* 91:94–98.

McRitchie, D. I., Girotti, M. J., Glynn, M.F.X., Goldberg, J. M., and Rotstein, O. D. (1991) Effect of systematic fibrinogen depletion on intraabdominal abscess formation. *J. Lab. Clin. Med.* 118:48–55.

Miles, L. A., and Plow, E. F. (1987) Receptor mediated binding of the fibrinolytic components, plasminogen and urokinase, to peripheral blood cells. *Thromb. Haemost.* 58:936–942.

Miller, L. J., Bainton, D. F., Borregaard, N., and Springer, T. A. (1987) Stimulated mobilization of monocyte Mac-1 and p150, 95 from an intracellular vesicular compartment to the cell surface. *J. Clin. Invest.* 80:535–544.

Min, H. Y., Semnani, R., Mizukami, I. F., Watt, K., Todd, R. F., III, and Liu, D. Y. (1992) cDNA for Mo3, a monocyte activation antigen, encodes the human receptor for urokinase plasminogen activator. *J. Immunol.* 148:3636–3642.

Mochan, E., and Keler, T. (1984) Plasmin degradation of cartilage proteoglycan. *Biochem. Biophys Acta* 800:312–315.

Naldini, A., Carney, D. H., Bocci, V., Klimpel, K. D., Asuncion, M., Soares, L. E., and Klimpel, G. R. (1993) Thrombin enhances T-cell proliferative responses and cytokine production. *Cell Immunol.* 147:367–377.

Nathan, C., Srimal, S., Farber, C., Sanchez, E., Kabbash, L., Asch, A., Gailit,, and Wright, S. D. (1989). Cytokine J.-induced respiratory burst of human neutrophils: Dependence on extracellular matrix proteins and CD11/CD18 integrins. *J. Cell Biol.* 109:1341–1349.

Nawroth, P. P., McCarthy, D., Kisiel, W., Handley, D., and Stern, D. M. (1985) Cellular processing of bovine factors X and Xa by cultured bovine aortic endothelial cells. *J. Exp. Med.* 162:559–572.

Ng-Sikorski, J., Andersson, R., Patarroyo, M., and Andersson, T. (1991) Calcium signaling capacity of the CD11b/CD18 integrin on human neutrophils. *Exp. Cell Res.* 195:504–508.

Nicholson, A. C., Nachman, R. L., Altieri, D. C., Summers, B. D., Ruf, W., Edgington, T S., and Hajjar, D. P. (1996) Effector cell protease receptor-1 is a vascular receptor for coagulation factor Xa. *J. Biol. Chem.* 271:28407–28413.

Noda-Heiny, H., and Sobel, B. E. (1995) Vascular smooth muscle cell migration mediated by thrombin and urokinase receptor. *Am. J. Physiol.* 268:C1195–C1201.

Nykjaer, A., Moller, B., Todd, R. F., III, Christensen, T., Andreasen, P. A., Gliemann, J., and Petersen, C. M. (1994) Urokinase receptor. An activation antigen in human T lymphocytes. *J. Immunol.* 152:505–516.

Ossowski, L. (1988) In vivo invasion of modified chorioallantoic membrane by tumor cells: The role of cell surface-bound urokinase. *J. Cell Biol.* 107:2437–2445.

Papapetropoulos, A., Piccardoni, P., Cirino, G., Bucci, M., Sorrentino, R., Cicala, C., Johnson, K., Zachariou, V., Sessa, W. C., and Altieri, D. C. (1998) Hypotension and inflammatory cytokine gene expression triggered by factor Xa-nitric oxide signaling. *Proc. Natl. Acad. Sci. USA* 95:4738–4742.

Paysant, J., Vasse, M., Soria, J., Lenormand, B., Pourtau, J., Vannier, J. P., and Soria, C. (1998) Regulation of the uPAR/uPA system expressed on monocytes by the deactivating cytokines, IL-4, IL-10 and IL-13: consequences on cell adhesion to vitronectin and fibrinogen. *Br. J. Haematol.* 100:45–51.

Perez, R. L., and Roman, J. (1995) Fibrin enhances the expression of IL-1β by human peripheral blood mononuclear cells. Implications in pulmonary inflammation. *J. Immunol.* 154:1879–1887.

Plescia, J., Conte, M. S., VanMeter, G., Ambrosini, G., and Altieri, D. C. (1998) Molecular identification of the cross-reacting epitope on αMβ2 integrin I domain recognized by anti-αIIbβ3 monoclonal antibody 7E3 and its involvement in leukocyte adherence. *J. Biol. Chem.* 273: 20372–20377.

Plesner, T., Ploug, M., Ellis, V., Ronne, E., Hoyer-Hansen, G., Wittrup, M., Lindhart Petersen, T., Tscherning, T., Dano, K., and Hansen, N. E. (1994) The receptor for urokinase-type plasminogen activator and urokinase is translocated from two distinct intracellular compartments to the plasma membrane on stimulation of human neutrophils. *Blood* 83:808–815.

Ploug, M., Ronne, E., Behrendt, N., Jensen, A. L., Blasi, F., and Danø, K.. (1991) Cellular receptor for urokinase plasminogen activator. Carboxyl-terminal processing and membrane anchoring by glycosyl-phosphatidylinositol. *J. Biol. Chem.* 266:1926–1933.

Plow, E. F., Freaney, D. E., Plescia, J., and Miles, L. A. (1986) The plasminogen systems and cell surfaces: Evidence for plasminogen and urokinase receptors on the same cell type. *J. Cell Biol.* 103:2411–2420.

Pober, J. S., Gimbrone, M. A., Jr., Lapierre, L. A., Mendrick, D. L., Fiers, W., Rothlein, R., and Springer, T. A. (1986) Overlapping patterns of activation of human endothelial cells by interleukin-1, tumor necrosis factor and immune interferon. *J. Immunol.* 137:1893–1896.

Pöllänen, J. J. (1993) The N-terminal domain of human urokinase receptor contains two distinct regions critical for ligand recognition. *Blood* 82:2719–2729.

Poston, R. N., Haskard, D. O., Coucher, J. R., Gall, N. P., and Johnson-Tidey, R. R. (1992) Expression of intercellular adhesion molecule-1 in atherosclerotic plaques. *Am. J. Pathol.* 140: 665–673.

Rao, N. K., Shi, G.-P., and Chapman, H. A. (1995) Urokinase receptor is a multifunctional protein. Influence of receptor occupancy on macrophage gene expression. *J. Clin. Invest.* 96: 465–474.

Rodgers, G. M., and Shuman, M. A. (1983) Prothrombin is activated on vascular endothelial cells by factor Xa and calcium. *Proc. Natl. Acad. Sci. USA* 80:7001–7005.

Rogers, C., Edelman, E. R., and Simon, D. I. (1998) A mAb to the beta2-leukocyte integrin Mac-1 (CD11b/CD18) reduces intimal thickening after angioplasty or stent implantation in rabbits. *Proc. Natl. Acad. Sci. USA* 95:10134–10139.

Roldan, A. L., Cubellis, M. V., Masucci, M. T., Behrendt, N., Lund, L. R., Danø, K., Appella, E., and Blasi, F. (1990) Cloning and expression of the receptor for human urokinase plasminogen activator, a central molecule in cell surface, plasmin dependent proteolysis. *EMBO J.* 9: 467–474.

Ross, R. (1993) The pathogenesis of atherosclerosis: a perspective for the 1990s. *Nature* 362:801–809.

Salo, T., Liotta, L. A., Keski-Oja, J., and Turpeenniemi-Hujanen, T. (1982) Secretion of basement membrane collagen degrading enzyme and plasminogen activator by transformed cells: role in metastasis. *Int. J. Cancer* 30:669–673.

Schwartz, M. A., Schaller, M. D., and Ginsberg, M. H. (1995) Integrins: emerging paradigms of signal transduction. *Annu. Rev. Dev. Biol.* 11:549–599.

Senden, N.H.M., Jeunhomme, T.M.A.A., Heemskerk, J.W.M., Wagenvoord, R., van't Veer, C., Hemker, H. C., and Buurman, W. A. (1998) Factor Xa induces cytokine production and expression of adhesion molecules by human umbilical vein endothelial cells. *J. Immunol* 161: 4318–4324.

Shankar, R., de la Motte, C. A., Poptic, E. J., and DiCorleto, P. E. (1994) Thrombin receptor-activating peptides differentially stimulate platelet-derived growth factor production, monocytic cell adhesion, and E-selectin expression in human umbilical vein endothelial cells. *J. Biol. Chem.* 269:13936–13941.

Sherman, L., and Lee, J. (1977) Specific binding of soluble fibrin to macrophages. *J. Exp. Med.* 145:76–85.

Shetty, S., Kumar, A., Pueblitz, S., Emri, S., Gungen, Y., Johnson, A. R., and Idell, S. (1996) Fibrinogen promotes adhesion of monocytic to human msothelioma cells. *Thromb. Haemost.* 75:782–790.

Simmons, D., Makgoba, M. W., and Seed, B. (1988). ICAM, an adhesion ligand of LFA-1, is homologous to the neural cell adhesion molecule NCAM. *Nature* 331:624–627.

Simon, D. I., Rao, N. K., Xu, H., Wei, Y., Majdic, O., Ronne, E., Kobzik, L., and Chapman, H. A. (1996) Mac-1 (CD11b/CD18) and the urokinase receptor (CD87) form a functional unit on monocytic cells. *Blood* 88:3185–3194.

Simon, D. I., Xu, H., Ortlepp, S., Rogers, C., and Rao, N. K. (1997). 7E3 monoclonal antibody directed against the platelet glycoprotein IIb/IIIa cross-reacts with the leukocyte integrin Mac-1 and blocks adhesion to fibrinogen and ICAM-1. *Arterioscler. Thromb. Vasc. Biol.* 17:528–535.

Sitrin, R. G., Shollenberger, S. B., Strieter, R. M., and Gyetko, M. R. (1996a). Endogenously produced urokinase amplifies tumor necrosis factor-α secretion by THP-1 mononuclear phagocytes. *J. Leukoc. Biol.* 59:302–311.

Sitrin, R. G., Todd, R. F. III, Petty, H. R., Brock, T. G., Shollenberger, S. B., Albrecht, E., and Gyetko, M. R. (1996b). The urokinase receptor (CD87) facilitates CD11b/CD18-mediated adhesion of human monocytes. *J. Clin. Invest.* 97:1942–1951.

Sitrin, R. G., Pan, P. M., Srikanth, S., and Todd R. F., III (1998). Fibrinogen activates NF-kappa B transcription factors in mononuclear phagocytes. *J. Immunol.* 161:1462–1470.

Skogen, W. F., Senior, R. M., Griffin, G. L., and Wilner, G. D. (1988). Fibrinogen-derived peptide Bβ1-42 is a multidomained neutrophil chemoattractant. *Blood* 71:1475–1479.

Sower, L. E., Froelich, C. J., Carney, D. H., Fenton, J. W., II, and Klimpel, G. R. (1995). Thrombin induces IL-6 production in fibroblasts and epithelial cells. Evidence for the involvement of the seven-transmembrane domain (STD) receptor for α-thrombin *J. Immunol.* 155:895–901.

Sower, L. E., Froelich, C. J., Allegretto, N., Rose, P. M., Hanna, W. D.,and Klimpel, G. R. (1996). Extracellular activities of human granzyme A. Monocyte activation by granzyme A versus α-thrombin. *J. Immunol.* 156:2585–2590.

Springer, T. A. (1990) Adhesion receptors of the immune system. *Nature* 346:425–434.

Springer, T. A. (1994). Traffic signals for lymphocyte recirculation and leukocyte emigration: The multistep paradigm. *Cell* 76:301–314.

Sriramarao, P., Languino, L. R., and Altieri, D. C. (1996). Fibrinogen mediates leukocyte–endothelium bridging *in vivo* at low shear forces. *Blood* 88:3416–3423.

Stahl, A., and Mueller, B. M. (1995). The urokinase-type plasminogen activator receptor, a GPI-linked protein, is localized in caveolae. *J. Cell. Biol.* 129:335–344.

Staunton, D. E., Dustin, M. L., Erickson, H. P., and Springer, T. A. (1990). The arrangement of of the immunoglobulin-like domains of ICAM-1 and the binding sites for LFA-1 and rhinovirus. *Cell* 61:243–254.

Sugama, Y, Tiruppathi, C., Janakidevi, K., Andersen, T. T., Fenton, J. W., II, and Malik, A. B. (1992). Thrombin-induced expression of endothelial P-selectin and intercellular adhesion molecule-1: A mechanism for stabilizing neutrophil adhesion. *J. Cell Biol.* 119:935–944.

Tang, L., and Eaton, J. W. (1993) Fibrin (ogen) mediates acute inflammatory responses to biomaterials. *J. Exp. Med.* 178:2147–2156.

Tang, L., Ugarova, T. P., Plow, E. F., and Eaton, J. W. (1996) Molecular determinants of acute inflammatory responses to biomaterials. *J. Clin. Invest* 97:1329–1334.

Tang, L., Jennings, T. A., and Eaton, J. W. (1998) Mast cells mediate acute inflammatory responses to implanted biomaterials. *Proc. Natl. Acad. Sci. USA* 95:8841–8846.

Todd, R. F. III, Alvarez, P. A., Brott, D. A., and Liu, D. Y. (1985) Bacterial lypopolysaccharide, phorbol myristate acetate and muramyl dipeptide stimulate the expression of a human monocyte surface antigen Mo3. *J. Immunol.* 135:3869–3877.

Toothill, V. J., Van Mourik, J. A., Niewenhuis, H. K., Metzelaar, M. J., and Pearson, J. D. (1990) Characterization of the enhanced adhesion of neutrophil leukocytes to thrombin-stimulated endothelial cells. *J. Immunol.* 145:283–291.

Tordai, A., Fenton, J. W., II, Anderson, T., and Gelfand, E. W. (1993) Functional thrombin receptors on human T lymphoblastoid cells. *J. Immunol..* 150:4876–4886.

Tracy, P. B., Rohrbach, M. S., and Mann, K. G. (1983) Functional prothrombinase complex assembly on isolated monocytes and lymphocytes. *J. Biol. Chem.* 258:7264–7267.

Tracy, P. B., Nesheim, M. E., and Mann, K. G. (1992) Platelet factor Xa receptor. *Meth. Enzymol.* 215:329–360.

Tracy, P. B., Robinson, R. A., Worfolk, L. A., and Allen, D. H. (1993) Procoagulant activities expressed by peripheral blood mononuclear cells. *Meth. Enzymol.* 222:281–299.

Trezzini, C., Jungi, T. W., Kuhnert, P., and Peterhans, E. (1988) Fibrinogen association with human monocytes: Evidence for constitutive expression of fibrinogen receptors and for involvement of Mac-1 (CD18, CR3) in the binding. *Biochem. Biophys. Res. Commun.* 156:477–484.

Trezzini, C., Schüepp, B., Maly, F. E., and Jungi, T. W. (1991) Evidence that exposure to fibrinogen or to antibodies directed against Mac-1 (CD11b/CD18; CR3) modulates human monocyte effector functions. *Br. J. Haematol* 77:16–24.

Ueno, A., Murakami, K., Yamanouchi, K., Watanabe, M., and Kondo, T. (1996) Thrombin stimulates production of interleukin-8 in human umbilical vein endothelial cells. *Immunol.* 88:76–81.

van der Poll, T., Levi, M., Hack, C. E., ten Cate, H., van Deventer, S.J.H., Eerenberg, A.J.M., de Groot, E. R., Jansen, J., Gallati, H., Buller, H. R., ten Cate, J. W., and Aarden, L. A. (1994) Elimination of interluekin-6 attenuates coagulation in experimental endotoxemia in chimpanzees. *J. Exp. Med.* 179:1253–1259.

van de Stolpe, A., Jacobs, N., Hage, W. J., Tertoolen, L., v. K. Y., Novakova, I.R.O., and de Witte, T. (1996) Fibrinogen binding to ICAM-1 on EA.hy 926 endothelial cells is dependent on an intact cytoskeleton. *Thromb. Haemost.* 75:182–189.

van der Wal, A. C., Das, P. K., Tigges, A. J., and Becker, A. E. (1992) Adhesion molecules on the endothelium and the mononuclear cells in human atherosclerotic lesions. *Am. J. Pathol.* 141: 1427–1433.

Vedder, N. B., and Harlan, J. M. (1988) Increased surface expression of CD11b/CD18 (Mac-1) is not required for stimulated neutrophil adherence to cultured endothelium. *J. Clin. Invest.* 81:676–682.

Vu, T.-K.H., Hung, D. T., Wheaton, V. I., and Coughlin, S. R. (1991) Molecular cloning of a functional thrombin receptor reveals a novel proteolytic mechanism of receptor activation. *Cell* 64:1057–1068.

Walters, T. K., Gorog, D. A., and Wood, R. F. (1994) Thrombin generation following arterial injury is a critical initiating event in the pathogenesis of the proliferative stages of the atherosclerotic process. *J. Vasc. Res.* 31:173–177.

Waltz, D. A., Sailor, L. Z., and Chapman, H. A. (1993) Cytokines induce urokinase-dependent adhesion of human myeloid cells. A regulatory role for plasminogen activator inhibitors. *J. Clin. Invest.* 91:1541–1552.

Weber, C., and Springer, T. A. (1997) Neutrophil accumulation on activated, surface-adherent platelets in flow is mediated by interaction of Mac-1 with fibrinogen bound to αIIbβ3 and stimulated by platelet-activating factor. *J. Clin. Invest.* 100:2085–2093.

Wei, Y., Lukashev, M., Simon, D. I., Bodary, S. C., Rosenberg, S., D.M.V., and Chapman, H. A. (1996) Regulation of integrin function by the urokinase receptor. *Science* 273:1551–1555.

Wright, S. D., and Meyer, B. C. (1986) Phorbol esters cause sequential activation and deactivation of complement receptors on polymorphonuclear leukocytes. *J. Immunol.* 136:1759–1764.

Wright, S. D., Weitz, J. I., Huang, A. J., Levin, S. M., Silverstein, S. C., and Loike, J. D. (1988) Complement receptor type three (CD11b/CD18) of human polymorphonuclear leukocytes recognizes fibrinogen. *Proc. Natl. Acad. Sci. USA* 85:7734–7738.

Wu, X., Helfrich, M. H., Horton, M. A., Feigen, L. P., and Lefkowith, J. B. (1994) Fibrinogen mediates platelet–polymorphonuclear leukocyte cooperation during immune-complex glomerulonephritis in rats. *J. Clin. Invest.* 94:928–936.

Xue, W., Kindzelskii, A. L., Todd, R. F., III, and Petty, H. R. (1994) Physical association of complement receptor type 3 and urokinase-type plasminogen activator receptor in neutrophil membranes. *J. Immunol.* 152:4630–4640.

Zhou, L., Lee, D.H.S., Plescia, J., Lau, C. Y., and Altieri, D. C. (1994) Differential ligand binding specificities of recombinant CD11b/CD18 integrin I-domain. *J. Biol. Chem.* 269:17075–17079.

Zimmerman, G. A., McIntyre, T. M., and Prescott, S. M. (1985) Thrombin stimulates the adherence of neutrophils to endothelial cells in vitro. *J. Clin. Invest.* 76:2235–2246.

Zimmerman, G. A., McIntyre, T. M., and Prescott, T. M. (1992) Endothelial cell interactions with granulocytes: tethering and signaling molecules. *Immunol. Today* 13:93–100.

20

Coagulation and Fibrinolysis During Endotoxemia and Gram-Negative Sepsis

TOM VAN DER POLL, MARCEL LEVI,
and SANDER J. H. VAN DEVENTER

Severe gram-negative infections are sometimes associated with the clinical syndrome of disseminated intravascular coagulation (DIC). The derangement of the hemostatic mechanism not only comprises enhanced activation of coagulation, but also depression of inhibitory mechanism for coagulation and for the fibrinolytic system. Furthermore, depletion of platelets and clotting factors, primarily due to ongoing activation of the coagulation system, may induce severe bleeding complications. As a consequence, DIC can give rise to concurrent thrombosis and bleeding. Many, if not all, of the pro-inflammatory responses observed during gram-negative infection are induced by endotoxin, the lipopolysaccharide part of the outer membrane of gram-negative bacteria. In recent years, knowledge of the pathogenesis of procoagulant changes in sepsis has markedly increased, in large part due to investigations in humans and nonhuman primates injected with endotoxin or live *Escherichia coli*. In this chapter we will present a brief overview of the in vivo studies that have examined a number of mechanisms in the pathogenesis of hemostatic disorders in sepsis and endotoxemia.

Endotoxin and Endotoxin-Binding Proteins

Endotoxin is a lipopolysaccharide (LPS) and a major component of the outer membrane of gram-negative bacteria. Endotoxin has strong pro-inflammatory properties and can activate multiple inflammatory cascades. It is therefore considered to play a key role in the toxic sequelae of gram-negative sepsis (Manthous et al., 1993). LPS is composed of a lipid moiety, designated lipid A, and a hydrophilic polysaccharide chain. The polysaccharide portion of LPS consists of the O chain that protrudes from the bacterial membrane, and a "core part" that connects the O chain with lipid A. Whereas the O chain consists of a series of structurally and antigenically diverse oligosaccharides that determine the many different O-specific serotypes, the core part is identical for many different bacteria. Lipid A is highly conserved among gram-negative bacteria and is responsible for the biological effects of LPS.

Three cloned molecules expressed on the surface of mononuclear cells have been documented to bind the lipid A part of LPS: CD14, the β_2 leukocyte integrins (CD11a/CD18, CD11b/CD18, and CD11c/CD18), and the macrophage scavenger receptor (SR; Fenton and Golenbock, 1998). Binding of LPS to CD14 or CD11/CD18 eventually results in a cellular effect, whereas SR does not seem to function as a signaling receptor. Spontaneous binding of LPS to CD14 occurs at very slow rates. LPS–CD14 binding is greatly accelerated in the presence of LPS binding protein (LBP), an acute phase reactant mainly derived from the liver and present in blood at concentrations in the microgram permilliliter range (Ulevitch and Tobias, 1994; Fenton and Golenbock, 1998). LBP can also bind intact gram-negative bacteria via LPS in the outer membrane, and facilitate attachment of bacteria to CD14. LBP shows amino acid sequence homology with bactericidal permeability-increasing protein (BPI), a product of neutrophilic granulocytes. Like LBP, BPI binds to isolated LPS and to gram—negative bacteria via lipid A. However, the effect of BPI on LPS activity is opposite to the effect of LBP: whereas BPI neutralizes the effects of LPS on cells, LBP enhances them. Interestingly, LBP can also transfer LPS to lipoproteins, in particular, high-density lipoproteins, an interaction that results in inhibition of LPS activity. CD14 is present in serum in a soluble form. Cell types that do not express membrane-bound CD14 can be rendered LPS responsive by a mechanism that involves soluble CD14 and LBP (Ulevitch and Tobias 1994; Fenton and Golenbock, 1998). A role for LBP in the interaction between LPS and CD11/CD18 has not been identified.

It was recognized many years ago that CD14, which is a glycosylphosphatidylinositol (GPI)-anchored membrane protein and does not have an intracellular domain, is not the LPS receptor signaling element. Recent research has identified Toll-like receptor 4 as a signaling receptor for LPS (Ulevitch, 1999). (Fig. 20.1). The notion that Toll-like receptor 4 may play an important role in LPS signaling is supported by the finding that the LPS hyporesponsive mouse strains C3H/HeJ and C57BL/10ScCr have a defective Toll-like receptor 4 gene (Poltorak et al., 1998).

Regulation of Hemostasis

The generation and degradation of fibrin, the end product of blood coagulation, is tightly regulated by a number of closely cooperating systems that include both cellular elements and plasma proteins. In the current concept of the coagulation system, the coagulation cascade is viewed as one series of interrelated reactions that are driven by the generation of the factor VIIa–tissue factor complex (Van der Poll et al., 1997c; Fig. 20.2). This enzyme complex not only is able to activate factor X, but can also catalyze the conversion of factor IX to factor IXa, providing an additional route by which

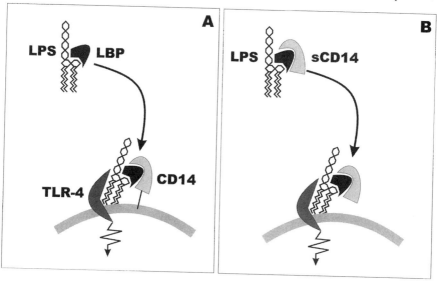

Fig. 20.1. Endotoxin-induced signal transduction: A. Endotoxin (LPS) complexed with LPS binding protein (LBP) binds to cell-associated CD14, which functions as a pattern recognition receptor but by itself does not induce cell activation. The LPS–CD14 complex then activates the Toll-like 4 receptor (TLR-4). B Cell types that do not express CD14 at their surface use soluble CD14, present in plasma, to activate TLR-4.

factor X activation can occur. Historically, the tissue factor–VIIa driven pathway was termed the *extrinsic route*, which existed next to the intrinsic route of the coagulation system. In the current concept of hemostasis, the contact system does not contribute to the initiation of coagulation, but, as will be outlined in the following, is considered to be of importance in the pathogenesis of hypotension during sepsis.

Cell types involved in hemostasis include platelets, endothelial cells, and monocytes. Platelets can provide a catalytic surface for clotting reactions by increasing the activation rates of factors IX, X, and prothrombin. The vascular endothelium also plays a major role in the regulation of the local hemostatic balance (Gerlach et al., 1990). Endothelial cells can express adhesion molecules that enable entrapping of leukocytes at sites of inflammation, and produce a number of factors that are actively involved in coagulant and anticoagulant mechanisms, including tissue-type plasminogen activator (tPA) urokinase—type plasminogen activator (uPA), plasminogen activator inhibitor-1 (PAI-1), thrombomodulin, tissue factor, and tissue factor pathway inhibitor (TFPI). Monocytes also express tissue factor at their surface upon stimulation with various stimuli. In addition, monocytes are a major source of cytokines.

The host can utilize several mechanisms to control and localize the for-

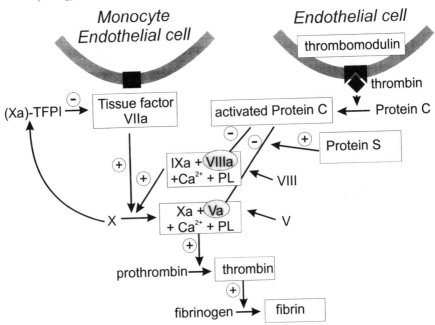

Fig. 20.2. Current concept of the coagulation system: Enhanced expression of tissue factor at the surface of endothelial cells and monocytes plays a central role in coagulation activation during systemic infection. The tissue factor–VIIa complex can be inhibited by tissue factor pathway inhibitor (TFPI) complexed with factor Xa. Activated protein C is an important endogenous anticoagulant by virtue of its capacity to inhibit factors VIIIa and Va (see text for further details).

mation of fibrin clots, including antithrombin III (AT-III), the protein C–protein S system, TFPI, and the fibrinolytic system. AT-III inhibits the activity of many proteases, including the activity of clotting factors IXa, Xa, and thrombin. The protein C–protein S system inhibits activation of coagulation factors Va and VIIIa (Esmon, 1987). Thrombin mediates the activation of protein C after binding to thrombomodulin, a receptor at the surface of endothelial cells. Protein S serves as a cofactor for activated protein C. The activity of the factor VIIa–tissue factor complex can be inhibited by TFPI, which can bind factor Xa, and thereafter inhibit factor VIIa–tissue factor activity by forming a quaternary Xa–TFPI–VIIa complex, although at high concentrations, TFPI may also inhibit VIIa–tissue factor activity in the absence of factor Xa (Rappaport, 1991). Plasmin is the key protease of the fibrinolytic system. The generation and activity of plasmin are controlled by plasminogen activators (tPA and uPA), plasminogen activator inhibitor (PAI) and α_2-antiplasmin.

Activation of Coagulation and Fibrinolysis in Models of Systemic Infection

Experimental studies in primates have been extremely useful for unraveling the pathogenetic mechanisms of DIC. In many studies, baboons have been used to determine the efficacy of potential therapeutic agents by assessing their ability to survive after a lethal *E coli* infusion (discussed later). In such animal models, the effect of the therapeutic intervention on the coagulopathy induced by sepsis can be denoted by using well-defined end points, such as the amount of fibrinogen consumption and deposition (Taylor et al., 1991d). In addition, studies in which either healthy humans or healthy chimpanzees were injected with low-dose LPS derived from *E coli* have also shed light on the early dynamics and route of coagulation activation during a systemic inflammatory response (Levi et al., 1993).

Injection of endotoxin into humans induces a transient stimulation of the common pathway of the coagulation system, as reflected by rises in the plasma concentrations of the prothrombin fragment F1+2 and of thrombin–AT-III (TAT) complexes, and is evident from 2 hours postinjection (Van Deventer et al., 1990). It is of considerable interest that in this model a transient activation of fibrinolysis precedes activation of coagulation (Van Deventer et al., 1990). Thus, intravenous injection of LPS results in an early and transient

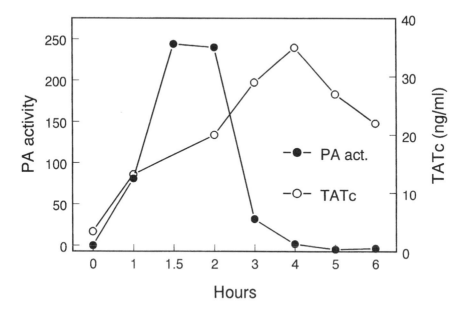

Fig. 20.3. Activation of fibrinolysis precedes activation of coagulation during human endotoxemia: Endotoxin (2 ng/kg) administered intravenously at t = 0 induces an early and transient rise in plasma plasminogen activator (PA) activity, followed by a more sustained increase in the plasma concentrations of thrombin–antithrombin III (TAT) complexes.

release of tPA into the circulation, followed by a brisk increase in PAI-1 levels, indicating that the fibrinolytic response to endotoxin is highly regulated (Suf-fredini et al., 1989; Van Deventer et al., 1990). Three hours after LPS injection, while coagulation activation is still proceeding, fibrinolysis is completely offset, suggesting that the net result of transient endotoxemia is a procoagulant state (Fig. 20.3). The kinetic pattern of early transient activation of fibrinolysis, and more sustained activation of coagulation, also emerges from studies in baboons infused with a lethal dose of live *E coli* (De Boer et al., 1993).

Route of Coagulation Activation and Interplay with Other Inflammatory Pathways

Several lines of evidence indicate that activation of the coagulation system during sepsis is driven by the extrinsic tissue factor-mediated route. First, a number of different strategies interfering with the activation of this pathway prevent the activation of the common pathway of coagulation in endotoxemic chimpanzees and septic baboons. These strategies include antibodies directed against tissue factor or factor VII/VIIa, active site inhibited factor VIIa (Dansyl–Glu–Gly–Arg chloromethylketone or DEGR–VIIa) and TFPI (Taylor et al., 1991c; Creasey et al., 1993; Levi et al., 1994; Biemond et al., 1995b; Carr et al., 1995; Taylor et al., 1998). Activation of the contact system does not contribute to the activation of the coagulation system during sepsis. Indeed, infusion of an antibody directed against factor XII did not prevent DIC in baboons with lethal *E coli* sepsis, as manifested by unchanged decreases in the plasma concentrations of fibrinogen and factor V (Pixley et al., 1993). Instead, anti-factor XII reversed the severe hypotension seen in untreated bacteremic animals, and extended survival time, arguing for a role of contact system products (i.e., bradykinin) in the development of shock during generalized infection (Pixley et al., 1993).

It should be noted that interventions inhibiting the tissue factor pathway in lethal *E coli* sepsis in baboons not only prevented DIC, but also resulted in an increased rate of survival (Taylor et al., 1991c; Creasey et al., 1993; Carr et al., 1995; Taylor et al., 1998). Of considerable interest, more downstream intervention in the coagulation system by administration of factor Xa blocked in its active center (DEGR-Xa), failed to influence lethality of bacteremic baboons, while completely inhibiting the development of DIC (Taylor et al., 1991b). Hence, it is unlikely that elimination of the tissue factor pathway protects against death merely by an effect on the coagulation system. It is therefore conceivable that the tissue factor—VIIa pathway exerts effects on inflammatory responses different from the procoagulant response. Several experimental findings support this hypothesis. Bacteremic baboons treated with TFPI or DEGR–VIIa demonstrated significantly lower interleukin-6 (IL-6) and IL-8 levels than baboons not infused with these compounds (Creasey et al., 1993; Carr et al., 1995; Jansen et al., 1997; Taylor et al., 1998). In addition, TFPI also reduced the release of interferon-γ, IL-10, and soluble Fas, but did not influence the plasma concentrations of tumor necrosis factor (TNF) or IL-1β (Jansen et al., 1997). In vitro, TFPI has been found to bind LPS, thereby blocking LPS effects on cells by interference with LPS transfer to CD14 (Park et al., 1997). Interestingly, inhibition of the contact system, although not influencing the activation of the coagulation system (Pixley et al., 1993), did affect a number of other inflammatory pathways. Indeed, anti-XIIa administration to septic baboons inhibited IL-6 release, complement activation, fibrinolytic activation, and neutrophil degranulation (Jansen et al., 1996).

Studies in baboons have established that activation of protein C represents an important host defense mechanism against excessive fibrin formation. Infusion of activated protein C into septic baboons prevented hypercoagulability and death, whereas inhibition of activation of endogenous protein C by a monoclonal antibody exacerbated the response to a lethal *E coli* infusion and converted a sublethal model produced by an LD_{10} dose of *E coli* into a severe shock response associated with DIC and death (Taylor et al., 1987). Interference with the bioavailability of protein S, the cofactor for protein C, resulted in similar changes. In plasma, 60% of protein S is complexed to a complement regulatory protein, C4b binding protein (C4bBP); the anticoagulant capacity of protein C is enhanced only by the free fraction of protein S. Administration of C4bBP, which causes a decrease in free protein S levels, converted a nonlethal acute phase response to a sublethal dose of live *E coli* into a lethal shock response with rapid consumption of fibrinogen and systemic organ damage (Taylor et al., 1991a). Hence, like the tissue factor mediated pathway, the protein C–protein S system may have other effects on host responses apart from its role in the coagulation system. Both activated protein C and recombinant thrombomodulin protected rats against LPS-induced lung injury by inhibition of leukocyte activation, not by an effect on the coagulation system (Uchiba et al., 1995; Murakami et al., 1996). One mechanism that may contribute to anti-inflammatory properties of the protein C–protein S–thrombomodulin system, is the capacity of protein C and protein S to inhibit LPS-induced production of TNF, IL-1β, and IL-6 by monocytes in vitro, and the ability of activated protein C to attenuate TNF release during endotoxemia in rats in vivo (Hancock et al., 1992; Grey et al., 1994).

Interestingly, in vitro studies indicate that end products of the coagulation cascade can initiate inflammatory responses. Coagulating blood has been found to produce IL-8, but not IL-6, in vitro. Addition of endotoxin to coagulating blood resulted in a synergistic enhancement of IL-8 production, which could be attenuated by the thrombin inhibitor hirudin or TFPI (Johnson et al., 1996). In addition, factor Xa, thrombin, and fibrin can elicit the synthesis of IL-6 and/or IL-8 by various cell types in vitro (Sower et al., 1995; Qi et al., 1997; Senden et al., 1998). At present, the relevance of these in vitro findings for the interplay between coagulation and inflammation in vivo is unknown.

Cytokines and Activation of the Hemostatic Mechanism

Cytokines are peptides with molecular weights below 80 kDa that can exert a wide variety of biological effects at picomolar concentrations. Proinflammatory cytokines, such as TNF and IL-1, facilitate inflammation. The production of these cytokines can be inhibited by so-called anti-inflammatory cytokines, of which IL-10 has been implicated in the pathogenesis of sepsis syndrome. The activity of pro-inflammatory cytokines can be further modulated by naturally occurring inhibitors, such as soluble TNF receptors and IL-1 receptor antagonist (IL-1ra). IL-6 is a cytokine with both pro- and anti-inflammatory properties.

Cytokines potentially involved in the altered vascular hemostatic properties in infection and inflammation in vivo are TNF, IL-1, IL-6, and IL-10. Both clinical and experimental studies have documented the enhanced production of these cytokines during systemic infection (Van der Poll and Van Deventer, 1999). The kinetics of cytokine release have been studied in experimental models of infection and inflammation. In those models, TNF is the first cytokine appearing in the circulation. Infusion of either a relatively low dose of LPS into healthy humans, or a lethal dose of live *E coli* into baboons resulted in transient release of TNF peaking after 90 minutes (Fong et al., 1989; Van der Poll et al., 1994c, 1997a; Van der Poll and Van Deventer, 1999). A close correlation exists between the magnitude of the bacterial challenge and the extent of TNF release; the levels of TNF detected in the lethal dose baboon studies were much higher than in the mild dose human volunteer studies. Shortly after the appearance of TNF, IL-6 and IL-10 can be detected during experimental sepsis and endotoxemia, but the detection of IL-1β (like IL-6 and IL-10 secreted shortly after TNF) is confined to lethal sepsis models (Fong et al., 1989; Van der Poll et al., 1994c, 1997a; Van der Poll and Van Deventer, 1999). Interestingly, the release of IL-1β, IL-6, and, to a lesser extent, IL-10 during experimental sepsis and endotoxemia is, at least in part, mediated by TNF because passive immunization against TNF attenuated the systemic appearance of the former cytokines (Fong et al., 1989; Van der Poll et al., 1994a). Inhibition of TNF or IL-1 was highly protective against lethality when given before intravenous infusion of a LD_{100} dose of endotoxin or live bacteria (Tracey et al., 1987; Hinshaw et al., 1990; Ohlsson et al., 1990; Fischer et al., 1992). IL-10 may serve a protective function during endotoxemia, at least in part related to its capacity to inhibit the production of pro-inflammatory cytokines. Thus, elimination of endogenous IL-10 enhanced mortality in mice exposed to high-dose LPS, and administration of recombinant IL-10 protected mice against LPS-induced lethality (Howard et al., 1993; Marchant et al., 1994). IL-6 does not play a significant role in the pathogenesis of toxicity associated with systemic LPS administration (Fattori et al., 1994).

A number of studies indicate that although TNF can induce activation of the coagulation system in vivo, it is not essential for the procoagulant response during endotoxemia. A single intravenous bolus injection of recombinant TNF into normal humans induced a sustained activation of the common pathway of the coagulation system, as reflected by elevated plasma levels of F1+2 for 6 to 12 hours (Van der Poll et al., 1990). TNF induced a profound activation of the fibrinolytic system in the first hour postinjection, mediated by tPA, followed by a fast inhibition, mediated by PAI-1, thereby mimicking the kinetics of fibrinolytic and coagulation activation during endotoxemia (Van der Poll et al., 1991). However, neutralization of TNF activity did not affect LPS-induced coagulation activation in healthy humans or chimpanzees, as reflected by unaltered rises in the plasma concentrations of both F1+2 and TAT complexes (Van der Poll et al., 1994c, 1997a; DeLa Cadena et al., 1998). In baboons infused with a lethal dose of *E. coli*, treatment with an anti-TNF antibody had little or no effect on fibrinogen consumption (Hinshaw et al., 1990). Importantly, in the chimpanzee and human models of low-grade endotoxemia, anti-TNF strategies strongly inhibited the activation of the fibrinolytic system, and virtually completely prevented the LPS-induced increase in tPA, PAI-1, and plasmin–α2-antiplasmin (PAP) complexes (Van der Poll et al., 1994c; Biemond et al., 1995a; Van der Poll et al., 1997a; DeLa Cadena et al., 1998).

Besides TNF, IL-1 can also activate the hemostatic mechanism in vivo. Infusion of IL-1α into baboons, at a dose that causes a transient shock-like state, elicited an early activation of the fibrinolytic system followed by activation of the common pathway of the coagulation system (Jansen et al., 1995). Similar to results obtained after LPS or TNF administration, fibrinolytic activation is tightly regulated after injection of IL-1; fibrinolysis was initiated by tPA, and subsequently offset by PAI-1. Consequently, the imbalance between coagulant and fibrinolytic responses observed after administration of endotoxin, live *E coli*, or TNF is also found after infusion of IL-1. The role of endogenously produced IL-1 in the hemostatic disorders during sepsis has been examined by administration of recombinant IL-1ra in baboons with lethal bacteremia (Jansen et al., 1995). In these animals, IL-1ra significantly attenuated coagulation activation. Plasma levels of PAP complexes were not influenced by IL-1ra, presumably because PAP levels were already maximal (after 1.0–1.5 hours) before IL-1 appears in the circulation in this model.

Other cytokines implicated in the regulation of hemostasis during severe infection are IL-6 and IL-10. In patients with renal cell carcinoma, intravenous administration of recombinant IL-6 was associated with rises in the plasma concentrations of F1+2 and TAT complexes, while leaving fibrinolysis unaffected (Stouthard et al., 1996). In chimpanzees exposed to low-dose LPS, treatment with an anti–IL-6 antibody prevented coagulation activation, but did not influence the activation of the fibrinolytic system (Van der Poll et al., 1994b). It remains to be established how IL-6 affects coagulation; IL-6 has not been reported to influence the hemostatic properties of vascular endothelium or monocytes in vitro. IL-10 potentially can inhibit coagulation activation by inhibiting the expression of tissue factor by monocytes (Pradier et al., 1993). Indeed, recombinant IL-10 (25 μ/kg) given to normal humans attenuated the procoagulant response induced by low-dose *E coli* LPS (4 ng/kg; Pajkrt et al., 1997). However, infusion of recombinant IL-10 at a much higher dose (500 μ/kg), did not influence activation of the coagulation system in baboons challenged with high-dose *Salmonella* LPS (500; gm/kg), despite a strong inhibition of pro-inflammatory cytokine release (Van der Poll et al., 1997b). Hence, further studies are required to define the potency of exogenous IL-10 and the role of endogenous IL-10 in coagulation activation during sepsis.

After administration of LPS, *E coli*, TNF, or IL-1 to humans or nonhuman primates, activation of the fibrinolytic system preceded that of the coagulation system, suggesting that fibrinolytic activation is initiated independently from coagulation activation. This hypothesis has been recently confirmed in chimpanzees, in which blockade of coagulation activation by antibodies against either tissue factor or factor VII/VIIa did not influence the activation of the fibrinolytic system (Levi et al., 1994; Biemond et al., 1995b). It should be noted, however, that during lethal bacteremia other mechanisms may contribute to the activation of the fibrinolytic system; treatment with either TFPI or antifactor XII reduced the fibrinolytic response in baboons infused with high-dose *E coli* (Jansen et al., 1996, 1997).

Conclusion

Knowledge of the mechanisms involved in activation of the hemostatic system has increased considerably in recent years. Experiments in humans and nonhuman primates have unraveled distinct pathways that mediate activation of either the coagulation system and/or the fibrinolytic system. It is clear now that systemic infection initiates activation of coagulation via the extrinsic-tissue factor mediated pathway. Although activation of the contact system can be documented during severe infection, this system does not contribute to DIC. Inhibition of coagulation in sublethal endotoxemia models does not result in inhibition of fibrinolysis, whereas an attenuated coagulant response during lethal bacteremia is associated with some inhibition of fibrinolysis, suggesting that coagulation and fibrinolysis are at least in part unlinked phenomena. The tissue factor–VIIa pathway not only contributes to coagulation activation, but probably has effects on other inflammatory systems yet to be defined. The protein C–protein S system probably also influences other inflammatory cascades besides its function as an important anticoagulant mechanism. Although TNF can induce the coagulation cascade in humans in vivo, and is a crucial factor in the lethality associated with infusion of live *E coli* in baboons, this cytokine is not involved in DIC, nor does it mediate coagulation activation in low-grade endotoxemia in chimpanzees and humans. Endogenously produced TNF is important, however, for LPS-induced activation of the fibrinolytic system. IL-1 is involved in both activation of the coagulation system and the fibrinolytic system during sepsis, whereas IL-6 is a possible mediator of coagulation activation. The regulation of the activation and inhibition of hemostasis in vivo is highly complex and the result of extensive cross-talk among many different inflammatory mediator cascades.

References

Biemond, B. J., ten Cate, H., Levi, M., Soule, H. R., Morris, L. D., Foster, D. L.., Bogowitz, C. A., van der Poll, T., Büller, H. R., and ten Cate, J. W. (1995b) Complete inhibition of endotoxin-induced coagulation activation in chimpanzees with a monoclonal Fab fragment against factor VII/VIIa. *Thromb. Haemostas.* 73:223–230.

Biemond, B. J., Levi, M., ten Cate, H., van der Poll, T., Büller, H. R., Hack, C. E., and ten Cate, J. W. (1995a) Plasminogen activator and PAI-1 release during experimental endotoxemia in chimpanzees: effects of various interventions in the cytokine and coagulation cascades. *Cli. Sci.* 88:587–594.

Carr, C., Bild, G. S., Chang, A.C.K., Peer, G. T., Palmier, M. O., Frazier, R. B., Gustafson, M. E., Wun, T. C., Creasey, A. A., and Hinshaw, L. B. (1995) Recombinant *E coli*-derived tissue factor pathway inhibitor reduces coagulopathic and lethal effects in the baboon gram-negative model of septic shock. *Circ. Shock* 44:126–137.

Creasey, A. A., Chang, A.C.K., Feigen, L., Wün, T. C., Taylor, F. B., Jr., and Hinshaw, L. B. (1993) Tissue factor pathway inhibitor reduces mortality from *Escherichia coli* septic shock. *J. Clin. Invest.* 91:2850–2860.

De Boer, J. P., Creasy, A. A., Chang, A., Roem, D., Brouwer, M. C., Eerenberg, A.J.M., Hack, C. E., and Taylor, F. B., Jr. (1993) Activation patterns of coagulation and fibrinolysis in baboons following infusion with lethal or sublethal dose of *Escherichia coli*. *Circ. Shock* 39:59–67.

DeLa Cadena, R. A., Majluf-Cruz, A., Stadnicki, A., Tropea, M., Reda, D., Agosti, J. M., Colman, R. W., and Suffredini, A. F. (1998) Recombinant tumor necrosis factor receptor p75 fusion protein (TNFR:Fc) alters endotoxin-induced activation of the kinin, fibrinolytic, and coagulation systems in normal humans. *Thromb. Haemostas.* 80:114–118.

Esmon, C. T. (1987) The regulation of natural anticoagulant pathways. *Science* 235:1348–1352.

Fattori, E., Cappelletti, M., Costa, P., Sellitto, C., Cantoni, L., Carelli, M., Faggioni, R., Fantuzzi, G., Ghezzi, P., and Poli, V. (1994) Defective inflammatory response in interleukin-6–deficient mice. *J. Exp. Med.* 180:1243–1250.

Fenton, M. J., and Golenbock, D. T. (1998) LPS-binding proteins and receptors. *J. Leukoc. Biol.* 64:25–32.

Fischer, E., Marano, M. A., Van Zee, K. J., Rock, C. S., CS, Hawes, A. S., Thompson, W. A., DeForge, L., Kenney, J. S., Remick, D. G., Bloedow, D. C., et al. (1992) Interleukin-1 receptor blockade improves survival and hemodynamic performance in *Escherichia coli* septic shock, but fails to alter host responses to sublethal endotoxemia. *J. Clin. Invest.* 89:1551–1557.

Fong, Y., Tracey, K. J., Moldawer, L. L., Hesse, D. G., Manogue, K. R., Kenney, J. S., Lee, A. T., Kuo, G. C., Allison, A. C., Lowry, S. F., and Cerami, A. (1989) Antibodies to cachectin/tumor necrosis factor reduce interleukin-1β and interleukin-6 appearance during lethal bacteremia. *J. Exp. Med.* 170:1627–1633.

Gerlach, H., Esposito, C., and Stern, D. M. (1990) Modulation of endothelial hemostatic properties: an active role in the host response. *Annu. Rev. Med.* 41:15–24.

Grey, S. T., Tsuchida, A., Hau, H., Orthner, C. L., Salem, H. H., and Hancock, W. W. (1994) Selective inhibitory effects of the anticoagulant activated protein C on the responses of human mononuclear phagocytes to LPS, IFN-γ, or phorbol ester. *J. Immunol.* 153:3664–3672.

Hancock, W. W., Tsuchida, Hau, H., Thomson, N. M., and Salem, H. H, (1992) A.The anticoagulants protein-C and protein-S display potent antiinflammatory and immunosuppressive effects relevant to transplant biology and therapy. *Transplant. Proc.* 24:2302–2303.

Hinshaw, L. B., Tekamp-Olson, P., Chang, A.C.K., Lee, P. A., Taylor, F. B., Jr., Murray, C. K., Peer, G. T., Emerson, T. E., Jr., Passey, B., and Kuo, G. C. (1990) Survival of primates in LD100 septic shock following therapy with antibody to tumor necrosis factor (TNF). *Circ. Shock* 30:279–292.

Howard, M., Muchamuel, T., Andrade, S., and Menon, S. (1993) Interleukin-10 protects mice from lethal endotoxemia. *J. Exp. Med.* 177:1205–1208.

Jansen, P. M., Boermeester, M. A., Fischer, E., de Jong, I. W., van der Poll, T., Moldawer, L. L., Hack, C. E., and Lowry, S. F. (1995) Contribution of interleukin-1 to activation of coagulation and fibrinolysis, to neutrophil degranulation and the release of sPLA$_2$ in sepsis. Studies in non-human primates following interleukin-1α administration and during lethal bacteremia. *Blood* 86:1027–1034.

Jansen, P. M., Pixley, R. A., Brouwer M, M., de Jong, I. W., Chang, A.C.K., Hack, C. E., Taylor F. B., Jr., and Colman, R. W. (1996) Inhibition of factor XII in septic baboons attenuates the activation of complement and fibrinolytic systems and reduces the release of interleukin-6 and neutrophil elastase. *Blood* 87:2337–2344.

Jansen, P. M., van Lopik, T., Lubbers Y, Y., de Jong, I. W., Brouwer, M., Chang, A.C.K., Johnson, K., Taylor, F. B., Jr., Aarden, L. A., Hack, C. E., and Creasey, A. A. (1997) The coagulant–inflammatory axis in the baboon response to *E coli*: Effects of tissue factor pathway inhibitor on hemostatic balance, the cytokine network and the release of the apoptosis marker sFas. In *Inflammatory Mediators in Primate Sepsis.* P. M. Jansen, ed. Free University of Amsterdam Amsterdam: (Academic Thesis), pp. 95–107.

Johnson, K., Aarden, L. A., Choi, Y., De Groot, E., and Creasey, A. (1996) The proinflammatory cytokine response to coagulation and endotoxin in whole blood. *Blood* 87:5051–5060.

Levi, M., ten Cate, H., van der Poll, T., and van Deventer, S.J.H. (1993) New insights in the pathogenesis of disseminated intravascular coagulation in sepsis. *JAMA* 270:975–979.

Levi, M., Ten Cate, H., Bauer, K. A., Van der Poll, T., Edgington, T. S., Büller, H. R., Van Deventer, S.J.H., Hack, C. E., Ten Cate, J. W., and Rosenberg, R. D. (1994) Inhibition of endotoxin-induced activation of coagulation and fibrinolysis by pentoxifylline or by a monoclonal anti-tissue factor antibody in chimpanzees. *J. Clin. Invest.* 93:114–120.

Manthous, C. A., Hall, J. B., and Samsel, R. W. (1993) Endotoxin in human disease. Part 1: Biochemistry, assay, and possible role in diverse disease states. *Chest* 104:1572–1581.

Marchant, A., Bruyns, C., Vandenabeele, P., Ducarme, M., Gérard, C., Delvaux, A., de Groote, D., Abramowicz, D., Velu, T., and Goldman, M. (1994) IL-10 controls IFN-γ and TNF production during experimental endotoxemia. *Eur. J. Immunol.* 24:1167–1171.

Murakami, K., Okajima, K., Uchiba, M., Johno, M., Nakagaki, T., Okabe, H., and Takatsuki, K. (1996) Activated protein C attenuates endotoxin-induced pulmonary vascular injury by inhibiting activated leukocytes in rats. *Blood* 87:642–647.

Ohlsson, K., Björk, P., Bergenfeldt, M., Hageman, R., and Thompson, R. C. (1990) Interleukin-1 receptor antagonist reduces mortality from endotoxin shock. *Nature* 348:550–552.

Pajkrt, D., van der Poll, T., Levi, M., Cutler, D. L., Affrime, M. B., van den Ende, A., ten Cate, J. W., and van Deventer, S.J.H. (1997) Interleukin-10 inhibits activation of coagulation and fibrinolysis during human endotoxemia. *Blood* 89:2701–2705.

Park, C. T., Creasey, A. A., and Wright, S. D. (1997) Tissue factor pathway inhibitor blocks cellular effects of endotoxin by binding to endotoxin and interfering with transfer to CD14. *Blood* 89:4268–4274.

Pixley, R. A., De La Cadena, R., Page, J. D., Kaufman, N., Wyshock, E. G., Chang, A., Taylor F. B., Jr., and Colman.,R. W. (1993) The contact system contributes to hypotension but not to disseminated intravascular coagulation in lethal bacteremia. *J. Clin. Invest.* 91:61–68.

Poltorak, A., Xialong, H., Sminova, I., Liu, M. Y., Van Huffel, C., Du, X., Birdwell, D., Alejos, E., Silva, M., Galanos, C. (1998) Defective LPS signaling in C3H/HeJ and C57BL/10ScCr mice: mutations in tlr4 gene. *Science* 282:2085–2088.

Pradier, O., Gérard, C., Delvaux, A., Lybin, M., Abramowicz, D., Capel, P., Velu, T., and Goldman, M. (1993) Interleukin-10 inhibits the induction of monocyte procoagulant activity by bacterial lipopolysaccharide. *Eur. J. Immunol.* 23:2700–2703.

Qi, J., Goranlnick, S., and Kreutzer D. L. (1997) Fibrin regulation of interleukin-8 gene expression in human vascular endothelial cells. *Blood* 90:3595–3602.

Rappaport, S. I. (1991) The extrinsic pathway inhibitor: a regulator of tissue factor-dependent blood coagulation. *Thromb. Haemostas.* 66:6–15.

Senden, N.M.H., Jeunhomme, T.M.A.A., Heemskerk, J.W.M., Wagenvoord, R., Van't Veer, C., Hemker, H. C., and Buurman, W. A. (1998) Factor Xa induces cytokine production and expression of adhesion molecules by human umbilical vein endothelial cells. *J. Immunol.* 161: 4318–4324.

Sower, L. E., Froelich, C. J., Fenton, J. W., and Klimpel, G. R. (1995) Thrombin induces IL-6 production in fibroblasts and epithelial cells. Evidence for the involvement of the seven-transmembrane domain (STD) receptor for alpha thrombin. *J. Immunol.* 155:895–901.

Stouthard, J.M.L., Levi, M., Hack, C. E., Veenhof, C.H.N., Romijn, J. A., Sauerwein, H. P., and van der Poll T. (1996) Interleukin-6 stimulates coagulation, not fibrinolysis, in humans. *Thromb. Haemostas.* 76:738–742.

Suffredini, A. F., Harpel, P. C., and Parrillo, J. E. (1989) Promotion and subsequent inhibition of plasminogen activation after administration of intravenous endotoxin to normal subjects. *N. Engl. J. Med.* 320:1165–1172.

Taylor, F. B. Jr., Chang, A., Esmon, T., D'Angelo, A., Vigano-D'Angelo, S., and Blick, K. E. (1987) Protein C prevents the coagulopathic and lethal effects of *Escherichia coli* infusion in the baboon. *J. Clin. Invest.* 79:918–925.

Taylor, F. B. Jr., Chang, A., Ferrell, G., Mather, T., Blick, K., and Esmon, C. T. (1991a) C4b-binding protein exacerbates the host response to *Escherichia coli*. *Blood* 78:357–363.

Taylor, F. B. Jr., Chang, A., Peer, G. T., Mather, T., Blick, K., Catlett, R., Lockhart, M. S., and Esmon, C. T. (1991b) DEGR-factor Xa blocks disseminated intravascular coagulation initiated by *Escherichia coli* without preventing shock or organ damage. *Blood* 78:364–368.

Taylor, F. B. Jr., Chang, A., Ruf, W., Morrissey, J. H., Hinshaw, L., Catlett, R., Blick, K., and Edgington, T. S. (1991c) Lethal *E coli* septic shock is prevented by blocking tissue factor with monoclonal antibody. *Circ. Shock* 33:127–134.

Taylor, F. B. Jr., Esmon, C. T., and Hishaw, L. B. (1991d) Summary of staging mechanism and intervention studies in the baboon model of *E. coli* sepsis. *J. Trauma* 12:197–204.

Taylor, F. B. Jr., Chang, A.C.K., Peer, G., Ezban, M., and Hedner, U. (1998). Active site inhibited factor VIIa (DEGR VIIa) attenuates the coagulant and interleukin-6 and -8, but not tumor necrosis factor, responses of the baboon to LD100 *Escherichia coli*. *Blood* 91: 1609–1615.

Tracey, K. J., Fong, Y., Hesse, D. G., Manogue, K. R., Lee, A. T., Kuo, G. C., Lowry, S. F., and Cerami, A. (1987) Anti-cachectin/TNF monoclonal antibodies prevent septic shock during lethal bacteraemia. *Nature* 330:662–664.

Uchiba, M., Okajima, K., Murakami, K., Nawa, K., Okabe, H., and Takatsuki, K. (1995) Recombinant human soluble thrombomodulin reduces endotoxin-induced pulmonary vascular injury via protein C activation in rats. *Thromb. Haemostas.* 74:1265–1270.

Ulevitch, R. J., and Tobias, P. S. (1994) Recognition of endotoxin by cells leading to transmembrane signaling. *Curr. Opin. Immunol.* 6:125–130.

Ulevitch, R. J. (1999) Toll gates for pathogen selection. *Nature* 401:755–756.

Van der Poll, T., Büller, H. R., Ten Cate, H., Wortel, C. H., Bauer, K. A., Van Deventer, S.J.H., Hack, C. E., Sauerwein, H. P., Rosenberg, R. D., and ten Cate, J. W. (1990) Activation of coagulation after administration of tumor necrosis factor to normal subjects. *N. Engl. J. Med.* 322:1622–1627.

Van der Poll, T., Levi, M., Büller, H. R., Van Deventer, S.J.H., De Boer, J. P., Hack, C. E., and Ten Cate, J. W. (1991) Fibrinolytic response to tumor necrosis factor in healthy subjects. *J. Exp. Med.* 174:729–732.

Van der Poll, T., Jansen, J., Levi, M., ten Cate, H., ten Cate, J. W., and van Deventer, S.J.H. (1994a) Regulation of interleukin-10 release by tumor necrosis factor in humans and chimpanzees. *J. Exp. Med.* 180:1985–1988.

Van der Poll, T., Levi, M., Hack, C. E., Ten Cate, H., Van Deventer, S.J.H., Eerenberg, A.J.M., De Groot, E. R., Jansen, J., Gallati, H., Büller, H. R., Ten Cate, J. W., and Aarden, L. A. (1994b) Elimination of interleukin-6 attenuates coagulation activation in experimental endotoxemia in chimpanzees. *J. Exp. Med.* 179:1253–1259.

Van der Poll, T., Levi, M., van Deventer, S.J.H., ten Cate, H., Haagmans, B. L., Biemond, B. J., Büller, H. R., Hack, C. E., and ten Cate, J. W. (1994c) Differential effects of anti-tumor necrosis factor monoclonal antibodies on systemic inflammatory responses in experimental endotoxemia in chimpanzees. *Blood* 83:446–451.

Van der Poll, T., Coyle, S. M., Levi, M., Jansen, P. M., Dentener, M., Barbosa, K., Buurman, W. A., Hack, C. E., ten Cate, J. W., Agosti, J. M., and Lowry, S. F. (1997a) Effect of a recombinant dimeric tumor hecrosis factor receptor on inflammatory responses to intravenous endotoxin in normal humans. *Blood* 89:3727–3734.

Van der Poll, T., Jansen, P. M., Montegut, W. J., Braxton, C. C., Calvano, S. E., Stackpole, S. A., Smith, S. M., Swanson, S. W., Hack, C. E., Lowry, S. F., and Moldawer, L. L. (1997b) Effects of IL-10 on systemic inflammatory responses during sublethal primate endotoxemia. *J. Immunol.* 158:1971–1975.

Van der Poll, T., Levi, M., and van Deventer, S.J.H. (1997c) Coagulopathy: disseminated intravascular coagulation. In: *Sepsis and Multiorgan Failure.* A. M. Fein, E. M. Abraham, R. A. Balk, G. R. Bernard, R. C. Bone, D. R. Dantzker, and M. P. Fink, eds. Baltimore: William & Wilkins, pp. 255–265.

Van der Poll, T., and van Deventer, S.J.H. (1999) Cytokines and anticytokines in the pathogenesis of sepsis. *Infect. Dis. Clin. North Am.* 13:413–426.

Van Deventer, S.J.H., Büller, H. R., Ten Cate, J. W., Aarden, L. A., Hack, C. E., and Sturk, A. (1990) Experimental endotoxemia in humans: analysis of cytokine release and coagulation, fibrinolytic and complement pathways. *Blood* 76:2520–2526.

21

Oxygen Radicals in Inflammation

NORMAN R. HARRIS and D. NEIL GRANGER

Oxygen radicals have been implicated as mediators of inflammatory responses associated with a number of disease states including rheumatoid arthritis, inflammatory bowel disease, pancreatitis, and ischemia and reperfusion (I/R) injury. The goal of this chapter is to define the nature of the involvement of oxygen radicals in the initiation and perpetuation of an inflammatory response. We (a) provide a brief overview of the biochemistry of oxygen radicals; (b) describe sources, biological targets, and mechanisms for neutralization of these reactive oxygen species; and (c) define the role of these radicals in the recruitment and activation of leukocytes into inflamed tissues. Particular attention will be given to the contribution of oxygen radicals to the pathobiology of I/R injury, a condition that is associated with markedly enhanced production of oxygen radicals by endothelial cells, neutrophils, and various auxiliary cells (mast cells) that also contribute to the overall injury process.

Physiological Chemistry of Oxygen Radicals

Definition and Chemistry

Most unreactive molecules have an even number of electrons that permits the pairing of electrons with opposite spins. Oxygen radicals, on the other hand, contain an unpaired electron that seeks to be paired, and therefore tends to be highly reactive. Stability of oxygen radicals is attained by the gain or loss of an electron through an oxidation/ reduction reaction, which often leaves target molecules with an unpaired electron. Therefore, generation of a single radical can initiate a series of oxidation/ reduction reactions when the intermediate species are sufficiently reactive.

Molecular oxygen is a biradical whose relatively low reactivity can be attributed to parallel spin of its two unpaired electrons in the outer orbital. The more reactive superoxide radical (O_2^-) can be formed when oxygen obtains one electron, leaving only one electron free. In physiological solutions, superoxide dismutase (SOD) can catalyze the formation of hydrogen peroxide (H_2O_2) from O_2^-. *Hydrogen peroxide* is considered to be a reactive oxygen species despite its even number of electrons; however, neither O_2^- nor H_2O_2 are as unstable and reactive as a product of their reaction, the hydroxyl radical (•OH).

The reaction between O_2^- and H_2O_2 to form •OH does not proceed at a significant rate in physiological solutions (Morris et al., 1995) unless iron is present:

$$Fe^{2+}$$
$$O_2^- + H_2O_2 \rightarrow O_2 + \bullet OH + {}^-OH.$$

This reaction is known as either the iron-catalyzed Haber–Weiss reaction or the Fenton reaction. Because of its instability, •OH reacts with virtually any molecule in close proximity; however, because the formation of •OH is dependent on the presence of iron, the target molecule often contains or binds iron (Morris et al., 1995).

A more inclusive nomenclature for reactive oxygen-containing molecules is *reactive oxygen species* (ROS). This term not only refers to radicals such as O_2^- and •OH, but also nonradicals such as H_2O_2, singlet oxygen, hypochlorous acid, peroxide, hydroperoxide, and others (Kehrer, 1993) that are still somewhat reactive despite having paired electrons. Several of these nonradical ROS play significant roles in various inflammatory conditions.

Sources of ROS

Phagocytes, mitochondrial and microsomal electron transport systems, cytosolic oxidases, transition metals, cigarette smoke, and radiation are all potential sources of ROS (Kehrer, 1993; Maxwell, 1995). Phagocytes can produce both O_2^- and H_2O_2 from which the more reactive •OH can be formed. These three ROS are used by neutrophils to kill bacteria and other invading organisms. However, an excessive production of these ROS may also inflict collateral damage to surrounding cells and/or initiate signal transduction pathways that can produce undesired secondary effects.

The electron transport systems of mitochondria and microsomes are capable of generating ROS through the cycling of NADH. The production of O_2^- and H_2O_2 from these systems is typically low under resting conditions, but can reach significant levels under conditions such as hypoxia, ischemia, and xenobiotic challenge (Kehrer, 1993). As with phagocytes, excessive production of ROS through electron transport systems can result in deleterious effects on the surrounding tissue.

A soluble enzyme that is known for its ability to oxidize substrates during inflammation is xanthine oxidase. This enzyme can catalyze both the univalent (O_2^-) and divalent (H_2O_2) reduction of molecular oxygen. The ROS generated by xanthine oxidase can also react in the presence of catalytically active iron to produce •OH. Xanthine oxidase (XO) has been implicated in the pathogenesis of I/R injury in a variety of tissues (Granger, 1988). Other ROS-producing enzymes that are potentially involved in tissue injury include dopamine-β-hydroxylase, D-amino acid oxidase, urate oxidase, and fatty acyl CoA oxidase (Kehrer, 1993); however, these enzymes have not been shown to contribute to inflammatory responses.

Biological Targets of ROS

Cellular injury resulting from inflammation can occur through ROS-mediated alterations in lipids, proteins, and DNA. Cell membrane function can be compromised directly by lipid peroxidation and membrane damage can alter ion gradients that control various enzyme systems (Kehrer, 1993). The effects of protein oxidation include fragmentation, cross-linking, and aggregation, resulting in dysfunctional ion channels and receptors, and failure of oxidative phosphorylation (Maxwell, 1995). Oxygen radicals can also impair DNA, causing single- or double-strand breaks (Birnboim and Kanabus-Kominska, 1987; Aruoma et al., 1989), or affect DNA function by activating transcription factors that regulate gene expression (Kehrer, 1993).

Antioxidants

Whereas oxygen radicals are routinely involved in beneficial cellular processes, their uncontrolled availability can be harmful to the extent of toxicity. Cells produce molecules that are able to either restrict the action of certain oxidants or even eliminate them. These so-called antioxidants can be classified into three categories: enzymes, metal ion sequesters, and scavenging agents (Maxwell, 1995).

Enzymes

The dismutation of superoxide allows for the elimination of this radical species by forming H_2O_2 and O_2^-. The spontaneous rate of superoxide dismutation is largely determined by the concentration of superoxide; it has been estimated that the half-life of O_2^- increases from 5 ms at 1 mM, to 5 s at 1 μM, and to 5000 s (83 min) at 1 nM (Fridovich, 1998). The enzyme superoxide dismutase (SOD) accelerates the dismutation reaction and reduces the half-life of O_2^- at any concentration to 17 μs (Fridovich, 1998), or by a factor of 300 million compared with the spontaneous dismutation of 1 nM O_2^-. Mammalian cells are endowed with three types of SOD: (a) cytosolic Cu, ZnSOD; (b) mitochondrial MnSOD; and (c) extracellular Cu, ZnSOD (ECSOD). The latter form of the enzyme binds to the glycocalyx found on the blood surface of endothelial cells, where it can detoxify superoxide generated by adherent leukocytes and/or endothelial cells. Another enzyme, catalase, serves to detoxify the H_2O_2 that is generated from the dismutation of superoxide. Catalase is conveniently localized in peroxisomes, a major site of H_2O_2-producing enzymes (Fridovich, 1998). Glutathione peroxidase (GSH-Px) is another enzyme, involved in the detoxification of H_2O_2.

GSH-Px reduces H_2O_2 while oxidizing reduced glutathione (GSH) to its oxidized form, glutathione disulfide (GSSG):

$$\text{GSH-Px}$$
$$2GSH + H_2O_2 \rightarrow GSSG + 2H_2O$$

A selenocysteine is found at the active site of GSH-Px, which accounts for the close relationship between GSH-Px antioxidant potential and selenium bioavailability (Winklhofer-Roob, 1994). Transgenic mice that overexpress either Cu, ZnSOD, MnSOD, ECSOD, catalase, or GSH-Px are now available.

Metal Ion Sequesters

Iron and copper have unpaired electrons, which allow these metals to participate actively in ROS-mediated reactions. The majority of iron and copper within the body is sequestered, rather than free, which minimizes their ability to participate in oxidation-reduction reactions. Ceruloplasmin is a naturally occurring copper chelator. Whereas transferrin, lactoferrin, hemosiderin, hemoglobin, and ferritin are involved in the sequestration of iron. The antioxidative abilities of metal ion sequesters can be overridden in certain circumstances. For example, transferrin and lactoferrin release their bound iron when pH drops below 5.6 (transferrin) or 4.0 (lactoferrin), which might occur in the immediate vicinity of activated phagocytes (Morris et al., 1995) or in severely ischemic tissues. Furthermore, the O_2^- produced by inflammatory cells can release iron from ferritin (Nelson and McCord, 1998), which enables phagocytes to generate •OH via the Fenton reaction.

Scavenging Agents

Oxidation/reduction reactions often represent a chain of reactions, with each step producing another radical that may have either more or less reactivity than its predecessor. This chain-reaction can be broken if the oxidized molecule that is generated has extremely low reactivity. Agents that scavenge radicals can therefore prevent tissue damage that might result from further oxidation. Radical scavengers can be grouped into those that are water soluble, such as ascorbate and urate, and those that are lipid soluble, such as the tocopherols and carotenoids (Maxwell, 1995).

Inflammatory Actions of Oxygen Radicals

Radical-Mediated Production of Inflammatory Mediators

There is a large body of evidence indicating that ROS can elicit the formation of substances that attract and activate leukocytes to sites of inflammation. For example, oxidants can interact with specific components of extracellular fluid to generate substances that are chemotactic for neutrophils. It has been demonstrated that chemotactic activity is generated in plasma treated with an oxidant-generating system (hypoxanthine-xanthine oxidase), an effect that is attenuated by superoxide dismutase but not catalase. Injection of superoxide-treated plasma or hypoxathine-xanthine oxidase into the dermis induces massive neutrophil infiltration, effects that are blocked by superoxide dismutase (Granger and Korthuis, 1995).

Hydrogen peroxide can elicit the formation of chemoattactants in extracellular fluid. Normal human serum exposed to H_2O_2 concentrations as low as 70 µM (activated neutrophils can produce H_2O_2 concentrations that approach 300 µM) produces chemotactic activity for human neutrophils. The fact that the chemotactic activity of plasma exposed to H_2O_2 is reduced by the addition of antibodies directed against C5, coupled with the observation that the addition of purified C5 to H_2O_2 generates chemotactic activity, suggests that H_2O_2 generates a C5a-like chemotactic factor through hydrolysis of C5. The ability of H_2O_2 to activate complement and generate a chemotactic agent in plasma is enhanced by the presence of catalytically active iron (e.g., Fe EDTA, hemoglobin), suggesting that the process of complement activation is not brought about by H_2O_2 per se, but by an oxidant derived from H_2O_2 (Granger and Korthuis, 1995).

Exposure of endothelial cells to certain ROS (e.g., H_2O_2, organic hydroperoxides) can also elicit the formation of platelet-activating factor (PAF), a powerful phospholipid that can attract and activate leukocytes. McIntyre et al. (1997) have demonstrated that high concentrations (1 mM) of H_2O_2 can activate phospholipase A_2 (PLA_2), which in turn can catalyze the formation of lyso-PAF, a precursor for PAF biosynthesis. Because PLA_2 prefers phospholipids that have arachidonic acid at the 2-position, many cells that produce PAF also produce arachidonic acid metabolites. Neutrophils, for example, may synthesize both PAF and leukotriene B_4 (LTB_4) when activated. Hence, PLA_2 has the capacity to promote the formation of two potent lipid mediators of inflammation, PAF and LTB_4. Although H_2O_2 leads to rapid and prolonged biosynthesis of PAF by endothelial cells, the physiological relevance of the high H_2O_2 levels required to elicit PAF production remains unclear (Grisham et al., 1998).

Radical-Mediated Activation of Nuclear Transcription Factors

Binding sites for oxidant-sensitive nuclear transcription factors, such as nuclear factor kappa-B (NF-κB) and activation protein-1 (AP-1), have been identified in the promoter region of different cytokines (e.g., interleukin-8) and endothelial cell adhesion molecules. Hydrogen peroxide and oxidant stresses (e.g., anoxia–reoxygenation) have been shown to activate NF-κB and AP-1 in endothelial cell monolayers, and these responses are accompanied by a subsequent increase in the biosynthesis and surface expression of E-selectin and inter cellular adhesion molecule-1 (ICAM-1) (Panes and Granger, 1998). Similarly, antioxidants and iron chelators have been shown to prevent the activation of NF-κB (Grisham et al., 1998). This linkage among ROS, nuclear transcription factors, and the expression of endothelial cell adhesion molecules may explain reports that describe an attenuating action of vitamin E treatment on ischemia–reperfusion-induced up-regulation of E-selectin and ICAM-1 on vascular endothelial cells (Formigli et al., 1997).

Oxidants and Mobilization of Preformed Adhesion Molecules

In addition to stimulating the de novo synthesis of endothelial cell adhesion molecules such as E-selectin, vascular cell adhesion molecule-1 (VCAM-1), and ICAM-1, oxidants are capable of stimulating the mobilization of pre-formed pools of adhesion glycoproteins to the surface of both leukocytes and endothelial cells. For example, incubation of naive neutrophils with hydrogen peroxide or monochloramine (NH_2Cl) increases the expression of CD11b/CD18, which is normally stored in intracellular granules. The fusion of these granules with the cell membrane allows for the rapid (within minutes) surface expression of β_2 integrins, and a comparably rapid induction of leukocyte–endothelial cell adhesion. Endothelial cells also manifest a rapid mobilization of P-selectin to the cell surface after exposure to an oxidant stress (McIntyre et al., 1997; Panes and Granger, 1998). This adhesion molecule, which is normally stored in granules (Weibel–Palade bodies), fuses to the blood surface of endothelial cells during an oxidant stress, thereby allowing for leukocyte–endothelial cell adhesion. Both in vitro and in vivo experiments have provided support for an oxidant-dependent, rapid up-regulation of P-selectin on vascular endothelial cells. For example, exposure of mesenteric venules to a superoxide-generating system results in an enhanced recruitment of rolling leukocytes, which is prevented in animals receiving a P-selectin–specific monoclonal antibody. In addition, exposure of monolayers of cultured endothelial cells to anoxia–reoxygenation (A/R) results in the rapid surface expression of P-selectin, a response that is significantly blunted by catalase or allopurinol, suggesting that xanthine-oxidase–derived oxidants mediate the rapid P-selectin mobilization elicited by A/R (Panes and Granger, 1998).

Interactions Between Reactive Metabolites of Oxygen and Nitrogen

There are several lines of evidence that implicate superoxide as a mediator of leukocyte–endothelial cell adhesion: (a) exposure of cultured endothelial cells or venules to superoxide promotes leukocyte–endothelial cell adhesion: (b) intravenously administered superoxide dismutase (SOD) attenuates the leukocyte–endothelial cell adhesion in postcapillary venules exposed to ischemia–reperfusion or PAF; and (c) transgenic mice that overexpress Cu, Zn-SOD show a blunted leukocyte–endothelial cell adhesion response in terminal hepatic venules after ischemia–reperfusion. There are also studies that describe an anti-adhesion action of intravenously administered catalase, supporting the view that hydrogen peroxide is also a physiologic mediator of leukocyte adhesion (Granger and Kubes, 1994).

The mechanism(s) involved in superoxide-mediated leukocyte adherence remain unclear; however, it has been suggested that nitric oxide (NO) may contribute to this response. Nitric oxide, which reacts avidly with superoxide, is normally produced by vascular endothelium (see Chapter 22). Inhibition of nitric oxide production with analogues of L-arginine (e.g., L-NAME, L-NMMA) results in an intense leukocyte adherence response in mesenteric venules (Granger and Kubes, 1994), suggesting that nitric oxide is an endogenous inhibitor of leukocyte–endothelial cell adhesion. Consequently, one would predict that inflammatory conditions associated with an enhanced formation of superoxide (e.g., I/R) should lead to increased leukocyte adherence because of superoxide's ability to render nitric oxide biologically inactive. The contention that nitric oxide attenuates leukocyte–endothelial cell adhesion is supported by reports that demonstrate a reduced adhesion response to different inflammatory mediators following the administration of nitric oxide donors (Granger and Kubes, 1994; Grisham et al., 1998). Endothelial cell production of nitric oxide appears to fall following I/R, and agents that spontaneously release nitric oxide have been shown to attenuate the endothelial barrier dysfunction (increased vascular permeability) that is frequently associated with ischemia and reperfusion (Granger and Kubes, 1994; Grisham et al., 1998). Additional considerations regarding nitric oxide include: (a) the potential production of peroxynitrite and hydroxyl radical following its reaction with superoxide; and (b) its ability to nitrosylate protein sulfhydryls as part of various regulatory reactions.

Role of Oxygen Radicals in Ischemia–Reperfusion Injury

Ischemia followed by reperfusion (I/R) is a phenomenon that has been implicated in the pathogenesis of a number of disorders, including stroke, myocardial infarction, multiple organ failure, arthritis, and inflammatory bowel disease. The organ dysfunction that accompanies this condition is generally associated with increased microvascular permeability, interstitial edema, impaired vasoregulation, inflammatory cell infiltration, and parenchymal cell dysfunction and necrosis (Granger and Korthuis, 1995). Although several mechanisms have been invoked to explain I/R-induced inflammation and tissue injury, considerable attention has been devoted to the contribution of reactive oxygen species. The observation that the reintroduction of molecular oxygen at reperfusion is required to produce postischemic cellular injury and dysfunction is consistent with the view that I/R injury may be due to the generation of ROS. There are several direct lines of evidence that support a role of ROS in I/R injury: (a) the production of oxidant species in postischemic tissues has been detected using electron spin resonance (ESR) spectroscopy and ESR spin trapping; (b) an oxidant stress in endothelial cells of postcapillary venules has been demonstrated after I/R using oxidant-sensitive fluorochromes (e.g., dihydrorhodamine); (c) by-products of oxidant-induced lipid peroxidation (e.g., malondialdehyde, lipid hydroperoxides, and conjugated dienes) are formed in postischemic tissues; (d) structural and functional changes that closely mimic those noted in postischemic tissues can be induced by local administration of exogenous oxidant-generating systems (in the absence of ischemia and reperfusion), (e) treatment with agents that limit either the production (e.g., xanthine oxidase inhibitors such as allopurinol) or accumulation (e.g., superoxide dismutase, catalase) of ROS attenuates I/R-induced leukocyte infiltration and tissue injury; and (f) mice that genetically overexpress the gene for SOD exhibit attenuated inflammatory and injury responses to I/R (Granger, 1988; Grisham et al., 1998).

Studies of the small intestine indicate that there are two phases of oxygen radical production after I/R: an early rise that precedes the influx of activated-leukocytes, and a slower, more profound rise in oxygen radical production that parallels the accumulation of leukocytes (Granger, 1988). Inhibitors of xanthine oxidase (allopurinol, oxypurinol) are often effective in preventing or blunting the initial component of oxygen radical production in postischemic tissues (particularly in the splanchnic circulation) and in monolayers of cultured endothelial cells, whereas interventions directed at limiting the accumulation of leukocytes tend to blunt the later phase of oxygen radical production. Although there is evidence for two distinct phases of oxygen radical production in postischemic tissues, the two phases appear to be linked by inflammatory signals that are generated as a consequence of xanthine-oxidase–derived oxidants. It has been demonstrated that inhibitors of xanthine oxidase and different oxygen radical scavengers significantly attenuate the adhesion of leukocytes in postischemic microvessels and reduce the accumulation of neutrophils (assessed by myeloperoxidase determination) in postischemic tissues (Granger, 1988; Panes and Granger, 1998). These observations have led to the proposal that xanthine-oxidase–derived superoxide and/or hydrogen peroxide in the early postischemic period results in the generation of inflammatory mediators that initiate the recruitment and activation of neutrophils, which directly contribute to the microvascular dysfunction and parenchymal cell necrosis observed after I/R. Reagents that interfere specifically with the production of oxygen radicals or inflammatory mediators, or that suppress leukocyte recruitment and/or activation, suggest that the initial burst of oxygen radicals formed by xanthine oxidase plays a more important role in recruiting and activating blood cells, rather than acting as a direct mediator of I/R injury. Hence, the proposed linkage between xanthine-oxidase–derived oxidants, inflammatory mediators, and leukocytes provides a basis for the shared protective actions of a diverse assortment of reagents in some models of I/R injury.

Conclusions

Oxygen radicals appear to contribute to different steps in the genesis of an inflammatory response. Although the initial focus of research on oxygen radical involvement in inflammation was directed to the cytotoxic potential of these unstable molecules, recent evidence ascribes an equal or more important role to oxygen radicals as intracellular and transcellular signaling agents (Fig. 21.1). Oxygen radicals are capable of stimulating the production

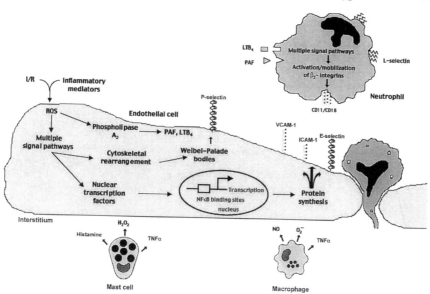

Fig. 21.1. Contributions of reactive oxygen species (ROS) to the endothelial responses to inflammation: ROS generation can be elicited by stimuli such as ischemia—reperfusion (I/R) and inflammatory mediators. The ROS can cause the activation of lipid mediators of inflammation such as platelet-activating factor (PAF) or leukotriene B_4 (LTB_4), which in turn can interact with receptors on neutrophils and produce leukocyte activation and adhesion molecule expression (e.g., β_2 integrins). ROS can also elicit the rearrangement of cytoskeletal elements in endothelial cells, resulting in the mobilization of storage granules for P-selectin (Weibel–Palade bodies) to the cell surface. The cell surface expression of P-selectin can sustain leukocyte rolling. ROS also can promote the activation of nuclear transcription factors (e.g., NF-κB) that bind to, and activate, the promoter region of genes for specific endothelial cell adhesion molecules (e.g., VCAM-1, E-selectin). The resultant enhancement of protein synthesis allows for a time-dependent expression of these adhesion molecules to the endothelial cell surface where they sustain the rolling and firm adhesion of leukocytes.

of inflammatory mediators (e.g., PAF, C5a, and LTB_4), which in turn can rapidly initiate the recruitment of leukocytes. In addition, oxygen radicals can help sustain inflammatory responses by activating transcription factors that promote the biosynthesis of endothelial cell adhesion molecules. Oxygen radicals are also likely to contribute to the increased vascular permeability and parenchymal cell dysfunction that often accompanies inflammation. Ischemia–reperfusion elicits an acute inflammatory response characterized by enhanced oxygen radical production and activation of neutrophils. Additional work is needed to define the contribution of oxygen radicals to other acute and chronic forms of inflammation.

References

Aruoma, O. I., Halliwell, B., and Dizdaroglu, M. (1989) Iron ion-dependent modification of bases in DNA by the superoxide radical generating system hypoxanthine/xanthine oxidase. *J. Biol. Chem.* 264:13024–13028.

Birnboim, H. C., and Kanabus-Kominska, M. (1987) The production of DNA strand breaks in human leukocytes by superoxide may involve a metabolic process. *Proc. Natl. Acad. Sci. USA* 82:6820–6824.

Formigli, L., Ibba Manneschi, L., Tani, A., Gandini, E., Adembri, C., Pratesi, C., Novelli, G. P., and Zecchi Orlandini, S. (1997) Vitamin E prevents neutrophil accumulation and attenuates tissue damage in ischemic-reperfused human skeletal muscle. *Histol. Histopathol.* 12:663–669.

Fridovich, I. (1998) An overview of oxyradicals in medical biology. In: *Oxyradicals in Molecular Biology.* J. M. McCord, ed. Greenwich, CT: JAI Press, pp. 1–14.

Granger, D. N. (1988) Role of xanthine oxidase and granulocytes in ischemia–reperfusion injury. *Am. J. Physiol.* 255:H1269–H1275.

Granger, D. N., and Kubes, P. (1994) The microcirculation and inflammation: modulation of leukocyte–endothelial cell adhesion. *J. Leukoc. Biol.* 55:662–675.

Granger, D. N., and Korthuis, R. J. (1995) Physiological mechanisms of postischemic tissue injury. *Annu. Rev. Physiol.* 57:311–332.

Grisham, M. B., Granger, D. N., and Lefer, D. J. (1998) Modulation of leukocyte–endothelial interactions by reactive metabolites of oxygen and nitrogen: Relevance to ischemic heart disease. *Free Rad. Biol. Med.* 25:404–433.

Kehrer, J. P. (1993) Free radicals as mediators of tissue injury and disease. *Crit. Rev. Toxicol.* 23: 21–48.

Maxwell, S.R.J. (1995) Prospects for the use of antioxidant therapies. *Drugs* 49:345–361.

McIntyre, T. M., Modur, V., Prescott, S. M., and Zimmerman, G. A. (1997) Molecular mechanisms of early inflammation. *Thromb. Haemost.* 78:302–305.

Morris, C. J., Earl, J. R., Trenam, C. W., and Blake, D. R. (1995) Reactive oxygen species and iron—a dangerous partnership in inflammation. *Int. J. Biochem. Cell. Biol.* 27:109–122.

Nelson, S. K., and McCord, J. M. (1998) Iron, oxygen radicals, and disease. In: *Oxyradicals in Molecular Biology.* J. M. McCord, ed. Greenwich, CT: JAI Press, pp. 157–183.

Panes, J., and Granger, D. N. (1998) Leukocyte–endothelial cell interactions: Molecular mechanisms and implications in gastrointestinal disease. *Gastroenterol.* 114:1066–1090.

Winklhofer-Roob, B. M. (1994) Oxygen free radicals and antioxidants in cystic fibrosis: the concept of an oxidant–antioxidant imbalance. *Acta Paediatr. Suppl.* 395:49–57.

22

Nitric Oxide in Inflammation

ALLAN M. LEFER and ROSARIO SCALIA

Overview of Nitric Oxide

Biosynthesis of Nitric Oxide

During the past few years, an enormous amount of research has been conducted on the vascular L-arginine/nitric oxide (NO) system. Alterations of NO production and/or bioavailability have been shown to occur both in experimental animal models (Osborne et al., 1989b; Tsao et al., 1990; Gauthier et al., 1995; Scalia et al., 1996) and in humans (Chester et al., 1990; Boger et al., 1997) in diverse settings such as hypertension, hypercholesterolemia, diabetes, ischemia–reperfusion, and heart failure.

Nitric oxide is synthesized by an enzyme termed *nitric oxide synthase* (NOS) that exists in three isoforms: endothelial NOS (eNOS), neural NOS (nNOS), and inducible NOS (iNOS). All three isoforms of NOS convert the semiessential amino acid L-arginine to L-citrulline, thereby releasing NO (Moncada et al., 1991). Calcium-calmodulin and tetrahydrobiopterin are essential cofactors in this reaction (Gross and Levi, 1992; Klatt et al., 1995; Su et al., 1995). The substrate for NOS is the basic amino acid L-arginine, with a K_m (Michaelis constant) of approximately 5 μmol/L (Venema et al., 1996). L-arginine is synthesized as a product of the urea cycle and circulates in the blood in concentrations nearly equal to 100 μmol/L (Boger et al., 1997). In endothelial cells, however, the concentration of L-arginine has been estimated to be in the several hundred micromolar to the low millimolar range (Arnal et al., 1995). L-arginine is actively transported into the endothelium (Bogle et al., 1996) through a process subject to regulation by cytokines (Cendan et al., 1995). Even in the absence of extracellular L-arginine, the endothelium can resynthesize this amino acid from L-citrulline by using a recently described novel biosynthetic pathway (Hecker et al., 1995). Binding of calmodulin to eNOS and nNOS appears to act as a "molecular switch" to enable electron flow from flavin prosthetic groups in the NADPH reductase to heme, thereby facilitating the conversion of O_2 and L-arginine to NO and L-citrulline (Su et al., 1995). Calmodulin is incorporated into the molecular structure of iNOS.

Tetrahydrobiopterin is a critical cofactor for NOS and appears to contribute to the ability of the enzyme to bind L-arginine. Interestingly, in the absence of tetrahydrobiopterin, the enzyme transfers electrons to molecular oxygen to produce the superoxide anion (Pou et al., 1992). Although several studies have suggested that levels of L-arginine, L-citrulline, and tetrahydrobiopterin may be deficient in acute and chronic inflammatory states (Cooke et al., 1992; Pieper, 1997; Stroes et al., 1997), future work to examine the manner in which various disease states affect the biosynthesis of NO is needed.

Physiological Versus Supraphysiological Concentrations of Nitric Oxide

Considerable research has focused on the physiological, biochemical, and molecular actions of NO in normal physiological processes and during pathological conditions. At low nanomolar concentrations, NO is cytoprotective in a number of experimental vascular diseases including ischemia–reperfusion injury (Aoki et al., 1990; Johnson et al., 1991; Siegfried et al., 1992a; Pabla et al., 1996), respiratory distress syndromes (Rossaint et al., 1993), intimal hyperplasia associated with vessel injury (Guo et al., 1995), atherosclerosis (Cooke et al., 1992), and vascular thrombosis (Groves et al., 1993). However, other experimental studies have suggested that high micromolar concentrations of NO are cytotoxic and contribute to cell injury in a variety of disease states including disorders of the lung (Wizemann et al., 1994), endotoxic and hypovolemic shock states (Nava et al., 1991), ischemia–reperfusion injury (Schulz and Wambolt, 1995), and anoxia–reoxygenation injury (De May and Vanhoutte, 1983). These cytotoxic effects of NO have been attributed mainly to the inducible form of NOS (iNOS), which is normally inactive, but can be induced by a variety of cytokines and other pathophysiologic agents including bacterial lipopolysaccharide (LPS) endotoxin (Cunha et al., 1994). Over a period of marked cytokine stimulation (i.e., 6–24 hours following stimulation of iNOS), suprapharmacologic concentrations of NO potentially may be produced, which are thought to contribute to cell and tissue injury (Robbins et al., 1994). More recently, it has been suggested that the purported toxic effects of NO are a result of the formation of a free radical species formed through the interaction between NO and superoxide, which has been reported to be peroxynitrite ($ONOO^-$; Pryor and Squadrito, 1995).

Biological Effects of Nitric Oxide

Nitric oxide is a gas [molecular mass, 30 daltons (D)] that is highly soluble in lipids and thus readily diffuses across cell membranes (Ignarro et al., 1987). Nitric oxide has a half-life of only 10 to 20 seconds in physiologic media, including blood (Palmer et al., 1987; Moncada et al., 1989). The vascular endothelium produces nitric oxide, which is basally released at concentrations of about 2 to 20 nmol/L. This nitric oxide diffuses to the subjacent vascular smooth muscle where it regulates vascular tone. However, the endothelium-derived NO also diffuses to the luminal surface of the endothe-

Table 22.1. Important Effects of Physiological Concentrations of Nitric Oxide

Preserves endothelial integrity

Dilates arterial blood vessels, participates in autoregulation of blood flow to vital organs

Inhibits leukocyte–endothelium interaction by suppressing expression of cell adhesion molecules

Inhibits platelet adherence and aggregation

Prevents microvascular fluid leakage

Maintains renal glomerular function

Promotes endothelial regeneration following injury

Inhibits vascular smooth muscle cell proliferation

No significant effects on myocardial contractility

lium where it exerts a number of important physiological effects (Table 22.1) including: (a) scavenging of superoxide radicals (Gryglewski et al., 1986; Rubanyi and Vanhoutte, 1986); (b) inhibition of platelet adherence and aggregation (Radomski et al., 1987a, 1990); (c) modulation of endothelial layer permeability (Kubes and Granger, 1992); and (d) attenuation of leukocyte–endothelium interaction (Kubes et al., 1991; Davenpeck et al., 1994a).

Against this backdrop of important effects of physiological concentrations of NO, effective NO levels are decreased in a variety of circulatory disorders, including myocardial ischemia–reperfusion (Tsao and Lefer, 1990; Pearl et al., 1994), circulatory shock and trauma (Lefer and Lefer, 1993; Scalia et al., 1996), hypercholesterolemia and atherosclerosis (Freiman et al., 1986; Osborne et al., 1989a). The decrease in nitric oxide levels occurs in the early stages of hypercholesterolemia before the development of atherosclerotic plaques (Freiman et al., 1986; Lefer and Ma, 1993; Scalia et al., 1998), and is clearly due to reduced basal release of NO (Lefer and Ma, 1993) in addition to diminished agonist-mediated NO release. It is therefore not surprising that replacement therapy to restore the NO deficit has been considered in several of these disease states.

Nitric Oxide Synthases

Nitric oxide is synthesized in mammalian cells by a family of three NO synthases (NOS; Moncada and Palmer, 1991). It is not known whether additional mammalian NOS isoforms exist, but the failure of homology-based molecular cloning approaches to identify novel NOS cDNA makes it unlikely that newly discovered members of the mammalian NOS gene family will bear significant structural similarity to the current trio of isoforms. A widely accepted nomenclature, which will be used in this chapter, identifies the three mammalian enzyme isoforms as nNOS, iNOS, and eNOS, reflecting the cell of origin for the original protein and cDNA isolates (Moncada et al., 1997). The human genes for the NOS isoforms are categorized in order of their isolation and characterization. Thus, the human genes encoding nNOS, iNOS, and

Table 22.2. Isoforms of Nitric Oxide Synthase (NOS)

Isoform	Regulation	Molecular Mass	Tissue/Cell
I (nNOS)	Ca²⁺-calmodulin	160 000	Brain Skeletal muscle
II (iNOS)	Unknown, inducible by cytokines	130 000	Macrophages Vascular smooth muscle Cardiac myocytes Glial cells
III (eNOS)	Ca²⁺-calmodulin	135 000	Endothelial cells Platelets Cardiac myocytes

eNOS are termed *NOS 1, NOS 2,* and *NOS 3,* respectively. Table 22.2 summarizes the main characteristics and tissue distribution for the three isoforms of NOS.

The eNOS and nNOS forms of the enzyme are important physiologically in maintaining a variety of homeostatic responses. The nNOS isoform of the enzyme is important as a neurotransmitter in the gastrointestinal tract (e.g., gastric emptying, defecation) and in central nervous system integration. The iNOS isoform of the enzyme is normally inactive, or functioning at low levels of expression, but can be induced by a variety of cytokines and bacterial endotoxin. However, the same NOS isoform may play entirely distinct biological roles when expressed in different tissues, and must not be assumed that pathways outlined in one tissue necessarily pertain when the same isoform is expressed in a different cell. For example, differential tissue-specific splicing of nNOS mRNA generates structurally distinct protein molecules when the enzyme is expressed in neurons versus skeletal muscle (Silvagno et al., 1996).

Physiological Roles of Nitric Oxide Relevant to Inflammation

Injury or activation of the endothelium changes its regulatory functions and results in abnormal endothelial function. The dysfunction of the endothelium has been functionally defined as an imbalance between relaxing and contracting factors, between procoagulant and anticoagulant mediators, or growth-inhibiting and growth-promoting substances. The endothelium undergoes phenotypic modulation in response to injury or activation. A role of the endothelial cells in cardiovascular diseases might then be dependent on these phenotypic alterations, rather then on actual damage per se.

One of the important early events in the pathophysiology of endothelial dysfunction is the loss of ability to release endothelium-derived NO (Lefer et al., 1991). There are several varieties of acute and chronic circulatory diseases that produce a marked degree of endothelial dysfunction characterized by a significant reduction of endothelium-derived NO. These include ische-mia–reperfusion of heart, kidney, splanchnic organs, and brain, in which a rapid increase in oxygen-derived free radicals is a major factor contributing to loss of effective concentrations of NO over a period of about 2.5 to 5 minutes (Tsao and Lefer, 1990; Tsao et al., 1990). Hemorrhage and traumatic shock also result in reduced NO within 5 minutes (Scalia et al., 1996), whereas congestive heart failure, atherosclerosis, and hypertension produce a gradual loss of NO over a period of weeks or months (Cohen et al., 1988; Freiman et al., 1996).

Effects on Vascular Smooth Muscle

Nitric oxide produced by the vascular endothelium regulates vascular tone by relaxing vascular smooth muscle cells (Furchgott and Vanhoutte, 1989). This effect of NO was shown to be inhibited by hemoglobin, methylene blue, and other agents such as dithiothreitol and hydroquinone and to be medi-ated by stimulation of guanylate cyclase with the consequent elevation of intracellular cyclic guanosine monophosphate (cGMP; Moncada et al., 1991). Endothelium-dependent relaxation, which has been shown in many vascular preparations, including veins, arteries, and microvessels, occurs in response to a variety of humoral agents, such as acetylcholine, adenine nucleotides, thrombin, substance P, the calcium ionophore A23187, and bradykinin (Moncada et al., 1991). Other stimuli such as hypoxia, increase in flow, and electrical stimulation, can also cause endothelium-dependent relaxation of vascular tissue in vitro. It has been extensively demonstrated that a contin-uous release of NO maintains dilator tone, thus regulating systemic blood pressure and endothelial function (Moncada et al., 1991). It is likely that NO-dependent vasodilator tone is locally regulated and, as such, is one of the simplest and yet most fundamental adaptive mechanisms in the cardiovas-cular system. Therefore, it is possible that the loss of NO-mediated vasodilator tone is at least as important in essential hypertension, atherosclerosis, and in vasospastic phenomenona as those observed in the irreversible phases of cir-culatory shock.

Inotropic Actions on Cardiac Muscle

Over the past 5 years, the explosion of reports on the role of nitric oxide in the regulation of cardiac energetics has generated much discussion. As in the case of vascular physiology and biology, the discovery and characteriza-tion of myocardial NO-dependent signaling pathways have clarified many aspects of specific signal transduction cascades in cardiac muscle while gen-erating apparent paradoxes and new hypotheses to be tested.

A number of cellular constituents of cardiac muscle can express iNOS in response to LPS and specific cytokines, including the endothelium and smooth muscle of the cardiac microvasculature, the endocardial endothe-lium, tissue macrophages, and cardiac myocytes (Kelly et al., 1996). However, the physiological roles and pathophysiological consequences following induction of this high-output NOS in these cells are less clear. The most convincing evidence for an important pathophysiological role for iNOS to date has come from experimental animal models of systemic inflammatory response syndrome (Ungureanu-Longrois et al., 1995) and cardiac allograft transplantation (Worrall et al., 1996). However, Thoenes et al. (1996) could find no evidence of increased iNOS expression in patients with heart failure from specimens obtained postmortem, although iNOS was present in the hearts of most of the patients who succumbed to systemic sepsis.

Because of this limited availability of information, much of our understanding of the inotropic effects of NO on cardiac myocytes is based on actions of pharmacological NO donors or agents that mimic some actions of cGMP. Nitric oxide donors do not appear to exert any significant effect on myocardial contractility up to and including rather high concentrations. Only when cardiac muscle is stimulated with β-adrenergic agents, do nitric oxide donors exert a negative inotropic effect, and that is small, averaging only 5%–7% decrease from control values (Brady et al., 1992; Balligand et al., 1993). Nitric oxide donors fail to exert a significant negative inotropic effect in isolated cardiac myocytes, or in isolated ventricular papillary muscles even at concentrations far above those that result in maximal vasorelaxation of vascular rings isolated from the same animal (i.e., 500 nmol; Weyrich et al., 1994). Nitric oxide donors also fail to induce a significant inotropic effect even in the intact animal (Pennington et al., 1979; Lefer et al., 1993; Crystal, and Gurevicius, 1996). Moreover, NOS inhibitors exacerbate the cardiodepression observed in dogs subjected to cardiac stunning (Hasebe et al., 1993). These and other data using authentic NO gas in isolated cardiac preparations fail to show a significant direct cardiodepressant effect of NO. This is not surprising because the high myoglobin levels in cardiac myocytes sequester the NO before it is able to exert any significant inotropic effect on the heart.

Effects on Leukocyte–Endothelium Interaction

Effective NO levels are decreased in a variety of acute inflammatory disorders of the cardiovascular system, including myocardial ischemia–reperfusion, circulatory shock, trauma, hypercholesterolemia, and atherosclerosis. Under these conditions, circulating leukocytes marginate, adhere to the microvascular endothelium, and emigrate through the endothelial monolayer where many of them infiltrate into the interstitial space, and migrate toward the source of inflammation (Fig. 22.1).

The first clear demonstration that nitric oxide can regulate leukocyte–endothelium interaction is the now classic study of Kubes et al. (1991), who showed that NOS inhibition enhanced leukocyte adherence to the mesenteric vascular endothelium in the cat, which could be blocked by a monoclonal antibody directed against the β₂ integrins. This was a seminal finding that pointed toward nitric oxide deficiency as being important in the pathophysiology of inflammation. Further studies demonstrated that this inhibitory effect on leukocyte behavior by NO has several components. First, nitric

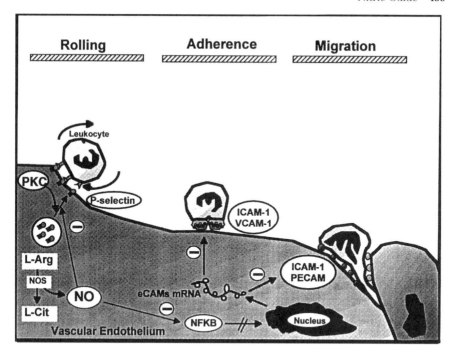

Fig. 22.1. Neutrophil–endothelial cell interactions in the microvasculature: Under normal conditions nitric oxide (NO) generated from L-arginine within the endothelial cell controls leukocyte rolling, adherence, and transmigration, thus protecting against inflammatory insult. Physiological NO levels in the endothelium modulate expression of cell adhesion molecules and the nuclear transcription factor (NF-κB); activation of NF-κB results in increased surface expression of endothelial cell adhesion molecules (eCAMs). Increased expression of P-selectin (P-sel) on the endothelial cell surface promotes PMN rolling via its high affinity P-selectin glycoprotein ligand-1 (PSGL-1) on the neutrophil (PMN) surface. Increased intercellular adhesion molecule-1 (ICAM-1) and vascular cell adhesion molecule-1 (VCAM-1) expression regulates firm adhesion. Finally, ICAM-1 and PCAM permits PMN transmigration across the vascular endothelium (PKC = protein kinase C; L-Arg-L-arginine; L-Cit = L-citrulline).

oxide markedly attenuates leukocyte rolling along the endothelium by inhibiting the expression of P-selectin on the vascular endothelium (Davenpeck et al., 1994b). Second, nitric oxide inhibits the firm adherence of leukocytes to the endothelium (Gauthier et al., 1994, 1995), partially by inhibition of ICAM-1 and VCAM-1 expression (De Caterina et al., 1995). Down-regulation of these cell adhesion molecules by NO occurs through inhibition of protein kinase C activation (Murohara et al., 1996) and by prevention of activation of the nuclear transcription factor NF-κB (De Caterina et al., 1995), which usually induces expression of the mRNA for these adhesion molecules. Third, NO inhibits leukocyte action by inhibiting the cytoassembly of NADPH oxidase (Clancy et al., 1992), thereby attenuating the release of superoxide radicals by activated leukocytes, particularly granulocytes (Moilanen et al., 1993).

The initial step in leukocyte recruitment during the inflammatory response is leukocyte rolling along the endothelium of postcapillary venules (Fig. 22.1). Leukocyte rolling is largely mediated by P-selectin, a member of the selectin family of adhesion glycoproteins. P-selectin is believed to be one of the earliest endothelial cell adhesion molecules involved in leukocyte recruitment to the site of inflammation. Davenpeck et al. (1994b) extensively studied the interrelationship between NO and P-selectin and its correlation to ischemia–reperfusion phenomena. They demonstrated that ischemia–reperfusion of the mesenteric circulation, a condition that has been shown to reduce dramatically endothelial NO, resulted in a rapid increase in leukocyte rolling and adherence to the venular endothelium within the first 30 minutes following reperfusion. This clearly indicates that the critical reduction in NO release 30 minutes after reperfusion is correlated with an increased upregulation of P-selectin on the endothelium (Davenpeck et al., 1994b). Moreover, Gauthier et al. (1994) showed that in the same model of ischemia–reperfusion of the rat mesenteric circulation, infusion of a nitric oxide donor markedly attenuated postreperfusion rolling and adherence of leukocytes to the venular endothelium. This clearly demonstrated that restoration of physiological NO levels in the systemic circulation during microcirculatory perturbations results in a reduced leukocyte–endothelial cell interaction with amelioration of the associated circulatory shock. In order to investigate this interrelationship between NO and adhesion molecules further, Davenpeck et al. (1994b) also showed that exposure of the rat mesenteric microvasculature to NOS inhibitors mimics many of the effects of ischemia–reperfusion; the main results from that study are depicted in Figure 22.2. The number of adherent leukocytes in the microvasculature is very low during normal physiological conditions. However, exposure of the rat mesentery to increasing concentrations of L-N^G-nitroarginine methyl ester (L-NAME) resulted in a consistent and concentration-dependent increase in leukocyte adherence. Equimolar concentrations of L-arginine, but not D-arginine, were able to overcome L-NAME–induced leukocyte adherence, thus suggesting the specific NO-mediated mechanism of L-NAME–induced leukocyte–endothelium interaction. In this regard, leukocyte adherence could be completely abolished by administration of a monoclonal antibody directed against P-selectin. Furthermore, immunohistochemical localization of P-selectin was upregulated in the rat mesenteric microvasculature following direct inhibition of NO synthase by L-NAME, confirming the important interaction between P-selectin and nitric oxide.

Similar results were obtained with leukocyte adherence. The expression of immunoglobulin superfamily members (i.e., intercellular adhesion molecule-1, or ICAM-1 and vascular cell adhesion molecule-1, or VCAM-1) on the microvascular endothelium has been recently correlated to inhibition of nitric oxide synthesis and release from endothelial cells during hypercholesterolemia (Scalia et al., 1998), and in experimental models of inflammation

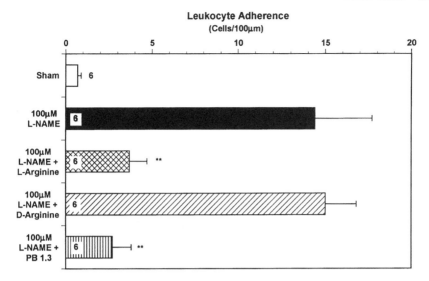

Fig. 22.2. L-NAME–induced inhibition of nitric oxide synthase increases leukocyte adherence along the venular endothelium of the rat mesenteric microcirculation. This phenomenon was inhibited by equimolar concentration of L-arginine and was also blocked by the systemic administration of an antibody against P-selectin (PB 1.3). Therefore, loss of endogenous nitric oxide release up-regulates leukocyte adherence, the prelude to leukocyte infiltration into inflamed tissues (from Davenpeck et al., 1994b).

induced by superfusion of the rat mesentery with either L-NAME, thrombin, or hydrogen peroxide (Scalia et al., 1997; Scalia and Lefer, 1998). In particular, ICAM-1 expression on endothelial cells was found to be up-regulated during induction of hypercholesterolemia in animals fed a high cholesterol diet (Gauthier et al., 1995; Scalia et al., 1998). More recently, nitric oxide was also found to be able to reduce cytokine-induced expression of another cell adhesion molecule characteristic of endothelial activation during atherogenesis (i.e., VCAM-1; De Caterina et al., 1995). Nevertheless, in chronic gastrointestinal inflammatory states, high concentrations of NO may be pro-inflammatory by being converted to nitrogen dioxide (NO_2) or nitrogen trioxide (N_2O_3; Miller and Sandoval, 1999).

Adhered leukocytes exit the microcirculation and emigrate into the extravascular space (Fig. 22.1). The process of extravasation requires a complex interaction between leukocyte adherence glycoproteins and their counter-receptors on the venular endothelial cells in response to chemotactic stimuli present within inflamed tissues. This process has also been shown to be modulated by NO released by the vascular endothelium, as confirmed by the increase in extravasated leukocytes in mesenteric tissue of L-NAME–superfused rat mesenteries (Scalia and Lefer, 1998).

Finally, selective gene deletion has been accomplished for all three isoforms of NOS (see Table 22.2). Recently, microvascular responses to thrombin stimulation have been studied in eNOS and nNOS gene-deleted mice (Lefer et al., 1999). Both eNOS and nNOS gene-deleted mice showed marked increases in both leukocyte rolling and adherence in thrombin-stimulated mouse peri-intestinal venules. These increased leukocyte–endothelium interactions were on the order of three to seven-fold, and were in large part due to up-regulation of P-selectin on the venular endothelium.

These findings, taken together, clearly point to a dynamic interaction between endothelium-derived nitric oxide and leukocyte–endothelial cell interaction in vivo. Reduced nitric oxide release from the microvascular endothelium, during abnormal pathological conditions, leads to increased adhesion molecule expression on the endothelial cell surface. This phenomenon plays a significant role in the margination and emigration of leukocytes from the blood stream and their subsequent accumulation into injured tissues.

Antiplatelet Effects of Nitric Oxide

One important anti-inflammatory property of NO is inhibition of platelet aggregation (Radomski et al., 1987a). NO inhibits platelet aggregation via a cGMP-dependent mechanism (Mellion et al., 1981). Together with prostacyclin, NO inhibits platelet aggregation and disaggregates platelets, suggesting that the release of NO by the vascular endothelium plays an important homeostatic role by maintaining thromboresistance of the endothelium.

In addition, NO inhibits platelet adhesion to collagen fibrils, endothelial cell matrix, and endothelial cell monolayers (Radomski et al., 1987b, 1987c). In contrast, prostacyclin has only a weak inhibitory effect on platelet adhesion (Higgs et al., 1978). This suggests a key role for NO in the process of platelet adhesion and repair of the vessel wall during physiological and pathophysiological conditions. In this regard, a recent study has reported that treatment of isolated platelets with nitric oxide donors attenuates expression of P-selectin induced by activation of protein kinase C (Murohara et al., 1996). Thus, NO exerts antiplatelet functions by both blocking platelet aggregation and inhibiting P-selectin expression on the platelet cell surface.

Nitric Oxide and Transcription Factors

Although it is clear that nitric oxide exerts significant anti-inflammatory effects in the intestinal microvasculature and epithelium, the precise mechanisms of these effects are not fully elucidated. The up-regulation of E-selectin, ICAM-1, and VCAM-1 in endothelial cells requires de novo synthesis of proteins, and therefore requires about 2 hours. De Caterina et al. (1995) recently showed that, in cytokine-stimulated human saphenous vein endothelial cells, several NO donors inhibit VCAM-1 expression by 35%–55%, and also reduce E-selectin and ICAM-1 expressions to a lesser extent under similar conditions. In the case of VCAM-1, nitric oxide attenuated VCAM-1 gene transcription, in part, by inhibiting NF-κB.

In cultured human endothelial cells, L-NAME markedly up-regulated P-selectin mRNA and protein expression (Armstead et al., 1997b), which led to significantly increased leukocyte adherence to cultured human endothelial monolayers. Moreover, this up-regulation of P-selectin could be reversed by co-incubation with the nitric oxide donor, SPM-5185 (Armstead et al., 1997b), but not by its non-NO donating control compound lacking the NO moiety. One of the messengers in the up-regulation of P-selectin, and other endothelial cell adhesion molecules in some species is NF-κB (De Caterina et al., 1995). Recently, NF-κB up-regulation (i.e., binding of a P-selectin–specific NF-κB element to nuclear extracts) was found in organs of rats subjected to traumatic shock (Armstead et al., 1997a). The mechanism of this enhanced P-selectin mRNA appears to relate to IκB-α promoter activity (Spiecker et al., 1998) because nitric oxide donors reduced endothelial cell adhesion molecule expression up to 70% through induction of IκB-α promoter activity. IκB-α is a functional inhibitor of NF-κB, and thus effectively diminishes P-selectin and other adhesion molecules' (e.g., ICAM-1) adhesive action on endothelial cells.

Actions of Supraphysiologic Concentrations of Nitric Oxide

Although NO exerts a variety of important homeostatic effects at nanomolar concentrations, NO is purported to exert cytotoxic effects at high concentrations (i.e., in the high micromolar range). These effects are somewhat controversial because it is not clear whether (a) these concentrations can ever occur in vivo, (b) all of these cytotoxic effects are detrimental to the host organism, and (c) the data pointing to cytotoxic effects of NO really are direct effects of NO, or are due to the actions of other substances. We will review the salient features of this area relevant to the role of NO in inflammation.

Antimicrobial Actions of Nitric Oxide

Nitric oxide was originally discovered in biological systems from two very different directions. The first insight was as an endothelium-derived relaxing factor (EDRF) by pharmacologists (Furchgott and Zawadski, 1990). However, in a parallel manner, NO was discovered by microbiologists as an endogenous bactericidal agent (Hibbs, 1991; Nathan and Hibbs, 1991). Thus, NO released by certain lymphocytes and macrophages can act as an anti-infective agent by killing invading bacteria. This works very well in murine leukocytes, but human leukocytes produce much lower levels of NO, which puts in doubt the clinical relevance of this mechanism in humans (Denis, 1991). The antimicrobial effects of NO appear to include a variety of viruses as well as bacteria and fungi (Mannick et al., 1994). In this case, both latent and lytic viruses, normally suppressed by endogenous NO, can reactivate and reinfect when NO synthesis is inhibited by conventional NOS inhibitors (i.e., L-NMMA). This raises an important question regarding the clinical usefulness of NOS inhibitors in situations like septic shock.

Potential Role of Nitric Oxide in Septic or Endotoxic Shock

The potential role of NO in endotoxemic or septic shock has been, and continues to be, controversial. Bacterial endotoxin is known to stimulate iNOS in vascular smooth muscle cells and in macrophages, generating large amounts of NO (Shears and Billiar, 1995). Whether these high levels actually occur in vivo is problematic and unproven at present. In fact, there is abundant evidence that vascular NO levels assessed by measuring endothelium-derived nitric oxide is uniformly reduced following endotoxemic shock (Lefer, 1998). If nitric oxide levels markedly increase in endotoxemic or septic shock, they would have to be elevated by three or four orders of magnitude in order to induce shock. It is highly unlikely that localized NO would spill over into the circulation, an event that is a prerequisite for the propagation of the hypotension occurring in septic shock (Lefer, 1998).

One of the main pillars of the hypothesis that NO is a key mediator of endotoxic or septic shock is that inhibition of nitric oxide synthases is beneficial in these forms of shock states. This topic has received considerable attention by many investigators since the provocative report of Petros et al. in 1991. That group treated two patients in septic shock with an NOS inhibitor. Of the two shock patients receiving L-NMMA, one lived and one died, rendering this study rather inconclusive because the usual mortality rate of septic shock is about 50%. Kilbourn and Griffith (1992) advanced the hypothesis that inhibition of NOS is a potentially important treatment in endotoxemic or septic shock, although others (Wright et al., 1992) have cautioned that inhibition of both constitutive and inducible NOS during endotoxemia may be undesirable.

Cobb and Danner (1996) reviewed the endotoxic shock literature related to the effects of NOS inhibitors on hemodynamics and survival in large animals and humans; of the 26 animal and 4 human studies, only 5 actually measured survival (i.e., dog and pig studies). Two of those studies showed that NOS inhibitors actually reduced survival and 3 showed no change in survival rates. Furthermore, deleterious effects of NOS inhibitors were found to contribute to increased mortality in endotoxemic rabbits (Pastor et al., 1994) and endotoxemic mice (Minnard et al., 1994). NOS inhibitors have deleterious hemodynamic effects in several species including dogs, sheep, pigs, and humans (Cobb and Danner, 1996). This relates to the vasoconstrictor effect of NOS inhibitors; of the 28 studies in which systemic vascular resistance was measured, 26 reported a marked increase in vascular resistance and 2 found no change (Cobbs and Danner, 1996). Coupled with cardiac output measurements in 29 studies, 22 showed a significant decrease and 7 exhibited no change in cardiac output during endotoxic shock. An increase in cardiac output—an essential compensatory response in circulatory shock states like endotoxemic shock—has never been observed following administration of a NOS inhibitor.

These latter findings suggest that by shutting off endogenous production of NO by the endothelium, one causes marked vasoconstriction, increasing arterial blood pressure at the expense of blood flow. NOS inhibitors also aggravate pulmonary hypertension and reduce oxygen delivery to the tissues. It is clear that circulatory shock is a consequence of a sustained and marked reduction in blood flow to the vital organs, which if not reversed, usually leads to cardiovascular collapse (i.e., circulatory shock) and eventually to death (Lefer, 1994). Thus, reducing cardiac output even further with NOS inhibitors is counterproductive in endotoxemic and other forms of circulatory shock.

As a further cautionary note, recent studies have shown that in iNOS-deficient mice, there is a significantly enhanced leukocyte–endothelium interaction that promotes local tissue inflammation (Hickey et al., 1997). This is consistent with the report that iNOS exerts vasculoprotective effects in the coronary circulation of pigs (Fukumoto et al., 1997). Thus, the increase in iNOS activity in sepsis may actually be a compensatory effect due to the decrease in eNOS activity.

In summary, there is reasonable doubt that NOS inhibition can significantly protect in endotoxic shock. Moreover, it is very difficult to obtain a selective iNOS inhibitor that does not also inhibit eNOS. The selectivity is blurred at doses that are necessary to dramatically inhibit iNOS. In fact, a recent class of "selective" iNOS inhibitors was found to be cardiotoxic and had to be discontinued as potential drug candidates (Southan et al., 1995). Moreover, when NOS inhibitors block nitric oxide production, they also expose the host to latent virus infections that can be extremely dangerous (Mannick et al., 1994) because nitric oxide functions normally to attenuate viral infections.

Peroxynitrite as a Toxic Mediator of Nitric Oxide Effects

Nitric oxide and superoxide radicals can interact to form the highly reactive species, peroxynitrite (ONOO$^-$; Radi et al., 1991; Pryor and Squadrito, 1995), which is reported to be cytotoxic at high concentrations (Radi et al., 1991). Peroxynitrite has been invoked as a mediator of myocardial and parenchymal cell injury resulting from ischemia–reperfusion or shock states (Szabo et al., 1995; Yasmin et al., 1997). These investigators found that concentrations of 30–100 μmol ONOO$^-$ cause myocardial injury in isolated perfused rat hearts subjected to ischemia–reperfusion, and that nitrotyrosine, a purported "footprint" of peroxynitrite, is detectable in these rat hearts as evidence of the presence of peroxynitrite.

There are several serious problems with accepting peroxynitrite as a major mediator of inflammatory states like reperfusion injury. First, circulating concentrations of NO are normally 1–10 nmol/L (Kelm and Schrader, 1990), and ONOO$^-$ levels, even at maximal iNOS activation, are only in the low micromolar range (i.e., 0.4–5.0 µmol; Grisham et al., 1998). These findings, coupled with the ultrashort half-life of ONOO$^-$ (< 1 second) make it highly unlikely that ONOO$^-$ occurs in vivo at concentrations above 1–2 µmol. In fact, when measured by electron spin resonance (ESR) techniques, peroxynitrite levels in the ischemic–reperfused rat heart were only 100 nmol (Wang et al., 1996). Second, NO and superoxide form peroxynitrite only when they both exist in close proximity at equimolar concentrations. When there is a significant imbalance between these two reactants, the excess reactant exerts a feedback inhibition that curtails ONOO$^-$ formation (Miles et al., 1996). Moreover, one cannot measure authentic peroxynitrite in vivo. One must resort to immunohistochemical measurement of the so-called footprint of ONOO$^-$, nitrotyrosine. Unfortunately, nitrotyrosine can be formed from a variety of substances other than ONOO$^-$, including chloride ions, hypochlorous acid, myeloperoxidase, and other nitrogenous radicals (Eiserich et al., 1996, 1998). Even more troubling, Pfeiffer and Mayer's (1998) landmark study showed that peroxynitrite failed to nitrate tyrosine at physiological pH, casting grave doubts about nitrotyrosine as a valid marker of peroxynitrite at all. Physiologically relevant concentrations of ONOO$^-$ (i.e., in the range of 400 nmol to 2 µmol) actually protect against myocardial ischemia–reperfusion injury in the rat (Lefer et al., 1997) and the cat (Nossuli et al., 1997). Moreover, these concentrations of ONOO$^-$ significantly attenuate leukocyte–endothelium interactions both in vitro and in vivo (Lefer et al., 1997; Nossuli et al., 1997). Finally, ONOO$^-$ in vivo releases NO in solution as an NO donor (Nossuli et al., 1998). Recently, Balazy et al. (1998) showed that ONOO$^-$ and glutathione (GSH) can react to generate S-nitroglutathione (GSNO$_2$), which decomposes to generate nitric oxide. Furthermore, NO can be transnitrosated onto carrier proteins in plasma, which acts as an NO carrier, thus transporting and protecting the circulating NO until it is released from the S-nitrosated carrier molecule (Stamler et al., 1992). Stamler et al. suggested that S-nitrosothiol protein adducts act as circulating carriers of NO. This mechanism could explain the cytoprotective and beneficial effects of ONOO$^-$ in vivo. Thus, a significant body of evidence exists that seriously questions the role of peroxynitrite as a mediator of ischemia–reperfusion injury or circulatory shock.

Nitric Oxide Modulating Agents in Inflammatory States

Nitric oxide can be applied or administered in several forms and by several routes. One should be aware that although NO has a half-life of about 5 to 10 seconds at physiological pH and temperature (Moncada et al., 1991), NO can be infused so that its effects can be sustained for hours or days. In the case of carotid artery endothelial denudation and subsequent restenosis of the artery, a nitric oxide donor was infused intravascularly for 7 days by an osmotic pump implanted in the neck of the rat (Guo et al., 1994). Under those conditions, the nitric oxide donor, but not a control molecule having the same organic backbone but lacking the NO moiety, prevented restenosis

Table 22.3. Methods of Administering Nitric Oxide to Intact Animals

Form of Administration	Advantages	Disadvantages
NO (breathing)	Authentic NO; regionally active	Dose must be carefully titrated
NO (in solution)	Authentic NO; can be injected at site desired	Transient
NO donors (e.g., nitroglycerin, sodium nitroprusside)	Eliminates problems with handling of gas; readily absorbed	Some induce tolerance; nonlinear release of NO
NO precursors (L-arginine, tetrahydrobiopterin)	Can be ingested in diet or given intravenously	Effective only if precursor activity is low
NO enhancers (e.g., SOD)	Reduces the inactivation of NO	Is not specific for NO
NOS gene transfection	Can exert a long-term effect	Difficult to transfect effectively

Note. NO = nitric oxide; NOS = nitric oxide synthase; SOD = superoxide dismutase.

of the artery and promoted endothelial regulation (Guo et al., 1994, 1995). These findings show that continuous administration of very low amounts of NO can be physiologically relevant.

Table 22.3 summarizes the potential forms of administration of NO in vivo. As can be seen, NO can be administered in a variety of forms including authentic NO gas and organic nitrates that release NO in solution. The different classes of nitric oxide donors and their biological effects have recently been reviewed (Lefer and Lefer, 1994). One can also promote the production of endogenous NO or retard the inactivation of endogenous NO. This can be done by administering the precursor of NO (i.e., L-arginine), or an essential cofactor (i.e., tetrahydrobiopterin, TB_4, or by utilizing recombinant human superoxide dismutase (rhSOD), which scavenges superoxide radicals and thus retards the inactivation of NO by this oxygen-derived free radical. Also, one can transfect blood vessels in vivo with the gene for eNOS and allow the endothelium to produce and release endogenous NO.

Nitric Oxide Gas

The first study to show that NO could protect against an inflammatory disorder like reperfusion injury was conducted by Aoki et al. (1990), who infused authentic NO gas into cats subjected to occlusion of the splanchnic circulation for 120 minutes. The NO gas was dissolved in physiologic saline and infused close to the site of ischemia starting just prior to reperfusion. Nitric oxide markedly attenuated the postreperfusion circulatory collapse, retarded plasma proteolysis, and inhibited the formation of a cardiotoxic peptide known as myocardial depressant factor (MDF Lefer, 1987). These salutary effects of physiologic levels of NO led to a significant improvement in survival time and severity of splanchnic ischemia shock. This report was closely followed by a study using authentic NO in feline myocardial ischemia reperfusion (Johnson et al., 1991). In these experiments, NO gas in solution was infused intravascularly just prior to coronary artery reperfusion, continuing over the entire 4.5-hour reperfusion period. The NO solution was also bioassayed on isolated cat aortic rings for vasorelaxant activity to ensure that the NO that was infused throughout the reperfusion period was biologically active. The beneficial effects of the NO infusion included a marked attenuation of cardiac necrosis and reduced neutrophil infiltration into the ischemic–reperfused myocardium (Johnson et al., 1991). Control solutions without NO were ineffective against these indices of cardioprotection. Thus, authentic NO in solution protected in two inflammatory situations.

In addition to using NO dissolved in aqueous media, NO gas can be inhaled. Zapol and colleagues (Frostell et al., 1991) pioneered the use of inhaled NO at low concentrations (i.e., 20–80 ppm) as a selective pulmonary vasodilator in hypoxic pulmonary hypertension. The beneficial effects of NO occurred in the absence of any systemic hemodynamic effects. Furthermore, inhaled NO attenuates leukocyte adherence in distant nonischemic microvascular beds during regional ischemia–reperfusion in the cat (Fox-Robichaud et al., 1998), clearly an anti-inflammatory effect. Thus, inhaled NO gas may be a useful means for delivering physiologically useful concentrations of NO to the heart and lungs, and perhaps other more distant organs. Presumably, the NO nitrosates plasma proteins and is transported in that manner to the site of action (Stamler et al., 1992). This may account for the effects of NO beyond the lungs.

Nitric Oxide Donors

A wide variety of nitrogenous compounds can release NO in solution. These NO-generating compounds are commonly known as NO donors. Virtually all of them are organic nitrates, but a substance as simple as sodium nitrite $NaNO_2$ at acidic pH (i.e., pH 2.0) can spontaneously release significant quantities of free nitric oxide in solution. The major classes of organic NO donors are the sydnonimines (e.g., SIN-1), cysteine-containing NO donors (e.g., SPM-5185), the NONOates (e.g., DEA/NO, SPER/NO), and of course the well-known organic nitrates widely used clinically for many years (e.g., nitroglycerin, sodium nitroprusside). The use of these NO donors in cardiovascular disease was reviewed in Lefer and Lefer (1994).

The earliest study showing that an NO donor is effective in reperfusion injury is that of Johnson et al. (1990) who employed acidified $NaNO_2$ in myocardial ischemia–reperfusion. The $NaNO_2$ significantly attenuated reperfusion-induced myocardial necrosis and cardiac infiltration of neutrophils demonstrating an anti-inflammatory effect. $NaNO_2$ also inhibited cat platelet aggregation in vitro. Later studies were conducted employing two sydnonimine NO donors including a control substance (i.e., the same organic backbone of the NO donor molecule minus the NO moiety). These NO donors (i.e., SIN-1, C87-3754) both attenuated cardiac necrosis by 65%–70%, confirming their effectiveness and supplying proof of concept. Importantly, the cardioprotective effect of these agents occurred at infusion rates that did not affect systemic hemodynamics. Furthermore, both SIN-1 and C87-3754 preserved the coronary endothelium, significantly attenuating the endothelial dysfunction observed in untreated ischemic–reperfused cats (Siegfried et al., 1992b). These NO donors also inhibited the inflammatory actions of activated PMNs by preventing their release of superoxide and its subsequent inactivation of endothelium-derived NO (Moilanen et al., 1993). These results are consistent with data obtained with a cysteine-containing NO donor employed in myocardial ischemia–reperfusion injury (Siegfried et al., 1992a).

In addition to myocardial ischemia–reperfusion, NO donors are effective in splanchnic ischemia (i.e., splanchnic artery occlusion/reperfusion, SAO/R) and in total body ischemia–reperfusion (i.e., hemorrhage–reinfusion). In the cat, the sydnonimine NO donor C87-3754 significantly protected against the lethality of SAO/R. Survival rate increased significantly from 0% in untreated SAO/R cats to 75% in cats given C87-3754 (Carey et al., 1992). Moreover, the plasma activities of two pro-inflammatory agents, cathepsin D (a lysosomal protease) and myocardial depressant factor (MDF; a cardiotoxic peptide; Carey et al., 1992), were significantly inhibited by the active NO donor. The results were confirmed by Gauthier et al. (1994), who reported that S-nitroso-N-acetylpenicillamine (SNAP), but not its NO-depleted form, exerted important salutary effects in SAO/R in rats. These beneficial effects included attenuating leukocyte–endothelium interaction at the microcirculatory level. SNAP, a well-known NO donor, had previously been shown to have potent antineutrophil effects (Ma et al., 1993), and to protect rats subjected to severe hemorrhage–reinfusion, resulting in shock (Symington et al., 1992). In the case of hemorrhagic shock (Symington et al., 1992; Kurose et al., 1994), SNAP increased survival from 0% to 88% and markedly attenuated PMN infiltration into splanchnic organs as well as attenuating endothelial dysfunction. This is consistent with NO donors, which have been shown to reduce microvascular protein leakage in splanchnic ischemia–reperfusion injury (Kurose et al., 1994).

These findings suggest that subvasodilator doses of NO donors are effective against reperfusion injury, and that major mechanisms of the tissue protection in reperfusion injury are endothelial preservation and reduced leukocyte–endothelium interaction (Siegfried et al., 1992a,b; Lefer et al., 1993). Moreover, these mechanisms are consistent with the results obtained using authentic NO in these same disease states (Lefer and Lefer, 1993).

Nitric Oxide Precursors

The substrate for NO biosynthesis, the amino acid L-arginine, has also been studied in different inflammatory states. L-arginine, but not its stereoisomer D-arginine, markedly attenuated myocardial necrosis in cats and dogs subjected to myocardial ischemia–reperfusion (Nakanishi et al., 1992; Weyrich et al., 1992). In both cases, L-arginine was infused intravascularly just prior to reperfusion and continued for several hours. In addition to the cardioprotection afforded by L-arginine, neutrophil infiltration into the reperfused myocardium was attenuated. Both studies also showed that L-arginine preserved coronary endothelial function, suggesting an effect on the vascular endothelium via generation of NO synthesis. This beneficial effect probably is mediated by antineutrophil effects on the dysfunctional endothelium because L-arginine infused into isolated rat hearts perfused with PMNs preserved left ventricular function and coronary flow in global ischemia–reperfusion (Pabla et al., 1996). Thus, L-arginine preserves the vascular endothelium, suppresses leukocyte–endothelium interaction, attenuates PMN infiltration, maintains cardiac integrity (i.e., reduces necrosis) and preserves cardiac contractility in the setting of myocardial ischemia–reperfusion. Similarly, tetrahydrobiopterin (TB_4) a cofactor in NO biosynthesis, also protects in myocardial reperfusion injury in the dog (Tiefenbacher et al., 1996).

In addition to myocardial ischemia–reperfusion, L-arginine infusion reduces reperfusion injury in rabbit skeletal muscle (Huk et al., 1997), in rat liver (Nilsson et al., 1997), and in rat skin (Cordeiro et al., 1997). Thus, L-arginine exerts cytoprotective effects in a wide variety of tissues when given parenterally just before reperfusion. Another advantage of L-arginine is that it can be given orally. This has been achieved in hypercholesterolemic rabbits by oral feeding of L-arginine (Cooke et al., 1992), which improved endothelial function and retarded atherogenesis over several months. More recently, humans ingesting L-arginine orally for 6 months experienced improved coronary vascular endothelial function associated with ameliorated symptoms of coronary artery disease (Lerman et al., 1998). These findings support the value of chronically enhancing endogenous NO production in coronary vascular disorders and other inflammatory diseases.

Nitric Oxide Snythase Gene Transfection

An interesting and new approach to augmenting physiologic quantities of NO in vivo is to transfect the gene encoding the endothelial form of nitric oxide synthase (eNOS). This has been achieved in the rat carotid artery subjected to intimal injury (von der Leyen et al., 1995). Transfection of this gene significantly attenuated the restenosis of the rat carotid artery and maintained vascular homeostasis in this important blood vessel. Thus, gene transfection may ultimately become a therapeutic modality to enable NO-deficient vessels to regain their NO synthetic capacity.

Summary

In summary, basal NO produced by the vascular endothelium in physiologic amounts results in circulating levels of 1–10 nmol/l and acts as a very important homeostatic agent. Nitric oxide formed by eNOS exerts a variety of anti-inflammatory effects including inhibition of leukocyte–endothelium interaction, attenuation of platelet aggregation, reduction in microvascular fluid leakage, and quenching of superoxide radicals.

Higher concentrations of NO in the low micromolar range can occur during activation of iNOS. Although high levels of NO are purported to be toxic to certain cells, micromolar concentrations of NO exert important bactericidal and antiviral effects that are important in preventing systemic and local infections. Indeed, NO formed from iNOS can replace the lost or reduced NO usually observed in inflammatory states like reperfusion injury and circulatory shock. Thus, more recent evaluation of the role of higher levels of NO tend to assign some positive value to these NO concentrations rather than the more classical negative view of higher NO concentrations.

This work was supported by research grant GM-45434 from the National Institutes of Health.

References

Aoki, N., Siegfried, M. and Lefer, A. M. (1989) Anti-EDRF effect of tumor necrosis factor in isolated perfused cat carotid arteries. *Am. J. Physiol.* 256:H1509–1512.

Aoki, N., Johnson, G. III, and Lefer, A. M. (1990) Beneficial effects of two forms of NO administration in feline splanchnic artery occlusion shock. *Am. J. Physiol.* 258:G275–G281.

Armstead, V. E., Minchenko, A. G., Campbell, B., and Lefer, A. M. (1997a) P-selectin is up-regulated in vital organs during murine traumatic shock. *FASEB J.* 11:1271–1279.

Armstead, V. E., Minchenko, A. G., Schuhl, R. A., Hayward, R., Nossuli, T. O., and Lefer, A. M. (1997b) Regulation of P-selectin expression in human endothelial cells by nitric oxide. *Am. J. Physiol.* 273:H740–H746.

Arnal, J. F., Munzel, T., Venema, R. C., James, N. L., Bai, C. L., Mitch, W. E., and Harrison, D. G. (1995) Interactions between L-arginine and L-glutamine change endothelial NO production. An effect independent of NO synthase substrate availability. *J. Clin. Invest.* 95:2565–2572.

Balazy, M., Kaminski, P. M., Mao, K., Tan, J., and Wolin, M. S. (1998) S-nitroglutathione, a product of the reaction between peroxynitrite and glutathione that generates nitric oxide. *J. Biol. Chem.* 273:32009–32015.

Balligand, J. L., Ungureanu, D., Kelly, R. A., Kobzik, L., Pimental, D., Michel, T., and Smith, T. W. (1993) Abnormal contractile function due to induction of nitric oxide synthesis in rat cardiac myocytes follows exposure to activated macrophage-conditioned medium. *J. Clin. Invest.* 91:2314–2319.

Boger, R. H., Bode-Boger, S. M., Thiele, W., Junker, W., Alexander, K., and Frolich, J. C. (1997) Biochemical evidence for impaired nitric oxide synthesis in patients with peripheral arterial occlusive disease. *Circ.* 95:2068–2074.

Bogle, R. G., Baydoun, A. R., Pearson, J. D., and Mann, G. E. (1996) Regulation of L-arginine transport and nitric oxide release in superfused porcine aortic endothelial cells. *J. Physiol. (Lond.)* 490:229–241.

Brady, A. J., Poole-Wilson, P. A., Harding, S. E., and Warren, J. B. (1992) Nitric oxide production within cardiac myocytes reduces their contractility in endotoxemia. *Am. J. Physiol.* 263:H1963–H1966.

Carey, C., Siegfried, M. R., Ma, X. L., Weyrich, A. S., and Lefer, A. M. (1992) Antishock and endothelial protective actions of a NO donor in mesenteric ischemia and reperfusion. *Circ. Shock* 38:209–216.

Cendan, J. C., Souba, W. W., Copeland, E. M., and Lind, D. S. (1995) Cytokines regulate endotoxin stimulation of endothelial cell arginine transport. *Surgery* 117:213–219.

Chester, A. H., O'Neil, G. S., Tadjkarimi, S., Palmer, R. M., Moncada, S., and Yacoub, M. H. (1990) The role of nitric oxide in mediating endothelium-dependent relaxations in the human epicardial coronary artery. *Intl. J. Cardiol.* 29:305–309.

Clancy, R. M., Leszczynska-Piziak, J., and Abramson, S. B. (1992) Nitric oxide, an endothelial cell relaxation factor, inhibits neutrophil superoxide anion production via a direct action on the NADPH oxidase. *J. Clin. Invest.* 90:1116–1121.

Cobb, J. P., and Danner, R. L. (1996) Nitric oxide and septic shock. *JAMA* 275:1192–1196.

Cohen, R. A., Zitnay, K. M., Haudenschild, C. C., and Cunningham, L. D. (1988) Loss of selective endothelial cell vasoactive functions caused by hypercholesterolemia in pig coronary arteries. *Circ. Res.* 63:903–910.

Cooke, J. P., Singer, A. H., Tsao, P., Zera, P., Rowan, R. A., and Billingham, M. E. (1992) Antiatherogenic effects of L-arginine in the hypercholesterolemic rabbit. *J. Clin. Invest.* 90:1168–1172.

Cordeiro, P. G., D. P., Mastorakos, Hu, Q.-Y., and Kirschner, R. E. (1997) The protective effect of L-arginine on ischemia–reperfusion injury in rat skin flaps. *Plast. Reconstr. Surg.* 100:1227–1233.

Crystal, G. J., and Gurevicius, J. (1996) Nitric oxide does not modulate myocardial contractility acutely in in situ canine hearts. *Am. J. Physiol.* 270:H1568–H1576.

Cunha, F. Q., Assreuy, J., Moss, D. W., Rees, D., Leal, L. M., Moncada, S., Carrier, M., O'Donnell, C. A., and Liew, F. Y. (1994) Differential induction of nitric oxide synthase in various organs of the mouse during endotoxaemia: role of TNF-alpha and IL-1β. *Immunol.* 81:211–215.

Davenpeck, K. L., Gauthier, T. W., Albertine, K. H., and Lefer, A. M. (1994a) Role of P-selectin in microvascular leukocyte–endothelial interaction in splanchnic ischemia–reperfusion. *Am. J. Physiol.* 267:H622–H630.

Davenpeck, K. L., Gauthier, T. W., and Lefer, A. M. (1994b) Inhibition of endothelial-derived nitric oxide promotes P-selectin expression and actions in the rat microcirculation. *Gastroenterol.* 107:1050–1058.

DeCaterina, C. R., Libby, P., Peng, H. B., Thannickal, V. J., Rajavashisth, T. B., Gimbrone, M.A.J., Shin, W. S., and Liao, J. K. (1995) Nitric oxide decreases cytokine-induced endothelial activation. Nitric oxide selectively reduces endothelial expression of adhesion molecules and proinflammatory cytokines. *J. Clin. Invest.* 96:60–68.

De May, M. J., and Vanhoutte, P. M. (1983) Anoxia and endothelium-dependent reactivity of the canine femoral artery. *J. Physiol. (Lond.)* 335:65–74.

Denis, M. (1991) Tumor necrosis factor and granulocyte macrophage colony-stimulating factor stimulate human macrophages to restrict growth of virulent *Mycobacterium avium* and to kill avirulent *M avium*: killing effector mechanism depends on the generation of reactive nitrogen intermediates. *J. Leuko. Biol.* 49:380–387.

Eiserich, J. P., Cross, C. E., Jones, A. D., Halliwell, B., and van der Vliet, A. (1996) Formation of nitrating and chlorinating species by reaction of nitrite with hypochlorous acid: a novel mechanism for nitric oxide-mediated protein modifications. *J. Biol. Chem.* 271:19199–19208.

Eiserich, J. P., Hristova, M., Cross, C. E., Jones, A. D., Freeman, B. A., Halliwell, B., and van der Vliet, A. (1998) Formation of nitric oxide-derived inflammatory oxidants by myeloperoxidase in neutrophils. *Nature* 391:393–397.

Fox-Robichaud, A., Payne, D., Hasan, S. U., Ostrovsky, L., Fairhead, T., Reinhardt, P., and Kubes, P. (1998). Inhaled NO as a viable antiadhesive therapy for ischemia/reperfusion injury of distal microvascular beds. *J. Clin. Invest.* 101:2497–2505.

Freiman, P. C., Mitchell, G. G., Heistad, D. D., Armstrong, M. L., and Harrison, D. G. (1996) Atherosclerosis impairs endothelium-dependent vascular relaxation to acetylcholine and thrombin in primates. *Circ. Res.* 58:783–789.

Frostell, C., Fratacci, M. D., Wain, J. C., Jones, R., and Zapol, W. M. (1991) Inhaled nitric oxide: a selective pulmonary vasodilator reversing hypoxic pulmonary vasocontraction. *Circ.* 83:2038–2047.

Fukumoto, Y., Shimokawa, H., Kozai, T., Kadokami, T., Kuwata, K., Yonemitsu, Y., Kuga, T., Egashira, K., Sueishi, K., and Takeshita, A. (1997) Vasculoprotective role of inducible nitric oxide synthase at inflammatory coronary lesions induced by chronic treatment with interleukin-1β in pigs in vivo. *Circ.* 96:3104–3111.

Furchgott, R. F., and Vanhoutte, P. M. (1989) Endothelium-derived relaxing and contracting factors. *FASEB J.* 3:2007–2018.

Furchgott, R. F., and Zawadski, J. V. (1990) The obligatory role of endothelial cells on the relaxation of arterial smooth muscle by acetylcholine. *Nature (Lond.)* 288:373–376.

Gauthier, T. W., Davenpeck, K. L., and Lefer, A. M. (1994) Nitric oxide attenuates leukocyte–endothelial interaction via P-selectin in splanchnic ischemia–reperfusion. *Am. J. Physiol.* 267: G562–G568.

Gauthier, T. W., Scalia, R., Murohara, T., Guo, J.-P., and Lefer, A. M. (1995) Nitric oxide protects against leukocyte–endothelium interactions in the early stages of hypercholesterolemia. *Arterioscler. Thromb. Vasc. Biol.* 15:1652–1659.

Grisham, M. B., Granger, D. N., and Lefer, D. J. (1998) Modulation of leukocyte–endothelial interactions by reactive metabolites of oxygen and nitrogen: relevance to ischemic heart disease. *Free Rad. Biol. Med.* 25:404–433.

Gross, S. S., and Levi, R. (1992) Tetrahydrobiopterin synthesis. An absolute requirement for cytokine-induced nitric oxide generation by vascular smooth muscle. *J. Biol. Chem.* 267:25722–25729.

Groves, P. H., Lewis, M. J., Cheadle, H. A., and Penny, W. J. (1993) SIN-1 reduces platelet adhesion and platelet thrombus formation in a porcine model of balloon angioplasty. *Circ.* 87: 590–597.

Gryglewski, R. J., Palmer, R. M., and Moncada, S. (1986) Superoxide anion is involved in the breakdown of endothelium-derived vascular relaxing factor. *Nature (Lond.)* 320:454–456.

Guo, J.-P., Milhoan, K. A., Tuan, R. S., and Lefer, A. M. (1994) Beneficial effect of SPM-5185, a cysteine-containing NO donor, in rat carotid artery intimal injury. *Circ. Res.* 75:77–84.

Guo, J.-P., Panday, M. M., Consigny, P. M., and Lefer, A. M. (1995) Mechanisms of vascular preservation by a novel NO donor following rat carotid artery intimal injury. *Am. J. Physiol.* 269: H1122–H1131.

Hasebe, N., Shen, Y. T., and Vatner, S. F. (1993) Inhibition of endothelium-derived relaxing factor enhances myocardial stunning in conscious dog. *Circ.* 88:2862–2871.

Hecker, M., Boese, M., Schini-Kerth, V. B., Mulsch, A., and Busse, R. (1995) Characterization of the stable L-arginine–derived relaxing factor released from cytokine-stimulated vascular smooth muscle cells as an NG-hydroxyl-L-arginine-nitric oxide adduct. *Proc. Natl. Acad. Sci. USA* 92:4671–4675.

Hibbs, J. Jr. (1991) Synthesis of nitric oxide from L-arginine: a recently discovered pathway induced by cytokines with antitumour and antimicrobial activity. *Res. Immunol.* 142:565–569.

Hickey, M., Sharkey, K. A., Sihota, E. G., Reinhardt, P. H., MacMicking, J. D., Nathan, C., and Kubes, P. (1997) Inducible nitric oxide synthase-deficient mice have enhanced leukocyte–endothelium interactions in endotoxemia. *FASEB J.* 11:955–964.

Higgs, E. A., Moncada, S., Vane, J. R., Caen, J. P., Michel, H., and Tobelem, G. (1978) Effect of prostacyclin (PG12) on platelet adhesion to rabbit arterial subendothelium. *Prostaglandins* 16: 17–22.

Huk, I., Nanobashvili, J., Neumayer, C., Punz, A., Mueller, M., Afkhampour, K., et al. (1997) L-arginine treatment alters the kinetics of nitric oxide and superoxide release and reduces ischemia/reperfusion injury in skeletal muscle. *Circ.* 96:667–675.

Ignarro, L. J., Buga, G. M., Wood, K. S., Byrns, R. E., and Chaudhuri, G. (1987) Endothelium-derived relaxing factor produced and released from artery and vein is nitric oxide. *Proc. Natl. Acad. Sci. USA* 84:9265–9269.

Johnson, G. III, Tsao, P. S., and Lefer, A. M. (1991) Cardioprotective effects of authentic nitric oxide in myocardial ischemia with reperfusion. *Crit. Care Med.* 19:244–252.

Johnson, G. III, Tsao, P. S., Mulloy, D., and Lefer, A. M. (1990) Cardioprotective effects of acidified sodium nitrite in myocardial ischemia with reperfusion. *J. Pharmacol. Exp. Therap.* 252: 35–41.

Jones, S. P., Girod, W. G., Palazzo, A. J., Granger, D. N., Grisham, M. B., Jourd'Heuil, D., Huang, P. L., and Lefer, D. J. (1999) Myocardial ischemia-reperfusion injury is exacerbated in absence of endothelial cell nitric oxide synthase. *Am. J. Physiol.* 276:H1567–H1573.

Kelly, R. A., Balligand, J. L., and Smith, T. W. (1996) Nitric oxide and cardiac function. *Circ. Res.* 79:363–380.

Kelm, M., and Schrader, J. (1990) Control of coronary vascular tone by nitric oxide. *Circ. Res.* 66:1561–1575.

Kilbourn, R. G., and Griffith, O. W. (1992) Overproduction of nitric oxide in cytokine-mediated and septic shock. *J. Natl. Cancer Inst.* 84:827–831.

Klatt, P., Schmidt, K., Lehner, D., Glatter, O., Bachinger, H. P., and Mayer, B. (1995) Structural analysis of porcine brain nitric oxide synthase reveals a role for tetrahydrobiopterin and L-arginine in the formation of an SDS-resistant dimer. *EMBO J.* 14:3687–3695.

Kubes, P., Suzuki, M., and Granger, D. N. (1991) Nitric oxide: an endogenous modulator of leukocyte adhesion. *Proc. Natl. Acad. Sci. USA* 88:4651–4655.

Kubes, P., and D. N. Granger (1992) Nitric oxide modulates microvascular permeability. *Am. J. Physiol.* 262:G575–G581.

Kurose, I., Wolf, R., Grisham, M. B., and Granger, D. N. (1994) Modulation of ischemia/reperfusion-induced microvascular dysfunction by nitric oxide. *Circ. Res.* 74: 376–382.

Lefer, A. M. (1987) Interaction between myocardial depressant factor and vasoactive mediators with ischemia and shock. *Am. J. Physiol.* 252:R193–R205.

Lefer, A. M., Tsao, P. S., Lefer, D. J., and Ma, X. L. (1991) Role of endothelial dysfunction in the pathogenesis of reperfusion injury after myocardial ischemia. *FASEB J.* 5:2029–2034.

Lefer, A. M., and Lefer, D. J. (1993) Pharmacology of the endothelium in ischemia–reperfusion and circulatory shock. *Annu. Rev. Pharmacol. Toxicol.* 33:71–90.

Lefer, A. M., and Ma, X. L. (1993) Decreased basal nitric oxide release in hypercholesterolemia increases neutrophil adherence to rabbit coronary artery endothelium. *Arterioscler. Thromb.* 13:771–776.

Lefer, A. M. (1994) Endotoxin, cytokines, and nitric oxide in shock: an editorial comment. *Shock* 1:79–80.

Lefer, A. M., and Lefer, D. J. (1994) Therapeutic role of nitric oxide donors in the treatment of cardiovascular disease. *Drugs of the Future* 19:665–672.

Lefer, A. M. (1998) Nitric oxide donors in endotoxic and septic shock: Evidence against nitric oxide as a mediator of shock. *Sepsis* 1:101–106.

Lefer, D. J., Nakanishi, K., Johnston, W. E., and Vinten-Johansen, J. (1993) Antineutrophil and myocardial protecting actions of a novel nitric oxide donor after acute myocardial ischemia and reperfusion of dogs. *Circ.* 88:2337–2350.

Lefer, D. J., Scalia, R., Campbell, B., Nossuli, T., Hayward, R., Salamon, M., Grayson, J., and Lefer, A. M. (1997) Peroxynitrite inhibits leukocyte–endothelial cell interactions and protects against ischemia–reperfusion injury in rats. *J. Clin. Invest.* 99:684–691.

Lefer, D. J., Jones, S. P., Girod, W. G., Baines, A., Grisham, M. B., Cockrell, A. S., Huang, P. L., and Scalia, R. (1999) Leukocyte–endothelial cell interactions in nitric oxide synthase deficient mice. *Am. J. Physiol.* 276:H1943–H1950.

Lerman, A., Burnett, J. C. Jr., Higano, S. T., McKinley, L. J., and Holmes, D. R. Jr. (1998) Long-term L-arginine supplementation improves small-vessel coronary endothelial function in humans. *Circ.* 97:2123–2128.

Ma, X. L., Lefer, A. M., and Zipkin, R. E. (1993) S-nitroso-N-acetylpenicillamine is a potent inhibitor of neutrophil–endothelial interaction. *Endothelium* 1:31–39.

Mannick, J. B., Asano, K., Izumi, K., Kieff, E., and Stamler, J. S. (1994) Nitric oxide produced by human B lymphocytes inhibits apoptosis and Epstein-Barr virus reactivation. *Cell* 79:1137–1146.

Mellion, B. T., Ignarro, L. J., Ohlstein, E. H., Pontecorvo, E. G., Hyman, A. L., and Kadowitz, P. J. (1981) Evidence for the inhibitory role of guanosine 3', 5'-monophosphate in ADP-induced human platelet aggregation in the presence of nitric oxide and related vasodilators. *Blood* 57: 946–955.

Miles, A. M., Bohle, D. S., Glassbrenner, P. A., Hansert, B., Wink, D. A., and Grisham, M. B. (1996) Modulation of superoxide-dependent oxidation and hydroxylation reactions by nitric oxide. *J. Biol. Chem.* 271:40–47.

Miller, M. J., and Sandoval, M. (1999) Nitric oxide. A molecular prelude to intestinal inflammation. *Am. J. Physiol.* 276:G795–G799.

Minnard, E. A., Shou, J., Naama, H., Cech, A., Gallagher, H., and Daly, J. M. (1994) Inhibition of nitric oxide synthesis is detrimental during endotoxemia. *Arch. Surg.* 129:142–148.

Moilanen, E., Vuorinen, P., Kankaanranta, H., Metsa-Ketela, T., and Vapaatalo, H. (1993) Inhibition by nitric oxide donors of human polymorphonuclear leucocyte functions. *Br. J. Pharmacol.* 109:852–858.

Moncada, S., Palmer, R. M., and Higgs, E. A. (1989) Biosynthesis of nitric oxide from L-arginine. A pathway for the regulation of cell function and communication. *Biochem. Pharmacol.* 38: 1709–1715.

Moncada, S., and Palmer, R. M. (1991) Biosynthesis and actions of nitric oxide. *Semin. Perinatol.* 15:16–19.

Moncada, S., Palmer, R. M., and Higgs, E. A. (1991) Nitric oxide: physiology, pathophysiology, and pharmacology. *Pharmacol. Rev.* 43:109–142.

Moncada, S., Higgs, A., and Furchgott, R. (1997) International union of pharmacology nomenclature in nitric oxide research. *Pharmacol. Rev.* 49:137–142.

Moro, M. A., Darley-Usmar, V. M., Lizasoain, I., Su, Y., Knowles, R. G., Radomski, M. W., and Moncada, S. (1995) The formation of nitric oxide donors from peroxynitrite. *Br. J. Pharmacol.* 116:1999–2004.

Murohara, T., Scalia, R., and Lefer, A. M. (1996) Lysophosphatidylcholine promotes P-selectin expression in platelets and endothelial cells. Possible involvement of protein kinase C activation and its inhibition by nitric oxide donors. *Circ. Res.* 78:780–789.

Nakanishi, K., Vinten-Johansen, J., Lefer, D. J., Zhao, Z., Fowler, W. C., III, McGee, D. S., et al. (1992) Intracoronary L-arginine during reperfusion improves endothelial function and reduces infarct size. *Am. J. Physiol.* 263:H1650–H1658.

Naseem, K. M., and Bruckdorfer, K. R. (1995) Hydrogen peroxide at low concentrations strongly enhances the inhibitory effect of nitric oxide on platelets. *Biochem. J.* 310:149–153.

Nathan, C. F., and Hibbs, J. Jr. (1991) Role of nitric oxide synthesis in macrophage antimicrobial activity. *Curr. Opin. Immunol.* 3:65–70.

Nava, E., Palmer, R. M., and Moncada, S. (1991) Inhibition of nitric oxide synthesis in septic shock: how much is beneficial? *Lancet* 338:1555–1557.

Nilsson, B., Yoshida, T., Delbro, D., Andius, S., and Friman, S. (1997) Pretreatment with L-arginine reduces ischemia/reperfusion injury of the liver. *Transplan. Proc.* 29:3111–3112.

Nossuli, T. O., Hayward, R., Scalia, R., and Lefer, A. M. (1997) Peroxynitrite reduces myocardial infarct size and preserves coronary endothelium after ischemia and reperfusion in cats. *Circ.* 96:2317–2324.

Nossuli, T. O., Hayward, R., Scalia, R., and Lefer, A. M. (1988) Mechanisms of cardioprotection by peroxynitrite in myocardial ischemia and reperfusion injury. *Am. J. Physiol.* 275:H509–H519.

Osborne, J. A., Lento, P. H., Siegfried, M. R., Stahl, G. L., Fusman, B., and Lefer, A. M. (1989a) Cardiovascular effects of acute hypercholesterolemia in rabbits. Reversal with lovastatin treatment. *J. Clin. Invest.* 83:465–473.

Osborne, J. A., Siegman, M. J., Sedar, A. W., Mooers, S. U., and Lefer, A. M. (1989b) Lack of endothelium-dependent relaxation in coronary resistance arteries of cholesterol-fed rabbits. *Am. J. Physiol.* 256:C591–C597.

Pabla, R., Buda, A. J., Flynn, D. M., Blesse, S. A., Shin, A. M., Curtis, M. J., and Lefer, D. J. (1996) Nitric oxide attenuates neutrophil-mediated myocardial contractile dysfunction after ischemia and reperfusion. *Circ. Res.* 78:65–72.

Palmer, R. M., Ferrige, A. G., and Moncada, S. (1987) Nitric oxide release accounts for the biological activity of endothelium-derived relaxing factor. *Nature (Lond.)* 327:524–526.

Pastor, C., Teisseire, B., Vicaut, E., and Payen, D. (1994) Effects of L-arginine and L-nitro-arginine treatment on blood pressure and cardiac output in a rabbit endotoxin shock model. *Crit. Care Med.* 22:465–469.

Pearl, J. M., Laks, H., Drinkwater, D. C., Sorensen, T. J., Chang, P., Aharon, A. S., Byrns, R. E., and Ignarro, L. J. (1994) Loss of endothelium-dependent vasodilatation and nitric oxide release after myocardial protection with University of Wisconsin solution. *J. Thorac. Cardiovasc. Surg.* 107:257–264.

Pennington, D. G., Vezeridis, M. P., Geffin, G., O'Keefe, D. D., Lappas, D. G., and Daggett W. M. (1979) Quantitative effects of sodium nitroprusside on coronary hemodynamics and left ventricular function in dogs. *Circ. Res.* 45:351–359.

Petros, A., Bennett, D., and Valance, P. (1991) Effect of nitric oxide synthase inhibitors on hypotension in patients with septic shock. *Lancet* 338:1557–1558.

Pfeiffer, S., and Mayer, B. (1998) Lack of tyrosine nitration by peroxynitrite generated at physiological pH. *J. Biol. Chem.* 273:27280–27285.

Pieper, G. M. (1997) Acute amelioration of diabetic endothelial dysfunction with a derivative of the nitric oxide synthase cofactor, tetrahydrobiopterin. *J. Cardiovasc. Pharmacol.* 29:8–15.

Pou, S., Pou, W. S., Bredt, D. S., Snyder, S. H., and Rosen, G. M. (1992) Generation of superoxide by purified brain nitric oxide synthase. *J. Biol. Chem.* 267:24173–24176.

Pryor, W. A., and Squadrito, G. L. (1995) The chemistry of peroxynitrite: a product from the reaction of nitric oxide with superoxide. *Am. J. Physiol.* 268:L699–L722.

Radi, R., Beckman, J. S., Bush, K. M., and Freeman, B. A. (1991) Peroxynitrite-induced membrane lipid peroxidant: the cytotoxic potential of superoxide and nitric oxide. *Arch. Biochem. Biophys.* 288:481–487.

Radomski, M. W., Palmer, R. M., and Moncada, S. (1987a) Endogenous nitric oxide inhibits human platelet adhesion to vascular endothelium. *Lancet* 2:1057–1058.

Radomski, M. W., Palmer, R. M., and Moncada, S. (1987b) The anti-aggregating properties of vascular endothelium: interactions between prostacyclin and nitric oxide. *Br. J. Pharmacol.* 92: 639–646.

Radomski, M. W., Palmer, R. M., and Moncada, S. (1987c) The role of nitric oxide and cGMP in platelet adhesion to vascular endothelium. *Biochem. Biophys. Res. Commun.* 148:1482–1489.

Radomski, M. W., Palmer, R. M., and Moncada, S. (1990) An L-arginine/nitric oxide pathway present in human platelets regulates aggregation. *Proc. Natl. Acad. Sci. USA* 87:5193–5197.

Robbins, R. A., Springall, D. R., Warren, J. B., Kwon, O. J., Buttery, L. D., Wilson, A. J., Adcock, I. M., Riveros-Moreno, V., Moncada, S., and Polak, J. (1994) Inducible nitric oxide synthase is increased in murine lung epithelial cells by cytokine stimulation. *Biochem. Biophys. Res. Commun.* 198:835–843.

Rossaint, R., Falke, K. J., Lopez, F., Slama, K., Pison, U., and Zapol, W. M. (1993) Inhaled nitric oxide for the adult respiratory distress syndrome. *N. Engl. J. Med.* 328:399–405.

Rubanyi, G. M., and Vanhoutte, P. M. (1986) Superoxide anions and hyperoxia inactivate endothelium-derived relaxing factor. *Am. J. Physiol.* 250:H815–H821.

Scalia, R., Pearlman, S., Campbell, B., and Lefer, A. M. (1996) Time course of endothelial dysfunction and neutrophil adherence and infiltration during murine traumatic shock. *Shock* 6: 177–182.

Scalia, R., Salamon, M. G., and Lefer, A. M. (1997) Characterization of thrombin-induced leukocyte endothelial cell interaction in the rat mesenteric microvasculature. *Cardiovasc. Pathobiol.* 1:160–166.

Scalia, R., Appel, J. Z., and Lefer, A. M. (1998) Leukocyte–endothelium interaction during the early stages of hypercholesterolemia in the rabbit: role of P-selectin, ICAM-1, and VCAM-1. *Arterioscler. Thromb. Vasc. Biol.* 18:1093–1100.

Scalia, R., and Lefer, A. M. (1998) In vivo regulation of PECAM-1 activity during acute endothelial dysfunction in the rat mesenteric microvasculature. *J. Leuko. Biol.* 64:163–169.

Schulz, R., and Wambolt, R. (1995) Inhibition of nitric oxide synthesis protects the isolated working rabbit heart from ischaemia–reperfusion injury. *Cardiovasc. Res.* 30:432–439.

Siegfried, M. R., Carey, C., Ma, X. L., and Lefer, A. M. (1992a) Beneficial effects of SPM-5185, a cysteine-containing NO donor in myocardial ischemia-reperfusion. *Am. J. Physiol.* 263:H771–H777.

Siegfried, M. R., Erhardt, J., Rider, T., Ma, X. L., and Lefer, A. M. (1992b) Cardioprotection and attenuation of endothelial dysfunction by organic nitric oxide donors in myocardial ischemia–reperfusion. *J. Pharmacol. Exp. Ther.* 260:668–675.

Silvagno, F., Xia, H., and Bredt, D. S. (1996) Neuronal nitric-oxide synthase-mu, an alternatively spliced isoform expressed in differentiated skeletal muscle. *J. Biol. Chem.* 271:11204–11208.

Shears, L. L. and Billiar, T. R., (1995) Biochemistry and synthesis of NO in sepsis. In: Role of Nitric Oxide in Sepsis and ARDS. Edited by M. P. Fink and D. Payen. pp. 14–28. Springer-Verlag, Heidelberg.

Southan, G. J., Szabo, C., and Thiemermann, C. (1995) Isothioureas: potent inhibitors of nitric oxide synthases with variable isoform selectivity. *Br. J. Pharmacol.* 114:510–516.

Spiecker, M., Darius, H., Kaboth, K., Hubner, F., and Liao., J. K. (1998) Differential regulation of endothelial cell adhesion molecule expression by nitric oxide donors and antioxidants. *J. Leuko. Biol.* 63:732–739.

Stamler, J. S., Jaraki, O., Osbourne, J., Simon, D. I., Keaney, J. F. Jr., Vital, J., Singel, D., Valen C. R., and Loscalzo, J. (1992) Nitric oxide circulates in mammalian plasma primarily as an S-nitroso adduct of serum albumin. *Proc. Natl. Acad. Sci. USA* 89: 7674–7677.

Stroes, E., Kastelein, J., Cosentino, F., Erkelens, W., Wever, R., Koomans, H., Luscher, T., and Rabelink, T. (1997) Tetrahydrobiopterin restores endothelial function in hypercholesterolemia. *J. Clin. Invest.* 99:41–46.

Stuehr, D. J., Cho, H. J., Kwon, N. S., Weise, M. F., and Nathan, C. F. (1991) Purification and characterization of the cytokine-induced macrophase nitric oxide synthase: An FAD- and FMN-containing flavoprotein. *Proc. Natl. Acad. Sci. USA* 88:7773–7777.

Su, Z., Blazing, M. A., Fan, D., and George, S. E. (1995) The calmodulin-nitric oxide synthase interaction. Critical role of the calmodulin latch domain in enzyme activation. *J. Biol. Chem.* 270:29117–29122.

Symington, P. A., Ma, X.-L., and Lefer, A. M. (1992) Protective actions of S-nitroso-N-acetylpenicillamine (SNAP) in a rat model of hemorrhagic shock. *Meth. Find. Exp. Clin. Pharmacol.* 14:789–797.

Szabo, C., Salzman, A. L., and Ischiropoulos, H. (1995) Peroxynitrite-mediated oxidation of dihydrorhodamine 123 occurs in early stages of endotoxic and hemorrhagic shock and ischemia-reperfusion injury. *FEBS Lett.* 372: 229–232.

Thoenes, M., Forstermann, U., Tracey, W. R., Bleese, N. M., Nussler, A. K., Scholz, and Stein, B. (1996) Expression of inducible nitric oxide synthase in failing and non-failing human he H.art. *J. Mol. Cell Cardiol.* 28:165–169.

Tiefenbacher, C. P., Chilian, W. M., Mitchell, M., and DeFily, D. V. (1996) Restoration of endothelium-dependent vasodilation after reperfusion injury by tetrahydrobiopterin. *Circ.* 94: 1423–1429.

Tsao, P. S., Aoki, N., Lefer, D. J., Johnson, G., and Lefer, A. M. (1990) Time course of endothelial dysfunction and myocardial injury during myocardial ischemia and reperfusion in the cat. *Circ.* 82:1402–1412.

Tsao, P. S., and Lefer, A. M. (1990) Time course and mechanism of endothelial dysfunction in isolated ischemic- and hypoxic-perfused rat hearts. *Am. J. Physiol.* 259:H1660–H1666.

Ungureanu-Longrois, D., Balligand, J. L., Kelly, R. A., and Smith, T. W. (1995) Myocardial contractile dysfunction in the systemic inflammatory response syndrome: role of a cytokine-inducible nitric oxide synthase in cardiac myocytes. *J. Mol. Cell Cardiol.* 27:155–167.

Venema, R. C., Sayegh, H. S., Kent, J. D., and Harrison, D. G. (1996) Identification, characterization, and comparison of the calmodulin-binding domains of the endothelial and inducible nitric oxide synthases. *J. Biol. Chem.* 271:6435–6440.

von der Leyen, H. E., Gibbons, G. H., Morishita, R., Lewis, N. P., Zhang, L., Nakajima, M., Kaneda, Y., Cooke, J. P., and Dzau, V. J. (1995) Gene therapy inhibiting neointima vascular lesion: in vivo transfer of endothelial cell nitric oxide synthase gene. *Proc. Nat. Acad. Sci. USA* 92:1137–1141.

Wang, P., Samouilov, A., Kuppusamy, P., and Zweier, J. L. (1996) Quantitation of superoxide, nitric oxide, and peroxynitrite generation in the postischemic heart. *Circ.* 94:I 467 [Abstract].

Weyrich, A. S., Ma, X.-L., and Lefer, A. M. (1992) The role of L-arginine in ameliorating reperfusion injury after myocardial ischemia in the cat. *Circ.* 86:279–288.

Weyrich, A. S., Ma, X.-L., Buerke, M., Murohara, T., Armstead, V. E., Lefer, A. M., Nicolas, J. M., Thomas, A. P., Lefer, D. J., and Vinten-Johansen, J. (1994) Physiological concentrations of nitric oxide do not elicit an acute negative inotropic effect in unstimulated cardiac muscle. *Circ. Res.* 75:692–700.

Wizemann, T. M., Gardner, C. R., Laskin, J. D., Quinones, S., Durham, S. K., Goller, N. L., Ohnishi, S. T., and Laskin, D. L. (1994) Production of nitric oxide and peroxynitrite in the lung during acute endotoxemia. *J. Leuko. Biol.* 56:759–768.

Worrall, N. K., Chang, K., Suau, G. M., Allison, W. S., Misko, T. P., Sullivan, P. M., Tilton, R. G.,

Williamson, J. R., and Ferguson., T.B.J. (1996) Inhibition of inducible nitric oxide synthase prevents myocardial and systemic vascular barrier dysfunction during early cardiac allograft rejection. *Circ. Res.* 78:769–779.

Wright, C. E., Rees, D. D., and Moncada, S. (1992) Protective and pathological roles of nitric oxide in endotoxin shock. *Cardiovasc. Res.* 26:48–57.

Yasmin, W., Strynadka, K. D., and Schulz, R. (1997) Generation of peroxynitrite contributes to ischemia–reperfusion injury in isolated rat hearts. *Cardiovasc. Res.* 33:422–432.

23

Mast Cells in Inflammation

BRENT JOHNSTON and PAUL KUBES

Mammals have developed effective innate response mechanisms to rapidly identify and eliminate potentially harmful foreign particles or organisms. To be effective, these responses need a system to detect pathogens in the tissues, and a mechanism to destroy these foreign bodies. A deficiency in either detection or elimination of foreign particles leads to a compromised host. However, excessive or inappropriate activation of either aspect of the inflammatory response can also lead to debilitating or even fatal diseases. The mast cell is one detection system found in most tissues that can cause the effector phase of the inflammatory response to rapidly mobilize leukocytes from the vasculature to affected tissues. In this chapter, we will highlight evidence that mast cells can initiate the leukocyte recruitment cascade in response to allergens, infectious agents, oxidative stress, and other inflammatory mediators. Unexplored and controversial areas will also be highlighted.

Mast Cell Biology

Mast cells were initially identified in the 1870s by Paul Ehrlich on the basis of the metachromatic staining properties of their cytoplasmic granules, which are now known to contain a myriad of preformed inflammatory mediators (Riley and West, 1953; Gordon and Galli, 1990; Metcalfe et al., 1997; Welle, 1997). These cells are often found adjacent to blood vessels and lymphatics, or associated with nerve tissues (Stead et al., 1987; Raud et al., 1989b; Hukkanen et al., 1991; Kubes et al., 1993), and are abundant in most tissues including the skin, peritoneum, joints, and mucosal surfaces (Stead et al., 1987; Galli, 1990; Hukkanen et al., 1991; Crowe and Perdue, 1992; Metcalfe et al., 1997). This places the mast cell in an ideal position to influence vascular responses and leukocyte recruitment during inflammation. Indeed, mast cells have been shown to contribute to vascular alterations and leukocyte recruitment during immediate and late-phase hypersensitivity reactions (Raud et al., 1989a, 1989b; Wershil et al., 1991), ischemia–reperfusion injury (Kanwar and Kubes, 1994a; Kanwar et al. 1998), and the clearance of microbial pathogens (Echtenacher et al., 1996; Malaviya et al., 1996). Alterations in mast cell numbers and reactivity have also been associated with chronic

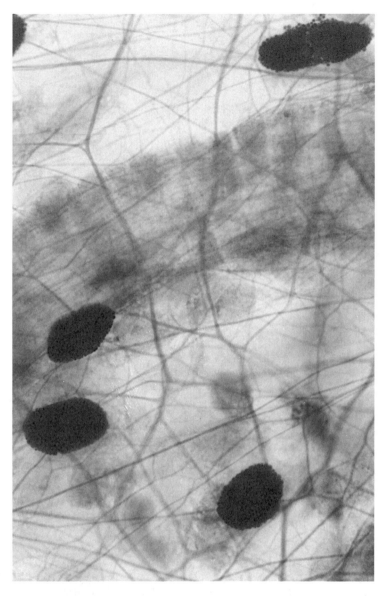

Fig. 23.1. Intact (panel A) and activated (panel B) mast cells adjacent to blood vessels in the connective tissue of the rat mesentery. Mast cells were stained with safranine in control preparations (panel A), and 45 minutes after stimulation with compound 48/80 (panel B). Activated mast cells can be seen to extrude their granules into the surrounding environment (magnification X585).

B

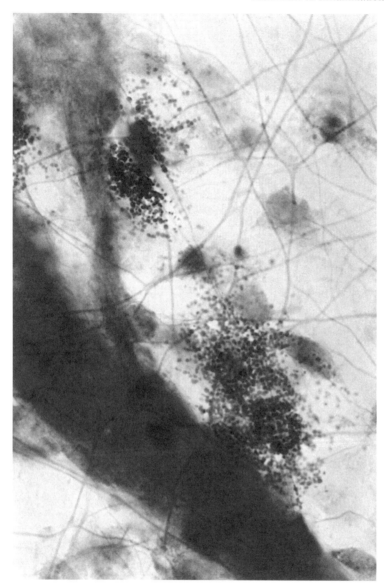

inflammatory diseases (Bridges et al., 1991; Fox et al., 1993; Atkinson et al., 1994), suggesting a potential contribution to chronic disease processes.

Mast cell precursors originate in the bone marrow from pluripotent precursor cells and circulate as nongranulated mononuclear cells (Kitamura et al., 1977). These immature mast cell progenitors leave the circulation and enter tissues, where they differentiate and mature under the influence of microenvironmental factors (Galli, 1990; Longley et al., 1997; Metcalfe et al.,

1997; Welle, 1997; Lee et al., 1998). It is important to note that mast cells in different tissue sites respond differently to activating stimuli, and can release different inflammatory mediators (Galli, 1990; Metcalfe et al., 1997; Welle, 1997).

Figure 23.1 shows mast cells in the rat mesentery stained with safranine: panel A shows intact mast cells in the mesentery, adjacent to a blood vessel; panel B shows degranulating mast cells with granules impacting directly upon the venular wall. These micrographs emphasize the extensive granular content of these cells and the potential interplay between mast cells and blood vessels. The constituents released from activated mast cells can initiate and modulate biologic responses of the vascular endothelium.

Table 23.1 summarizes some of the many mediators released by mast cells, ranging from vasoactive mediators and permeabilizing agents to cytokines and chemotactic molecules. Mast cells store a plethora of inflammatory mediators including preformed vasoactive amines (histamine and serotonin), proteases, and cytokines (TNF-α) (Riley and West, 1953; Gordon and Galli, 1990; Metcalfe et al., 1997; Welle, 1997). Additionally, they can synthesize lipid mediators (leukotrienes, prostaglandins, and platelet-activating factor), cytokines (TNF-α, IFN-α, IL-4, IL-5, etc.), and many other factors upon activation (Gordon and Galli, 1990; Gaboury et al., 1995; Metcalfe et al., 1997; Welle, 1997). However, some of these mediators have only been examined using cell lines, and the expression of many cytokines has only been shown at the mRNA level. Therefore, the roles of many cytokines are uncertain.

The approaches available to study the importance of mast cells in vivo have not been as simple as the study of other cells such as neutrophils. Neutrophils are easily isolated, and can be depleted with antineutrophil sera or other chemical reagents. Mast cells reside in tissues for prolonged periods of time and the drugs that deplete these cells from the tissues almost certainly have other biological effects. For example, it is well appreciated that topical glucocorticoids dramatically reduce mast cell numbers within the skin (Finotto et al., 1997). However, glucocorticoid treatments have many other effects that could interfere with in vivo assays. An alternative approach has been to treat animals with mast cell degranulating agents, such as compound 48/80, which cause mast cells to release their mediators (Gaboury et al., 1995). Inflammatory responses can then be elicited in these mast cell degranulated animals at later time points. However, three problems exist with this approach: (a) the initial degranulation of mast cells causes inflammation in its own right; (b) it is unclear how quickly the mast cells can resynthesize their constituents in vivo; and (c) there are mediators like leukotrienes and platelet-activating factor that do not require protein synthesis for production. Regardless, mast cell degranulating agents like compound 48/80 have been useful tools to demonstrate that degranulation of mast cells can indeed cause inflammation and leukocyte recruitment, as will be summarized in the next section.

Investigators have also made use of mast cell stabilizers that prevent mast cells from releasing their products. However, caution must be exercised with

Table 23.1. Compounds Released by Activated Mast Cells

Amines (performed)
   Histamine
   Serotonin

Lipids (synthesized)
   Platelet-activating factor (PAF)
   Leukotrienes (LTB$_4$, LTC$_4$)
   Prostaglandins (PGE$_2$)

Cytokines (performed and synthesized)
   TNF-α, IL-4, IL-6, TGF-β (have been detected performed and synthesized)
   IL-1, IL-3, IL-5, IL-10, IL-12, IL-13, IFN-γ (synthesized)
   Chemokines (MCP-1, MIP-1α, MIP-1β, IL-8, RANTES, eotaxin)
   Stem cell factor (SCF)

Proteases (performed)
   Chymase
   Tryptase
   Cathepsin G
   Carboxypeptidase

Others
   Proteogycans (heparin sulfate, chrondroitin sulfates)
   Oxidants (superoxide)
   Neutrophil chemotactic factor (NCF-A)
   Eosinophil chemotactic factor (ECF-A)

these molecules as they may impact on the function of other cells and may not inhibit the release of all mediators. Mast cell stabilizers may also exhibit species-specific properties so that a reagent such as cromoglycate (cromolyn) works well in rats but is less effective in other species including mice and humans. Probably the most effective approach to studying mast cell biology is to use mast cell deficient and mast cell-reconstituted mice. The defect in mast cell deficient mice is related to either a deficiency in expression of stem cell factor receptor (known as W/W^v mice), a tyrosine-kinase membrane receptor also known as *c-Kit*, or a deficiency in the soluble form of stem cell factor (*Sl/Sld* mice), also known as the *steel factor* (summarized in Valent, 1994; Metcalfe et al., 1997). However, in addition to an almost complete absence of tissue mast cells, these mice have other deficiencies. Some of the identified problems include sterility and modest anemia. An interesting approach to ascertain whether a particular inflammatory response is indeed related to mast cells is to use mast cell-deficient mice reconstituted with bone marrow derived mast cells (Kitamura et al, 1977). This method clearly demonstrates that the biological effect is mast cell-dependent, and also helps overcome problems that may be related to other phenotypical features of these animals. Although some approaches to mast cell function are more direct than others, all of the aforementioned tools have been used to demonstrate that mast cells do indeed recruit leukocytes in a variety of inflammatory conditions.

Mast Cells Recruit Leukocytes

Many studies have implicated mast cells as important cells in the initiation of inflammatory responses and the recruitment of leukocytes to sites of injury (Raud et al., 1989b; Gaboury et al., 1995; Malaviya et al., 1996; Kanwar et al., 1998). In vivo, direct mast cell degranulation with compound 48/80 impacts upon the vasculature to recruit leukocytes from the mainstream of blood. This agent induced an early (1–2 hours) neutrophilic influx and a delayed mononuclear infiltrate (24 hours) when injected into the skin of rats (Tannenbaum et al., 1980). Similarly, purified granules released from peritoneal mast cells treated with compound 48/80 elicited a comparable cellular infiltrate when injected into rat skin (Tannenbaum et al., 1980). These authors concluded that mast cell degranulation results in the release of various mediators that can mimic inflammatory events including initial neutrophil recruitment followed by the later mononuclear cell infiltration. Whether it was the early recruitment of neutrophils or mediators from the degranulating mast cells that were responsible for the delayed mononuclear cell recruitment was not examined. Similar experiments have been repeated in the rat mesenteric tissue and hamster cheek pouch, models that allow leukocyte behavior to be visualized directly within the microvasculature of these optically clear tissues. Superfusion of these tissues with compound 48/80 caused rapid increases in microvascular permeability and the number of rolling and adherent leukocytes within postcapillary venules (Raud et al., 1989a, 1989b; Thorlacius et al., 1994; Gaboury et al., 1995).

In Gaboury et al. (1995), the vital dye ruthenium red was used to monitor mast cell reactivity continuously in the rat mesentery. The charge and size of this molecule make ruthenium red relatively membrane-impermeable, but the stain selectively enters into mast cells following activation. An electron microscopic study revealed that ruthenium red did not stain granules in unstimulated, nonsecreting mast cells, whereas cells avidly bound this vital stain in cases where granules made contact with the extracellular space via fusion pores in the membrane (Lagunoff, 1972). The ruthenium red uptake in vivo (mast cell activation) correlated closely with the increased leukocyte rolling and adhesion, suggesting that mast cell activation was responsible for the increased leukocyte recruitment. Stabilization of mast cells with sodium cromoglycate or ketotifen prior to the addition of compound 48/80 reduced both mast cell activation and leukocyte recruitment (Gaboury et al., 1995). Similarly, chronic depletion of mast cell granules in vivo prevented the subsequent recruitment of leukocytes with compound 48/80 (Gaboury et al., 1995). In an in vitro experiment, Gaboury et al. (1995) incubated neutrophils with cultured endothelium in the presence of compound 48/80, unactivated mast cells, or compound 48/80-activated mast cells. Neutrophils only adhered at significant levels to endothelium in wells that had compound 48/80-activated mast cells. These data strongly support the view that compound 48/80-induced neutrophil recruitment was mast cell dependent. Additionally, the in vitro experiment excludes the possibility that compound 48/80 was directly activating neutrophils and/or endothelium.

Since the increases in leukocyte rolling and adhesion were observed almost immediately after superfusion with compound 48/80, these data suggest that presynthesized adhesion molecules were utilized. Indeed, a blocking monoclonal antibody directed against P-selectin as well as a selectin-binding carbohydrate, fucoidan, completely inhibited leukocyte rolling (Gaboury et al., 1995; Kubes and Gaboury, 1996). This indicates that substances released from mast cells mobilized preformed P-selectin from endothelial granules to support leukocyte rolling. The mediator responsible for the early compound 48/80-induced leukocyte rolling appeared to be histamine, but the histamine receptor (H_1 or H_2) remains somewhat controversial. In our laboratory, diphenhydramine (an H_1-receptor antagonist) inhibited the mast cell-associated leukocyte rolling (Gaboury et al., 1995), whereas Thorlacius et al. (1994) reported that the compound 48/80-induced leukocyte rolling was not inhibitable by an H_1-receptor antagonist (mepyramine) alone or in combination with an H_2-receptor antagonist (cimetidine). The discrepancy between these two studies must be related to the use of different histamine-receptor antagonists in as much as the preparations were otherwise identical. Inhibitors of other mediators were unremarkable in their ability to prevent the rise in mast cell-induced leukocyte rolling; inhibitors of leukotrienes, PAF, or serotonin did not reduce the increased leukocyte rolling observed after compound 48/80 superfusion (Gaboury et al., 1995; Kubes and Gaboury, 1996).

The firm adhesion was dependent on platelet-activating factor (PAF) because a PAF receptor antagonist blocked the mast cell-induced neutrophil adhesion (Gaboury et al., 1995). In contrast, a leukotriene synthesis inhibitor had no impact upon the neutrophil adhesion (Gaboury et al., 1995). Because mast cells can produce PAF, it seemed reasonable to conclude that the mast cells were releasing histamine to induce rolling, and PAF to cause adhesion. An alternative explanation was that histamine released from the mast cell caused the endothelium to produce PAF to induce neutrophil adhesion. However, mast cell-induced neutrophil adhesion to endothelium or to protein-coated coverslips without endothelium in vitro were both blocked by a PAF receptor antagonist (Gaboury et al. 1995). This experiment supports the view that the mast cells were producing a biologically significant amount of PAF. Finally, a CD18 antibody and antineutrophil serum prevented compound 48/80-induced adhesion in vivo, consistent with the view that the β_2 integrin (CD11/CD18) was responsible for firm adhesion of neutrophils in response to mast cell activation (Gaboury et al., 1995). The mechanism of mononuclear cell recruitment observed by Tannenbaum et al. (1980) after more prolonged exposure to compound 48/80 has not been examined in further detail. Because mast cells are able to generate a large number of cytokines and chemokines during activation, it is difficult to predict which mediator(s) are involved.

Table 23.2 summarizes some of the mediators that may activate mast cells, leading to leukocyte recruitment. For example, substance P has been shown to induce mast cell degranulation in tissue cultures (Matis et al., 1990) and induce leukocyte infiltration in normal mice (Yano et al., 1989). Substance

Table 23.2. Mast Cell Activators

Antigen
   cross-linking of antigen-specific IgE bound to FcεR1

Complement Components
   C3a
   C5a

Neuropeptides
   Substance P
   Vasoactive intestinal peptide (VIP)
   Somatostatin
   Calcitonin gene-related peptide (CGRP)

Oxidants
   Superoxide

Lipids
   Platelet-activating factor (PAF)
   Leukotrienes LTC$_4$, LTB$_4$
   Prostaglandin D$_2$

Cytokines
   IL-1
   MCP-1
   MIP-1α
   Stem cell factor (SCF)

Microbial Products
   Lipopolysaccharide (LPS)
   Bordetalla pertussis toxin
   Vibrio cholera Toxin B
   Clostridium difficile Toxin A
Escherichia coli Fim H, hemolysin
   Helicobacter pylori toxin
   Listeria monocytogenes hemolysin

Secretagogues
   Compound 48/80
   Calcium ionophore A23187
   Morphine sulfate

Others
   Bee venom (mellitin)
   Bradykinin

P does not induce leukocyte recruitment in mast cell-deficient mice, suggesting that mast cells are involved in the substance P-induced leukocyte recruitment (Yano et al., 1989). Smith et al. (1993) demonstrated that intradermal injection of substance P induced a significant increase in neutrophil accumulation into normal human skin. This was associated with enhanced P-selectin (early) and E-selectin (4–8 hours post injection) expression on dermal vessels. Although a direct role for mast cells up-regulating these selectins in response to substance P was not shown in that study, Matis et al. (1990) reported that cromoglycate prevented mast cell-induced E-selectin expression in human tissues in response to substance P.

Some oxidants can also activate mast cells. Xanthine oxidase is an enzyme that generates both superoxide and hydrogen peroxide. When applied to in vivo preparations (Del Maestro et al., 1982; Gaboury et al., 1994), it caused rapid leukocyte recruitment that could be inhibited by superoxide dismutase (scavenges superoxide) but not catalase (detoxifies hydrogen peroxide), suggesting that sufficient amounts of superoxide, but not hydrogen peroxide, were generated to cause increased leukocyte recruitment. Interestingly, superoxide-dependent increases in leukocyte recruitment could be inhibited by ketotifen, a mast cell stabilizer (Kubes et al., 1993). These data suggest that superoxide induces leukocyte recruitment via mast cells. In contrast, hydrogen peroxide was still able to induce neutrophil adhesion in the presence of mast cell stabilizers in vivo (Johnston et al., 1996), and also induced adhesion in vitro in the absence of mast cells (Patel et al., 1991). These data are also consistent with unpublished in vitro work from our laboratory showing that hydrogen peroxide, H_2O_2 is a very weak stimulus for mast cell degranulation (histamine release), whereas the hypoxanthine and xanthine oxidase system is a potent activator of histamine release from mast cells. Collectively, these data suggest that superoxide, but not hydrogen peroxide, activates mast cells to cause leukocyte recruitment.

Many other factors, including bacterial products, chemokines, and complement components (C3a and C5a) have been shown to induce mast cell degranulation in certain situations (Table 23.2). However, some mediators have only been tested with mast cell lines, and other mediators have conflicting reports in the literature that need to be resolved. Monocyte chemotactic protein-1 (MCP-1) illustrates some of the controversy. Rat peritoneal mast cells are responsive to human MCP-1 and release histamine and serotonin in vitro (Conti et al., 1995). Similarly, injection of human MCP-1 into footpads of mice has been shown to induce partial mast cell degranulation in vivo (Alam et al., 1994). However, human MCP-1 did not activate human skin mast cells to release histamine (Petersen et al., 1996), raising the possibility that rodent, but not human, mast cells respond to human MCP-1. Taub and colleagues (1995) demonstrated that bone marrow-derived murine mast cells migrated in response to murine MCP-1 but did not degranulate. Our own work has suggested that rat mast cells do not become activated (ruthenium red uptake) in response to rat MCP-1 (B. J. and P. K., unpublished observation), but we have not examined mast cell chemotaxis. Clearly, a number of issues are highlighted by these studies: (a) some mediators may play a role as potential mast cell chemoattractants rather than mast cell-degranulating agents; (b) the use of reagents that cross species may activate mast cells differently than reagents from the same species; and (c) mast cell responses may differ depending on the species and the tissue from which the mast cells were obtained. Similar discrepancies presently exist for other activators including the chemokines RANTES and IL-8.

Mast Cells in Ischemia–Reperfusion Injury

Reperfusion injury of ischemic tissues is thought to be associated with increased oxidative stress, which leads to leukocyte recruitment and microvascular and tissue dysfunction (Blum et al., 1986 Granger et al., 1989). If oxidants such as superoxide can activate mast cells to induce leukocyte recruitment, then it is conceivable that mast cells play a role in ischemia–reperfusion. Indeed, mast cells become activated during ischemia–reperfusion as determined by both histological and biochemical methods. In the rat system, a protease exclusive to mucosal mast cells, rat mast cell protease II (RMCP II), is released during mast cell degranulation. The level of this protease was shown to increase significantly in the systemic circulation following intestinal ischemia–reperfusion (Kanwar and Kubes, 1994b), supporting the view that mast cells degranulate in this inflammatory condition. Kurose et al. (1994c) reported a significant increase in degranulated mast cells in postischemic rat mesentery that coincided closely with increased leukocyte recruitment.

To address directly the issue of whether mast cell degranulation contributes to leukocyte recruitment during ischemia–reperfusion, a number of strategies have been used, including mast cell stabilizers. Pretreatment with these reagents prevented the rise in RMCP II levels, and also reduced myeloperoxidase (MPO) activity in the postischemic intestine (Kanwar and Kubes, 1994b), an index of neutrophil infiltration. To determine which phase of leukocyte recruitment was affected by mast cells during ischemia–reperfusion, intravital microscopy was performed to assess leukocyte rolling, adhesion, and emigration in the postischemic mesenteric microvasculature of the cat (Kanwar and Kubes, 1994a). Within 2–3 minutes of reperfusion, a very significant increase in leukocyte rolling was noted in postischemic cat venules. In cromolyn-pretreated animals however, the flux of rolling leukocyte was reduced by 60%. It should be noted that leukocyte rolling needs to be inhibited by more than 90% to have any impact on leukocyte adhesion (Kubes et al., 1995). In cromolyn-treated animals, there was only a subtle decrease in leukocyte adhesion. However, mast cell stabilization appeared to have the greatest impact on leukocyte emigration. In untreated cats, approximately 1 leukocyte emigrated from the postischemic vasculature in the field of view every 2 minutes. In comparison, 1 leukocyte emigrated from the postischemic field of view every 10 minutes in animals that received cromoglycate. This is an 80% reduction in reperfusion-induced leukocyte migration from the vasculature. Clearly, there were other factors contributing to the induction of leukocyte rolling and adhesion, but mediators released from mast cells were important regulators of leukocyte emigration.

Although work from mast cell-deficient mice supports a role for mast cells in ischemia–reperfusion, the use of these mice has revealed an important caveat with respect to tissue differences. In the intestinal tract, leukocyte recruitment in response to ischemia–reperfusion was dependent upon mast cells. In wild-type animals, ischemia–reperfusion induced approximately an eight-fold increase in tissue MPO activity and a three-fold increase in tissue wet-to-dry weight ratio (Kanwar et al., 1998), a measure of microvascular fluid leakage (dysfunction). However, ischemia–reperfusion did not induce increases in MPO activity and wet-to-dry weight ratio in mast cell-deficient animals, suggesting that mast cells were critical mediators of ischemia–reperfusion injury in the intestine. In addition, the epithelial barrier that protects the internal milieu from the luminal contents of the intestine became leaky to radioactive tracers in the wild-type, but not mast cell-deficient mice, again highlighting the importance of these cells in intestinal ischemia–reperfusion. In contrast, when ischemia–reperfusion was induced in skeletal muscle, similar increases in leukocyte infiltration and tissue wet-to-dry weight ratio were observed in both wild-type animals and mast cell-deficient animals. This suggests that mast cells did not play a role in reperfusion-induced injury in this tissue. Clearly, the intestine and skeletal muscle are both susceptible to ischemia–reperfusion injury, but mast cells contributed to neutrophil recruitment in the intestine but not in skeletal muscle. A recent article has reported a two to three fold increase in P-selectin expression in the intestinal tract of both wild-type and mast cell-deficient mice 10 minutes following ischemia–reperfusion (Eppihimer et al., 1997), but later time points were not examined.

Although mast cell-derived histamine, cysteinyl leukotrienes, and PAF have all been postulated to be involved in leukocyte recruitment during ischemia–reperfusion of the intestine, the role of these mediators is somewhat unclear. Histamine release from the postischemic intestine has been reported (Boros et al., 1989). Although the cellular source of the histamine was not identified, mast cells are known to be a primary source of this pro-inflammatory mediator in the small bowel (Crowe and Perdue, 1992). However, antihistamines did not attenuate microvascular dysfunction in intestinal ischemia–reperfusion, suggesting that this mediator may not be the only molecule involved. Lehr et al. (1991) reported that selective inhibition of LTC_4/LTD_4 reduced reperfusion-induced microvascular permeability, whereas leukocyte recruitment was attenuated only when total leukotriene synthesis was blocked with an inhibitor of 5-lipoxygenase. In a separate study, an inhibitor of 5-lipoxygenase was also able to block P-selectin expression in the postischemic intestine (Eppihimer et al., 1997). Therefore, if mast cells are thought to contribute to leukocyte recruitment in reperfusion, then there must be some association between these cells and leukotriene production. Presently, it is thought that mast cells produce cysteinyl leukotrienes, but very little LTB_4, the molecule more apt to induce leukocyte–endothelium interactions during ischemia–reperfusion. PAF released from mast cells may also contribute to ischemia–reperfusion-induced leukocyte recruitment. Although the evidence is indirect, the effects of PAF inhibition were very similar to results obtained when mast cells were stabilized. Like cromolyn treatment, leukocyte adhesion was only affected marginally by a PAF receptor antagonist, whereas leukocyte emigration was reduced by 90% during reperfusion (Kubes et al., 1990). Based on these data, it is conceivable that PAF released from mast cells is responsible for the early leukocyte emigration seen during reperfusion of the ischemic intestine.

If mast cell degranulation causes leukocyte infiltration into postischemic tissue, then some factor(s) must be activating the mast cells. Based on the fact that superoxide is known to activate mast cells (Kubes et al., 1993), the generation of oxidants at the onset of reperfusion may be responsible for mast cell activation during ischemia–reperfusion. In order to test the hypothesis that oxidants are involved in ischemia–reperfusion induced mast cell degranulation, animals were pretreated with the oxidant scavengers superoxide dismutase and catalase (Kanwar and Kubes, 1994b). This protocol prevented the release of RMCP II from mast cells and the subsequent leukocyte infiltration, suggesting that superoxide and/or hydrogen peroxide were indeed instrumental in mast cell degranulation. Although the source of the oxidants remains unknown, Boros et al. (1989) demonstrated that allopurinol blocked histamine release from postischemic gut by 87%. This experiment suggests an important role for the oxidant-generating enzyme xanthine oxidase in ischemia–reperfusion induced mast cell activation.

Another family of mediators known to activate mast cells are the anaphylatoxins, including C3a and C5a (Johnson et al., 1974; Hachfeld del Balzo et al., 1985). Because C3a and C5a have also been shown to play a role in ischemia–reperfusion injury (Weisman et al., 1993), it is possible that the anaphylatoxins may contribute to leukocyte recruitment by stimulating mast cells to release pro-inflammatory mediators. Indeed, complement blockade has been shown to reduce injury and mast cell activation during intestinal ischemia–reperfusion (Kimura et al., 1998). It should be pointed out, however, that anaphylatoxins can recruit leukocytes directly—independent of mast cells—as they are strong chemoattractants.

Mast Cells in Hypersensitivity Reactions

Mast cells and IgE are known to play important roles in allergic diseases including atopic dermatitis and asthma. The cross-linking of antigen-specific IgE bound to the high-affinity IgE receptor (FcεR1) on mast cells initiates an immediate hypersensitivity response associated with mast cells activation and release of performed and newly synthesized inflammatory mediators. These mediators can elicit enhanced microvascular permeability (histamine, serotonin, leukotrienes, and prostaglandins), alter vasoactivity (adenosine, leukotrienes, and prostaglandins), and up-regulate the adhesion molecules required for the recruitment of leukocytes (PAF, LTB_4, LTC_4 and histamine). In vivo, IgE-dependent activation of mast cells has been shown to elicit leukocyte rolling, adhesion, and emigration from postcapillary venules of the hamster cheek pouch (Raud et al. 1989a, 1989b). The onset of this process was rapid, with elevated leukocyte rolling and adhesion observed within 5–10 minutes, and some leukocyte emigration noted within 40–50 minutes.

In addition to the rapid recruitment of leukocytes during immediate hypersensitivity responses, mast cells have also been implicated in the leukocyte infiltration observed during the late-phase response that occurs several hours after the initial hypersensitivity response. IgE cross-linking with antigen caused profound leukocyte infiltration into the skin of normal mice, reaching maximal levels 6–12 hours after challenge (Wershil et al., 1991). However, leukocyte infiltration was virtually undetectable in genetically mast cell-deficient mice. The leukocytic infiltrate observed 6 hours after antigen challenge in normal mice could be reduced approximately 50% with an antiserum against TNF-α, suggesting that this cytokine partially contributes to the delayed leukocyte infiltration in this IgE-dependent mast cell degranulation system. Indeed, mast cells have been shown to synthesize as well as store preformed pools of TNF-α in their granules (Table 23.1), which can be released by IgE-dependent stimulation (Gordon and Galli, 1990, 1991).

The release of TNF-α from mast cells could contribute to the late-phase response by up-regulating the expression of endothelial adhesion molecules including E-selectin, vascular cell adhesion molecule-1 (VCAM-1) and intercellular adhesion molecule-1 (ICAM-1) (Klein et al., 1989; Meng et al., 1995). Indeed, mast cell degranulation in vitro has been shown to up-regulate these molecules on cultured endothelium (Meng et al., 1995; van Haaster et al., 1997). For example, Klein et al. (1989) demonstrated that chemical and IgE-dependent activation of human mast cells induced E-selectin expression on endothelium 6 hours after stimulation, an event that was blocked by a TNF-α antiserum. Based on the fact that this endothelial adhesion molecule supports leukocyte rolling (Abbassi et al., 1993), Klein et al. (1989) proposed a scenario in which IgE-dependent mast cell degranulation stimulates leukocyte–endothelial cell interactions via TNF-α and E-selectin.

In addition to TNF-α, mast cells can also synthesize and release other cytokines that enhance leukocyte recruitment (IL-1, IL-8, MIP1α, IL-5, and MCP-1), and influence immune responses (IL-3, Il-4, IL-12, IL-13, and IFNγ) (Burd et al., 1989; Williams and Coleman 1995; Metcalfe et al., 1997, Moller et al., 1998). As many of these cytokines have only been demonstrated with mast cell lines, or in vitro cultures, there is little direct evidence that these mast cell-derived mediators contribute to the expression of endothelial adhesion molecules in models of inflammation. One approach to test the role of individual mediators directly would be to reconstitute mast cell-deficient mice with mast cells from mice lacking specific cytokines or other mediators. For example, to establish directly that mast cell-derived TNF-α is responsible for selectin expression in antigen-induced leukocyte recruitment, mast cell-deficient mice would need to be reconstituted with mast cells from TNF-α deficient mice.

In a chimeric severe combined immunodeficiency (SCID) mouse model, Christofidou-Solomidou et al. (1996) illustrated that a monoclonal antibody against human E-selectin significantly reduced leukocyte migration into human skin grafts 4 hours after mast cell degranulation was induced. In contrast, mutant mice lacking E-selectin had no leukocytic impairment in delayed-type hypersensitivity responses, a process that could be reduced with a P-selectin antibody (Labow et al., 1994). More recently, de Mora et al. (1988) reported that neutrophil recruitment in an IgE/mast cell-dependent model of cutaneous late phase hypersensitivity in mice was dependent upon both E-selectin and P-selectin. Inhibition of either selectin alone was not sufficient to block leukocyte recruitment. It appears that there may be species differences as there is a role for both P-selectin and E-selectin in mouse skin, whereas E-selectin alone may support leukocyte recruitment into human skin.

Using intravital microscopy, we have developed a model of late phase hypersensitivity (4–8 hours) in both murine striated muscle and skin (Hickey et al., 1999). Four hours after antigen challenge, there was an increase in leukocyte rolling, adhesion, and emigration in venules of the cremaster muscle. Leukocyte recruitment in the muscle was dependent almost exclusively upon P-selectin as an antibody against P-selectin inhibited all leukocyte rolling in this model. In direct contrast, leukocyte recruitment in skin was not reduced unless both E-selectin and P-selectin were blocked. It should be noted that a caveat exists when using the selectin knockout mice. At 4 hours of antigen challenge in muscle, P-selectin antibody blocked all leukocyte rolling in wild-type mice, whereas there was still ample rolling in the P-selectin–deficient mouse (Kanwar, et al., 1997, Hickey et al., 1999). Indeed, we have shown that antigen challenge increases E-selectin in the P-selectin–deficient mouse, whereas E-selectin is not up-regulated in wild-type mice (Kanwar et al., 1997).

Eight hours after antigen challenge, when many cells are observed rolling in the microcirculation of the cremaster muscle, administration of an antibody directed against the α_4 integrin ($\alpha_4\beta_1$) reduced leukocyte rolling by 50% (Kanwar et al., 1997). However, the fact that P-selectin antibody eliminated all rolling suggests that the α_4 integrin-associated rolling was dependent upon initial leukocyte–endothelial cell interactions via P-selectin. This is not entirely surprising based on in vitro experiments using parallel plate flow chambers (Alon et al., 1995). The α_4 integrin could not support tethering to its ligand, VCAM-1, at shear rates where tethering occurred via the selectins. Once tethered, however, the α_4 integrin could support leukocyte rolling at high shear. Therefore, there may be an initial requirement for selectin-dependent tethering for integrin-dependent leukocyte rolling to occur.

L-selectin on leukocytes may also contribute significantly to the pathology of hypersensitivity reactions. However, this contribution may be more important at later time points. L-selectin–deficient mice, or mice treated with an L-selectin antibody, had about a 60% reduction in leukocyte rolling at 4, 8, and 24 hours of antigen challenge (Kanwar et al., 1999). However, the adhesion and emigration were not impaired in these mice. Interestingly, the emigrated leukocytes in L-selectin–deficient mice remained stationary near the vessels rather than migrating toward an extravascular chemotactic agent. Whether this altered leukocyte behavior contributes to the ultimate tissue dysfunction remains unknown.

Mast Cells in Host Defense

A role for mast cells in innate IgE-independent responses to infectious pathogens and sepsis has been clearly demonstrated using mice genetically deficient in mast cells. Malaviya et al. (1996) demonstrated that mast cells were critical for the clearance of virulent strains of *Klebsiella pneumoniae* from the lungs and peritoneum of mice. Indeed, mast cell-deficient mice exhibited greater mortality associated with experimental infection. Similarly, Echtenacher et al. (1996) showed that there was a greatly enhanced rate of mortality in mast cell-deficient mice following caecal ligation and puncture, a standard model of sepsis. In both these studies, increased mortality could be prevented by reconstituting mast cell-deficient mice by adoptive transfer of cultured bone marrow-derived mast cells. These experiments provide direct evidence for the importance of mast cells in mediating protective responses to infection and sepsis.

Another important feature of these two studies was that the cytokine TNF-α played an important role in mast cell-dependent protection. In the caecal ligation and puncture model, the protection afforded by mast cell reconstitution was abolished by the administration of a neutralizing antibody against TNF-α (Echtenacher et al., 1996). Similarly, the injection of TNF-α into mast cell-deficient mice (instead of mast cells) was also protective, but only at certain concentrations (Echtenacher et al., 1996). Early release of TNF-α from mast cells also played an important role in the clearance of *K pneumoniae* infections (Malaviya et al., 1996). In this model, TNF-α released after mast cell activation was associated with the recruitment of neutrophils and the clearance of bacteria (Malaviya et al., 1996). Treatment with TNF-α antibodies reduced neutrophil recruitment in this model by 70%. These studies illustrate a real benefit for preformed TNF-α which is rapidly secreted upon mast cell activation (Gordon and Galli, 1990, 1991).

In the *K pneumoniae* infection model, it is thought that mast cell activation was induced directly by an interaction of mast cells with the type 1 fimbriae (Fim H) as nonvirulent Fim H$^-$ bacteria did not induce the release of TNF-α from mast cells (Malaviya et al., 1996). Indeed, direct mast cell responses to Fim H proteins have been demonstrated in vitro (Malaviya et al. 1994a, 1994b). In contrast, mast cell activation in the caecal ligation and puncture model may be more indirect. Prodeus et al. (1997) demonstrated that mice deficient in the C3 or C4 complement components (C3$^{-/-}$ and C4$^{-/-}$ mice) were more sensitive to caecal ligation and puncture than wild-type mice. These mice exhibited reduced degranulation of peritoneal mast cells, reduced TNF-α production, and reduced neutrophil recruitment. This suggests that the classical complement pathway may play a role in activating the mast cells in this model of sepsis.

An interrelationship between mast cells and immune complexes may also exist. Zhang et al. (1992) demonstrated that immune complex-induced peritonitis was attenuated in mast cell-deficient mice. This was associated with reduced TNF-α activity, particularly at the early time points. As immune complexes are known to activate complement, this pathway may be involved in up-regulating mast cell responses in this model.

Mast cells have also been shown to react with other bacterial products (Table 23.2; Abraham and Malaviya, 1997). However, some of these responses can be detrimental. For example, pseudomembranous colitis, which can result from antibiotic therapy, is thought to be a response to two protein exotoxins released from the gram-negative anaerobic bacillus *Clostridium diffi-cile*: toxin A and toxin B. Based on animal studies, it is thought that toxin A mediates the excess fluid secretion and inflammation associated with exper-imental *C difficile* enterocolitis (Pothoulakis et al., 1993; Wershil et al., 1998). Mast cells have been implicated in the pathobiology of toxin A-induced mu-cosal dysfunction as mast cell degranulation has been observed in gut mu-cosa within 15 minutes of toxin A exposure. Pretreatment of animals with the mast cell stabilizer ketotifen attenuated toxin A-induced leukocyte infil-tration and tissue necrosis (Pothoulakis et al., 1993). Similarly, mast cell-deficient mice had reduced responses to toxin A (Wershil et al., 1998). Toxin A is thought to activate mast cells indirectly by inducing the release of sub-stance P as a substance P receptor antagonist also attenuated toxin A-induced enteritis in mice (Wershil et al., 1998).

Utilizing intravital video microscopy, it has been shown that toxin A causes increased leukocyte adhesion and emigration, enhanced albumin leakage in postcapillary venules, and the degranulation of perivenular mast cells in the rat mesentery (Kurose et al., 1994b). The recruitment of leukocytes elicited by toxin A was blocked by a P-selectin antibody, or a soluble form of sialyl-Lewis$^\times$ (sLe$^\times$), a carbohydrate counterreceptor for the selectins. These treat-ments also reduced the albumin leakage normally elicited by toxin A, sug-gesting that the recruitment of leukocytes was an essential prerequisite for the microvascular alteration. Lodoxamide, a mast cell stabilizer, effectively prevented toxin A-induced mast cell degranulation in rat mesentery, and also attenuated leukocyte recruitment and albumin leakage. Similar protective effects were noted following treatment with either a histaminase (diamine oxidase) or an H$_1$-receptor antagonist (hydroxyzine). These observations sug-gest that histamine represents an important mast cell-derived mediator for toxin A-induced leukocyte recruitment. Based on these data, it seems likely that toxin A induces substance P-dependent mast cell degranulation, leading to the release of histamine into the perivenular compartment. Histamine would engage H$_1$-receptors on endothelial cells to increase the expression of P-selectin, which mediates leukocyte recruitment.

A second toxin that may recruit leukocytes via mast cells is from *Helicobacter pylori*, a bacterium responsible for the pathogenesis of chronic gastritis and gastric ulceration. The role of mast cells in response to *H pylori* has also been demonstrated using intravital microscopic techniques (Kurose et al., 1994a). Exposure of the rat mesentery to a water extract of *H pylori* leads to leukocyte recruitment and emigration into the adjacent interstitial compartment. The *H pylori*-induced leukocyte recruitment is accompanied by mast cell degran-ulation and enhanced albumin leakage in mesenteric venules. The mast cell degranulation induced by *H pylori* occurred as early as 10 minutes after ex-posure to the extract and was largely prevented by prior treatment with the mast cell stabilizer ketotifen. Although this mast cell stabilizer had no effect on *H pylori*-induced leukocyte adhesion, it significantly attenuated the leu-kocyte emigration and albumin leakage responses. The lack of effect of ke-totifen on *H pylori*-induced adhesion in vivo is consistent with the view that the bacterium promotes the adhesion of isolated human neutrophils to monolayers of human umbilical endothelial cells in the absence of mast cells in vitro (Yoshida et al., 1994). Interestingly, comparable inflammatory responses were not elicited by exposure of the rat mesentery to a water extract of *E coli*, suggesting that not all toxins cause mast cell degranulation. However, *E coli* and other microbes can induce mast cell degranulation by direct contact (ie., Fim H; Table 23.2).

Mast Cells In Chronic Inflammation

The role of mast cells in the development and maintenance of more persistent or chronic inflammatory responses is less clear. Mast cell proliferation has been associated with many inflammatory disease states, including rheumatoid arthritis (Bridges et al., 1991), inflammatory bowel disease and other bowel disorders (Fox et al., 1993), and atherosclerosis (Atkinson et al., 1994). Mast cell proliferation and activation has also been noted in animal models of disease. In fibrotic tight skin mice (TSK), much of the inflammation is associated with chronic mast cell degranulation (Walker et al., 1987). In a mouse model of collagen-induced arthritis, mast cell-deficient mice had reduced parameters of injury (van den Broek et al., 1988), suggesting mast cell involvement in the joint. Similarly, mast cell activation has been observed in the joints of rats during the onset of adjuvant-induced arthritis (Gryfe et al., 1971). Clearly, there is a need to characterize the contribution of mast cells to the onset, pathology, and leukocyte recruitment in these chronic disease states.

Mast cells may also play a role in the initiation of ($HgCl_2$-induced necrotizing vasculitis in the caecum of Brown Norway rats (Oliveira et al., 1995). Mast cells from Brown Norway rats were activated by $HgCl_2$ and up-regulated the expression of IL-4, whereas mast cells from resistant Lewis rats did not generate IL-4 in response to $HgCl_2$. The generation of IL-4 by mast cells may contribute to the autoimmunity in these animals, which is mediated by Th2 lymphocytes.

In a model of adjuvant-induced vasculitis and arthritis, mast cell activation was noted in the mesentery 4, but not 12, days after immunization (Johnston et al., 1998). Mast cell stabilization with cromolyn during the first 4 days after immunization reduced vasculitis and joint swelling at days 4 and 12, suggesting that the mast cells play a critical role at an early time point in the initiation and development of adjuvant-induced vasculitis (Johnston et al., 1998). In this model, it is possible that mast cells may contribute to the early inflammatory cascade or initiation of the immune response that permits the full progression of chronic vasculitis. It is known that adjuvant arthritis is dependent on the early recruitment and activation of CD4[+] T lymphocytes because antibodies directed against these cells prevented the development of disease, even when the antibodies were given only during the first several days after immunization (Curry and Ziff, 1968; Pelegri et al., 1995). If mast cells stabilization prevented the early recruitment of helper T lymphocytes critical for disease progression, then subsequent leukocyte recruitment at day 12 would also be impaired. This would be consistent with the observation that skin mast cells become activated and migrate to draining lymph nodes during immunogenic sensitization in the dinitrofluorobenzene model of contract hypersensitivity (Wang et al., 1998). In the lymph nodes, mast cells contributed to the recruitment of T lymphocytes and the initiation of the immune response through their production of chemotactic cytokines (Wang et al., 1998).

Anti-Inflammatory Roles of Mast Cells

In addition to producing many pro-inflammatory mediators, mast cells are also known to release numerous molecules that may inhibit leukocyte function or recruitment, including nitric oxide (Salvemini et al., 1990), IL-10 and IL-13 (Marietta et al. 1996), TGF-β (Bissonnette et al., 1997), and heparan sulfate (Nelson et al., 1993). Therefore, it is possible that mast cells may act as anti-inflammatory cells in chronic inflammatory disease. In a model of chronic adjuvant-induced vasculitis, leukocyte infiltration into the extravascular space was enhanced when mast cells were stabilized with cromolyn 9–12 days after disease onset (Johnston et al., 1998). Although this may be a case of mast cells dampening the recruitment of leukocytes in an inappropriate inflammatory response, an alternative explanation may be nonspecific effects of cromolyn.

Mast cells also release mediators, such as tryptase and TGF-β (Bissonnette et al., 1997; Gruber et al., 1997), which play roles in wound healing and angiogenesis. This function could act to repair damage done by inflammatory leukocytes. However, it is also possible that repair mechanisms may contribute to the pathogenesis of disease, as in the arthritic joint where fibroblast proliferation is associated with pannus formation and cartilage destruction (Kobayashi and Ziff, 1975; Shiozawa et al., 1983).

Conclusion

Although the mast cell has been known for many years to play a central role in immediate hypersensitivity reactions, evidence is growing to suggest that mast cells also play critical roles in other inflammatory responses. Many stimuli induce mast cells to release compounds that regulate the expression of endothelial adhesion molecules and initiate the recruitment of circulating leukocytes. Our knowledge is increasing in terms of the type of mediators that are released from the mast cells and the types of leukocytes that are recruited by those mediators, but direct links between specific mast-derived mediators and the recruitment of different leukocyte subpopulations remains a poorly explored area. With the advent of mediator-deficient mice and the ability to reconstitute mast cell-deficient mice with mast cells from these animals, the importance of individual mast cell-derived mediators in leukocyte recruitment can be determined. Mast cells have different secretory profiles in different tissues and during different inflammatory conditions, suggesting the possibility of varied and specific responses. It would not be surprising if mast cells turn out to be central figures in numerous inflammatory conditions, releasing key mediators to recruit selective populations of leukocytes.

References

Abbassi, O., Kishimoto, T. K., McIntire, L. V., Anderson, D. C., and Smith, C. W. (1993). E-selectin supports neutrophil rolling in vitro under conditions of flow. *J. Clin. Invest.* 92:2719–2730.

Abraham, S. N., and Malaviya, R. (1997) Mast cells in infection and immunity. *Infect. Immun.* 65: 3501–3508.

Alam, R., Kumar, A., Anderson-Walters, D., and Forsythe, P. (1994) Macrophage inflammatory protein-1α and monocyte chemoattractant peptide-1 elicit immediate and late cutaneous reactions and activate murine mast cells in vivo. *J. Immunol.* 152:1298–1303.

Alon, R., Kassner, P. D., Carr, M. W., Finger, E. B., Hemler, M. E., and Springer, T. A. (1995) The integrin VLA-4 supports tethering and rolling in flow on VCAM-1. *J. Cell Biol.* 128:1243–1253.

Atkinson, J. B., Harlan, C. W., Harlan, G. C., and Virmani, R. (1994) The association of mast cells and atherosclerosis: A morphologic study of early atherosclerotic lesions in young people. *Hum. Pathol.* 25:154–159.

Bissonnette, E. Y., Enciso, J. A., and Befus, A. D. (1997) TGF-β1 inhibits the release of histamine and tumor necrosis factor-α from mast cells through an autocrine pathway. *Am. J. Respir. Cell Mol. Biol.* 16:275–282.

Blum, H., Summers, J. J., Schnall, M. D., Barlow, C., Leigh, J. S., Chance, B., and Buzby, G. P. (1986) Acute intestinal ischemia studies by phosphorous nuclear magnetic resonance spectroscopy. *Ann. Surg.* 204:83–88.

Boros, M., Kaszaki, J., and Nagy, S. (1989) Oxygen free radical-induced histamine release during intestinal ischemia and reperfusion. *Eur. Surg. Res.* 21:297–304.

Bridges, A. J., Malone, D. G., Jicinsky, J., Chen, M., Ory, P., Engber, W., and Graziano, F. M. (1991) Human synovial mast cell involvement in rheumatoid arthritis and osteoarthritis. Relationship to disease type, clinical activity and antirheumatic therapy. *Arthritis Rheum.* 34:1116–1124.

Burd, P. R., Rogers, H. W., and Gordon, J. R. (1989) Interleukin 3-dependent and- independent mast cells stimulated with IgE and antigen express multiple cytokines. *J. Exp. Med.* 170:245–257.

Christofidou-Solomidou, M., Murphy, G. F., and Albelda, S. M. (1996) Induction of E-selectin–dependent leukocyte recruitment by mast cell degranulation in human skin grafts transplanted on SCID mice. *Am. J. Pathol.* 148:177–188.

Conti, P., Boucher, W., Letourneau, R., Feliciani, C., Reale, M., Barbacane, R. C., Vlagopoulos, P., Bruneau, G., Thibault, J., and Theoharides, T. C. (1995) Monocyte chemotactic protein-1 provokes mast cell aggregation and [3H]5HT release. *Immunol.* 86:434–440.

Crowe, S. E., and Perdue, M. H. (1992) Gastrointestinal food hypersensitivity: Basic mechanisms of pathophysiology. *Gastroenterol.* 103: 1075–1095.

Curry, H.L.F., and Ziff, M. (1968) Suppression of adjuvant disease in the rat by heterologous antilymphocyte globulin. *J. Exp. Med.* 127:185–203.

de Mora, F., Williams, C. M., Frenette, P. S., Wagner, D. D., Hynes, R. O., and Galli, S. J. (1998) P- and E-selectins are required for the leukocyte recruitment, but not the tissue swelling, associated with IgE-and mast cell-dependent inflammation in mouse skin. *Lab. Invest.* 78:497–505.

Del Maestro, R. F., Planker, M., and Arfors, K. E. (1982) Evidence for the participation of superoxide anion radical in altering the adhesive interaction between granulocytes and endothelium, in vivo. *Int. J. Microcirc. Clin. Exp.* 1:105–120.

Echtenacher, B., Mannel, D. N., and Hultner, L. (1996) Critical protective role of mast cells in a model of acute septic peritonitis. *Nature* 381:75–77.

Eppihimer, M. J., Russell, J., Anderson, D. C., Epstein, C. J., Laroux, S., and Granger, D. N.

(1997) Modulation of P-selectin expression in the postischemic intestinal microvasculature. *Am. J. Physiol.* 273:G1326–G1332.

Finotto, S., Mekori, Y. A., and Metcalfe, D. D. (1997) Glucocorticoids decrease tissue mast cell number by reducing the production of the c-Kit ligand, stem cell factor, by resident cells: in vitro and in vivo evidence in murine systems. *J. Clin. Invest.* 99:1721–1728.

Fox, C. C., Lichtenstein, L. M., and Roche, J. K. (1993) Intestinal mast cell responses in idiopathic inflammatory bowel disease. Histamine release from human intestinal mast cells in response to gut epithelial proteins. *Dig. Dis. Sci.* 38:1105–1112.

Gaboury, J., Anderson, D. C., and Kubes, P. (1994) Molecular mechanisms involved in superoxide-induced leukocyte–endothelial cell interactions in vivo. *Am. J. Physiol.* 266:H637–H642.

Gaboury, J. P., Johnston, B., Niu, X.-F., and Kubes, P. (1995) Mechanisms underlying acute mast cell-induced leukocyte rolling and adhesion in vivo. *J. Immunol.* 154:804–813.

Galli, S. J. (1990) New insights into "the riddle of the mast cells": microenvironmental regulation of mast cell development and heterogeneity. *Lab. Invest.* 62:5–33.

Gordon, J. R., and Galli, S. J. (1990) Mast cells as a source of both performed and immunologically inducible TNF hα/cachectin. *Nature* 346:274–276.

Gordon, J. R., and Galli, S. J. (1991) Release of both performed and newly synthesized tumor necrosis factor-α (TNF-α)/ cachectin by mouse mast cells stimulated via the FcεRI. A mechaism for the sustained action of mast cell-derived TNF-α during IgE-dependent biological responses. *J. Exp. Med.* 174:103–107.

Granger, D. N., Benoit, J. N., Suzuki, M., and Grisham, M. B. (1989) Leukocyte adherence to venular endothelium during ischemia–reperfusion. *Am. J. Physiol.* 257:G683–G688.

Gruber, B. L., Kew, R. R., Jelaska, A., Marchese, M. J., Garlick, J., Ren, S., Schwartz, L. B., and Korn, J. H. (1997) Human mast cells activate fibroblasts: tryptase is a fibrogenic factor stimulating collagen messenger ribonuclei acid synthesis and fibroblast chemotaxis. *J. Immunol.* 158:2310–2317.

Gryfe, A., Sanders, P. M., and Gardner, D. L. (1971) The mast cell in early rat adjuvant arthritis. *Ann. Rheum. Dis.* 30:24–30.

Hachfeld del Balzo, U., Levi, R., and Polley, M. J. (1985) Cardiac dysfunction caused by purified human C3a anaphylatoxin. *Proc. Natl. Acad. Sci. USA* 82:886–890.

Hickey, M. J., Kanwar, S., McCafferty, D., Granger, D. N., Eppihimer, M. J., and Kubes, P. (1999) Varying roles of E-selectin and P-selectin in different microvascular beds in response to antigen. *J. Immunol.* 162:1137–1143.

Hukkanen, M., Gronblad, M., Rees, R., Konttinen, Y. T., Gibson, S. J., Hietanen, J., Polak, J. M., and Brewerton, D. A. (1991) Regional distribution of mast cells and peptide containing nerves in normal and adjuvant arthritic rat synovium. *J. Rheumatol.* 1991:177–183.

Johnson, A. R., Hugli, T. E., and Muller-Eberhard, H. J. (1974) Release of histamine from rat mast cells by the complement peptides C3a and C5a. *J. Immunol.* 28:1067–1080.

Johnston, B., Kanwar, S., and Kubes, P. (1996) Hydrogen peroxide induces leukocyte rolling: modulation by endogenous antioxidant mechanisms including nitric oxide. *Am. J. Physiol.* 40:614–621.

Johnston, B., Burns, A. R., Niu, X.-F., and Kubes, P. (1998) A role for mast cells in the development of adjuvant-induced vasculitis and arthritis. *Am. J. Pathol.* 152:555–563.

Kanwar, S., and Kubes, P. (1994a) Ischemia/reperfusion-induced granulocyte influx is a multistep process mediated by mast cells. *Microcirc.* 1:175–182.

Kanwar, S., and Kubes, P. (1994b) Mast cells contribute to ischemia/reperfusion-induced granulocyte infiltration and intestinal dysfunction. *Am. J. Physiol.* 267:G316–G321.

Kanwar, S., Bullard, D. C., Hickey, M. J., Smith, C. W., Beaudet, A. L., Wolitzky, B. A., and Kubes, P. (1997) The association between α₄ integrin, P-selectin, and E-selectin in an allergic model of inflammation. *J. Exp. Med.* 185:1–11.

Kanwar, S., Hickey, M. J., and Kubes, P. (1998) Postischemic inflammation: a role for mast cells in intestine but not in skeletal muscle. *Am. J. Physiol.* 275:G212–G218.

Kanwar, S., Steeber, D. A., Tedder, T. F., Hickey, M. J., and Kubes, P. (1999) Overlapping roles for L-selectin and P-selectin in antigen-induced immune responses in the microvasculature. *J. Immunol.* 162:2709–2716.

Kimura, T., Andoh, A., Fujiyama, Y., Saotome, T., and Bamba, T. (1998) A blockade of complement activation prevents rapid intestinal ischemia–reperfusion injury by modulating mucosal mast cell degranulation in rats. *Clin. Exp. Immunol.* 111:484–490.

Kitamura, Y., Shimada, M., Hatanaka, K., and Miyano, Y. (1977) Development of mast cells from grafted bone marrow cells in irradiated mice. *Nature* 268:442–443.

Klein, L. M., Lavker, R. M., Matis, W. L., and Murphy, G. F. (1989) Degranulation of human mast cells induces an endothelial antigen central to leukocyte adhesion. *Proc. Natl. Acad. Sci. USA* 86:8972–8976.

Kobayashi, I., and Ziff, M. (1975) Electron microscopic studies of the cartilage–pannus junction in rheumatoid arthritis. *Arthritis Rheum.* 18:475–483.

Kubes, P., Ibbotson, G., Russell, J. M., Wallace, J. L., and Granger, D. N. (1990) Role of platelet-activating factor in ischemia/reperfusion-induced leukocyte adherence. *Am. J. Physiol.* 259: G300–G305.

Kubes, P., Kanwar, S., Niu, X.-F., and Gaboury, J. (1993) Nitric oxide synthesis inhibition induces leukocyte adhesion via superoxide and mast cells. *FASEB J.* 7:1293–1299.

Kubes, P., Jutila, M. A., and Payne, D. (1995) Therapeutic potential of inhibiting leukocyte rolling in ischemia/reperfusion. *J. Clin. Invest.* 95:2510–2519.

Kubes, P., and Gaboury, J. (1996) Rapid mast cell activation causes polymorphonuclear leukocyte and independent permeability alterations in postcapillary venules. *Am. J. Physiol.* 271:H2438–H2446.

Kurose, I., Granger, D. N., Evans, D. J., Evans, D. G., Graham, D. Y., Anderson, D. C., Wolf, R. E., and Kvietys, P. R. (1994a) Helicobacter pylori induced microvascular protein leakage in rats: role of neutrophils, mast cells and platelets. *Gastroenterol.* 107:70–79.

Kurose, I., Pothoulakis, C., Lamont, J. T., Anderson, D. C., Paulson, J. C., Miyasaka, M., Wolf, R., and Granger, D. N. (1994b) Clostridium difficile toxin A-induced microvacular dysfunction: role of histamine. *J. Clin. Invest.* 94:1919–1926.

Kurose, I., Wolf, R., Grisham, M. B., and Granger, D. N. (1994c) Modulation of ischemia/reperfusion-induced microvascular dysfunction by nitric oxide. *Circ. Res.* 74:376–382.

Labow, M. A., Norton, C. R., Rumberger, J. M., Lombard-Gillooly, K. M., Shuster, D. J., Hubbard, J., Bertko, R., Knaack, P. A., Terry, R. W., Harbison, M. L., et al. (1994) Characterization of E-selectin–deficient mice: demonstration of overlapping function of the endothelial selectins. *Immun.* 1:709–720.

Lagunoff, D. (1972) Vital staining of mast cells with ruthenium red. *J. Histochem. Cytochem.* 20: 938–944.

Lee, Y. M., Jippo, T., Kim, D. K., Katsu, Y., Tsujino, K., Moril, E., Kim, H. M., Adachi, S., Nawa, Y., and Kitamura, Y. (1998) Alteration of protease expression phenotype of mouse peritoneal mast cells by changing the microenvironment as demonstrated by in situ hybridization histochemistry. *Am. J. Pathol.* 153:931–936.

Lehr, H. A., Guhlmann, A., Nolte, D., Keppler, D., and Messmer, K. (1991) Leukotrienes as mediators in ischemia–reperfusion injury in a microcirculation model in the hamster. *J. Clin. Invest.* 87:2036–2041.

Longley, B. J., Tyrell, L., Lu, S., Ma, Y., Klump, V., and Murphy, G. F. (1997) Chronically KIT-stimulated clonally derived human mast cells show heterogeneity in different tissue microenvironments. *J. Invest. Dermatol.* 108:792–796.

Malaviya, R., Ross, E., Jakschik, B. A., and Abraham, S. N. (1994a) Mast cell degranulation induced by type 1 fimbriated *Escherichia coil* in mice. *J. Clin. Invest.* 93:1645–1653.

Malaviya, R., Ross, E. A., MacGregor, J. I., Ikeda, T., Little, J. R., Jakschik, B. A., and Abraham, S. N. (1994b) Mast cell phagocytosis of FimH-expressing enterobacteria. *J. Immunol.* 152: 1907–1914.

Malaviya, R., Ikeda, T., Ross, E., and Abraham, S. N. (1996) Mast cell modulation of neutrophil influx and bacterial clearance at sites of infection through TNF-α. *Nature* 381:77–79.

Marietta, E. V., Chen, Y., and Weis, J. H. (1996) Modulation of expression of anti-inflammatory cytokines interleukin-13 and interleukin-10 by interleukin-3. *Eur. J. Immunol.* 26:49–56.

Matis, W. L., Lavker, R. M., and Murphy, G. F. (1990) Substance P induces the expression of an endothelial–leukocyte adhesion molecule by microvascular endothelium. *J. Invest. Dermatol.* 94:492–495.

Meng, H., Tonnesen, M. G., Marchese, M. J., Clark, R.A.F., Bahou, W. F., and Bruber, B. L. (1995) Mast cells are potent regulators of endothelial cell adhesion molecule ICAM-1 and VCAM-1 expression. *J. Cell. Physiol.* 165:40–53.

Metcalfe, D. D., Baram, D., and Mekori, Y. A. (1997) Mast cells. *Physiol. Rev.* 77:1033–1079.

Moller, A., Henz, B. M., Grutzkau, A., Lippert, U., Aragane, Y., Schwarz, T., and Kruger-Krasagakes, S. (1998) Comparative cytokine gene expression: regulation and release by human mast cells. *Immunol.* 93:289–295.

Nelson, R. M., Cecconi, O., Roberts, W. G., Aruffo, A., Linhardt, R. J., and Bevilacqua, M. P. (1993) Heparin oligosaccharides bind L- and P-selectin and inhibit acute inflammation. *Blood* 82:3253–3258.

Oliveira, D.B.G., Gillespie, K., Wolfreys, K., Mathieson, P. W., Qasim, F., and Coleman, J. W. (1995) Compounds that induce autoimmunity in the brown Norway rat sensitize mast cells for mediator release and interleukin-4 expression. *Eur. J. Immunol.* 25:2259–2264.

Patel, K. D., Zimmerman, G. A., Prescott, S. M., McEver, R. P., and McIntyre, T. M. (1991) Oxygen radicals induce human endothelial cells to express GMP-140 and bind neutrophils. *J. Cell Biol.* 112:749–759.

Pelegri, C., Morante, M. P., Castellote, C., Castell, M., and Franch, A. (1995) Administration of a non-depleting anti-CD4 monoclonal antibody (W3/25) prevents adjuvant arthritis, even upon rechallenge: parallel administration of a depleting anti-CD8 monoclonal antibody (OX8) does not modify the effect of W3/25. *Cell. Immunol.* 165:177–182.

Petersen, L. J., Brasso, K., Pryds, M., and Skov, P. S. (1996) Histamine release in intact human skin by monocyte chemoattractant factor-1, RANTES, macrophage inflammatory protein-1 alpha, stem cell factor, anti-IgE, and codeine as determined by an ex vivo skin microdialysis technique. *J. Allergy Clin. Immunol.* 98:790–796.

Pothoulakis, C., Karmeli, F., Kelly, C. P., Eliakim, R., Joshi, M. A., O'Keane, C. J., Castagliulo, I., and Lamont, J. T. (1993) Ketotifen inhibits *Clostridium difficile* toxin A induced enteritis in rat ileum. *Gastronenterol.* 105:701–707.

Prodeus, A. P., Zhou, X., Maurer, M., Galli, S. J., and Carroll, M. C. (1997) Impaired mast cell-dependent natural immunity in complement C3-deficient mice. *Nature* 390:172–175.

Raud, J., Dahlen, S.-E., Smedegard, G., and Hedqvist, P. (1989a) An intravital microscopic model for mast cell-dependent inflammation in the hamster cheek pouch. *Acta. Physiol. Scand.* 135: 95–105.

Raud, J., Lindbom, L., Dahlen, S.-E., and Hedqvist, P. (1989b) Periarteriolar localization of mast cells promotes oriented interstitial migration of leukocytes in the hamster cheek pouch. *Am. J. Pathol.* 134:161–169.

Riley, J. F., and West, G. B. (1953) The presence of histamine in tissue mast cells. *J. Physiol. Lond.)* 120:528–537.

Salvemini, D., Masini, E., Anggard, E., Mannaioni, F., and Vane, J. (1990) Synthesis of nitric oxide-like factor from L-arginine by rat serosal mast cells: stimulation of guanylate cyclase and inhibition of platelet aggregation. *Biochem. Biophys. Res. Commun.* 169: 596–601.

Shiozawa, S., Shiozawa, K., and Fujita, T. (1983) Morphologic observations in the early phase of the cartilage–pannus junction. Light and electron microscopic studies of active cellular pannus. *Arthritis Rheum.* 26:472–478.

Smith, C. H., Barker, J.N.W.N., Morris, R. W., MacDonald, D. M., and Lee, T. H. (1993) Neuropeptides induce rapid expression of endothelial cell adhesion molecules and elicit granulocyte infiltration in human skin. *J. Immunol.* 151:3274–3282.

Stead, R. H., Tomioka, M., Quinnonez, G., Simons, G. T., Felten, S. Y., and Bienenstock, J. (1987) Intestinal mucosal mast cells in normal and nematode infected rat intestines are in intimate contact with peptidergic nerves. *Proc. Natl. Acad. Sci. USA* 84:2975–2949.

Tannenbaum, S., Oertel, H., Henderson, W., and Kaliner, M. (1980) The biologic activity of mast cell granules. I. elicitation of inflammatory responses in rat skin. *J. Immunol.* 125:325–335.

Taub, D., Dastych, J., Inamura, N., Upton, J., Kelvin, D., Metcalfe, D., and Oppenheim, J. (1995) Bone marrow-derived murine mast cells migrate, but do not degranulate, in response to chemokines. *J. Immunol.* 154:2393–2402.

Thorlacius, H., Raud, J., Rosengren-Beesley, S., Forrest, M. J., Hedqvist, P., and Lindbom, L.

(1994) Mast cell activation induces P-selectin–dependent leukocyte rolling and adhesion in postcapillary venules in vivo. *Biochem. Biophys. Res. Commun.* 203:1043–1049.

Valent, P. (1994) The riddle of the mast cell: Kit (CD117)-ligand as the missing link? *Immunol. Today* 15:111–114.

van den Broek, M. F., van den Berg, W. B., and van de Putte, L.B.A. (1988) The role of mast cells in antigen induced arthritis in mice. *J. Rheumatol.* 15:544–551.

van Haaster, C. M., Derhaag, J. G., Engels, W., Lemmens, P.J.M.R., Gijsen, A. P., Hornstra, G., van der Vusse, G. J., and Duijvestijin, A. M. (1997) Mast cell-mediated induction of ICAM-1, VCAM-1 and E-selectin in endothelial cells in vitro: constitutive release of inducing mediators but no effect of degranulation. *Pflugers Arch.* 435:137–144.

Walker, M. A., Harley, R. A., and Leroy, E. C. (1987) Inhibition of fibrosis in TSK mice by blocking mast cell degranulation. *J. Rheumatol.* 14:299–301.

Wang, H.-W., teldla, N., Lloyd, A. R., Wakefield, D., and McNeil, H. P. (1998) Mast cell activation and migration to lymph nodes during induction of an immune response in mice. *J. Clin. Invest.* 102:1617–1626.

Weisman, H. F., Bartow, T., Leppo, M. K., Marsh, H. C., Carson, G. R., Concino, M. F., Boyle, M. P., Roux, K. H., Weisfeldt, M. L., and Fearon, D. T. (1993) Soluble human complement receptor type 1: in vivo inhibitor of complement suppressing post-ischemic myocardial inflammation and necrosis. *Science* 249:146–151.

Welle, M. (1997) Development, significance, and heterogeneity of mast cells with particular regard to the mast cell-specific proteases chymase and tryptase. *J. Leukoc. Biol.* 61:233–245.

Wershil, B. K., Wang, Z. S., Gordon, J. R., and Galli, S. J. (1991) Recruitment of neutrophils during IgE-dependent cutaneous late phase reactions in the mouse is mast cell-dependent. *J. Clin. Invest.* 87:446–453.

Wershil, B. K., Castagliulo, I., and Pothoulakis, C. (1998) Direct evidence of mast cell involvement in *Clostridium difficile* toxin A-induced enteritis in mice. *Gastroenterol.* 114:956–964.

Williams, C.M.M., and Coleman, J. W. (1995) Induced expression of mRNA for IL-5, IL-6, TNF-alpha, MIP-2 and IFN-gamma in immunologically activated rat peritoneal mast cells: inhibition by dexamethasone and cyclosporin A. *Immunol.* 86:244–249.

Yano, H., Wershil, B. K., Arizono, N., and Galli, S. J. (1989) Substance P-induced augmentation of cutaneous vascular permeability and granulocyte infiltration in mice is mast cell dependent. *J. Clin. Invest.* 84:1276–1286.

Yoshida, N., Granger, D. N., Evans, D. J., Evans, D. G., Graham, D. Y., Anderson, D. C., Wolf, R. E., and Kvietys, P. R. (1994) Mechanisms involved in *Helicobacter pylori* induced inflammation. *Gastroenterol.* 107:70–79.

Zhang, Y., Ramos, B. F., and Jakschik, B. A. (1992) Neutrophil recruitment by tumor necrosis factor from mast cells in immune complex peritonitis. *Science* 258:1957–1959.

24

Resolution of Inflammation

JOHN SAVILL and CHRIS HASLETT

Inflammation evolved as a beneficial, self-limited response to tissue injury or infection; "successful" inflammatory responses resolve completely. Driven by the recognition that the inflammatory response is a key component of many diseases, however, research into inflammation has concentrated on molecular and cellular mechanisms that mediate the initiation and amplification of the response. This impressive body of work has led to characterization of a number of key therapeutic targets, with demonstrated or anticipated improvements in the treatment of inflammatory conditions.

Nevertheless, therapies for inflammatory conditions often run the hazard of unacceptable toxicity and display limited efficacy, especially where there is a need to control persistent inflammatory responses or prevent postinflammatory scarring from leading to permanent loss of organ function. These deficiencies in the therapeutic approach to inflammatory disease reflect very limited knowledge of the mechanisms that normally mediate safe resolution of inflammatory responses. Indeed, it would seem particularly important to characterize resolution mechanisms in order to explore whether these go awry in situations in which inflammation becomes persistent.

Excitingly, the last decade has seen a number of new discoveries in the resolution phase of inflammation that suggest new therapeutic approaches. This chapter is not intended to serve as an exhaustive description of the field; instead, our aim is to provide a selection of growth points.

Prerequisites For Resolution of Inflammation

As will become apparent in the following, by concentrating on mechanisms involved in the resolution of the simplest "type" of inflammatory response, acute granulocytic inflammation, investigators have been able to define resolution mechanisms of wide general relevance. If one considers the resolution of a simple model of self-limited granulocytic inflammation, as occurs when bacteria are deliberately instilled into the lung, it is evident that there are a number of prerequisites for resolution of the response, which will now be considered briefly.

Cessation of Initiating Stimuli

In the case of an obvious inciting stimulus, such as infection with gram-negative bacteria releasing potent inflammatory mediators such as ƒMLP or endotoxin, uptake and degradation of bacteria by neutrophils will obviously lead to removal of the primary initiating stimuli. Furthermore, it is notable that many of the mediators that predominate in acute inflammatory responses are either unstable and liable to spontaneous degradation (e.g., nitric oxide) or are rapidly inactivated by neutralizing enzyme systems (e.g., platelet-activating factor, or PAF). Indeed, mediator inactivation may be accomplished by simple dissipation of a "pulse" of mediator released into the tissues; in experimental arthritis induced by the chemoattractant complement product C5a, transfer of joint fluid showed that declining capacity to incite inflammation in a normal joint was closely correlated with a rapid fall in the concentration of the administered stimulus (Haslett et al., 1989).

These and other observations have encouraged therapeutic approaches based on the targeting and inactivation of key pro-inflammatory mediators, the spectacular but time-limited effects of anti–TNF-α antibodies in rheumatoid arthritis being an exciting example. However, even if this can be achieved, much more remains before the inflammatory response can resolve.

Cessation of Leukocyte Influx

Clearly, a further prerequisite for safe resolution of inflammation is that leukocytes should stop entering the perturbed site. However, although a number of contributions in this volume emphasize that a great deal is now known of the sequential interactions between chemoattractants and endothelial cell adhesion molecules, which mediate emigration of leukocytes from the microvasculature into inflamed sites, much less is known of the mechanisms by which these events are "turned off."

Although the mechanisms responsible will need further characterization, there is intriguing evidence that time-limited expression of leukocyte recruitment systems is "programmed" into the inflammatory response. Thus, in experimental kidney injury induced in rats by administration of antibodies to glomerular basement membrane, Tam and colleagues (1996) found that neurophil infiltration very closely tracked expression of the chemokine MIP-2, with both falling rapidly after 6 hours, whereas the slower kinetics of monocyte accumulation followed expression of MCP-1. A candidate mechanism for down-regulation of chemokine expression might be the programmed production of IL-6 in inflammatory responses because (a) local and systemic levels of IL-6 typically rise later in inflammatory responses than those of pro-inflammatory cytokines (Kishimoto, 1989); (b) IL-6 plays important roles in both decreasing macrophage production of, and responsiveness to, inflammatory mediators (Kishimoto, 1989); and (c) administration of exogenous IL-6 reduced neutrophil infiltration in antibody-mediated glomerular injury (Karkar et al., 1993). Similar "built-in" controls may also govern the time-limited expression of endothelial adhesion molecules such as E-selectin (Springer, 1990). This will be a rich area for future research.

However, in seminal studies of the kinetics of neutrophil influx in experimental inflammation, using the tool of radiolabeled cells, it was remarkable that neutrophil influx ceased within a few hours of the induction of self-limited inflammation of the skin, joint, or lungs (Haslett et al., 1989; Haslett, 1992). The speed with which this occurs hints at local generation of "stop" signals at the inflamed site, and there are exciting data to suggest that lipoxins may be endogenously produced inhibitors of leucocyte recruitment to inflamed sites. Lipoxins are produced by metabolism of arachidonic acid catalyzed by 15-lipoxygenase, an enzyme induced by anti-inflammatory cytokines, such as IL-4 and IL-13. Detectable at inflamed sites, lipoxins inhibit neutrophil chemotaxis, adhesion, and transmigration (Brady et al., 1995, Serhan et al., 1995) induced by various mediators including the alternate pro-inflammatory products of arachidonic acid, leukotrienes, that are generated by 5-lipoxygenase. Indeed, it is intriguing that these candidate stop signals may also have the additional proresolution property of promoting macrophage clearance of dying leukocytes (see the following). Clearly, dissection of the biological roles of lipoxins will be of great interest.

Clearance of Extravasated Material

The mechanisms by which leukocytes are cleared from inflamed sites will be covered in the following as the major focus of this contribution. However, it is important to remember that extravasation of plasma components and fluid is an important component of the inflammatory response. Although the main "drainage" job is done by the lymphatics in the resolution phase, macrophages may also play an important role in clearance of fluid phase debris through extremely active pinocytosis, which may occur at rates such that 25% of the cell surface is "re-used" per minute (Steinmann et al., 1976). Furthermore, it is self-evident that fluid clearance will only be effective if there is restoration of normal microvascular permeability, an area in which more research is needed.

Clearance of Leukocytes

Leukocyte Death at Inflamed Sites

Necrosis Versus Apoptosis

Once the neutrophil has left the bloodstream, this archetypal inflammatory leukocyte usually appears to meet its fate at the inflamed site. Death in situ seems almost inevitable in "closed" sites such as solid organs or serosal cavities, because there is no evidence that extravasated neutrophils return to the blood, and at most, there is only minimal emigration via lymphatics (Haslett, 1992).

Until recently, it was widely assumed that neutrophils usually died at inflamed sites by undergoing necrosis, with inevitable release of histotoxic granule contents (Hurley, 1983). Although there are potent defense mechanisms against neutrophil contents, such as irreversible inactivation of neutrophil elastase by α_1 antiprotease inhibitor, there is also compelling evidence that these defenses can be overcome in inflammatory disease, with the result that neutrophil contents directly injure tissue (Campbell and Campbell, 1988). Indeed, neutrophil necrosis is only prominent when the outcome of inflammation is tissue destruction and abscess formation, rather than safe resolution. Furthermore, histotoxic contents are not possessed by neutrophils alone; eosinophils, monocytes, and lymphocytes (especially CD8-positive cytotoxic cells) all contain potent injurious agents from which, it would appear, appropriate to shield the perturbed tissue of the infected site. As if the threat of direct injury were not enough, the contents of dying leukocytes can also promote inflammatory tissue injury indirectly by stimulating macroplages to release pro-inflammatory mediators (Stern et al., 1996).

These deleterious consequences of leukocyte necrosis emphasize that this form of cell death is rarely physiological. Instead, necrosis is widely viewed as an "accidental" form of cell death in which exposure to noxious stimuli (such as severe hypoxia, extremes of temperature, or high doses of ionizing radiation) leads to fields of cells losing the ability to regulate membrane permeability so that the stricken cells swell and rapidly disintegrate (Wyllie, 1980). At first glance, it would seem most unlikely that such a messy and dangerous form of cell death would play a significant role in leukocyte detection during safe resolution of inflammation.

By contrast, there is a strong prima facie case to invoke apoptosis, the other major form of cell death (Kerr et al., 1972; Wyllie, 1980), in removal of leukocytes from the inflamed sites. *Apoptosis* (a word coined in 1972, derived from the ancient Greek for "falling, as of leaves from a tree") is a physiological and programmed form of death first defined on the grounds of typical and stereotypical morphological changes including cell shrinkage, condensation of nuclear chromatin, and, in many cases, fragmentation of the nucleus and other cellular elements into membrane-bound "apoptotic bodies." Intense activity over the last few years has shown that these changes reflect stereotypical biochemical changes including mitochondrial permeability transition (Zamzani et al., 1996), activation of a family of cysteine proteases termed *caspases* (Martin and Green, 1995), and cleavage of many cellular proteins and consequent activation of endonucleases that cleave internucleosomal DNA (Enari et al, 1998). However, the key feature of apoptosis and the reason to invoke this death program in safe leukocyte deletion is that this form of cell death marks intact unwanted cells for swift, efficient, and non-inflammatory clearance by phagocytes (Savill, 1997). These may be neighboring cells of the same type, acting as "semiprofessional" phagocytes, but where the clearance task is large, this job is done by the body's professional phagocytes, cells of the macrophage line. Indeed, this is exemplified by the thymus in which over 90% of would-be lymphocytes fail selection and die. However, this huge load of dying cells is safely eliminated by apoptosis and phagocytosis by thymic macrophages without inciting inflammation, even though such macrophages can be seen to be "stuffed" with large numbers of apoptotic cells (Surh and Sprent, 1994).

Before going on to explore the role of apoptosis in clearance of neutrophils and other leucocytes from inflamed sites, it is important to emphasize the speed with which apoptotic cells are cleared by phagocytes. Various approaches (reviewed in Savill, 1997) indicate that cell clearance by apoptosis is rapid; in general, it takes little over an hour for a cell to display the first morphological features of apoptosis, progress through the program, undergo uptake by a phagocyte, and then be degraded beyond histological recognition. These kinetics result in apoptosis being a histologically inconspicuous form of cell clearance; in a hypothetical tissue in which there is no cell birth by mitosis, if 1% of cells appear apoptotic one can predict that, on the basis of a clearance time of 1 hour, 24% of cells will be deleted in a day. Clearly, in removal of unwanted cells, visible apoptosis is merely the tip of the iceberg of cell death.

Leukocyte Clearance by Apoptosis in Vitro and in Vivo

Neutrophil clearance from inflamed sites by macrophage uptake of the senescent cell was described in the 19th century by the great pathologist Elie Metchnikoff (1893). However, the mechanisms responsible for phagocyte recognition of "senescent-self" remained obscure for nearly a century until it was discovered that neutrophils are constitutively programmed to undergo apoptosis (Savill et al., 1989b). Typically, around 50% of normal human neutrophils undergo apoptosis after overnight culture, the proportion increasing with time so that all cells have undergone this form of death by 48 hours in the culture. Furthermore, by using approaches such as elutriation to purify apoptotic cells from populations "aging" in vitro, it was confirmed that apoptosis in the neutrophil rendered the senescent cell susceptible to swift recognition and phagocytosis by macrophages (Savill et al., 1989b) and semi-professional phagocytes such as glomerular mesangial cells (Savill et al., 1992) and fibroblasts (Hall et al., 1994).

Clearly, a key question was whether neutrophil deletion by apoptosis and phagocyte clearance was a major mechanism for neutrophil removal from inflamed sites in vivo during natural resolution of the response. As will be explained later, it has not yet been possible to perform the definitive experiment to address this issue: block the uptake of apoptotic cells in vivo so that it can be determined that all extravasated neutrophils undergo apoptosis at the inflamed site. However, there is now a compelling circumstantial case, including careful time-course studies, that apoptosis does indeed direct the removal of extravasated neutrophils from the inflamed lung (Cox et al., 1995), peritoneum (Sanui et al., 1982), and kidney (Savill et al., 1992a) (Hughes et al., 1997a). Nevertheless, it should be noted that extravasated neutrophils can be removed by other mechanisms, such as direct expulsion in sputum, feces, or urine where this is possible (discussed later). However, in such situations, neutrophil apoptosis and uptake by macrophages can still be prominent in the inflammatory exudate (Grigg et al., 1991).

It rapidly became apparent that this clearance mechanism first defined for neutrophils was also important in the deletion of other leukocyte types. In vitro, eosinophils (Stern et al., 1992) undergo apoptosis constitutively (albeit with slower kinetics than neutrophils, the half time of apoptosis in culture being 48–72 hours), whereas activated monocytes (Mangan et al., 1991) and lymphocytes (Akbar et al., 1993) only do so if deprived of cytokine survival factors. Nevertheless, there is now growing evidence that apoptosis leading to phagocytic clearance in situ at the inflamed site is available to eosinophils (Tsuyuki et al., 1995), monocyte/macrophages (Atkins, 1995), and lymphocytes (Milik et al, 1997), even though emigration may be the more usual fate for the latter two cell types (discussed later). What might be the consequences of leukocyte deletion by apoptosis?

Leukocyte Deletion by Apoptosis: Safe—But Not Always?
There is strong evidence that neutrophil clearance by apoptosis is likely to limit injury at inflamed sites. First, by mechanisms including down-regulation of surface receptors for chemoattractants, apoptotic neutrophils lose the ability to respond to receptor-mediated stimuli that normally incite injurious release of granules or reactive oxygen species (Whyte et al., 1993). Second, neutrophils undergoing apoptosis do not spontaneously release dangerous granule contents such as myeloperoxidase (Savill et al., 1989b) and remain demonstrably intact until taken up by phagocytes (Fig. 24.1). Third, the uptake by unstimulated macrophages and semiprofessional phagocytes of intact apoptotic cells of neutrophil and other lineages failed to stimulate increased release from phagocytes of a range of pro-inflammatory mediators including eicosanoids, granule enzymes, or chemokines (Meagher et al., 1992; Hughes et al., 1997b). Indeed, uptake of apoptotic leukocytes by macrophages often induced a small but statistically significant suppression of mediator release when compared to unstimulated macrophages (Meagher et al., 1992). Brisk release of pro-inflammatory mediators from macrophages taking up apoptotic cells deliberately opsonized with immunoglobulin and complement demonstrated that the teleologically attractive "neutral" response of unstimulated macrophages to the uptake of apoptotic cells was conditioned by the molecular recognition mechanisms involved, rather than the apoptotic cell being inherently "poisonous" (Meagher et al., 1992).

A particularly exciting recent development is evidence that the clearance of apoptotic cells by activated macrophages may be positively "anti-inflammatory" rather than merely "silent." In the most detailed study available, Fadok and colleagues (1998a) showed that release of TNF-α from endotoxin-stimulated macrophages was actively inhibited by the uptake of apoptotic cells. The mechanisms responsible involved a complex paracine-autocrine signaling loop mediated by macrophage release of the immuosuppressive cytokine-transforming growth factor β_1 (TGF-β_1) and the eicosanoids prostaglandin E_2 and plaletet-activating factor (Fadok et al., 1998a). Comparable data were described contemporaneously by Voll and colleagues (1997), but their report that uptake of apoptotic cells triggered endotoxin-stimulated macrophages to release IL-10 was not confirmed by Fadok et al. (1998a). It is possible that this reflects some loss of viability by apoptotic cells

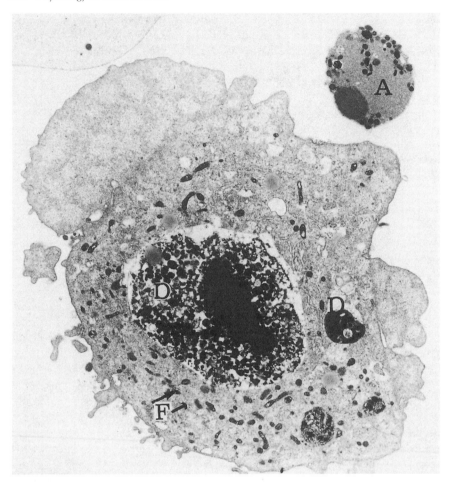

Fig. 24.1. Safe clearance of apoptotic contents: Electron micrograph (X 12 500) of myofibroblast-like glomerular mesangial cell (phenotype evident from microfilaments at F), which has ingested in vitro two apoptotic granulocytes (D). On the left is a recently ingested cell with a full complement of granules; on the right the ingested material is at an advanced stage of degradation; a non-ingested granulocyte-derived apoptotic body is present (A).

in the system employed by Voll et al. (1997), because Gao et al. (1998) recently reported that lymphoid cells undergoing apoptosis mediated by ligation of the Fas death receptor unexpectedly synthesize the immunosuppressive cytokine IL-10. Indeed, a particularly fascinating finding was that, by contrast, with antigen-coupled apoptotic cells from wild-type animals, which upon instillation into the immunologically privileged mouse eye resulted in systemic tolerization to the antigen (Griffith et al., 1996), antigen-coupled apoptotic cells from IL-10$^{-/-}$ knockout mice failed to induce tolerization.

These data emphasize that phagocyte clearance of apoptotic cells would normally be expected to suppress inflammatory and immune responses, representing an ideal route of disposal for leukocytes during resolution of inflammation.

However, recent experiments suggest that there are routes by which leukocyte apoptosis may trigger apparently undesirable immune responses. By contrast with administration to the eye, Mevorach and colleagues (1998b) found that intravenous administration to normal mice of 10 million syngeneic thymocytes irradiated so as to trigger apoptosis stimulated transient appearance in the blood of nuclear autoantibodies, antisingle-stranded DNA and anticardiolipin autoantibodies. Furthermore, although these animals did not develop proteinuria, a high proportion exhibited immunoglobulin deposition in renal glomeruli. This could represent a nonspecific immunostimulatory effect of oligonucleosomes released from apoptotic cells that eluded safe clearance (Bell and Morrison, 1991) because, if cells engaging the apoptotic program are not cleared by phagocytes, the dying cells eventually undergo secondary necrosis and disintegrate. However, a more alarming possibility is that these autoantibodies might have arisen following presentation by dendritic cells to T lymphocytes of antigen derived from apoptotic cells, as has been demonstrated recently in vitro (Albert et al., 1998a, 1998b). These data emphasize that phagocyte clearance of apoptotic leukocytes may not be safe in all circumstances.

Nevertheless, despite the risks inherent in professional antigen-presenting cells being capable of phagocytic clearance of apoptotic cells, which may be exacerbated by the probable generation of neo/autoantigens by caspase cleavage of proteins in the dying cells (Casciola-Rosen et al., 1995, 1996), there are controls on this process. First, intriguing in vitro studies indicate that dendritic cell presentation of apoptotic leukocyte-derived antigen to T cells was only observed when a large "load" of apoptotic cells was "fed" to immature dendritic cells, as uptake of lesser numbers of apoptotic cells failed to incite production of IL-1β or TNF-α from these phagocytes, thereby limiting maturation of the phagocytes to fully efficient antigen-presenting cells (Rovere et al., 1998). Second, if macrophages were also present, then dendritic cell presentation to T cells of apoptotic cell-derived antigen was markedly impaired (Albert et al., 1998b), perhaps because the macrophages cleared apoptotic cells so efficiently that dendritic cell access to the "meal" was denied, or because macrophages ingesting apoptotic cells released immunosuppressive cytokines such as TGF-β_1 that inhibited dendritic cell maturation–antigen presentation. Therefore, it appears probable that dendritic cell presentation of apoptotic cell-derived antigens is only likely to occur when a large load of dying cells eludes clearance by macrophages.

To conclude, although dendritic cell phagocytosis of apoptotic leukocytes could pose a threat to safe resolution of inflammation, there is a weight of in vitro evidence to indicate that clearance of apoptotic leukocytes by macrophages or semiprofessional phagocytes may not only be silent, but could also be actively anti-inflammatory. Because a definitive test of the significance of phagocyte clearance of apoptotic leukocytes would require the specific

Table 24.1. "Eat-Me" Markers on Cells Dying by Apotosis

Marker	Reference(s)
Carbohydrate changes	Duvall et al., 1985; Dini et al., 1992; Hall et al., 1994
Phosphatidylserine exposure	Fadok et al., 1992
Thrombospondin binding sites	Savill et al., 1992a
ICAM-3	Moffatt et al., 1999
Clq binding sites	Korb and Ahern, 1997; Botto et al., 1998

blockade of this event, it is now important to focus on the molecular mechanisms responsible for phagocytosis of apoptotic cells.

Mechanisms by Which Phagocytes Ingest Apoptotic Leukocytes

It is only recently that the study of cell culture systems in vitro has provided insights into the key issue of how apoptotic cells are recognized by phagocytes as "unwanted" self ripe for clearance (Savill, 1997, 1998). However, it should be evident from Figure 24.2 that in vivo studies will need to take account of possible roles for many different cell surface molecules, both "eat-me" molecules on the dying cell (Table 24.1) and receptors on phagocytes (Table 24.2). Furthermore, studies of genetic mutations in the nematode *Caenorhabditis elegans*, that impair clearance by nonprofessional neighbors of

Table 24.2. Phagocyte Surface Molecules Mediating Ingestion of Apoptotic Cells

Molecule (class/example)	Reference
Lectins	
unclassified	Duvall et al., 1985; Hall et al., 1994
asialoglycoprotein receptor	Dini et al., 1992
Integrins	
$\alpha_v\beta_3$	Savill et al., 1990
$\alpha_v\beta_5$	Albert et al., 1998a
$\alpha_m\beta_2$	Mevorach et al., 1998a
Class B Scavenger Receptors	
CD36	Savill et al., 1992a; Ren et al., 1995
CD68/macrosialin	Sambrano and Steinberg, 1995
SRB1 (CD36 homologue)	Fukasawa et al., 1996
Croquemort (CD36 homologue)	Franc et al., 1996, 1999
Class A Scavenger Receptor	Platt et al., 1996
ABC Transporters	
ABC 1 (mouse)	Luciani and Chimini 1996
CED-7 (*C elegans*)	Wu and Horvitz, 1998b
Endotoxin Receptor CD14	Devitt et al., 1998

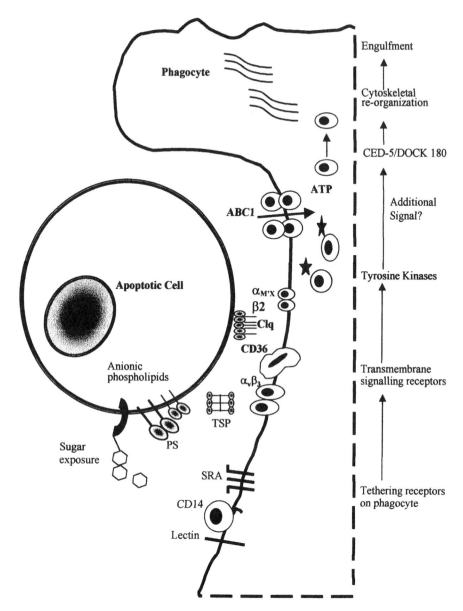

Fig. 24.2. Schema for recognition of apoptotic cells (see, also, text and Tables 24.1 and 24.2): The apoptotic cell is depicted as displaying three "eat-me" signals, exposed sugars, exposed phosphatidylserine (PS), and anionic phospholipids that may serve as receptors for "bridging" thrombospondin (TSP), C1q is also shown as a bridging molecule. It is speculated that lectins, CD14 and the class A scavenger receptor (SRA) on phagocytes serve to tether apoptotic cells, before transmembrane receptors ($\alpha_v \beta_3$, CD36, and possibly the complement receptors $\alpha_m \beta_2$ and $\alpha_x \beta_2$), capable of signaling and activating tyrosine kinases, come into play. Because ABC1 is an ATP-dependent transporter, this molecule may provide an additional signal for cytoskeletal reorganization, in which CED-5, a *C elegans* homologue of DOCK-180, participates (Wu and Horvitz, 1998a) prior to engulfment (adapted from Savill, 1998).

cells dying apoptosis-like developmental deaths have so far tended to define roles for intracellular signaling molecules rather than cell surface molecules (Wu and Horvitz, 1998a, Liu and Hengartner, 1998), emphasizing the importance of understanding how the phagocytic machinery is engaged within scavenging cells. Indeed, there is not a full understanding of the molecular basis of either of the two cases in which specific molecular defects account for failed clearance of apoptotic cells in higher organisms. In mammalian cells, our own experiments identified the class B scavenger receptor CD36 as a high-efficiency receptor for apoptotic cells employed by macrophages in partnership with the $\alpha_v\beta_3$ vitronectin receptor integrin to bind bridging thrombospondin (Savill et al., 1992b, Ren et al. 1995). Excitingly, Franc et al. (1996, 1999) have recently obtained definitive evidence in *Drosophila*, including specific rescue of a genetic defect, that the CD36 homologue Croquemort mediates clearance of apoptotic cells by this organism's professional phagocytes. However, this does not tell us whether CD36 has important roles in man, nor how CD36 homologues bind apoptotic cells or govern their ingestion and the subsequent phagocyte response. Thus, in addition to partnering the $\alpha_v\beta_3$ integrin, there is new evidence that CD36 may partner the yet-to-be characterized receptor for phosphatidylserine exposed on apoptotic cells (Fadok et al., 1998b). Furthermore, although the capacity of CD36 to signal the suppressive effects of thrombospondin on angiogenesis (Greenwalt et al., 1992) indicates that CD36 is an attractive candidate for directing the anti-inflammatory responses made by macrophages ingesting apoptotic cells, especially as ligation of CD36 inhibits TNF-α secretion from stimulated macrophages (Voll et al., 1997), this inhibitory signaling role is called into question by the likely role for CD36 in partnering the $\alpha_v\beta_3$ integrin in phagocytosis of apoptotic cells by dendritic cells so that apoptotic cell-derived antigens are presented to T cells (Albert et al., 1998a).

Similarly, although there is exciting in vivo evidence that C1q, the first component of complement, may be involved in clearance of apoptotic cells from inflamed sites, many details remain to be worked out. A body of evidence (Duvall et al., 1985; Dini et al., 1992, 1995; Hall et al., 1994) indicating that cell-surface sugar changes flag the "eat-me" status of apoptotic cells to phagocyte lectins, which then mediate their clearance, was available to underpin the intriguing finding by Korb and Ahearn (1997) that lectin-like C1q could bind apoptotic cells. However, before the details of how C1q might bridge apoptotic cells to phagocytes were defined, Botto et al (1998) observed a marked excess of apoptotic cells (strongly suggestive of impaired clearance) in the normal and inflamed kidneys of C1q knockout mice—a model of C1q deficiency in humans—that almost invariably leads to the severe multisystem autoimmune disorder, systemic lupus erythematosus (SLE). Preliminary data gained from deliberate administration of apoptotic cells to C1q$^{-/-}$ mice (M. Botto, personal communication, oral, 1999) support a defect in clearance and allow one to speculate that this contributes to perpetuation (and perhaps initiation) of immune and inflammatory responses to the contents of dying cells in autoimmune inflammatory diseases. Furthermore, similar defects are seen in triple knockout mice also deficient in C2 and factor B (T. Cook, personal communication, oral, 1999). Since such mice cannot fix complement, these data suggest that C1q binds directly to phagocyte receptors, rather than leading to the generation of opsonic complement fragments such as iC3b. Indeed, although Mevorach and colleagues (1998a) implicated iC3b in tethering apoptotic cells to phagocyte β_2 integrins we found no defect in uptake of apoptotic cells by macrophages taken either from humans with β_2 integrin deficiency (Davies et al., 1991) or from mice knocked out for such molecules (Ren et al., 2000).

Clearly, understanding the mechanisms by which apoptotic cells are cleared by phagocytes will be a growth point in the field. Although it is possible that the multiple mechanisms implicated so far merely represent redundancy, there is evidence that particular phagocytes employ particular predominant mechanisms to ingest apoptotic cells (Fadok et al., 1992), and hints that different clearance systems may operate in different organs or microenvironments (Savill, 1997; Botto et al, 1998). Furthermore, there is growing evidence that as cells dying by apoptosis progress through the program, they may engage a temporal hierarchy of clearance mechanisms, some preferring either early or late apoptotic cells, for example (Savill, 1997). Thus, although human monocyte-derived macrophages and murine peritoneal inflammatory macrophages recognize apoptotic neutrophils via mechanisms mediated by CD36 and phosphatidylserine receptors (PSRs), respectively (Savill et al. 1989b; Fadok et al 1992), late apoptotic neutrophils (characterized by nuclear resorption or "evanescenece"; Herbert et al., 1996) are recognized by both macrophage types via a CD36-and PSR-independent mechanism involving thrombospondin and $\alpha_v\beta_3$ (Ren et al., 2000) Nevertheless, no release of chemokines was incited, suggesting that this is a last line of tissue defence against dying neutrophils, clearing the cells before they eventually undergo secondary necrosis (see Fig. 24.3).

Perturbation of Safe Clearance

In addition to C1q deficiency, in vitro data suggest that low pH (Savill et al., 1989a), charged molecules (Savill et al 1989a), and fragments of extracellular matrix molecules (Savill et al., 1990, 1992a) could impair phagocyte uptake of apoptotic cells (see Fig. 24.3). More subtly, antiphospholipid (aPL) autoantibodies present in a number of autoimmune states including SLE, can bind phosphatidylserine exposed by apoptotic cells (Price et al., 1996) and opsonize the dying cells for phagocyte Fc receptors, triggering release of pro-inflammatory TNF-α from macrophages (Manfredi et al, 1998) and promoting presentation of apoptotic cell-derived antigens by dendritic cells (Rovere et al, 1998). Further research is obviously needed to seek defects in safe phagocyte clearance of apoptotic cells in disease, but before moving on from mechanisms employed to clear leukocytes dying in situ at inflamed sites, it is important to emphasize that leukocytes can also be cleared by emigration.

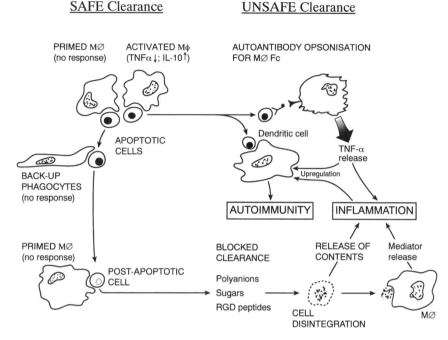

Fig. 24.3. Safe versus unsafe clearance of apoptotic cells: Safe clearance of apoptotic cells is achieved by primed macrophages (MØ) and semiprofessional "back-up" phagocytes such as mesangial cells; indeed, uptake of apoptotic cells by activated Mφ results in responses likely to suppress inflammation. Furthermore, apoptotic cells eluding clearance to reach a postapoptotic or late apoptotic state can still be cleared by primed Mφ without a pro-inflammatory response. However, if clearance is blocked then unsafe clearance ensues, apoptotic cells undergo secondary necrosis and disintegrate, and release contents that are directly pro-inflammatory, and that stimulate macrophages to release further pro-inflammatory mediators. Unsafe clearance also occurs if apoptotic cells are taken up by dendritic cells: the risk of autoantigen presentation would be exacerbated by inflammation because this promotes dendritic cell maturation. Opsonization of apoptotic cells by antiphospholipid autoantibodies stimulates Mφ release of TNF-α and other pro-inflammatory mediators (reproduced from Ren and Savill, 1998, with permission).

Emigration of Leukocytes from Inflamed Sites

Active Emigration as a Means of Leukocyte Clearance

Since the seminal studies of Gowans, Ford, and others, in the 1950s and 1960s it has been known that lymphocytes not only traffic through normal tissues, passing from the blood through tissues to emigrate via lymph vessels and regional lymph nodes before returning to the blood, but also move through inflamed or injured tissues at increased rates. Indeed, despite evidence of in situ clearance of apoptotic lymphocytes from inflamed sites, it appears most likely that the reductions in expanded lymphocyte populations, which are known to occur by apoptosis during resolution of lymphocytic infiltration, occur in such a way that unwanted cells move to the lymph nodes before dying and being ingested by "tingible body" macrophages (Akbar et al., 1994).

Similar principles apply to clearance of inflammatory macrophages, which, by contrast with freshly isolated monocytes, are remarkably resistant to pro-apoptotic stimuli such as survival factor deprivation in vitro. Using a fluorescent label to tag inflammatory macrophages in experimental peritonitis, Bellingan et al. (1996) discovered that most macrophages emigrate from the inflamed site to reach draining lymph nodes. This route of clearance was also reported for inflammatory macrophages present in the inflamed kidney (Lan et al., 1993), although in this organ in situ clearance of macrophages by apoptosis can occur (Atkins, 1995). Nevertheless, these findings highlight our almost complete ignorance of the cues and molecular mechanisms mediating macrophage emigration from inflamed sites, identifying this area is an important growth point for research.

Passive Leukocyte Emigration

When inflammatory responses occur in tissues that are in contact with the "outside world," passive leukocyte emigration may be an important clearance mechanism. Thus, neutrophils in particular may leave the inflamed lung via sputum, the urinary tract via urine, the gut via feces, and the skin via inflammatory exudate. The quantitative importance of this route of clearance is difficult to assess and will obviously vary on a case-by-case basis.

However, we have observed a more subtle form of passive leukocyte emigration in studies of immune complex-mediated injury of the glomerulus (Hughes et al., 1997a). In keeping with observations in humans with this type of microvascular injury, nearly all the neutrophils localizing to the tissue remained adherent to the damaged endothelium rather than migrating across the vessel wall, perhaps because the highest concentration of chemoattractant factors is present at the endothelial level. Neutrophils undergoing apoptosis could be observed in the capillary lumen and clearance by intravascular macrophages was prominent in those severely injured capillaries occluded by fibrin. By using radiolabeling techniques to track the fate of recruited neutrophils, we found that only 29% of neutrophils present at 4 hours remained in the kidney at 24 hours: 71% had already departed. The techniques available were not suitable for tracking neutrophil emigration quantitatively. However, although occasional labeled cells were seen within macrophages reaching draining lymph nodes, there was a strong likelihood that most neutrophils had emigrated by returning to the blood stream, either de-adhering to die later or losing adherence by reason of apoptosis (Hughes et al, 1992a) These data emphasize that leukocytes that have not crossed the endothelium could be passively cleared through the blood, a further point at which new treatments could be targeted.

Remodeling of the Inflamed Organ

So far, we have concentrated on mechanisms underlying resolution of an obvious and pathognomonic feature of inflammation, leukocyte infiltration. However, this is but part of a triad of histological features evident in inflammatory responses: proliferation and phenotypic change of resident cells so that these frequently resemble myofibroblasts, and deposition of extracellular matrix are also key features of inflammation, particularly where this becomes persistent. Therefore, if the response is to resolve mechanisms by which these changes in resident cells and extracellular matrix are remodeled should be considered.

Restoration of the Normal Population of Resident Cells

Proliferation of Myofibroblastic and Other Resident Cells
In many organs including the skin (Darby et al., 1990; Desmoulière et al., 1993), kidney (Johnson et al., 1991), liver (Iredale et al., 1998), and lung (Polunovsky et al 1993), wounding or inflammatory injury of the organ results in local accumulation of myofibroblast-like cells that appear to promote healing or resolution by repairing tissue defects and laying down a temporary extracellular matrix. Myofibroblasts may arise by phenotypic change of resident cells, such as mesangial cells in the renal glomerulus (Johnson et al., 1991), or hepatic stellate cells in the liver (Iredale et al., 1998). Alternatively, there is evidence that they may migrate into the area of tissue damage from expandable reservoirs in the walls of neighboring microvessels (Hugo et al, 1997). Whatever their source, myofibroblasts share features of smooth muscle cells (such as expression of the useful marker protein α-smooth muscle actin) and fibroblasts (such as the capacity to lay down interstitial collagens).

Although the accumulation of myofibroblasts in an inflamed tissue is widely regarded as a threat for later scarring, it is also a key event in repair. A compelling example of the repair function of myofibroblasts is provided by the anti-Thy 1.1 antibody model of self-limited glomerular injury in the rat (Bagchus et al., 1986). Administration of this antibody, which binds to cell surface Thy 1.1 antigen normally expressed by rat glomerular mesangial cells, triggers their complement-mediated death so that virtually all the mesangial cells disappear. However, myofibroblasts arising from the walls of supplying blood vessels undergo intensive division and migrate to repopulate the glomerulus (Hugo et al., 1997). Initially there is an "overshoot" such that by 2 weeks, the mesangial cell complement is double the normal size, but these excess mesangial cells are deleted (see the following) and the glomerulus regains normal structure by 4–5 weeks (Bagchus et al., 1986).

Because expanded myofibroblast populations are often seen as a "bad thing," there has been extensive study of the mechanisms governing myofibroblast proliferation. This has been most successful in glomerular injury for which there is compelling evidence that mitosis of myofibroblast-like mesangial cells is driven by platelet-derived growth factor (PDGF): (a) PDGF stimulates mesangial cell proliferation in vitro (Abboud, 1993); (b) is expressed in vivo at levels that correlate closely with the frequency of mesangial cell division (Floege et al., 1993); and (c) when administered by infusion (Floege et al., 1993) or gene transfer (Isaka et al, 1993) to rats, can induce mesangial cell proliferation. Furthermore, in the Thy 1.1 model described in the previous paragraph, mesangial cell proliferation is attenuated by neutralizing antibody to PDGF (Johnson et al., 1992). As a consequence, there is considerable interest in PDGF antagonist drugs that might limit accumulation of myofibroblasts and the attendant threat of irreversible deposition of excess, abnormal extracellular matrix.

Furthermore, depending on the site and nature of the tissue injury and inflammatory response, there is a growing interest in determining to what extent normal versus abnormal proliferation of cell types other than myofibroblasts governs whether inflammation resolves successfully or leads to scarring. A growth point will be research into mechanisms controlling angiogenesis and other events regulating pattern formation in the injured organ; further discussion of this area is beyond the scope of this chapter.

Deletion of Resident Cells: A Double-Edged Sword?

Given the power of apoptosis to mediate safe deletion of unwanted leukocytes, it should come as no surprise that in self-limited inflammatory injury of the kidney (Baker et al., 1994) (Shimizu et al., 1995), liver (Iredale et al., 1998), and skin (Desmoulière et al., 1995), there is compelling evidence that beneficial deletion of excess myofibroblast-like cells appears to be achieved by this programmed form of cell death. This conclusion is based on "area-under-the-curve" estimates (Savill et al., 1996a) of the rate of cell deletion in careful time-course studies of experimental models of reversible myofibroblast proliferation; definitive experiments await an understanding of how to block, highly selectively, apoptosis in the cell population under study.

However, at least in the example of glomerular inflammation and scarring, apoptosis in resident cells such as myofibroblasts may be a double-edged sword that is both beneficial and dangerous (Savill et al., 1996b). This concept arises because there is growing evidence that unscheduled apoptosis in resident glomerular cells is a final common pathway by which the inflamed, injured glomerulus progresses to hypocellular, functionless scar tissue (Sugiyama et al., 1996b): the deleterious edge of the apoptosis sword. Clearly, therefore, it is critical to develop an understanding of how the survival or death of resident cells such as myofibroblasts is regulated.

Control of Myofibroblast Survival

At present, in vitro experiments indicate that a wide range of stimuli (both specific and nonspecific) can trigger apoptosis in myofibroblast-like mesangial cells (e.g., see Table 24.3). However, in most cases there is a problem in determining how the stimulus might selectively trigger apoptosis in myofibroblastic cells, and there are no data to indicate whether such stimuli are relevant in vivo. Notable exceptions are the capacity of anti-Thy 1.1 antibodies to trigger acute complement-dependent apoptosis of normal glomerular mesangial cells in rats, and a report that ligation of the Fas death receptor

Table 24.3. Triggering of Apoptosis in Myofibroblast-like Glomerular Mesangial Cells

Stimulus	Selected References
Nonspecific	
Serum starvation	Baker et al., 1994; Mooney et al., 1997
Detachment	Singhal et al., 1998
Shear stress	Singhal et al., 1998
Hydrostatic pressure	Singhal et al., 1998
DNA damage	Singhal et al., 1998
Reactive oxygen species	Ishikawa et al., 1997; Sugiyama et al., 1996b; Yokoo and Kiamura, 1997
Ionizing radiation	Cha et al., 1996
Cytotoxic drugs	Baker et al., 1994; Cha et al., 1996
Specific	
Anti-Thy 1.1 antibodies	Sato et al., 1996, 1997
Anti-Fas antibodies	Gonzalez-Cuadrado et al., 1997
TNF-α	Liu et al., 1996; Guo et al., 1998
IL-1α	Liu et al., 1996
IL-1β	Guo et al., 1998
C1q	Sato et al., 1996
Anti-ds DNA antibodies	Tsai et al., 1993
LDL	Sharma et al., 1996
Lovastatin	Ghosh et al., 1997
Nitric oxide	Mühl et al., 1996; Sandau et al., 1997; Nitsch et al., 1997
Superoxide	Sandau et al., 1997
cAMP	Mühl et al., 1996

Note. TNF, tumor necrosis factor; IL-1, interleukin-1; LDL, low-density lipoprotein; cAMP, cyclic odenosine monophosphate.

(Nagata and Golstein, 1995) by administration of agonistic anti-Fas antibody to mice not only induces catastrophic hepatocellular injury, but also triggers golmerular cell apoptosis (Gonzalez-Cuadrado et al., 1996). However, in neither case are the mesangial cells triggered into apoptosis known to have the myofibroblastic phenotype, so these data should be viewed with caution. Nevertheless, the idea that myofibroblastic populations might be reduced in size by homeostatic "death" factors gains credence from the demonstration by Polunovsky et al. (1993) that bronchial lavages obtained from patients with resolving fibroblastic granulation tissue in the lung had the capacity to induce death of cultured fibroblasts and other lung cells.

Despite the potential importance of prodeath factors in regulating myofibroblast populations, it is also important to note that site-and lineage-specific control of cell number can be achieved by altering supply of so-called survival factors, agents that promote cell survival by inhibiting apoptosis. Raff (1992) formulated the important hypothesis that all cells in the adult body will inevitably undergo apoptosis unless they receive a sufficient supply of survival factors that are integrated to provide spatially localized and exquisitely lineage-specific signals to ensure that cells that wander from their correct home are automatically deleted. In cultures of myofibroblastic glomerular mesangial cells, we found that insulin-like growth factor-1 (IGF-1) and IGF-2 were able to inhibit apoptosis induced by a range of stressful stimuli, such as serum deprivation, etoposide-mediated DNA damage, or cycloheximide-mediated inhibition of protein synthesis (Mooney et al., 1997). However, the likely specificity of survival factor control of myofibroblast fate and numbers in vivo was emphasized by the failure of PDGF, a potent mitogen for myofibroblastic cells (as discussed previously) and a survival factor for oligodendrocytes, to promote survival of mesangial cell-derived myofibroblasts. Similarly, no protective effect was observed with epidermal growth factor (EGF), which is a survival factor for kidney tubule epithelial cells. Interestingly, we also obtained evidence of paracine survival signaling mediated by IGF-1 which might sustain expanded populations of myofibroblasts because medium conditioned by healthy mesangial cells was able to inhibit apoptosis in stressed cells, a property specifically abrogated by neutralizing antibody to IGF-1. Nevertheless, despite the capacity of IGF-1 to inhibit a range of pro-apoptotic influences, there is clear evidence that survival signals can be overridden in certain circumstances by death factors. Thus, in myofibroblastic mesangial cells sensitized to Fas-mediated death by exposure to interferon-γ (IFN-γ), IGF-1 failed to protect cells against the pro-apoptotic effects of Fas ligation (Mooney et al., 1997).

In a series of experiments addressing whether extracellular matrix (ECM) signaling of survival via integrins was relevant to myofibroblast-like mesangial cells, evidence was obtained that alterations in extracellular matrix might render myofibroblasts particularly susceptible to unscheduled deletion by apoptosis (Mooney et al., 1999). Thus, although normal constituents of the glomerular ECM (such as type IV collagen and laminin) supplied β_1 integrin-mediated survival signals to serum-starved and etoposide-treated myofibroblast-like mesangial cells, abnormal constituents of ECM that accumulate as glomerular inflammation progresses to scarring (i.e., type I collagen or plasma fibronectin) failed to provide survival signals.

The in vivo relevance of cytokine and matrix survival signals for myofibroblasts remains to be proven. Furthermore, intensive work is required to characterize the molecular mechanisms by which such exogenous factors suppress engagement of the apoptotic caspase cascade in this cell lineage. Perhaps surprisingly, in view of reports on other cell types (Zhang et al., 1995), neither cytokine nor matrix survival factors for myofibroblastic cells altered the balance of expression of anti-apoptotic and pro-apoptotic members of Bcl-2 family of death regulatory proteins (Mooney et al, 1997, 1999). However, at least in the specific case of apoptosis induced by TNF-α, but not a range of other pro-apoptotic stimuli, we were able to deploy a "superrepressor" mutant of IκBα to demonstrate a key prosurvival role for transcription factors of the NF-κB family, although the "downstream" NF-κB-regulated protective genes remain to be characterized.

It should be obvious that there has been, so far, a very limited attack on mechanisms regulating myofibroblast survival and population size. Nevertheless, it should be equally clear that this is an important growth point in research into resolution mechanisms in inflammation.

Removal of Excess/Abnormal Extracellular Matrix Components

The potential importance of successful remodeling of the extracellular matrix (ECM) for resolution of inflammation cannot be overemphasized, given the increasing appreciation that the ECM is an active structure capable of controlling gene expression in attached cells, directly by integrin and other adhesion receptors, or indirectly by modulating cytokine action (Nathan and Sporn, 1991). Exquisite and plastic control of cell function is to be expected as most cell types present at inflamed sites not only synthesize ECM components, but can also degrade established ECM by secretion of enzymes such as matrix metalloproteinases (MMPs). In turn, these can be activated by other proteases or oxidants, or inactivated by locally secreted molecules such as tissue inhibitors of metalloproteinases (TIMPs).

An example of the potential significance of persistence of an abnormal "inflammatory" ECM rich in interstitial collagens and plasma-type fibronectin has already been cited: a potential to render resident cells undesirably susceptible to apoptosis by denying them the correct ECM-derived survival signals (Mooney et al., 1999). Indeed, in a noninflammatory context it is notable that local activation of MMPs and degradation of normal ECM precedes loss of mammary epithelial cells by apoptosis during involution of the lactating breast (Talhouk et al., 1992). Nevertheless, regulation of the ECM during inflammatory responses is largely uncharted territory and the significance of events identified so far is uncertain. An example is an early study of Thy 1.1 nephritis (*described previously*) in which there is gross accumulation of abnormal ECM as myofibroblast-like mesangial cells proliferate. Lovett et al (1992) demonstrated a marked increase in local expression of MMP-2 (a 72-kD type IV collagenase) during this early phase of ECM remodeling, but the significance of the observation is uncertain. This is a further aspect of the resolution of inflammation in which much useful work could be done.

Control of Resolution

Endogenous Controls on Resolution of Inflammation

Control Points in Inflammatory Cell Disposal

Mention has already been made of the concept that expression of down-regulatory control molecules, such as IL-6 or lipoxins, can be programmed into the inflammatory response in such a manner that leukocyte recruitment is time limited. However, the subsequent discussion in this chapter highlights additional new control points

First, the rate at which infiltrating leukocytes undergo apoptosis could be regulated. Indeed, it is intriguing that some, but not all, inflammatory mediators involved in initiation of the response such as endotoxin or granulocyte macrophage colony-stimulating factor (GM-CSF), can delay the onset of constitutive apoptosis in leukocytes such as neutrophils, and may therefore govern resolution of inflammation (Lee et al., 1993). Teliologically, this might not only serve to delay deletion of the first wave of neutrophils until an increased phagocyte clearance capacity has developed at the inflamed site (see the following), but could also ensure that these inflammatory "storm troopers" remain viable long enough to kill and ingest invading bacteria (Haslett, 1992). In this regard it is intriguing that complement-mediated phagocytosis of particles (Coxon et al., 1996) or uptake of bacteria (Watson et al., 1996), a key job for infiltrating neutrophils, actually hastens deletion of these cells, rather like programmed retirement of a workforce that has done its job. However, the potential complexity of endogenous controls on leukocyte life span at inflamed sites is emphasized by the example of TNF-α, which can accelerate apoptosis in a subset of neutrophils while inhibiting the process in others (Murray et al., 1997).

Second, the capacity of phagocytes to remove apoptotic inflammatory cells has also been identified as a key control point in resolution of inflammation. Again, there is evidence of endogenous controls on this event being programmed into the inflammatory response. Monocytes must mature into macrophages before the capacity to ingest apoptotic cells is acquired (Newman et al., 1982; Savill et al., 1990). We found that the capacity of "semi-mature" macrophages to ingest apoptotic neutrophils was rapidly unregulated by cytokines, which can also slow neutrophil apoptosis, such as GM-CSF or IL-1β (Ren et al., 1995). Thus, cytokines that delay neutrophil deletion also simultaneously ready monocyte-derived macrophages for clearance of neutrophils once the granulocytes have done their job.

These two examples emphasize the obvious: resolution mechanisms are likely to be tightly programmed into inflammatory processes: however, if this is the case, we are still left with the problem of how the duration and outcome of inflammatory response is governed. A trivial inflammatory response in the skin caused by a pinprick and the severe inflammatory response that enabled the lung to eliminate pneumocci in the pre-antibiotic era are examples of dramatically different degrees of inflammation, that, nevertheless, are both successful in that complete resolution occurs. Clearly, there must be a "ringmaster" in control of the inflammatory circus.

The Inflammatory Macrophage as a Candidate for Ringmaster

The inflammatory macrophage is emerging as a potential ringmaster in inflammatory cell clearance by apoptosis. It is well-established that macrophages can elaborate cytokines likely to inhibit apoptosis of leukocytes (e.g., GM-CSF) and myofibroblasts (e.g. IGF-1), but the degree to which macrophages prolong the life span of such inflammatory cells is unknown.

Conversely, although various macrophage-derived cytokines (Ren and Savill, 1995) can promote monocyte/macrophage capacity for phagocytosis of inflammatory cells once these have undergone apoptosis, we know almost nothing of the extent to which the capacity for clearance of apoptotic cells is governed by such paracrine interactions between phagocytes. Indeed, dissection of such signaling could prove particularly profitable in understanding how presentation of apoptotic cell-derived antigens by dendritic cells fits into the picture, given the capacity of macrophages to inhibit this event (Albert et al., 1998b).

Developmental biology demonstrates a further, ringmaster-like role for the macrophage: the capacity to direct apoptosis in unwanted cells during tissue remodeling. This was demonstrated in seminal work by Lang and colleagues on elimination from the neonatal rodent eye of a leash of blood vessels behind the lens (Lang and Bishop, 1993; Lang, 1997) Careful observation coupled with definitive macrophage depletion–repletion studies in vivo showed that macrophage "locked on" to microvascular endothelial cells and triggered apoptosis, albeit by unknown mechanisms.

We now have evidence that macrophages can also direct apoptosis of leukocytes and myofibroblastic cells to promote remodeling of inflamed tissue. First, it was found that human monocyte-derived macrophages ingesting opsonized zymosan released Fas ligand and conditioned supernatants for Fas-mediated killing of neutrophils and monocytes (Brown and Savill, 1999). However, although uptake of latex beads also triggered macrophage release of Fas ligand, the supernatants did not accelerate leukocyte apoptosis, emphasizing that in this system an unidentified cofactor is required to enable Fas ligand to promote death of target cells. Nevertheless, the capacity of macrophages to act in a negative feedback control loop in inflammation was suggested by release of Fas ligand (and conditioning of the supernatants for leukocyte killing) from macrophages ingesting apoptotic neutrophils; as such cells are cleared, "bystander" leukocytes would also be triggered into apoptosis by macrophage-derived Fas ligand, hastening the clearance of infiltrating leukocytes. This hypothesis needs testing in vivo.

Second, macrophages (either human monocyte-derived or rodent bone marrow-derived) deliberately activated by agents such as interferon-γ can, when cocultured with the target cell type, direct apoptosis and inhibit mitosis of myofibroblast-like mesangial cells in vitro (Duffield et al., 2000). The use of inhibitors and macrophages from inducible nitric oxide synthase (iNOS) knockout mice demonstrated that products of this enzyme (presumably nitric oxide, but possibly other reactive species such as peroxynitrite) were critical in promoting apoptosis or inhibiting mitosis. Although priming mesangial cells with inflammatory cytokines rendered the myofibroblastic cells susceptible to Fas ligand-induced apoptosis and increased the capacity of activated macrophages to kill, we found that this additional kill was not mediated by macrophage release of Fas ligand: instead, there appears to be a role for TNFα. Further mechanistic work needs to be done in this system, and macrophage depletion–repletion experiments in vivo will, be essential to assess the importance of macrophage control of myofibroblast populations.

To conclude this section there are now exciting pointers to reinforce the concept, established by the seminal demonstration by Liebovich and Ross (1975) that macrophages are essential for wound healing, that the macrophage is a ringmaster in safe resolution and repair of inflammation.

Can Resolution of Inflammation Be Controlled for Therapeutic Benefit?

Directing Leukocyte Apoptosis

Although there is controversy over whether "fratricide" mediated by Fas–Fas ligand interaction between neighboring cells is important in constitutive apoptosis in granulocytes (Liles et al., 1996, Brown and Savill, 1999), an exciting report from Tsuyuki et al., (1995) suggests that the expression of the Fas death receptor by leukocytes could be exploited for therapeutic advantage. In a rabbit model of eosinophilic inflammation it was possible to direct eosinophil elimination by apoptosis by administering aerosolized Fas ligand into the airways, without apparent ill effects on resident tissues. Although recent data suggest that Fas ligand could damage airway epithelium (Matute-Bello et al., 1999), limiting the therapeutic usefulness of this approach, Tsuyuki et al.'s work is the first clear demonstration that mechanisms mediating resolution of inflammation can be modulated by exogenous factors and highlights the therapeutic potential of directed deletion of leukocytes by deliberately triggering apoptosis.

Elimination of eosinophils by apoptosis in vivo could also be achieved by the use of glucocorticoids because these potent anti-inflammatory agents were found to accelerate apoptosis in eosinophils in vivo (Meagher et al., 1996) in a manner entirely in keeping with observations made in animal models (Kawabori et al., 1991) and human cases (Woolley et al. 1996) of eosinophilic inflammation, which indicated that steroid treatment diminishes the life span of eosinophils at inflamed sites. However, although glucocorticoids could also direct lymphocyte apoptosis, it is intriguing that these agents have a modest inhibitory effect on constitutive apoptosis in neutrophils (Cox, 1995); further investigation is required.

Promoting Safe Phagocytic Clearance of Apoptotic Leukocytes

In keeping with the capacity of glucocorticoids to direct eosinophil death, Woolley et al., (1996) reported widespread apoptosis in pulmonary exudates from asthma patients receiving glucocorticoids. However, their study also demonstrated that apoptotic eosinophils were commonly inside macrophages. We wondered whether this might indicate that glucocorticoids also promote phagocyte ingestion of apoptotic leukocytes.

In studies of the phagocytosis of apoptotic neutrophils, eosinophils or lymphocytes by human/rodent macrophages and semiprofessional human mesangial cells, there was clear evidence that glucocorticoids could specifically induce up to four-fold increases in phagocyte capacity to ingest apoptotic cells (Liu et al., 1999). Importantly, this increased capacity was not gained at the cost of pro-inflammatory responses; steroid-treated phagocytes still failed to release chemokines after ingestion of apoptotic leukocytes. Work is in progress on the molecular mechanisms mediating this second, hitherto unrecognized proresolution effect of glucocorticoids, which appears likely to complement the capacity of these agents to trigger apoptosis in some leukocyte types. Our unpublished preliminary experiments in thioglycolate-induced peritonitis suggest that glucocorticoids can indeed promote macrophage clearance of apoptotic neutrophils in vivo.

This is exciting because further in vitro experiments point to other potentially less toxic means to promote phagocyte clearance of apoptotic cells from inflamed sites. First, ligation of macrophage CD44 induces a very rapid increase in capacity for phagocytes of apoptotic neutrophils without, intriguingly, promoting the uptake of apoptotic lymphocytes (Hart et al., 1997). Second, as mentioned previously, the lipoxin LXA_4 can also promote human monocyte-derived macrophage phagocytes of apoptotic neutrophils (Godson et al., 1998). Ongoing work in both systems is likely to reveal new approaches to therapy of inflammation.

Conclusion and Future Prospects

Despite the recent advances described here, remarkably little is understood of the mechanisms that mediate safe resolution of inflammation. This field will be a rich hunting ground for researchers seeking new therapeutic targets in inflammatory disease.

It should be equally obvious that the progress made so far has provided important new insights into why inflammatory responses may become persistent and lead to scarring and loss of function. Growth points will be the further definition of the mechanisms and consequences of perturbed phagocyte clearance of inflammatory cells undergoing apoptosis, dissection of controls upon the possible presentation of apoptotic cell-derived autoantigens by phagocyte dendritic cells, and detailed study of how the balance between survival and death of resident cells such as myofibroblasts determines successful remodeling or progression to hypocellular, functionless scar. There is clearly a need to move on from the culture dish to animal models of inflammation, but it will be important to develop genetic or other means by which to target and manipulate particular cell types during resolution of inflammatory responses.

Furthermore, the new insights gained are already pointing to new therapeutic approaches toward inflammatory disease that will be based on promoting safe resolution We already have animal model "proof of concept" for the utility of directed deletion of leukocytes by selective induction of apoptosis, and the $Clq^{-/-}$ mouse will be a useful test animal for agents that could promote safe phagocytic clearance of apoptotic inflammatory cells. Resolution of inflammation is clearly worthy of further attention.

We gratefully acknowledge long-term support from both the U.K. Medical Research Council and the Wellcome Trust. Mark Farquhar typed the manuscript.

References

Abboud, H. E. (1993) Nephrology forum: growth factors in glomerulonephritis. *Kidney Int.* 43: 252–267.

Akbar, A. N., Borthwick, N., Salmon, M., Gombert, W., Bofill, M., Shamsadeen, N., Pett, S., Grundy, J. E., and Janossy, G. (1993) The significance of low bcl-2 expression by CD45RO T cells, in normal individuals and patients with acute viral infection. The role of apoptosis in T cell memory. *J. Exp. Med.* 178:427–434.

Akbar, A. N., Savill, J., Gombert, W., Bofill, M., Borthwick, N. J., Whitelaw, F., Grundy, J., Janossy, G., and Salmon, M. (1994) The specific recognition by macrophages of CD8+, CD45RO+ T cells undergoing apoptosis: A mechanism for T cell clearance during resolution of viral infections. *J. Exp. Med.* 180:1943–1947.

Albert, M. L., Pearce, F. A., Francisco, L. M., Sauter, B., Roy, P., Silverstein, R. L., and Bhardwaj, N. (1998a) Immature dendritic cells phagocytose apoptotic cells via $\alpha_v\beta_3$ and cross-present antigens to cytotoxic T lymphocytes. *J. Exp. Med.* 188:1359–1368.

Albert, M. L., Sauter, B., and Bhardwaj, N. (1998b), Dendritic cells acquire antigen from apoptotic cells and induce class 1-restricted CTLs. *Nature* 392: 86–89.

Atkins, R. C. (1995) Interleukin-1 in crescentic glomerulonephritis. *Kidney Int.* 4:576–586.

Bagchus, W. M., Hoedemaeker, P. J., Rozing, J., and Bakker, W. W. (1986) Glomerulonephritis induced by monoclonal anti-Thyl. 1 antibodies. A sequential histological and ultrastructural study in the rat. *Lab. Invest.* 55:680–687.

Baker, A. J., Mooney, A., Hughes, J., Lombardi, D., Johnson, R. J., and Savill, J. (1994) Mesangial cell apoptosis: The major mechanism for resolution of glomerular hypercellularity in experimental mesangial proliferative nephritis. *J. Clin. Invest.* 94:2105–2116.

Bell, D. A., and Morrison, B. (1991) The spotaneous apoptotic death of normal human lymphocytes in vitro: The release of and immunoproliferative response to nucleosomes in vitro. *Clin. Immunol. Immunopathol.* 60:13–26.

Bellingan, G. J., Caldwell, H., Howie, S.E.M., Dransfield, I., and Haslett, C. (1996) In vivo fate of the inflammatory macrophage during the resolution of inflammation: Inflammatory macrophages do not die locally, but emigrate to the draining lymph nodes. *J. Immunol.* 157:2577–2585.

Botto, M., DellAgnola, C., Bygrave, A. E., Thompson, E. M., Cook, H. T., Petry, F., Loos, M., Pandolfi, P. P., and Walport, M. J. (1998) Homozygous C1q deficiency causes glomerulonephritis associated with multiple apoptotic bodies. *Nature Genetics* 19:56–59.

Brady, H. R., Lamas, S., Takata, S., Jimenez, W., Matsubara, M., and Marsden, P. A. (1995) Lipoxygenase product formation and cell adhesion during interactions of human neutrophils and glomerular endothelial cells. *Am J Physiol.* 37:F1–F12.

Brown, S. B., and Savill, J. S. (1999) Phagocytosis triggers macrophage release of fas ligand and induces apoptosis of bystander lymphocytes. *J. Immunol.* 162:480–485.

Campbell, E. J., and Campbell, M. A. (1988) Cellular proteolysis by neutrophils in the presence of proteinase inhibitors: effects of substrate opsonization. *J. Cell Biol.* 106:667–675.

Casciola-Rosen, L. A., Anhalt, G. J., and Rosen, A. (1995) DNA-dependent protein kinase is one of a subset of autoantigens specifically cleaved early during apoptosis. *J. Exp. Med.* 182:1625–1634.

Casciola-Rosen, L., Rosen, A., Petri, M., and Schlissel, M. (1996) Surface blebs on apoptotic cells are sites of enhanced procoagulant activity: Implications for coagulation events and antigenic spread in systemic lupus erythematosus. *Proc. Natl. Acad. Sci. USA* 93:1624–1629.

Cha, D. R., Feld, S. M., Nast, C., Lapage, J., and Adler, S. G. (1996) Apoptosis in mesangial cells induced by ionizing radiation and cytotoxic drugs. *Kidney Int.* 50:1565–1571.

Cox, G. (1995) Glucocorticoid treatment inhibits apoptosis in human neutrophils. *J. Immunol.* 154:4719–4725.

Cox, G. J., Crossley, J., and Xing, Z. (1995) Macrophage engulfment of apoptotic neutrophils contributes to the resolution of acute pulmonary inflammation in vivo. *Am. J. Respir. Cell Mol. Biol.* 12:232–237.

Coxon, A., Rieu, P., Barkalow, F. J., Askari, S. Sharpe, A. H., von Andrian, U. H., Arnaout, M. A., and Mayadas, T. N. (1996) A novel role for the β2 integrin CD11b/CD18 in neutrophil apoptosis: A homeostatic mechanism in inflammation. *Immun.* 5:653–666.

Darby, I., Skalli, O., and Gabbiani, G. (1990) Alpha-smooth muscle actin is transiently expressed by myofibroblasts during wound healing. *Lab. Invest.* 63:21–29.

Davies, K. A., Toothill, V. J., Savill, J., Hotchin, N., Peters, A. M., Pearson, J. D., Haslett, C., Burke, M., Law, S.K.A., Mercer, N.F.G., et al. (1991) A 19-year-old man with leucocyte adhesion deficiency. In vitro and in vivo studies of leucocyte function. *Clin. Exp. Immunol.* 84:223–231.

Desmoulière, A., Geinoz, A., Gabbiani, F., and Gabbiani, G. (1993) Transforming growth-factor β1 induces α-smooth muscle actin expression in granulation tissue myofibroblasts and in quiescent and growing cultured fibroblasts. *J. Cell Biol.* 122:103–111.

Desmoulière, A., Redard, M., Darby, I., and Gabbiani, G. (1995) Apoptosis mediates the decrease in cellularity during the transition between granulation tissue and scar. *Am. J. Pathol.* 146:56–66.

Devitt, A, Moffatt, O. D., Raykundalia, C., Capra, J. D., Simmons, D. L., and Gregory, C. D. (1998) Human CD14 mediates recognition and phagocytosis of apoptotic cells. *Nature* 392:505–509.

Dini, L., Autori, F., Lentini, A., Oliviero, S., and Piacentini, M. (1992) The clearance of apoptotic cells in the liver is mediated by the asialoglycoprotein receptor. *FEBS Lett.* 296:174–178.

Dini, L., Lentini, A., Diez, G. D., Rocha, M., Falasca, L., Serafino, L., and Vidal-Vanaclocha, F. (1995) Phagocytosis of apoptotic bodies by liver endothelial cells. *J. Cell Sci.* 108:967–973.

Duffield, J., Erwig, L. P., Wei, X., Liew, F. Y., Rees, A. J., and Savill, J. S., (2000) Macrophages activated in vivo and in vitro control glomerular mesangial cell number by induction of apoptosis and inhibition of mitosis. *J. Immunol.* 164:2110–2119.

Duvall, E., Wyllie, A. H., and Morris, R. G. (1985) Macrophage recognition of cells undergoing programmed cell death. *Immunol.* 56:351–358.

Enari, M., Sakahira, H., Yokoyama, H., Okawa, K., Iwamatsu, A., and Nagata, S. (1998) A caspase-activated DNase that degrades DNA during apoptosis, and its inhibitor ICAD. *Nature* 391:43–50.

Fadok, V., Savill, J. S., Haslett, C., Bratton, D. L., Doherty, D. E., Campbell, P. A., and Henson, P. M. (1992) Different populations of macrophages use either the vitronectin receptor or the phosphatidylserine receptor to recognise and remove apoptotic cells. *J. Immunol.* 149:4029–4035.

Fadok, V. A., Bratton, D. L., Konowal, A., Freed, P. W., Westcott, J. Y., and Henson, P. M. (1998a) Macrophages that have ingested apoptotic cells in vitro inhibit proinflammatory cytokine production through autocrine/paracrine mechanisms involving TGF-β PGE2 and PAF. *J. Clin. Invest.* 101:890–898.

Fadok, V. A., Warner, M. L., Bratton, D. L., and Henson, P. M. (1998b) CD36 is required for phagocytosis of apoptotic cells by human macrophages that use either a phosphatidyl serine receptor or the vitronectin receptor ($\alpha_v\beta_3$). *J. Immunol.* 161:6250–6257.

Floege, J., Eng, E., Young, B. A., Alpers, C. E., Barrett, T. B., Bowen-Pope, D. F., and Johnson, R. J. (1993) Infusion of PDGF or basic FGF induces selective glomerular mesangial cell proliferation and matrix accumulation in rats. *J. Clin. Invest.* 92:2952–2962.

Franc, N. C., Dimarcq, J.-L., Lagueux, M., Hoffmann, J., and Ezekowitz, R.A.B. (1996) Croquemort, a novel *Drosophila* hemocyte/macrophage receptor that recognises apoptotic cells. *Immun.* 4:431–433.

Franc, N. C., Heitzler, P. Ezekowitz, R. A., and White, K. (1999) Requirement for croquemort in phagocytosis of apoptotic cells in *Drosophila*. *Science* 18:284–5422.

Fukasawa, M., Adachi, H., Hirota, K., Tsujimoto, M., Arai, H., and Inoue, K. (1996) SRB1, a class B scavenger receptor, recognizes both negatively charged liposomes and apoptotic cells. *Exp. Cell Res.* 222:246–250.

Gao, Y., Herndon, J. M., Zhang, H., Griffith, T. S., and Ferguson, T. A. (1998) Antinflammatory effects of CD95 ligand (Fas-L)-induced apoptosis. *J. Exp. Med.* 188:887–896.

Ghosh, P. M., Mott, G. E., Choudhury, N., Radnik, R. A., Stapleton, M. I., Ghidoni, J. J., and Kreisberg, J. (1997) Lovastatin induces apoptosis by inhibiting mitotic and post-mitotic events in cultured mesangial cells. *Biochem. Biophys. Act* 1359: 13–24.

Godson, C., Mitchell, S., Harvey, K., Fokin, V., Petasis, N., and Brady, H. R. (1998) Lipoxins stimulate macrophage phagocytosis of apoptotic neutrophils. *J. Am. Soc. Nephrol.* 9:482A.

Gonzalez-Cuadrado, S., Lopez-Armada, M. J., Gomez-Guerrero, C., Subir, D., Garcia-Sahuquillo, A., Ortiz-Gonzalez, A., Neilson, E. G., Egido, J., and Ortiz, A. (1996) Anti-Fas antibodies induce cytolysis and apoptosis in cultured human mesangial cells. *Kidney Int.* 49:1064–1070.

Gonzalez-Cuadrado, S., Lorz, C., Garcia del Moral, R., O'Valle, F., Alsono, C., Ramiro, F., Ortiz-Gonzalez, A., Egido, J., and Ortiz, A. (1997) Agonisitic anti-Fas antibodies induce glomerular cell apoptosis in mice in vivo. *Kidney Int.* 51:1739–1746

Greenwalt, D. E., Lipsky, R. H., Ockenhouse, C. F., Ikeda, H., Tandon, N. N., and Johnson, G. A. (1992) Membrane glycoprotein CD36: A review of its role in adherence, signal transduction and transfusion medicine. *Blood* 80:1105–1115.

Griffith, T. S., Yu, X., Herndon, J. M., Green, D. R., and Ferguson, T. A. (1996) CD95-induced apoptosis of lymphocytes in an immune privileged site induces immunological tolerance. *Immun.* 5:7–16.

Grigg, J., Savill, J., Sarraf, C., Haslett, C., and Silverman, M. (1991) Neutrophil apoptosis and clearance from neonatal lungs. *Lancet* 338:720–722.

Guo, Y. I., Baysal, K., Kang, B., Yang, L-J., and Williamson, J. R. (1998) Correlation between sustained c-Jun N-terminal protein kinase activation and apoptosis induced by tumor necrosis factor-α in rat mesangial cells. *J. Biol. Chem.* 273:4027–4034.

Hall, S., Savill, J., Henson, P., and Haslett, C. (1994) Apoptotic neutrophils are phagocytosed by fibroblasts with participation of the fibroblast vitronectin receptor and involvement of a mannose/fucose-specific lectin. *J. Immunol.* 153:3218–3227.

Hart, S. P., Dougherty, G. J., Haslett, C., and Dransfield, I. (1997) CD44 regulates phagocytosis of apoptotic neutrophil granulocytes, but not apoptotic lymphocytes, by human macrophages. *J. Immunol.* 159:919–925.

Haslett, C., Jose, P. J., Giclas, P. C., Williams, T. J., and Henson, P. M. (1989) Cessation of neutrophil influx in C5a-induced acute experimental arthritis is associated with loss of chemoattractant activity from joint spaces. *J. Immunol.* 142:3510–3517.

Haslett, C. (1992) Resolution of acute inflammation and the role of apoptosis in the tissue fate of granulocytes. *Clin. Sci.* 83:639–648.

Herbert, M. I., Takano, T., and Brady, H. R. (1996) Sequential morphologic events during apoptosis of human neutrophils: modulation by lipoxygenase-derived eicosanoids. *J. Immunol.* 157: 3105–3115.

Hughes, J., Johnson, R. J., Mooney, A., Hugo, C., Gordon, K., and Savill, J. (1997a) Neutrophil fate in experimental glomerular capillary injury in the rat: Emigration exceeds in situ clearance by apoptosis. *Am. J. Pathol.* 150:223–234.

Hughes, J., Liu, Y., Van Damme, J., and Savill, J. (1997b) Human glomerular mesangial cell phagocytosis of apoptotic neutrophils: Mediation by a novel CD36-independent vitronectin receptor/thrombospondin recognition mechanism that is uncoupled from chemokine secretion. *J. Immunol.* 158:4389–4397.

Hugo, C., Shankland, S. J., Bowden, X. S., Pope, D. F., Couser, W. G., and Johnson, R. J. (1997) Extraglomerular origin of the mesangial cell after injury: A new role of the juxtaglomerular apparatus. *J. Clin. Invest.* 100:786–794.

Hurley, J. V. (1983) In *Acute Inflammation.* J. V. Hurley, ed London: Churchill Livingstone, pp. 109–117.

Iredale, J. P., Benyon, R. C., Pickering, J., McCullen, M., Northrop, M., Pawley, S., and Hovell, C. (1998) Mechanisms of spontaneous resolution of rat liver fibrosis–hepatic stellate cell apoptosis and reduced expression of metalloproteinase inhibitors. *J. Clin. Invest.* 102:538–549.

Isaka, Y., Fujiwara, Y., Ueda, N., Kaneda, T., and Imai, E. (1993) Glomerulosclerosis induced by in vivo transfection of transforming growth factor-á or platelet-derived growth factor gene into the rat. *J. Clin. Invest.* 92:2597–2601.

Ishikawa, Y., Yokoo, T., and Kitamura, M. (1997) c-Jun/AP-1, but not NF-κB, is a mediator for oxidant-initiated apoptosis in glomerular mesangial cells. *Biochem. Biophys. Res. Commun.* 240: 496–501.

Johnson, R. J., Iida, H., Alpers, C. E., Majesley, M. W., Schwartz, S. M., Pritzl, P., Gordon, K., and

Gown, A. M. (1991) Expression of smooth muscle cell phenotype by rat mesangial cells in immune complex nephritis. *J. Clin. Invest.* 87:847–858.

Johnson, R. J., Raines, E. W., Floege, J., Yoshimura, A., Pritzl, P., Alpers, C. E., and Ross, R. (1992) Inhibition of mesangial cell proliferation and matrix expansion in glomerulonephritis in the rat by antibody to platelet-derived growth factor. *J. Exp. Med.* 175:1413–1416.

Karkar, A. M., Tam, F. W., Proudfoot, A. E., Meager, A., and Rees, A. J. (1993) Modulation of antibody mediated glomerular injury in vivo by interleukin-6. *Kidney Int.* 44:967–973.

Kawabori, S., Soda, K., Perdue, M. H., and Bienenstock, J. (1991) The dynamics of intestinal eosinophil depletion in rats treated with dexamethasone. *Lab. Invest.* 64:224–232.

Kerr, J.F.R., Wyllie, A. H., and Curie, A. R. (1972) Apoptosis a basic biological phenomenon with widespread implications in tissue kinetics. *Br. J. Cancer* 26:239–257.

Kishimoto, T. (1989) The biology of interleukin-6. *Blood* 74:1–10.

Korb, L. C., and Ahern, J. M. (1997) C1q binds directly and specifically to surface blebs of apoptotic human keratinocytes. Complement deficiency and systemic lupus erythematosis revisited. *J. Immunol.* 158:4525–4528.

Lan, H. Y., Nikolic-Paterson, D. J., and Atkins, R. C. (1993) Trafficking of inflammatory macrophages from the kidney to draining lymph nodes during experimental glomerulonephritis. *Clin. Exp. Immunol.* 92:336–341.

Lang, R. A., and Bishop, J. M. (1993) Macrophages are required for cell death and tissue remodeling in the developing mouse eye. *Cell* 74:453–462.

Lang, R. A. (1997) Apoptosis in mammalian eye development lens morphogenesis, vascular regression and immune privilege. *Cell Death and Differ.* 4:12–20.

Lee, A., Whyte, M.K.B., and Haslett, C. (1993) Inhibition of apoptosis and prolongation of neutrophil functional longevity by inflammatory mediators. *J. Leukoc. Biol.* 54:283–288.

Leibovich, S. J., and Ross, R. (1975) The role of the macrophage in wound repair. *Am. J. Pathol.* 78:71–100.

Liles, W. C., Kiener, P. A., Ledbetter, J. A., Aruffo, A., and Klebanoff, S. J. (1996) Differential expression of Fas (CD95) and Fas ligand ligand on normal human phagocytes: Implications for the regulation of apoptosis in neutrophils. *J. Exp. Med.* 184:429–440.

Liu, Q. A., and Hengartner, M. O. (1998) Candidate adaptor protein CED-6 promotes the engulfment of apoptotic cells in C elegans. *Cell* 93:961–972.

Liu, Y., Cousin, J. M., Hughes, J., Van Damme, J., Seckl, J. R., Haslett, C., Dransfield, I., Savill, J., and Rossi, A. G. (1999) Glucocorticoids promote non-phlogistic phagocytosis of apoptotic leukocytes. *J. Immunol.* 162:3639–3646.

Liu, Z. H., Striker, G. E., Stetler-Stevenson, M., Fukushima, P., Patel, A., and Striker, L. J. (1996) TNF-α and IL-1β induce mannose receptors and apoptosis in glomerular mesangial but not endothelial cells. *Am. J. Physiol.* 270:1595–1560.

Lovett, D. H., Johnson, R. J., Marti, J., Davies, M., and Couser, W. G. (1992) Structural characterization of the mesangial cell type IV collagenase and enhanced expression in a model of immune complex-mediated glomerulonephritis. *Am. J. Pathol.* 141:85–98.

Luciani, M. E., and Chimini, G. (1996) The ATP binding cassette transporter ABC1, is required for engulfment of corpses generated by apoptotic cell death. *Embo J.* 15:226–235.

Manfredi, A. A., Rovere, P., Galati, G., Heltai, S., Bozzolo, E., Soldini, L., Davoust, J., Balestrieri, G., Tincani, A., and Sabbadini, M. G. (1998) Apoptotic cell clearance in systemic lupus erythematosus. *Arthritis Rheum.* 41:205–214.

Mangan, D. F., Welch, G. R., and Wahl, S. M. (1991) Lipopolysaccharide, tumour necrosis factor-α and interleukin-lβ prevent programmed cell death (apoptosis) in human peripheral blood monocytes. *J. Immunol.* 146:1541–1545.

Martin, S. J., and Green, D. R. (1995) Protease activation during apoptosis: death by a thousand cuts? *Cell* 82:349–352.

Matute-Bello, G., Liles, W. C., Steinberg, K. P., Kiener, P. A., Mongovin, S., Chi, E. Y., Jonas, M., and Martin, T. R. (1999) Soluble Fas ligand epithelial cell apoptosis in humans with acute lung injury (ARDS). *J. Immunol.* 163:2217–2225.

Meagher, L. C., Savill, J. S., Baker, A., and Haslett, C. (1992) Phagocytosis of apoptotic neutrophils does not induce macrophage release of Thromboxane B2. *J. Leukoc. Biol.* 52:269–273.

Meagher, L. C., Cousin, J. M., Seckl, J. R., and Haslett, C. (1996) Opposing effects of glucocorticoids on the rate of apoptosis in neutrophilic and eosinophilic granulocytes. *J. Immunol.* 156:4422–4428.

Metchnikoff, E. (1893) *Lectures on the comparative pathology of inflammation.* F. A. Starling and E. H. Starling, eds. and trans. London: Kegan, Paul, Trench and Trubner.

Mevorach, D., Mascarenhas, J. O., Gershov, D., and Elkon, K. B. (1998a) Complement-dependent clearance of apoptotic cells by human macrophages. *J. Exp. Med.* 188:2313–2320.

Mevorach, D., Zhou, J. L., Song, X., and Elkon, K. (1998b) Systemic exposure to irradiated apoptotic cells induces autoantibody production. *J. Exp. Med.* 188:387–392.

Milik, A. M., Buechner-Maxwell, V. A., Sonstein, J., Kim, S., Seitzman, G. D., Beals, T. F., and Curtis, J. L. (1997) Lung lymphocyte elimination by apoptosis in the murine response to intractracheal particulate antigen. *J. Clin. Invest.* 99:1082–1091.

Moffat, O. D., Devitt, A., Bell, E. D., Simmons, D. L., and Gregory, C. D. (1999) Macrophage recognition of ICAM-3 on apoptotic leukocytes. *J. Immunol.* 162:6800–6810.

Mooney, A., Jobson, T., Bacon, R., Kitamura, H., Ishizaki, M., Sugisaki, Y., and Yamanaka, N. (1997) Cytokines regulate glomerular mesangial cell survival by stimulus-dependent inhibition of apoptosis. *J. Immunol.* 159:3949–3960.

Mooney, A., Jackson, K., Bacon, R., Streuli, C., Edwards, G., Bassuk, J., and Savill, J. (1999) Type IV collagen and laminin regulate glomerular mesangial cell susceptibility to apoptosis via beat (1) integrin-mediated survival signals. *Am. J. Pathol.* 155:599–606.

Mühl, H., Sandau, K., Brüne, B., Briner, V. A., and Pfeilschifter, J. (1996) Nitric oxide donors induce apoptosis in glomerular mesangial cells, epithelial cells and endothelial cells. *Eur. J. Pharmacol.* 317:137–149.

Murray, J., Barbara, J.A.J., Dunkley, S. A., Lopez, A. F., van Ostade, X, Condliffe, A. M., Dransfield, I., Haslett, C., and Chilvers, E. R. (1997) Regulation of neutrophil apoptosis by tumor necrosis factor α. Requirement for TNFR55 and TNFR75 for induction of apoptosis in vitro. *Blood* 90:2772–2783.

Nagata, S., and Golstein, P. (1995) The Fas death factor. *Science* 267:1449–1456.

Nathan, C. and Sporn, M. (1991) Cytokines in context. *J. Cell Biol.* 113:981–984.

Newman, S. L., Henson, J., and Henson, P. M. (1982) Phagocytosis of senescent neutrophils by human monocyte-derived macrophages and rabbit inflammatory macrophages. *J. Exp. Med.* 156:430–442.

Nitsch, D. D., Ghilardi, N., Mühl, H., Nitsch, C., Pfeilschifter, J., and Pfeilschifter, J. (1997) Apoptosis and expression of inducible nitiric oxide sythase are mutually exclusive in renal mesangial cells. *Am. J. Pathol.* 150:889–900.

Platt, N., Suzuki, H., Kurihara, Y., Kodama, T., and Gordon, S. (1996) Role for the class A macrophage scavenger receptor in the phagocytosis of apoptotic thymocytes in vitro. *Proc. Natl. Acad. Sci. USA* 93:12456–12460.

Polunovsky, V. A., Chen, B., Henke, C., Snover, D., Wendt, C., Ingbar, D. H., and Bitterman, P. B. (1993) Role of mesenchymal cell death in lung remodelling after injury. *J. Clin. Invest.* 92:388–397.

Price, B. E., Rauch, J., Shia, M. A., Walsh, M. T., Lieberthal, W., Gilligan, H. M., O'Laughlin, T., Koh, J. S., and Levine, J. S. (1996) Anti-phospholipid autoantibodies bind to apoptotic, but not viable, thymocytes in a á(-2)-glycoprotein I-dependent manner. *J. Immunol.* 157:2201–2208.

Raff, M. C. (1992) Social controls on cell survival and cell death. *Nature* 356:397–400.

Ren, Y., and Savill, J. (1995) Pro-inflammatory cytokines potentiate thrombospondin-mediated phagocytosis of neutrophils undergoing apoptosis. *J. Immunol.* 154:2366–2374.

Ren, Y., Silverstein, R. L., Allen, J., and Savill, J. (1995) CD36 gene transfer confers capacity for phagocytosis of cells undergoing apoptosis. *J. Exp. Med.* 181:1857–1862.

Ren, Y., and Savill, J. (1998) Apoptosis: the importance of being eaten. *Cell Death Differ.* 5:563–568.

Ren, Y., Stuart, L., Lindberg, F. P., Rosenkranz, A. R., Chen, Y., Mayadas, T. N., and Savill, J. Thrombospondin and macrophage vitronectin receptor mediate efficient, non-phlogistic β2-integrin-independent phagocytosis of late apoptotic neutrophils. Submitted for publication.

Rovere, P., Vallinoto, C., Bondanza, A., Crosti, M. C., Rescigno, M., Ricciardi-Castagnoli, P., Rugarli, C., and Manfredi, A. A. (1998) Bystander apoptosis triggers dendritic cell maturation and antigen-presenting function. *J. Immunol.* 161:1215–1224.

Sambrano, G. R., and Steinberg, D. (1995) Recognition of oxidatively damaged and apoptotic cells by an oxidized low-density lipoprotein receptor on mouse peritoneal macrophages: role of membrane phosphatidylserine. *Proc. Natl. Acad. Sci. USA* 92:1396–1400.

Sandau, K, Pfeilschifter, J., and Brüne, B. (1997) The balance between nitric oxide and superoxide determines apoptotic and necrotic death of rat mesangial cells. *J. Immunol.* 158:4938–4946.

Sanui, H., Yoshida, S.-I., Nomoto, K., Ohhara, R., and Adachi, Y. (1982) Peritoneal macrophages which phagocytose autologous polymorphonuclear leucocytes in guinea-pigs. *Br. J. Exp. Pathol.* 63:278–285.

Sato, T., van Dixhoorn, M.G.A., Schroeijers, W.E.M. Huizinga, T.W.J., and Reutelingsperger, O.P.M. (1996) Apoptosis of cultured rat glomerular mesangial cells induced by IgG2a monoclonal anti-Thy-1 antibodies. *Kidney Int.* 49:403–412.

Sato, T., van Dixhoorn, M.G.A., Schroeijers, W.E.M., van Es, L. A., and Daha, M. R. (1997) Efficient induction of apoptosis in cultured rat glomerular mesangial cells by dimeric monoclonal IgA anti-Thy-1antibodies. *Kidney Int.* 51:173–81.

Savill, J. S., Henson, P. M., and Haslett, C. (1989a) Phagocytosis of aged human neutrophils by macrophages is medicated by a novel "charge sensitive" recognition mechanism. *J. Clin. Invest.* 84:1518–1527.

Savill, J. S., Wyllie, A. H., Henson, J. E., Walport, M. J., Henson, P. M., and Haslett, C. (1989b) Macrophage phagocytosis of aging neutrophils in inflammation. Programmed cell death in the neutrophil leads to its recognition by macrophages. *J. Clin. Invest.* 83:865–867.

Savill, J., Dransfield, I., Hogg, N., and Haslett, C. (1990) Vitronectin receptor mediated phagocytosis of cells undergoing apoptosis. *Nature* 343:170–173.

Savill, J., Hogg, N., Ren, Y., and Haslett, C. (1992a) Thrombospondin cooperates with CD36 and the vitronectin receptor in macrophage recognition of neutrophils undergoing apoptosis. *J. Clin. Invest.* 90:1513–1522.

Savill, J, Smith, J., Ren, Y., Sarraf, C., Abbott, F., Rees, A. J. (1992b) Glomerular mesangial cells and inflammatory macrophages ingest neutrophils undergoing apoptosis. *Kidney Int.* 42:924–936.

Savill, J., Mooney, A., and Hughes, J. (1996a) Apoptosis in acute renal inflammation. In *Immunologic Renal Diseases*. E. G. Neilson and W. G. Couser, eds. New York: Raven Press, pp. 309–330.

Savill, J., Mooney, A., and Hughes, J. (1996b) What role does apoptosis play in progression of renal disease? *Curr. Opin. Nephrol. Hypertens.* 5:369–374.

Savill, J. (1997) Recognition and phagocytosis of cells undergoing apoptosis. *Br. Med. Bull.* 53 (3):491–508.

Savill, J. (1998) Phagocytic docking without shocking. *Nature* 392:442–443.

Serhan, O. N., Maddox, J. F., Brady, H. R., Colgan, S. P., and Madara, J. L. (1995) Design of lipoxin A_4 stable analogues that block transmigration and adhesion of human neutrophils. *Biochem. J.* 34:14609–14615.

Sharma, P., Reddy, K., Franki, N., Sanwal, V., Sankaran, R., Ahuja, T. S., Gibbons, N., Mattana, J., and Singhal, P. C. (1996) Native and oxidized low density lipoproteins modulate mesangial cell apoptosis. *Kidney Int.* 50:1604–1611.

Shimizu, A., Kitamura, H., Masuda, Y., Ishizaki, M., Sugisaki, Y., and Yamanaka, N. (1995) Apoptosis in the repair process of experimental proliferative glomerulonephritis. *Kidney Int.* 47:114–121.

Singhal, P. C., Gibbons, N., Franki, N., Reddy, K., Sharma, P., and Mattana, J. (1998) Simulated glomerular hypertension promotes mesangial cell apoptosis and expression of cathepsin-B and SGP-2. *J. Invest. Med.* 46:42–50.

Springer, T. A., (1990) Adhesion receptors of the immune system.*Nature* 346:425–433.

Steinmann, R. M., Brodie, S. E., and Cohn, Z. A. (1976) Membrane flow during pinocytosis—a sterological analysis. *J. Cell Biol.* 68:665–687.

Stern, M., Meagher, L. C., Savill, J. S., and Haslett, C. (1992) Apoptosis in human eosinophils. Programmed cell death in the eosinophil leads to phagocytosis by macrophages and is modulated by IL-5. *J. Immunol.* 148:3543–3549.

Stern, M., Savill, J., and Haslett, C. (1996) Human monocyte-derived macrophage phagocytosis of senescent eosinophils undergoing apoptosis: Mediation by αvβ3/CD36/thrombospondin recognition mechanism and lack of phlogistic response. *Am. J. Pathol.* 149 (3):991–921.

Sugiyama, H., Kashihara, N., Makino, H., Yamasaki, Y., and Ota, Z. (1996a) Reactive oxygen species induce apoptosis in cultured human mesangial cells. *J. Am. Soc. Nephrol.* 7:2357–2363.

Sugiyama, H., Kashihara, N., Makino, H., Yamasaki, Y., and Ota, Z. (1996b) Apoptosis in glomerular sclerosis. *Kidney Int.* 49:103–111.

Surh, C. D., and Sprent, J. (1994) J. T-cell apoptosis detected in situ during positive and negative selection in the thymus. *Nature* 372:100–103.

Talhouk, R. S., Bissell, M. J., and Werb, Z. (1992) Co-ordinated expression of extracellular matrix-degrading proteinases and their inhibitors regular mammary epithelial function during involution. *J. Cell Biol.* 118:1271–1282.

Tam, F.W.K., Karkar, A. M., Smith, J., Yoshimura, T., Steinkasserer, A., Kurrle, R., Langner, K., and Rees, A. J. (1996) Differential expression of macrophage inflammatory protein-2 and monocyte chemoattractant protein-1 in experimental glomerulonephritis. *Kidney Int.* 49:715–721.

Tsai, C. Y., Wu, T. H., Sun, K. H., Liao, T. S., Lin, W. M., and Yu, C. L. (1993) Polyclonal IgG anti-dsDNA antibodies exert cytotoxic effect on cultured rat mesangial cells by binding to cell membrane and augmenting apoptosis. *Scand. J. Rheumatol.* 22:162–171.

Tsuyuki, S., Bertrand, C., Erard, F., Trifilieff, A., Tsuyuki, J., Wesp, M., Anderson, G. P., and Coyle, A. J. (1995) Activation of the Fas receptor on lung eosinophils leads to apoptosis and the resolution of eosinophilic inflammation of the airways. *J. Clin. Invest.* 96:2924–2931.

Voll, R. E., Herrmann, M., Roth, E. A., Stach, C., and Kalden, J. R. (1997) Immunosuppressive effects of apoptotic cells. *Nature* 390:350–351.

Watson, R.W.G., Redmond, H. P., Wang, J. H., Condron, C., and Bouchier-Hayes, D. (1996) Neutrophils undergo apoptosis following ingestion of *Escherichia coli*. *J. Immunol.* 156:3986–3992.

Whyte, M.K.B., Meagher, L. C., MacDermot, J., and Haslett, C. (1993) Impairment of function in aging neutrophils is associated with apoptosis. *J. Immunol.* 150:5124–5134.

Woolley, K. L., Gibson, P. G., Carty, K., Wilson, A. J., Twaddell, S. H., and Woolley, M. J. (1996) Eosinophil apoptosis and the resolution of airway inflammation in asthma. *Am. J. Respir. Crit. Care. Med.* 154:237–243.

Wu, Y. C., and Horvitz, R. (1998a) *C. Elegans* phagocytosis and cell-migration protein CED-5 is similar to human DOCK 180 *Nature* 392:501–504.

Wu, Y. C., and Horvitz, H. R. (1998b) The *C. Elegans* cell corpse engulfment gen *ced-7* encodes a protein similar to ABC transporters. *Cell* 93:951–960.

Wyllie, A. H. (1980) Glucocorticoid-induced thymocyte apoptosis is associated with endogenous endonuclease activation. *Nature* 284:555–556.

Yokoo, T., and Kitamura, M. (1997) IL-1β depresses expression of the 70-kilodalton heat shock protein and sensitises glomerular cells to oxidant-initiated apoptosis. *J. Immunol.* 159:2886–2892.

Zamzani, N., Susin, S. A., Marchetti, P., Hirsch, T., Gomez-Monterrey, I., Castedo, M., and Kroemer, G. (1996) Mitochondrial control of nuclear apoptosis. *J. Exp. Med.* 183:1533–1544.

Zhang, Z., Vuori, K., Reed, J. C., and Ruoslahti, E. (1995) The α5β 1 integrin supports survival of cells on fibronectin and up-regulates Bcl-2 expression. *Proc. Natl. Acad. Sci. USA* 92:6161–6165.

Index